T0231190

Clinical Management of Chronic Obstructive Pulmonary Disease

LUNG BIOLOGY IN HEALTH AND DISEASE

Executive Editor

Claude Lenfant

Former Director, National Heart, Lung, and Blood Institute
National Institutes of Health
Bethesda, Maryland

1. Immunologic and Infectious Reactions in the Lung, *edited by C. H. Kirkpatrick and H. Y. Reynolds*
2. The Biochemical Basis of Pulmonary Function, *edited by R. G. Crystal*
3. Bioengineering Aspects of the Lung, *edited by J. B. West*
4. Metabolic Functions of the Lung, *edited by Y. S. Bakhle and J. R. Vane*
5. Respiratory Defense Mechanisms (in two parts), *edited by J. D. Brain, D. F. Proctor, and L. M. Reid*
6. Development of the Lung, *edited by W. A. Hodson*
7. Lung Water and Solute Exchange, *edited by N. C. Staub*
8. Extrapulmonary Manifestations of Respiratory Disease, *edited by E. D. Robin*
9. Chronic Obstructive Pulmonary Disease, *edited by T. L. Petty*
10. Pathogenesis and Therapy of Lung Cancer, *edited by C. C. Harris*
11. Genetic Determinants of Pulmonary Disease, *edited by S. D. Litwin*
12. The Lung in the Transition Between Health and Disease, *edited by P. T. Macklem and S. Permutt*
13. Evolution of Respiratory Processes: A Comparative Approach, *edited by S. C. Wood and C. Lenfant*
14. Pulmonary Vascular Diseases, *edited by K. M. Moser*
15. Physiology and Pharmacology of the Airways, *edited by J. A. Nadel*
16. Diagnostic Techniques in Pulmonary Disease (in two parts), *edited by M. A. Sackner*
17. Regulation of Breathing (in two parts), *edited by T. F. Hornbein*
18. Occupational Lung Diseases: Research Approaches and Methods, *edited by H. Weill and M. Turner-Warwick*
19. Immunopharmacology of the Lung, *edited by H. H. Newball*
20. Sarcoidosis and Other Granulomatous Diseases of the Lung, *edited by B. L. Fanburg*

The opinions expressed in these volumes do not necessarily represent the views of the National Institutes of Health.

Clinical Management of Chronic Obstructive Pulmonary Disease

Second Edition

Edited by

Stephen I. Rennard
University of Nebraska Medical Center
Omaha, Nebraska, USA

Roberto Rodríguez-Roisin
Hospital Clínic, Servei de Pneumologia
Universitat de Barcelona
Barcelona, Spain

Gérard Huchon
Université Paris Descartes
Hôpital de l'Hôtel-Dieu, Paris, France

Nicolas Roche
Université Paris Descartes
Hôpital de l'Hôtel-Dieu, Paris, France

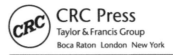

CRC Press
Taylor & Francis Group
Boca Raton London New York

CRC Press is an imprint of the
Taylor & Francis Group, an **informa** business

Informa Healthcare USA, Inc.
52 Vanderbilt Avenue
New York, NY 10017

© 2008 by Informa Healthcare USA, Inc.
Informa Healthcare is an Informa business

No claim to original U.S. Government works

International Standard Book Number-10: 0-8493-7587-8 (Hardcover)
International Standard Book Number-13: 978-0-8493-7587-3 (Hardcover)

Library of Congress Cataloging-in-Publication Data

Clinical management of chronic obstructive pulmonary disease / edited by Stephen
I. Rennard, Roberto Rodríguez-Roisin, Gérard Huchon, Nicolas Roche–2nd ed.
p. ; cm. – (Lung biology in health and disease ; 222)
Rev. ed. of: Clinical management of chronic obstructive pulmonary disease. c2002.
Includes bibliographical references and index.
ISBN-13: 978-0-8493-7587-3 (hardcover : alk. paper)
ISBN-10: 0-8493-7587-8 (hardcover : alk. paper) 1. Lungs–Diseases, Obstructive. I. Rennard,
Stephen I., 1954-. II. Rodríguez-Roisin, Roberto. III. Huchon, Gérard. IV. Roche, Nicolas.
V. Clinical management of chronic obstructive pulmonary disease. VI. Series.
[DNLM: 1. Pulmonary Disease, Chronic Obstructive–diagnosis. 2. Pulmonary Disease,
Chronic Obstructive–therapy. 3. Respiratory Muscles–physiology. W1 LU62 v.222 2007 /
WF 600 C6413 2007]
RC776.O3C525 2007
616.2'4–dc22   2007026210

Visit the Informa Web site at
www.informa.com

and the Informa Healthcare Web site at
www.informahealthcare.com

We are pleased to dedicate this second edition of
Clinical Management of Chronic Obstructive Pulmonary Disease
to four major contributors to the advancement
of COPD research and care:

Mitchell Friedman, Romain Pauwels,
Paul Vermeire, and Maurizio Vignola.

Each was deeply appreciated
and all will be missed.

Introduction

In 1978, one year after the initiation of this series of monographs, *Lung Biology in Health and Disease* presented a volume (#9) titled *Chronic Obstructive Pulmonary Disease*, edited by Dr. Thomas L. Petty. In the following three decades we have witnessed extraordinary successes in the fight against COPD—as it is globally called today.

Since the publication of the first volume on COPD, the series published no less than fifteen volumes on many aspects or topics about this disease. In addition, many other monographs were published which, in part, covered topics relevant to the understanding of COPD or to its treatment regimens, albeit palliative. The rationale behind so many volumes was simply to follow and report the very productive avenues for both fundamental and clinical research which were being pursued in the United States and abroad with the support of the respective governments and of the pharmaceutical industry. The many outcomes of this research have been augmenting our understanding of COPD at a very fast pace, and patients have started to receive very positive and significant benefits from this research. Of course, it was, and still is, recognized, that these benefits are temporary and that no cure is in sight. But, yet, so much can be of help to these patients. As per the slogan for World COPD Day, these patients are "Breathless, not Helpless."

Thus, it was inevitable that one of the volumes on COPD in this series would eventually focus on the *Clinical Management of Chronic Obstructive Lung Disease*. It appeared in 2002 and was edited by Thomas Similowski, William A. Whitelaw, and Jean-Philippe Derenne. But since, progress has marched on, actually at a faster pace, and it became evident that more research outcomes could be explained and comprehensively translated into a "practical" source that could help and enhance clinical practice. This is what led to this new volume, now titled *Clinical Management of Chronic Obstructive Pulmonary Disease*. This volume, edited by Stephen I. Rennard, Roberto Rodríguez-Roisin, Gérard Huchon, and Nicolas Roche, is more than just a second edition, it is a new phase in the journey of COPD. It is a tool to provide even better care to the patients.

COPD research today is a very global goal, simply because the disease has no frontiers and it affects all peoples and nations. The editors are well aware of this situation and, in response, they called on contributors of many nations so that all advances from can be presented to the readership.

As the Executive Editor of the series of monographs Lung Biology in Health and Disease, I am very proud to introduce this volume to our readers, and am very thankful to the editors and the contributors that they gave us the opportunity to include this volume in the series.

Claude Lenfant, MD
Gaithersburg, Maryland, U.S.A.

Foreword

The first edition of *Clinical Management of Chronic Obstructive Pulmonary Disease*, the 165th volume of the Lung Biology in Health and Disease series edited by Claude Lenfant, was published during the spring of 2002. The first letters to putative authors had been sent out by the editors, Jean-Philippe Derenne, William Whitelaw, and myself, early in 1998. The Global Initiative for Obstructive Lung Disease (GOLD) had been launched in 1997, and the first version of the Global Initiative for Obstructive Lung Disease guidelines was issued during the fall of 2001. In a way, the first edition of this book therefore marked the end of an era, during which COPD was the preoccupation of a minority of clinicians and researchers. In that era, the disease was considered in a rather nihilistic manner, and although pathophysiological studies had disentangled many of its mechanisms, few therapeutic approaches had been the object of "serious" studies (none of which would currently meet publication standards). Among other things, full realization of the inflammatory nature of the disease was lacking, as well as clear awareness of its systemic impact.

In a very few years, the COPD landscape has changed dramatically. The disease has become the focus of much attention. As underlined in the editors' preface, this enormous amount of attention has led to a better understanding of the epidemiology and burden of the disease, has permitted the dissection of the mechanisms of dyspnea, the main COPD–related symptom, and, beyond that, of the determinants of exercise limitation. It has made us realize that COPD is a global disease and not a mere set of lung and bronchi lesions, has provided us with a more complete image of what exacerbations are and represent from a prognostic point of view, and has led to the rationalization of available treatments and to the conception of new ones, among them practical tools soon to come from genetic research. Very clearly, there is still a long way to go, but, thanks to the Global Initiative for Obstructive Lung Disease, progress in the field of COPD is not going to stop in its tracks or be derailed. Thanks go to the Global Initiative for Obstructive Lung Disease, but thanks also go to the pharmaceutical industry, which has been investing colossal means in COPD research and has enabled academics and clinicians to conduct vast trials. This effort must continue, with scientific committees and agencies around the world securing the unbiased validity of the ensuing practice guidelines.

Nevertheless, there is one thing that has not changed about COPD, and is unfortunately not going to change so soon. COPD is a preventable disease that arises from self-inflicted tobacco abuse. Even though there are other factors, they must not obscure the picture or deflect attention. As, again, clearly outlined in the editors' preface, serious blows have been dealt to tobacco consumption in recent years in industrialized countries, but they are largely compensated by major "successes" of the tobacco industry in developing countries, where tobacco consumption is growing unabated. Despite the launch of the Global Alliance against Chronic Respiratory Diseases, the most recent forecasts from the World Health Organization indicate that in less than 20 years, tobacco consumption could kill close to 10 million people. Is that acceptable?

This new edition of *Clinical Management of Chronic Obstructive Pulmonary Disease* is thus more than welcome. It provides, in an academic sum that is also a practical bible, current knowledge on chronic obstructive pulmonary disease. It also gives a clear picture of what our next advances will be. Readers will derive great satisfaction from perusing this book, but they must keep in mind that identifying and adequately managing COPD is not the only goal. People must be persuaded to stop smoking. Youngsters must be prevented from starting the habit. Learned societies, medical associations, patient lobbies, international bodies have a common mission: to refuse fatalism ("people will continue to smoke") and fight, constantly, inflexibly, the spread of the smoking plague, hoping that governments will support them in the end, and that populations will have access to the information and resources that will allow them to make the right choices. David, albeit small, defeated Goliath. In the fight against tobacco smoking, the medical community must remember that it is anything but small.

Thomas Similowski, MD, PhD
Head of Respiratory Medicine and Intensive Care
Pitié-Salpêtrière Hospital
Paris, France

Foreword

I. Chronic Obstructive Pulmonary Disease, A Major Health Care Issue

Surely everyone already knows that chronic obstructive pulmonary disease is a major health care issue, but how that status was firmly established is, I suspect, much less well appreciated; part of the story, in fact, is inherent in the title of this book. This edition and its predecessor could have been entitled *Clinical Management of Chronic Obstructive* Lung *Disease*, which, with its abbreviation COLD, are recognizable but infrequently used terms; most of the book's chapters are headed by more familiar terminology, either "chronic obstructive *pulmonary* disease" or its acronym, "COPD." Actually, COLD is the progenitor expression, having been introduced in 1964 in the seminal paper by Charles Fletcher and Norman Jones from London, and Ben Burrows and Albert Niden from Chicago (1). These investigators were consummating a transatlantic partnership they had established to document the clinical and physiological manifestations that characterized British patients with what was then called "chronic bronchitis" and Americans who had been diagnosed with "emphysema." Occasional individual distinctions were identified, but—overall—the patients were found to be similar in all the key features: Fletcher, Jones, Burrows, and Niden concluded that the chief difference between the two groups was semantic, not medical.

Next, to clarify and simplify clinical understanding, the four authors introduced a new diagnostic designation that described more precisely what their patients were suffering from: chronic obstructive lung disease (COLD), a mixture of inflammatory disease of the airways (bronchitis) and destruction of the lung parenchyma (emphysema), both of which contributed to the physiological hallmark of the condition, expiratory airflow limitation. The term had great practical appeal and quickly caught on. Diagnostic standards and registry classifications were revised to include the new definition. Somehow during the process, the L, for lung, was changed to P, for pulmonary, perhaps because of COLD's alarming connotations with an upper respiratory infection or, worse yet, hypothermia; whatever the reason, P and pulmonary have clearly prevailed. But it didn't really matter whether the indicator term turned out to be lung or pulmonary. What counted was the availability of a comprehensive and workable definition: long-awaited meaningful epidemiological and clinical studies immediately followed.

Recognizing from the outset that COPD was nearly always a mixture of *both* airways and parenchymal involvement, in a companion article Burrows, Niden, Fletcher, and Jones (2) tried to further classify patients with the disorder into two physiological subtypes, A and B, which evolved into the much more colorful and clinically vivid descriptors, "pink puffers" and "blue bloaters." The puffers were patients who supposedly had mainly emphysema and who were a hearty pink because they puffed all the time, which pumped sufficient oxygen into their bloodstreams to maintain a deceptively healthy complexion, but which used up energy and created scrawniness. In contrast, the bloaters were patients who were thought to have mainly chronic bronchitis and who were dusky blue and edematous because they hypoventilated and, consequently, were hypoxic, cyanotic, and likely to develop cor pulmonale with heart failure.

This intriguing concept gradually languished because it proved impossible to find consistently identifiable anatomical and physiological differences between the two types of patients, and it was acknowledged that virtually every patient with COPD had elements of both inflammatory disease in large and small airways, and destruction of the lung parenchyma. But the search for ways of differentiating between these two components of COPD has once again recurred because, as discussed elsewhere in this book, of the current need to accurately identify suitable candidates for lung volume reduction surgery. Computed tomography, a modern imaging technique that can quantify the extent of lung destruction and the thickness of airways, plus diffusing capacity of the lung and exercise testing, two old fashioned physiological measurements, have proved helpful in selecting candidates for the operation.

A. Definition

The year 1964 bid welcome to two important declarations. In the first of these, Associate Justice Potter Stewart of the United States Supreme Court wrote that "pornography" was difficult to define, but that "I know it when I see it": this remains one of the most famous judicial statements ever made. At roughly the same time, Fletcher, Jones, Burrows, and Niden (1) announced that British chronic bronchitis and American emphysema comprised components of the same disease, which they called COLD, and that the defining physiologic abnormality was limitation of expiratory airflow; this innovative concept got the investigative ball rolling, but in contrast to Stewart's enduring pronouncement, has been modified, expanded, and otherwise revised over and over again: only the inclusion of airflow limitation remains.

The current last word on the subject comes from an assembly of international experts who wrote the National Heart, Lung, and Blood Institute/World Health Organization Global Initiative for Obstructive Lung Disease (GOLD): this group defines COPD as "a preventable and treatable disease with some significant extrapulmonary effects that may contribute to the severity in individual patients. Its pulmonary component is characterized by airflow limitation that is not fully reversible. The airflow limitation is usually progressive and associated with an abnormal inflammatory response of the lung to noxious particles or gases" (3). It remains to be seen how long this definition holds up, but at the moment it incorporates a tremendous amount of knowledge about many aspects of COPD that have come to light since Fletcher et al.'s breakthrough effort nearly half a century ago. These include the following:

- The definition of COPD no longer mentions either chronic bronchitis, the presence of usually productive cough for at least three months of the year and for at least two successive years, or emphysema, an anatomic diagnosis based on permanent abnormal enlargement and destruction of distal air spaces. Narrowing and closure of small airways contributes more to pathogenesis than chronic bronchitis of large airways, and emphysema is only one of several pathological abnormalities that may be present.
- COPD is now considered as a "preventable and treatable disease," an elaboration designed to correct the age-old pessimistic attitude about the fate of patients with the disease; the amendment also affirms the availability of long-acting pharmacological agents that improve symptoms and reduce the frequency of exacerbations, as well as the fact that lung volume reduction surgery in properly selected patients, in addition to long-term oxygen therapy, has been shown to prolong survival (4).
- COPD is not just a pulmonary disease but has "some significant extrapulmonary effects," such as severe muscle wasting and cachexia, which influence prognosis to a greater extent than the severity of the decrease in FEV_1; moreover, the statement attempts to account for the high frequency of COPD–associated cardiovascular complications, which are thought possibly to be mediated by low-grade systemic inflammation (5).
- The airflow limitation is associated with an abnormal inflammatory response of the lung "to noxious particles or gases," which is accurate in a general sense, but which dodges the real pathogenic issue: it seems to me that the authors should come right out and put the blame where it belongs—on cigarette smoke, by far the chief culprit—as well as on airborne hazards in the workplace or residence and air pollution.

The Global Initiative for Obstructive Lung Disease definition is a good one, but problems remain with staging of the disease; reliance on an FEV_1/FVC ratio of <0.70 may "substantially" underdiagnose COPD in the young and overdiagnose it in the elderly (6), though the latter concern seems to have been mitigated (7). Furthermore, no consensus has emerged on how to define the presence and severity of exacerbations, which are unquestionably the most common of the life-threatening complications faced by patients with COPD.

B. Health Care Burden

Despite the long-standing quibbles over the definition and staging of COPD, there has never been any doubt concerning its importance as a cause of death, an end point about which there is no debate. In the United States today COPD ranks as the fourth most common cause of death, up from fifth in the 1990s and slated to be third in 2020, unless cigarette smoking decreases drastically. This upsurge differs remarkably from what has happened to other top killers. An analysis of the trends in the six leading causes of death in America—in order, heart disease, all types of cancer, stroke, COPD, accidents, and diabetes mellitus—from 1970 to 2002 underscores the astounding growth of COPD in comparison with all the other conditions (8). Decreases in age-standardized death rates were observed from stroke (63%), heart disease (52%), and accidents (41%). Deaths from cancer increased until 1990, then decreased, whereas those from diabetes decreased until 1987, then increased. In striking contrast, deaths from COPD increased steadily during the entire 33-year interval and at the end of it had doubled.

The economic burden of the increasing prevalence of COPD has been compounded by the enormous rise in the costs of caring for individual patients. Estimates of the total expenditures vary, but a recent estimate by the National Heart, Lung, and Blood Institute puts the figure at $38.8 billion, of which well over half, $21.8 billion, was for direct patient care (9).

We used to think of COPD as a rich country disease, but that is no longer true: it is increasing virtually everywhere in the world. Deceitful advertising and political arm-twisting by the tobacco industry in low- and middle-income countries has resulted in a huge increase in cigarette smoking, which, when coupled with the increasing life expectancy that is occurring in many of the same countries, has caused more and more people throughout the world to develop COPD: an increase that shows no signs of stopping. In 2005, for example, more than three million people died of COPD, of whom almost 90% lived in nonindustrialized (poor) countries. The overall global prevalence of COPD in adults 40 years and older was recently calculated at 9% to 10%, but some regions have not been thoroughly studied, and methodological differences render the data somewhat shaky (10).

The World Health Organization has become increasingly concerned by the rising health burden from COPD and other chronic respiratory diseases, and has formed a new Global Alliance against Chronic Respiratory Diseases (GARD) to deal with the issue (11). One justification for this new mission is the estimate that 80 million people in the world have late-stage COPD, much of it undiagnosed and untreated (12). And mortality will worsen: from the fifth leading cause of death globally in 2002, COPD is projected to become the fourth leading cause by 2030 unless, as already stated, smoking and other underlying risk factors decrease enormously.

Sometimes it seems as though the more we learn about COPD the bigger the problem grows: the disease is undeniably a major health care issue today and its magnitude is clearly worsening. Preventive measures—particularly tobacco control and reducing exposure to airborne toxins—are of the highest priority and need to be strengthened immediately. But political weakness and industrial clout will dampen the rate of progress. Meanwhile, as detailed in this book, we need to apply the discoveries of recent decades that have greatly enhanced the clinical management of COPD: these improvements will lessen suffering and benefit the quality of life for the millions of people who have the disease now and those destined to develop it in the near future.

John F. Murray, MD, FRCP
Professor Emeritus of Medicine
University of California San Francisco
San Francisco, California, U.S.A.

References

1. Fletcher CM, Jones NL, Burrows B, Niden A. American emphysema and British bronchitis. A standardized comparative study. Am Rev Respir Dis 1964; 90:1–13.
2. Burrows B, Niden AH, Fletcher CM, Jones NL. Clinical types of chronic obstructive lung disease in London and in Chicago. A study of one hundred patients. Am Rev Respir Dis 1964; 90:14–27.
3. Global Strategy for the Diagnosis, Management, and Prevention of COPD. Gold Initiative for Chronic Obstructive Lung Disease (GOLD) 2006. Available from http://www.goldcopd.org. Accessed 24 May 2007.
4. Celli BR. Chronic obstructive pulmonary disease. From unjustified nihilism to evidence-based optimism. Proc Am Thorac Soc 2006; 3:58–65.
5. Mannino DM, Watt G, Hole D, et al. The natural history of chronic obstructive pulmonary disease. Eur Respir J 2006; 27:627–43.
6. Hnizdo E, Glindmeyer HW, Petsonk EL, Enright P, Buist AS. Case definitions for chronic obstructive pulmonary disease. COPD 2006; 3:95–100.
7. Mannino DM, Buist AS, Vollmer WM. Chronic obstructive pulmonary disease in the older adult: what defines abnormal lung function? Thorax 2007; 62:237–41.
8. Jemal A, Ward E, Hao Y, Thun M. Trends in the leading causes of death in the United States, 1970–2002. J Am Med Assoc 2005; 294:1255–9.
9. Foster TS, Miller JD, Marton JP, Caloyeras JP, Russell MW, Menzin J. Assessment of the economic burden of COPD in the U.S.: a review and synthesis of the literature. COPD 2006; 3:211–8.
10. Halbert RJ, Natoli JL, Gano A, Badadamgarav E, Buist AS. Global burden of COPD: systematic review and meta-analysis. Eur Respir J 2006; 28:523–32.
11. Bousquet J, Dahl R, Khaltaev N. Global alliance against chronic respiratory diseases. Eur Respir J 2007; 29:233–9.
12. World Health Organization. Chronic respiratory diseases: Burden. http://who.int/respiratory/copd/burden/en/index.html. Accessed 24 May 2007.

Preface

Since the publication of the first edition of *Clinical Management of Chronic Obstructive Pulmonary Disease*, the emerging awareness about chronic obstructive pulmonary disease as a public health issue that was ours then has become a major preoccupation. The burden of chronic obstructive pulmonary disease has continuously increased, in line with the predictions of the World Health Organization, and unfortunately this ominous trend is not waning. Indeed the enemy, tobacco smoking, although retreating on several fronts, has been winning enormous territories. In the often densely populated developing countries where health care resources are still focused on more basic issues, chronic obstructive pulmonary disease will undoubtedly become the main killer of the 2020s.

In parallel, our knowledge of the disease's determinants and correlates has progressed markedly; the results of several important large-scale therapeutic trials have become available; and international guidelines have been established, corrected, adapted, and rapidly evolving. The research on chronic obstructive pulmonary disease, long confined to pathophysiological studies and undervalued, is currently one of the most active in respiratory medicine. Therefore, updating *Clinical Management of Chronic Obstructive Pulmonary Disease* was mandatory to help clinicians to stay afloat in the maelstrom of new information that is bound to influence their everyday practice.

To begin with, many data have been published about the burden of chronic obstructive pulmonary disease. Gathering this information was difficult because of the requirement of mass-scale spirometry; most of the corresponding studies come from developed countries. They estimate a prevalence of chronic airflow obstruction of 4% to 10% among adults, and all agree on the marked under-diagnosis of the disease.

Finally, they unmask the potential role of environmental risk factors in addition to the main one, tobacco smoking, including some occupational exposures. Although data from developing countries are still scarce, these areas of the world have become the main targets of the tobacco industry, and may well be particularly plagued by other risk factors such as the exposure to domestic fumes.

While epidemiologists provided us with increasingly reliable data on the prevalence of chronic obstructive pulmonary disease and environmental risk factors, the knowledge about chronic obstructive pulmonary disease's pathophysiology and possible genetic risk factors improved constantly. In parallel, the physiological mechanisms of chronic obstructive pulmonary disease–related dyspnea have been identified with more accuracy; the clinical and prognostic importance of systemic components of the disease has been better understood; and the role of exacerbations in the natural history of the disease has been thoroughly investigated. As a consequence, new tools have been proposed to help us assess patients with chronic obstructive pulmonary disease in their entirety rather than solely on the basis of lung function. Altogether, these progresses will allow us to define more accurately the various phenotypes of the disease, leading to more rational and effective choices of therapeutic strategies.

Last, but not least, new treatments and strategies have been made available and very new directions, targeting specific pathophysiological mechanisms, are being investigated. More efficient and practical bronchodilators are now widely used. The target population of inhaled corticosteroids is more precisely defined. Molecules targeting specific pathophysiological mechanisms are reaching the stage of human trials. The effectiveness of several non-pharmacological interventions included in respiratory rehabilitation, such as education or exercise training, has been demonstrated or confirmed, putting this approach on top of therapeutic options.

However, despite these tremendous advances in the knowledge about chronic obstructive pulmonary disease and in the management of patients suffering from this disease, several challenges remain. Large-scale long-term studies are being performed to assess the effect of treatments on the natural history of the disease, as reflected not only by the decline of lung function but also by exacerbations, exercise capacity, quality of life, and, of course, mortality. Together with economical analysis, the results of such trials should help us define the most effective strategies to decrease the disease's burden. To achieve this goal, strategies for early diagnosis also have to be investigated, especially from a cost-effectiveness point of view. Indeed, detecting chronic obstructive pulmonary disease is not a job for respiratory physicians only; general practitioners are concerned in the first place, together with all possible preventive structures. In addition, the general population has to be informed, since many studies show a very poor knowledge of the disease. All these points are now carefully addressed in recent international and local guidelines, but significant work remains to be done to implement them.

The purpose of this book is to provide clinicians with practical tools to understand the disease and integrate this understanding in clinical practice. Therefore, a first section has been added and is dedicated to an overview of epidemiological and pathophysiological considerations, addressing both respiratory and systemic aspects of the disease. The other sections deal with diagnostic and therapeutic issues, including specific problems such as smoking cessation, comorbidities, clinical implications of systemic manifestations, and palliative treatments. Following comments on the first edition, some chapters have been combined to make the book more practical for readers. Indeed, the target is not restricted to specialists: the variety of themes and approaches intends to cover all aspects of the disease (except exacerbations, which warrant a whole book by themselves), providing all health care professionals with useful and immediately applicable information.

Stephen I. Rennard
Roberto Rodríguez-Roisin
Gérard Huchon
Nicolas Roche

Contributors

Alvar Agusti Hospital Universitario Son Dureta and Fundació Caubet-CIMERA, Palma, Mallorca, Spain

David H. Au Health Services Research and Development, Veterans Administration Puget Sound Health Care System, and Division of Pulmonary and Critical Care Medicine, Department of Medicine, University of Washington, Seattle, Washington, U.S.A.

Joan Albert Barberà Servei de Pneumologia, Hospital Clínic, Universitat de Barcelona, Barcelona, Spain

Catherine Beigelman-Aubry Department of Radiology, Pitié-Salpêtrière Hospital, Pierre and Marie Curie University, Paris, France

Pierre-Yves Brillet Department of Radiology, Avicenne Hospital, Bobigny Paris XIII University, Bobigny, France

Anne-Laure Brun Department of Radiology, Pitié-Salpêtrière Hospital, Pierre and Marie Curie University, Paris, France

Ketan Buch Division of Pulmonary, Critical Care, and Sleep Medicine, Department of Medicine, University of Kentucky, Lexington, Kentucky, U.S.A.

Chris Burtin Respiratory Rehabilitation and Respiratory Division, University Hospitals, and Faculty of Kinesiology and Rehabilitation Sciences, Katholieke Universiteit Leuven, Leuven, Belgium

Peter M. A. Calverley   Division of Infection and Immunity, Department of Respiratory Medicine, Clinical Sciences Center, University Hospital Aintree, Liverpool, U.K.

Matthieu Canuet   Service de Pneumologie, Hôpital Universitaire de Strasbourg, Strasbourg, France

Kevin M. Chan   Division of Pulmonary and Critical Care Medicine, Department of Internal Medicine, University of Michigan Health System, Ann Arbor, Michigan, U.S.A.

Andrew C. Chang   Section of Thoracic Surgery, Department of Surgery, University of Michigan Health System, Ann Arbor, Michigan, U.S.A.

Ari Chaouat   Service de Pathologie, Respiratoire, et Réanimation Respiratoire, Hôpital Universitaire de Nancy, Nancy, France

François Clergue   Service d'Anesthésiologie, Hôpitaux Universitaires de Genève, Genève, Suisse

J. Randall Curtis   Division of Pulmonary and Critical Care Medicine, Department of Medicine, University of Washington, Seattle, Washington, U.S.A.

Marc Decramer   Respiratory Rehabilitation and Respiratory Division, University Hospitals, and Faculty of Kinesiology and Rehabilitation Sciences, Katholieke Universiteit Leuven, Leuven, Belgium

Dennis E. Doherty   Division of Pulmonary, Critical Care, and Sleep Medicine, Respiratory Care Services, Department of Medicine, University of Kentucky, Veterans Administration Medical Center, Lexington, Kentucky, U.S.A.

M. W. Elliott   Department of Respiratory Medicine, St. James's University Hospital, Leeds, U.K.

Wen Qi Gan   Respiratory Division, University of British Columbia, and The James Hogg iCAPTURE Center for Cardiovascular and Pulmonary Research, St. Paul's Hospital, Vancouver, British Columbia, Canada

Mark A. Giembycz   Department of Pharmacology and Therapeutics, Faculty of Medicine, Institute of Infection, Immunity, and Inflammation, University of Calgary, Calgary, Alberta, Canada

Rik Gosselink   Respiratory Rehabilitation and Respiratory Division, University Hospitals, and Faculty of Kinesiology and Rehabilitation Sciences, Katholieke Universiteit Leuven, Leuven, Belgium

Philippe Grenier   Department of Radiology, Pitié-Salpêtrière Hospital, Pierre and Marie Curie University, Paris, France

Lisa M. Hepp   Department of Internal Medicine, University of Nebraska, Nebraska Medical Center, Omaha, Nebraska, U.S.A.

James C. Hogg Department of Pathology and Laboratory Medicine, University of British Columbia, McDonald Research Laboratories, St. Paul's Hospital, Vancouver, British Columbia, Canada

Gérard Huchon Pneumologie et Réanimation, Université Paris Descartes, Assistance Publique–Hôpitaux de Paris, Hôpital de l'Hôtel-Dieu, Paris, France

Christine Jenkins Woolcock Institute of Medical Research, University of Sydney, and Department of Thoracic Medicine, Concord Hospital, Sydney, Australia

Paul W. Jones Department of Respiratory Medicine, St. George's, University of London, London, U.K.

Romain Kessler Service de Pneumologie, Hôpital Universitaire de Strasbourg, Strasbourg, France

Yves Lacasse Centre de Pneumologie, Hôpital Laval, Ste-Foy, Quebec, Canada

Marc Licker Service d'Anesthésiologie, Hôpitaux Universitaires de Genève, Genève, Suisse

Donald A. Mahler Section of Pulmonary and Critical Care Medicine, Dartmouth Medical School, Dartmouth-Hitchcock Medical Center, Lebanon, New Hampshire, U.S.A.

François Maltais Centre de Pneumologie, Hôpital Laval, Ste-Foy, Quebec, Canada

S. F. Paul Man Respiratory Division, University of British Columbia, and The James Hogg iCAPTURE Center for Cardiovascular and Pulmonary Research, St. Paul's Hospital, Vancouver, British Columbia, Canada

Fernando J. Martinez Division of Pulmonary and Critical Care Medicine, Department of Internal Medicine, University of Michigan Health System, Ann Arbor, Michigan, U.S.A.

Véronique Pepin Centre de Pneumologie, Hôpital Laval, Ste-Foy, Quebec, Canada

Stephen I. Rennard Department of Internal Medicine, University of Nebraska, Nebraska Medical Center, Omaha, Nebraska, U.S.A.

Nicolas Roche Pneumologie et Réanimation, Université Paris Descartes, Assistance Publique–Hôpitaux de Paris, Hôpital de l'Hôtel-Dieu, Paris, France

Roberto Rodríguez-Roisin Servei de Pneumologia, Hospital Clínic, Universitat de Barcelona, Barcelona, Spain

Carme Santiveri Department of Respiratory Medicine, St. George's, University of London, London, U.K., and Dos de maig Hospital, Consorci Sanitari Integral, Barcelona, Spain

Jaume Sauleda   Servei de Pneumologia and Unidad de Investigación, Hospital Universitari Son Dureta, Palma de Mallorca, Mallorca, Illes Balears, Spain

Sanjay Sethi   Division of Pulmonary and Critical Care Medicine, Department of Medicine, State University of New York at Buffalo, and Department of Veterans Affairs, Western New York Healthcare System, Buffalo, New York, U.S.A.

Don D. Sin   Respiratory Division, University of British Columbia, and The James Hogg iCAPTURE Center for Cardiovascular and Pulmonary Research, St. Paul's Hospital, Vancouver, British Columbia, Canada

J. J. Soler-Cataluña   Unidad de Neumologia, Servicio de Medicina Interna, Hospital General de Requena, Requena, Valencia, Spain

Joan B. Soriano   Program of Epidemiology and Clinical Research, Fundació Caubet-CIMERA Illes Balears, International Centre for Advanced Respiratory Medicine, Mallorca, Illes Balears, Spain

Martijn A. Spruit   Department of Research, Development, and Education, Center for Integrated Rehabilitation of Organ Failure, Horn, The Netherlands

Ján Tkáč   The James Hogg iCAPTURE Center for Cardiovascular and Pulmonary Research, St. Paul's Hospital, Vancouver, British Columbia, Canada

Thierry Troosters   Respiratory Rehabilitation and Respiratory Division, University Hospitals, and Faculty of Kinesiology and Rehabilitation Sciences, Katholieke Universiteit Leuven, Leuven, Belgium, and Postdoctoral Fellow of the Research Foundation–Flanders, Brussels, Belgium

Emmanuel Weitzenblum   Service de Pneumologie, Hôpital Universitaire de Strasbourg, Strasbourg, France

Emiel F. M. Wouters   Center for Integrated Rehabilitation of Organ Failure, Horn, The Netherlands, and Department of Respiratory Medicine, University Hospital Maastricht, Maastricht, The Netherlands

Contents

PART III: PHARMACOLOGICAL TREATMENTS OF COPD

PART I: UNDERSTANDING COPD AND ITS IMPACT

1

The Burden of COPD

WEN QI GAN and DON D. SIN
Respiratory Division, University of British Columbia, and The James Hogg iCAPTURE
Center for Cardiovascular and Pulmonary Research, St. Paul's Hospital, Vancouver,
British Columbia, Canada

I. Introduction

Chronic obstructive pulmonary disease (COPD) is one of the leading causes of morbidity and mortality worldwide (1). COPD is a debilitating disease and is associated with poor health status and quality of life (2). COPD is also a very expensive disease, costing society billions of dollars every year in direct and indirect expenditures (3,4). COPD has been one of the fastest growing diseases in the world over the past three decades (5). In the United States the age-adjusted mortality for COPD increased by 103% between 1970 and 2002. In stark contrast, mortality rates for heart disease, stroke, and cancer decreased by 52%, 63%, and 3%, respectively, during the same period of time (5). The future looks no better. Owing to a variety of different reasons (e.g., aging population, the rising use of cigarettes especially in the developing countries), the health burden of COPD will continue to rise over the next 20 years (6). By 2020, COPD will be the third leading cause of mortality accounting for four to five million deaths per year (and representing 7% of all deaths) and the fifth leading cause of disability worldwide (7). Currently, COPD is the fourth leading cause of death and the 13th leading cause of disability (7). Although these data are clearly alarming, they are likely a gross underestimate of the true health burden of COPD in society, because reduced lung function contributes to morbidity and mortality related to ischemic heart disease, stroke, osteoporosis, cachexia, and even cancer (8–10). In this chapter, we review the epidemiology of COPD and its impact on society.

II. Definition and Clinical Features of COPD

The Global Initiative for Chronic Obstructive Lung Disease (GOLD) Scientific Committee defines COPD as "a disease state characterized by airflow limitation that is not fully reversible. The airflow limitation is usually both progressive and associated with an abnormal inflammatory response of the lungs to noxious particles or gases" (11). A physiologic hallmark of COPD is irreversible or poorly reversible airflow obstruction related to chronic inflammation from long-term exposure to toxic particles

1

or gases such as tobacco smoke, occupational dusts, or vapors, and indoor or outdoor air pollution. COPD has two main phenotypes, chronic bronchitis and emphysema. In a vast majority of patients, both phenotypes are present (12). Chronic bronchitis is defined clinically by a productive cough for at least three months per year for two successive years in the absence of other causes of a productive cough (e.g., bronchiectasis). Patients with chronic bronchitis also frequently complain of breathlessness at rest or during exertion. Physiologically, chronic bronchitis is characterized by airway inflammation and narrowing, and mucous hypersecretion and plugging. Emphysema, on the other hand, is defined pathologically and is characterized by destruction of alveolar tissue beyond the terminal bronchioles, which results in impairments in gas exchange. The damage to the alveolar units is usually irreversible and morphometrically appears as small "holes" in the lungs. With progressive destruction of alveolar tissue and the surrounding elastic matrix, the lungs gradually lose their elastic recoil pressure, resulting in premature collapse of the airways during expiration, which results in dynamic hyperinflation during exertion. As such, the predominant symptoms in patients with emphysema are breathlessness and limited exercise tolerance (11,12).

The clinical diagnosis of COPD is confirmed when standardized spirometry demonstrates airflow limitation, which is defined as forced expiratory volume in one second (FEV_1) to forced vital capacity (FVC) ratio of less than 0.7 after bronchodilation. Most patients with COPD also demonstrate reduced FEV_1 of less than 80% of predicted (11). COPD may be classified into four stages of severity: mild (Stage 1), moderate (Stage 2), severe (Stage 3), and very severe COPD (Stage 4) (Table 1) (11). A fifth stage (Stage 0, at risk) was previously included to emphasize that many individuals will have symptoms of cough and sputum. The most recent case definition of COPD adopted by the American Thoracic Society and the European Thoracic Society is very similar to that of GOLD (13). Other professional thoracic societies have

Table 1   GOLD Classification of COPD Severity

Stage	Symptom	Lung function[a]	
		FEV_1/FVC	FEV_1 (%)
0 (at risk)[b]	Cough, sputum	Normal	Normal
I (mild)	With or without symptoms (cough, sputum)	<0.7	>80
II (moderate)	With or without symptoms (cough, sputum, dyspnea)	<0.7	50–80
III (severe)	With or without symptoms (cough, sputum, dyspnea)	<0.7	30–50
IV (very severe)	Respiratory failure or right heart failure	<0.7	<30[c]

[a] Based on post-bronchodilator lung function.
[b] Included in previous GOLD classifications.
[c] A post-bronchodilator $FEV_1 < 30\%$ predicted or $FEV_1 < 50\%$ predicted with respiratory failure.
Abbreviations: COPD, chronic obstructive pulmonary disease; GOLD, global initiative for chronic obstructive lung disease; FEV_1, forced expiratory volume in one second; FVC, forced vital capacity.
Source: From Ref. 11.

used slightly different definitions. The Canadian Thoracic Society (CTS), for example, excluded from its case definition individuals whose FEV_1 is 80% of predicted or greater regardless of the FEV_1 to FVC ratio (14). Additionally, CTS defined mild COPD as FEV_1 less than 80% of predicted but greater or equal to 60% of predicted; moderate COPD was defined as FEV_1 less than 60% of predicted but greater or equal to 40% of predicted; and severe COPD was defined as FEV_1 less than 40% of predicted. Although the British Thoracic Society accepts the 0.7 cutoff for the ratio of FEV_1 to FVC, it defines mild COPD as $FEV_1 \geq 80\%$ of predicted; moderate as 30% to 79% of predicted; and severe as less than 30% of predicted (15).

There are other conditions such as bronchiectasis, cystic fibrosis, tuberculosis, or asthma that can produce irreversible or poorly reversible airflow limitation. Bronchiectasis may be distinguished from COPD by its characteristic radiographic appearance on high-resolution computed tomographic scans (e.g., bronchial wall thickening, bronchial ectasia or dilation, and "tram tracking"). Cystic fibrosis is usually discovered in childhood or adolescence and is characterized by extensive bronchiectasis. Tuberculosis is diagnosed by sputum examination or culture. Asthma may be associated with allergies and atopy. In chronic asthma, chronic airflow limitation may be observed; however, dissimilar to COPD, diffusion capacity is normal or near normal, even in advanced cases. However, in a small minority of cases, despite careful history, physical, laboratory, and physiologic examinations, accurate separation of asthma from COPD may not be possible.

III. The Prevalence of COPD

The worldwide prevalence of COPD is estimated to be 9.3 per 1000 men and 7.3 per 1000 women of all ages (1). The prevalence of COPD is dependent on the case definition used. A recent systematic review and meta-analysis showed that the average prevalence of COPD based on spirometry (using the GOLD, the 1995 American Thoracic Society, or the 1995 European Respiratory Society definitions of COPD) was 7.5% [95% confidence interval (CI), 6.0–9.2%]. When studies used self-report of COPD or physician diagnosis of COPD, the prevalence was reduced to 4.9% (95% CI, 2.8–8.3%) and 5.2% (95% CI, 3.3–7.9%), respectively (16). Even when using spirometric definition of COPD, there is considerable heterogeneity in the prevalence of COPD depending on the FEV_1 cutoff used to dichotomize COPD from non-COPD. For instance, in studies that used GOLD Stages 2 to 4 to define COPD (i.e., FEV_1 to FVC ratio of less than 0.7 and FEV_1 less than 80% of predicted), the prevalence of COPD was 5.5% (95% CI, 3.3–9.0%), while studies that also included Stage 1 disease reported a much higher prevalence of COPD of 9.1% (95% CI, 5.0–16.1%) (16). In general, the use of the 1995 American Thoracic Society's definition of COPD (12) (FEV_1 to FVC ratio of less than 0.75) produces higher prevalence estimates (21.8%), compared with the use of 1995 European Respiratory Society's definition (17) (FEV_1/ FVC less than 88% predicted in males and less than 89% of predicted in females) (9.9%) or the GOLD criteria (FEV_1 to FVC ratio less than 0.70) (9.1%) (16).

Since smoking is one of the leading risk factors for COPD, smoking status of subjects makes a material impact on prevalence estimates. Prevalence is lowest in lifetime nonsmokers (4.3%; 95% CI, 3.2–5.7%) and highest in current smokers (15.4%; 95% CI, 11.2–20.7%). The prevalence estimates among ex-smokers fall somewhere in between these two extremes (10.7%; 95% CI, 8.1–14.0%) (16). There is a dose-dependent relationship between smoking and occurrence of COPD. Compared to nonsmokers, smokers who consume fewer than five cigarettes per day are 78% more likely to develop COPD; smokers who consume 5 to 14 cigarettes per day have eight times the odds of developing COPD; and those who smoke 15 cigarettes or more per day have 8.8 times the odds of developing COPD (18).

As it takes several decades for susceptible individuals to develop impaired lung function and symptoms, the prevalence of COPD naturally increases with aging. Below 40 years of age, the prevalence of COPD in adults is 3.1%; whereas in those over 40 years of age, the prevalence is 9.9% (16). In the Third National Health and Nutrition Examination Survey (NHANES III), which was conducted between 1988 and 1994 in the United States, the prevalence of COPD (defined as pre-bronchodilator FEV_1/FVC of less than 0.7) in participants 25 to 74 years of age was 13.5% (16.5% in men and 10.7% in women) (19). The prevalence of Stage 2 or greater COPD (FEV_1 less than 80% of predicted and FEV_1 to FVC ratio less than 0.7) in different age categories is shown in Figure 1. In 2000, there were 10 million adults in the United States, who indicated that they were diagnosed with COPD by their physician. However, based on spirometry, there were at least 24 million adults who had airflow limitation ($FEV_1/FVC < 0.7$), which suggests that COPD is significantly underdiagnosed in the community.

Prevalence is generally higher in men than in women (9.8% vs. 5.6%), which may reflect differences in smoking habits between men and women. The prevalence also appears to be higher in urban than in rural areas (10.2% vs. 8.6%). Worldwide, the prevalence of COPD is highest in South East Asia (e.g., Thailand, India) at ∼11%, followed by the Western Pacific (e.g., Japan and China) at ∼9% and Europe at ∼7%. The lowest prevalence has been reported in the Americas (∼5%), though these differences may in part be related to differences in the way in which spirometric information was collected in these studies and the age distribution of the sample

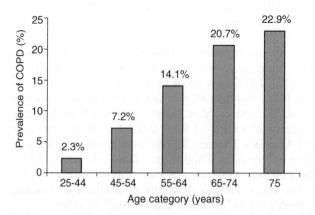

Figure 1   The prevalence of Stage 2 or greater COPD across different age groups in the United States. COPD here is defined as forced expiratory volume in one second (FEV_1) less than 80% of predicted and FEV_1 to forced vital capacity (FVC) ratio less than 0.7. *Abbreviation*: COPD, chronic obstructive pulmonary disease. *Source*: Data derived from Ref. 19.

population (16). Some specific examples of national estimates of COPD prevalence are provided in the following section.

As previously mentioned, the estimated prevalence of COPD in the United States is 13.5% in adults 25 to 74 years of age according to the NHANES III data (19). In Korea, a large national survey was conducted in 2002, which found a COPD prevalence (as defined by a pre-bronchodilator FEV_1/FVC of less than 0.7) of 7.8% (10.9% in men, 4.9% in women) in Korean adults 18 years and older. The prevalence was much higher when the analysis was restricted to Korean adults 45 years of age and older (17.2%; 25.8% in men and 9.6% in women). The majority of the COPD cases in this study had mild to moderate disease (pre-bronchodilator $FEV_1 > 50\%$); only 7.4% of the participants (10.0% in men and 1.3% in women) had an FEV_1 less than 50% of predicted (20). Notably, in this survey, three-quarters of the participants with spirometric evidence of COPD and one-third of participants with severe disease did not know that they had COPD. Only 13% of the participants with COPD were receiving treatment for their disease at the time of the survey (20).

Similar to the American and Korean national surveys, a multicenter study reported COPD prevalence (defined as FEV_1/FVC ratio < 0.88 of predicted in men or < 0.89 of predicted in women) of 9.1% (14.3% in men and 3.9% in women) in Spanish adults 40 to 69 years of age. When stratified by smoking status, the prevalence was 15%, 12.8%, and 4.1% in current, former, and never smokers, respectively. Of the COPD cases found, 78.2% did not know that they had COPD prior to the survey. Only 49.3% of the severe cases, 11.8% of the moderate cases, and 10% of the mild cases were receiving treatment for COPD at the time of the survey (21). Another study conducted in the northern part of Sweden reported a COPD prevalence (defined as a post-bronchodilator $FEV_1/FVC < 0.7$) of 14.3% (15.5% in men and 13.1% in women) in Swedish adults 45 years of age and older. Only 18% of COPD cases were known to have COPD prior to the survey (18).

The Proyecto Latinoamericano study determined the prevalence of COPD in five major Latin American cities including Sao Paulo (Brazil), Santiago (Chile), Mexico City (Mexico), Montevideo (Uruguay), and Caracas (Venezuela). There was a wide variation in COPD prevalence across these sites (defined by a post-bronchodilator $FEV_1/FVC < 0.7$) ranging from 7.8% (11.0% in men and 5.6% in women) in Mexico City to 19.7% (27.1% in men and 14.5% in women) in Montevideo. The median prevalence of these five cities was 15.8% (18.0% in men and 14.0% in women), which was in Sao Paulo (22). Adjustments for key risk factors including age, sex, and smoking could not fully explain the high rates of COPD in Montevideo. The vast majority of these patients with COPD did not know they had COPD at the time of the survey (22).

The totality of these studies indicates that COPD is a highly prevalent disease with an overall prevalence of $\sim 10\%$ in adults. There is considerable heterogeneity in the prevalences across regions and continents. While some of these differences can be attributed to known risk factors such as age, sex, and smoking patterns of the participants, much of the heterogeneity remains unexplained, suggesting that there are other (unmeasured) risk factors that are also relevant to COPD. Importantly, a large majority of patients do not know they have COPD and are not treated. Despite the growing awareness of COPD in the community, it remains a silent epidemic in many parts of the world. The full extent of COPD burden across the world is currently being studied by the Burden of Obstructive Lung Disease initiative. Within the next few years, this project is expected to generate population-based estimates of COPD prevalence across the world (23).

IV. Functional Impairment and Office Visits for COPD

Patients with COPD are major consumers of health care services because COPD is a debilitating disease, which places significant restrictions on patients' ability to work and perform common activities of living and reduces their quality of life. More than a third of COPD patients in the community report that their condition causes them to miss time at work or prevents them from participating in the workforce altogether (24). In the United States, COPD patients are $\sim 11\%$ less likely to be employed than individuals without COPD. A majority of patients with moderate to severe disease experience restrictions in their ability to engage in sporting or recreational activities or to perform household chores (24,25). COPD patients are over two times more likely to report limitations in physical activities compared with those without COPD. Indeed, there is a direct inverse relationship between FEV_1 and self-report of physical activities. Compared to individuals with $FEV_1 \geq 90\%$ of predicted, those with FEV_1 less than 60% of predicted reported a 22% reduction in their ability to perform physical activities (25). Interestingly, the relationship between FEV_1 and physical activities is fairly flat above FEV_1 of 90% of predicted, suggesting that limitations in physical activities become most apparent in GOLD Stages 2 to 4.

Not surprisingly given these symptoms, COPD patients frequently seek medical attention. In one survey, over 80% of COPD patients had at least one physician office visit per year (24). Nearly a quarter of the patients saw their doctor on a monthly basis for their disease. In 2003, there were over 10 million office visits for COPD in the United States. Although COPD is frequently considered a disorder of the aged, over 79% of these visits were incurred by patients under 75 years of age. The annual rate of COPD office visits is ~ 4.5 per 100 U.S. population 25 years of age and older (19).

V. Emergency Room Visits and Hospitalizations

In 2000, there were 1.5 million emergency room visits for COPD, which represents a 42% increase since 1992. These figures translate to 8.72 emergency room visits per 1000 U.S. population 25 years of age and older (19). In the same year, there were 726,000 hospitalizations for COPD in the United States. Approximately 38% of the hospitalizations occurred in patients who were 75 years of age or older. However, nearly 35% of hospitalizations were incurred by patients younger than 55 years of age, indicating that COPD is not just a disease of the aged (19). The annual rate of hospitalization for COPD in adults 25 years of age and older is ~ 4.1 per 1000 U.S. population. Dissimilar to other major causes of hospitalization in the United States, the hospitalization rates for COPD have risen substantially since 1990. Between 1990 and 2000, the age-adjusted hospitalization rates for COPD increased from 3.04 per 1000 (463,000) to 4.08 per 1000 population (726,000), representing a 34% increase in the annual rate. The hospitalization rates for COPD have increased among all age groups but have been particularly notable for those ≥ 65 years (19). The average length of hospitalization is ~ 10 days.

Other western nations have had similar experiences as the United States in terms of hospitalizations for COPD. In Canada, for example, between 1981 and 1994, the total number of hospitalization increased by 32% (from 42,102 to 55,785). The rise was particularly striking in women, who experienced a 67% increase; whereas in men, the rise was a more modest 14%. The age-adjusted rate of hospitalization in women increased by 25% during the same period of time; in men, the age-adjusted rate did not change significantly. Overall in 1994, the age-adjusted hospitalization rate in Canada was 1.9 per 1000 (2.5 per 1000 in men and 1.5 per 1000 in women) (26). In 2000, there were nearly 60,000 hospitalizations in Canada (27). In the United Kingdom, there were 109,000 hospitalizations for COPD in 2001 (28).

VI. Mortality

The Global Burden of Disease Study estimated that in 2002 there were 2.75 million people who died from COPD (1.41 million men, 1.34 million women), which represents 4.8% of all deaths in that year (1). COPD is currently the fourth leading cause of death worldwide and is projected to be the third leading cause of death by 2020 (1). In the United States alone 124,816 adults 25 years and older died from COPD in 2002 (19). Most patients who die from COPD are 60 years of age and older.

In the United States, overall, the age-adjusted mortality rate for COPD in 2000 was 66.9 per 100,000 population (82.6 per 100,000 in men and 56.6 per 100,000 in women). The annual mortality rate from COPD has been steadily rising since the early 1970s. Between 1980 and 2000, the age-adjusted mortality rate increased by 64.4% (19). This is in stark contrast to other major causes of mortality. The age-adjusted mortality rate for cardiovascular disease decreased by 30%, for cerebrovascular disease 40%, and cancer by 3% during the same time period (Fig. 2) (29,30). The increment in COPD mortality has been particular notable in women where the mortality rate increased by 182%. In contrast, the rate increased by a more modest 13.2% in men. A decade ago, experts predicted that the mortality rates in women would surpass that in men by the year 2000. At least in the United States, this prediction has been realized (Fig. 3). In Canada between 1980 and 1995, the age-adjusted mortality rate remained relatively stable at 45 per 100,000 in men, whereas in women, it jumped to 17.3 per 100,000 from 8.3 per 100,000 (26). In 1995, the overall age-adjusted mortality rate in Canada was 27 per 100,000 (26) and in 1998, 9042 people died of COPD in Canada, representing 4% of all deaths (27). In the United Kingdom, 30,000 people died from COPD in 1999, representing 5.1% of all deaths (28). In Italy, COPD claims the lives of ~18,000 people yearly (31).

VII. Economic Burden

Owing to the high rates of health services utilization, COPD places a substantial economic burden on the health care system. The total costs of COPD in the United States were $37.2 billion in 2004 (the direct costs being $20.9 billion and indirect costs being $16.3 billion) (32). In 1993, the total costs were $24 billion, 60% of which were driven by direct expenditures for hospital-based care. Prescription drug costs and outpatient clinic cost accounted for 12% and 15% of the direct expenditures,

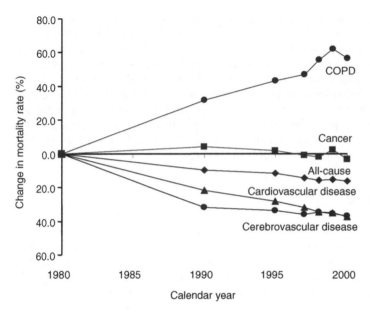

Figure 2 Change in age-adjusted mortality rates for select conditions between 1980 and 2000 in the United States. *Abbreviation*: COPD, chronic obstructive pulmonary disease. *Source*: Data derived from Ref. 29.

respectively (4). Over the past decade, the total costs for COPD have increased by 55.6%. Direct costs have increased by 29.7%, and indirect costs by 77.2% (4,32). COPD is a much more expensive disease compared with other common respiratory maladies. The total annual cost for asthma, for instance, in 1993 was $13 billion, and that for pneumonia was $8 billion. In Japan, the total annual direct cost of COPD was estimated to be 645 billion yen (~ $5.5 billion USD). Inpatient care accounted for 37% of the total direct costs and outpatient care accounted for 46% of the costs (32).

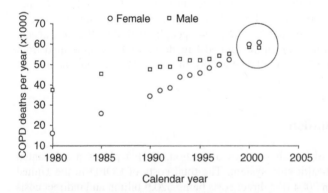

Figure 3 Mortality from COPD in the United States according to gender between 1980 and 2001. Circles represent women and squares represent men. *Abbreviation*: COPD, chronic obstructive pulmonary disease. *Source*: Data derived from Ref. 32.

Because COPD affects the working population, the indirect costs of COPD to society are substantial. Using the NHANES III data, Sin and colleagues estimated the impact of workforce nonparticipation and wage loss from COPD to be $9.9 billion in 1994 (33). Compared to individuals without COPD, patients with COPD were ~4% less likely to be in the workforce. Patients with severe COPD (defined as FEV_1 less than 30% of predicted) experienced the greatest reduction at 14.4%, followed by those with moderate disease at 3.9% (FEV_1 between 30% and 80% of predicted) and mild disease ($FEV_1 > 80%$ of predicted) at 3.4% (33). In Japan, the annual indirect costs of COPD are estimated to be 160 billion yen (~$1.4 billion) (32).

Direct and indirect costs of COPD can be calculated based on per patient basis. The Confronting COPD International Survey, which was conducted in seven countries in North America and Europe in 2000 (34), reported that the average annual direct costs were $4119 per patient in the United States, $3106 in Spain, $1258 in Canada, $1254 in the United Kingdom, $1245 in Italy, $606 in The Netherlands, and $522 in France. Approximately 52% to 84% of the direct costs resulted from inpatient hospitalizations. Indirect costs were also substantial. In the United States, the annual indirect costs per patient were estimated to be $1527, though it was lower in Italy at $47. Intriguingly, in France the indirect costs were nearly double the amount for direct expenditures. The total societal costs per patient, which includes both direct and indirect costs, were $6475 in Spain, $5646 in the United States, $4202 in Canada, $3511 in the United Kingdom, $2086 in France, $1871 in Italy, and $1361 in The Netherlands (all in U.S. dollars, currency exchanged based on 1997 Gross National Product Purchasing Power Parity) (34).

In Sweden, the average total annual costs of COPD were $1284 per patient representing $871 million of expenditures in 1999. The direct costs accounted for 42% and indirect costs accounted 58% of the total costs (35). The costs were directly related to the severity of the illness. The costs for severe COPD were three times higher than those for moderate COPD and more than 10 times higher than those for mild COPD.

A major methodogical limitation of these estimates was that they were generated from cross-sectional surveys. A more robust and reliable method would be to use a prospective longitudinal study design. This was done by the Miravitlles and colleagues (36). In their prospective follow-up study of 1510 patients with COPD, they found that the average annual direct cost for each COPD patient was $1760. The cost for mild disease was $1484 per patient, while the cost for severe disease was $2911. The main items of expenditure were hospitalization (43.8%), medications (40.8%), clinic visits, and diagnostic tests (15.4%) (36). Owing to the aging population and the high prevalence of smoking during the 1960s and 1970s, the economic burden from COPD will likely increase by 90% at constant prices between 1994 and 2015 (6). In a pessimistic model, the increase may be as high as 140% (6).

VIII. Natural History

In general, lung function in healthy subjects rises to its maximum between ages of 20 and 25 years. After a short plateau period, lung function starts to decline along an accelerating curvilinear trajectory (Fig. 4) (37). For lifetime male nonsmokers in their 30s and 40s, the average annual decline in FEV_1 is approximately 25 mL/yr; whereas it is 50 mL/yr for continued smokers. For some heavy smokers the annual decline in

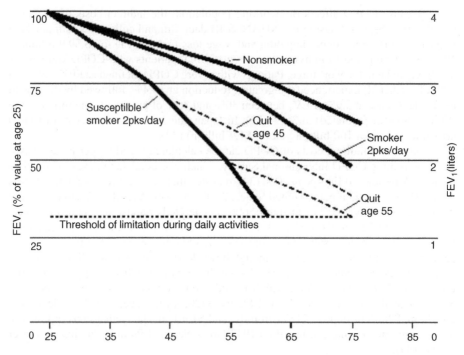

Figure 4 Fletcher–Peto diagram showing the natural history and the change over time of the FEV$_1$ in nonsmokers and smokers. *Abbreviation*: FEV$_1$, forced expiratory volume in one second. *Source*: Adapted from Ref. 37, figure from Ref. 2.

FEV$_1$ can be as large as 100 mL/yr. For COPD patients who quit smoking, the annual change in FEV$_1$ falls to near normal levels ($\sim$30 mL/yr for men and 21 mL/yr for women). For those who quit smoking but occasionally relapses, the FEV$_1$ decline is approximately 48 mL/yr. For COPD patients who continue to smoke, analogous to the data from the general population, the annual decline in FEV$_1$ is 66 mL/yr in men and 54 mL/yr in women (38). It is interesting that about a quarter of smokers with reduced FEV$_1$ do not have a chronic cough or sputum production and about 20% of smokers with chronic productive cough demonstrate normal FEV$_1$ (39). Thus, mucus hypersecretion is not necessarily associated with impaired lung function, though some but not all studies have demonstrated that chronic mucus hypersecretion may be associated with increased risk of hospitalization for COPD (40) and all-cause mortality (41).

IX. The Relevance of Stage 0 Disease

The clinical significance of Stages 0 and 1 COPD is uncertain and controversial. In the Copenhagen City Heart Study, which was a prospective epidemiologic study initiated in 1976–1978, chronic cough with mucous secretion (Stage 0) did not predict progression of disease to higher GOLD stages, though a more recent study suggests that chronic productive cough is indeed a risk factor for COPD (42). Interestingly, in the former study, nearly 40% of patients with Stage 0 disease after five years no longer had a productive cough, which suggests that the previously included GOLD Stage 0 is an unstable state and that patients do not necessarily progress in an orderly fashion from Stages 0 to 4 (43). Individuals who continued to smoke, however, had over nine times the risk for progressing to more severe COPD compared with individuals who did not smoke (44). Although in the Copenhagen Study, chronic productive cough was not significantly related to progression, recurrent wheeze, and breathlessness in patients with Stage 0 COPD predicted progression of disease to higher severity categories. In the study by de Marco et al., chronic productive cough was associated with increased risk of COPD in young adults (42). Individuals who reported chronic cough with mucous secretion were nearly three times more likely to develop COPD in this study.

X. Risk Factors

A. Tobacco Smoke

Cigarette smoking is the single most important risk factor for COPD (11). Cigarette smokers are more likely than nonsmokers to develop respiratory symptoms, respiratory tract infections, accelerated decline in lung function, and greater mortality from COPD (44–49). At the population level, smoking is probably responsible for 50% to 60% of incident cases of COPD. In one study, the population attributable risk for COPD (using the GOLD criteria) imposed by cigarette smoking in current and ex-smokers was ~61% (50). Thus, while cigarette smoking is undoubtedly a critical risk factor for COPD pathogenesis, there are other salient factors, which collectively contribute to the remaining 40% to 50% of the risk.

The traditional belief, which arose largely from the seminal work by Fletcher and Peto, is that approximately 15% of smokers develop COPD during their lifetime. However, this figure is likely to be a gross underestimate of the real risk incurred by smokers (37). It has been known for over 30 years that nearly all patients regardless of age who smoke long enough develop some pathological changes in the peripheral airways (51) and these patients develop some degree of airflow impairment (52). Only about 15% of long-term smokers develop what we now term "moderate to severe" airflow limitation; however, many more demonstrate mild airflow limitation (52). These patients with mild airflow limitation have cough and breathlessness with exertion (25). Moreover, these patients are at increased risk of lung cancer and cardiovascular morbidity and mortality (8,9). In summary, the so-called "15% rule" defines the incidence of moderate to severe COPD; many more develop milder airflow limitation. Airflow limitation related to cigarette smoking is not an "all or none" phenomenon but rather a continuous process (52) and nearly all smokers develop some degree of FEV_1 reduction if they smoke long enough (51).

Smoking cessation, therefore, is the single most effective therapy in modifying the natural history of COPD (53). Although smoking cessation cannot fully restore lung function in COPD patients, it can slow down disease progression. In fact, smoking cessation restores the rate of decline in FEV_1 to levels observed for lifetime nonsmokers especially in younger smokers (less than 45–55 years of age) (46). Moreover, within the first year of smoking cessation, FEV_1 increases by 50 to 100 mL

(54). This increase is associated with a marked improvement in patient symptoms (55). While smoking cessation clearly ameliorates the risk for COPD, smokers who quit and then restart may experience an accelerated decline in FEV_1, which may be greater than that experienced by continued smokers. In the Tucson Epidemiological Study, male restarters (i.e., individuals who were ex-smokers at the beginning of the study but took up smoking during follow-up or individuals who quit smoking in the study but took up smoking during later stages of follow-up) experienced a decline in FEV_1 of 56 mL/yr, while female restarters had a 43 mL/yr fall in FEV_1. In contrast, continued male smokers experienced a 19 mL/yr fall in FEV_1 and female continued smokers had a 18 mL/yr decline in FEV_1 (56). Smoking cessation reduces all-cause mortality by $\sim22\%$, which is largely driven by a reduction in deaths from cardiovascular disorders and lung cancer (57).

Cigar and pipe smoke are also independent risk factors for COPD morbidity and mortality, though the risk appears to be smaller than those associated with cigarette smoking (58,59). Using the Kaiser Permanente Health Plan data, Iribareen and colleagues showed that cigar smoking was associated with a 45% increase in the risk for COPD and related conditions in men (58). Cigar smoking elevated the risk for coronary heart disease [relative risk (RR), 1.27], and lung cancer (RR, 2.14). The more these men smoked cigars the higher the risks became. Men, who smoked five or more cigars per day, had a RR of 2.25 for COPD, RR of 1.56 for coronary heart disease, and RR of 3.24 for lung cancer; while men, who smoked fewer than five cigars per day, had a RR of 1.20 for coronary heart disease, RR of 1.30 for COPD, and 1.57 for lung cancer. Similarly, using data from the Cancer Prevention Study II, Henley and colleagues showed that smoking pipes increased the risk for all-cause mortality (RR, 1.33), lung cancer (RR, 5.00), coronary heart disease (RR, 1.30), and COPD (RR, 2.98) (59). Many cigar and pipe smokers switch to cigarette smoking later on in their life, which further increases their risk of COPD and other adverse outcomes. A large prospective study reported that cigar and pipe smokers who had switched from cigarettes over 20 years earlier were 51% more likely to die from the three smoking-related diseases: COPD, lung cancer, and ischemic heart disease, compared to lifelong pipe or cigar smokers (60).

The number of marijuana smokers is increasing in western society, especially in young adults and adolescents (61). Marijuana smoking is likely to become a major risk factor for COPD over the next decade as it is associated with similar respiratory symptoms and airway inflammation as those observed for cigarette smoking (61–63). However, there is a marked scarcity of epidemiologic studies that have quantified the risk estimates of COPD and lung cancer associated with marijuana exposure.

B. Environmental Tobacco Smoke (Passive Smoking)

Maternal smoking during pregnancy is associated with impaired lung function in young infants and childhood, which suggests that maternal smoking may impair in utero development of the lungs (64–67). Impairment in lung growth in utero, combined with subsequent exposure to cigarette smoke in infancy and childhood, may increase the risk of developing COPD in adulthood (68,69). In adults, environmental tobacco smoke exposure provokes respiratory symptoms (69,70). Although there is some heterogeneity in results, most epidemiological studies indicate that passive smoke exposure reduces lung function and increases the risk for COPD by $\sim70\%$ when compared with those with no or trivial exposure (69–71). Nonsmokers who live with a spouse, who smokes, have a 10% to 20% increase in the risk for all-cause mortality and 20% to 30% increase in the risk for ischemic heart disease (71,72), though not all studies have shown these associations (73).

C. Outdoor Air Pollution

The epidemiologic data linking acute air pollution to adverse health outcomes are dramatic and compelling. For example, during the London fog of December 1952, there were more than 4000 deaths that were directly related to this event. Most of the deaths were cardiorespiratory events (74).

More subtle day-to-day increases in air pollution may also produce deleterious effects in COPD patients. Several studies have linked day to day fluctuations in air quality with hospital admissions (75–78) and mortality for COPD (79–82). A five-year study in Spain reported that the daily number of emergency room admissions for COPD was significantly related to the concentrations of sulfur dioxide, black smoke, and carbon monoxide in the ambient air (76). In that study, a 25 $\mu g/m^3$ increase in sulfur dioxide levels increased the risk for emergency visits for COPD by 6% in winter and 9% in the summer (75,76). Another study showed that a 13 $\mu g/m^3$ increase in particulate sulfate concentrations in ambient air was associated with a 3.7% increase in respiratory admissions to hospitals (77). All-cause mortality and COPD-specific mortality have been associated with the concentrations of suspended particulate matter (PM) as well as sulfur dioxide in ambient air (79–82). One study suggests for every 100 $\mu g/m^3$ increase in total suspended PM, total mortality increases by 7%, and COPD mortality increases by 19% (79).

Long-term exposure to air pollution, irrespective of day-to-day variations, may also be deleterious. Several studies have shown a strong association between air pollution and occurrence of respiratory symptoms and illnesses (83–86). A cross-sectional study using a random population sample of adults aged 18 to 60 years in Switzerland reported that long-term exposure to air pollutants consisting of nitrogen dioxide, total suspended PM, and small PM with an aerodynamic diameter of less than 10 μm (PM10) was associated with a higher prevalence of respiratory symptoms. In never smokers, a 10 $\mu g/m^3$ increase in the annual mean concentration of PM10 was associated with a 27% increase in the frequency of chronic cough and sputum production, a 33% increase in breathlessness at rest, and a 32% increase in dyspnea on exertion (84).

Long-term exposure to air pollution reduces lung function (87,88). An eight-year-prospective study of 10-year-old schoolchildren in southern California demonstrated that exposure to air pollutants consisting of nitrogen dioxide, acid vapor, PM with an aerodynamic diameter of less than 2.5 μm (PM2.5), and elemental carbon was associated with a significant impairment in lung growth. At the lowest level of exposure to PM2.5, only 1.6% of the children had a FEV_1 less than 80% of predicted by the time they reached 18 years of age. In contrast, 7.9% of children who were in the highest exposure category to PM2.5 had FEV_1 less than 80% of predicted by the time they reached 18 years of age ($p = 0.002$), irrespective of other factors (87). Similar results were reported by other groups, even among never smokers (88,89).

D. Indoor Air Pollution

Indoor air pollution derived from combustion of biomass fuel for heating and cooking in poorly ventilated dwellings is an emerging, important risk factor for COPD in developing countries. Burning of biomass fuel generates a variety of respirable PMs, which range in size from 500 to 2000 $\mu g/m^3$ (90). Average 24-hour exposure for people in households that burn biomass fuel is ~ 90 $\mu g/m^3$ for those not involved in cooking and ~ 231 $\mu g/m^3$ for those who are the primary cooks. In contrast, exposure is ~ 82 $\mu g/m^3$ for households that use clean fuels (90). In developing countries, women and small children are disproportionately exposed to indoor air pollution.

Several high-quality studies have shown a significant relationship between indoor air pollution and the occurrence of respiratory symptoms and chronic airway diseases in nonsmoking women, who are exposed to biomass cooking (91–93). In rural Turkey, women who use biomass fuel have 2.5 times the risk of developing COPD, defined by FEV_1 to FVC ratio of less than 0.7, compared with women without such exposure (91). In Bogota, the use of biomass fuel increased the risk for COPD by over threefold (odds ratio, 3.4) (94). Similar findings have been reported in Mexico and elsewhere (95,96). Improving ventilation of stoves significantly reduces the risk of COPD. This was well exemplified in the study by Chapman and colleagues (95). In Xuanwei County, China, where $>90\%$ are farmers, the rates of COPD are over twice the national average. Although most women do not smoke, they cook over usually unvented household stoves that use coal or wood. In the 1990s, some households installed chimneys for better ventilation; others did not. The incidence of COPD decreased dramatically in households that installed these chimneys compared to households that did not (RR reduction in men 42% and 25% in women) (95).

E. Occupational Exposure

There is a growing body of scientific literature linking certain occupational exposure with COPD (97,98). Occupational exposures to grain, isocyanates, cadmium, coal, and other mineral dusts, or welding fumes have been implicated in COPD (97,98). The major industries where excess risks may be observed are rubber, plastic, leather, and textile mill manufacturing sectors (97). Several cohort studies have shown that occupational exposure is associated with an accelerated decline in FEV_1 (99–102). A 12-year follow-up study of 556 male workers in Paris demonstrated that occupational exposure to dust, gases, and heat was associated with an accelerated decline of FEV_1 in a dose-dependent fashion. After adjustments for age, smoking, and baseline FEV_1, the excess annual decline in FEV_1 ranged from 7 to 16 mL (100). A 13-year follow-up study in Cracow, Poland showed similar results. Occupational exposure to dusts, chemicals, or gases was associated with an accelerated decline in FEV_1. The magnitude of the effect was similar to those observed with cigarette smoking. Importantly, the deleterious effects on lung function related to occupational exposures and cigarette smoking were additive (101). A large prospective cohort study using a random sample of 1933 men aged 22 to 54 years in Bergen, Norway reported a dose–response relationship between the number of occupational agents that individuals were exposed to and the annual decline in the rate of FEV_1 (99). A 25-year population-based cohort study in Zutphen, Holland found that approximately 40% of the participants were occupationally exposed to various dusts, gases, or fumes. Their risk of developing nonspecific chronic lung disease during the follow-up period increased by 46%

compared with those unexposed (103). A recent study based on the NHANES III data estimated that 19% of the cases of COPD in the U.S. working population aged 30 to 75 years could be attributed to occupational exposures. For never smokers, the attributable risk related to occupational exposures was 31% (104).

A recent large nine-year follow-up study of young adults aged 20 to 45 years in the European Community Respiratory Health Survey found that occupational exposures to dusts, gases, and fumes were associated with increased incidence of chronic bronchitis. However, they failed to observe any significant differences in the decline of FEV_1 between individuals exposed and unexposed (102). This study had younger subjects, a shorter cumulative exposure period, and a cleaner working condition compared with the previous studies, which may have accounted for the differential results.

F. Genetic Factors

The only clearly established genetic risk factor for COPD is homozygosity for the Z allele in the α_1-antitrypsin gene (105–107). Individuals with severe deficiency for α_1-antitrypsin are more likely to develop COPD (106). When these individuals smoke cigarettes, they tend to develop severe early onset COPD usually in their 30s or 40s (107). Other environmental risk factors such as occupational gases may also interact with genetic factors to produce early onset COPD. There are likely to be other salient genetic factors that contribute to COPD. Even in the absence of α_1-antitrypsin deficiency, siblings of patients with severe early onset COPD are more likely to have COPD compared with subjects without a known family history of COPD (108–110). Other candidate genes for early onset COPD include α_1-antichymotrypsin, microsomal epoxide hydrolase, vitamin D-binding protein, glutathione S-transferase, heme oxygenase-1, tumor necrosis factor-α, α_2-macroglobulin, and blood group antigens (106).

G. Gender and Cigarette Smoke

Over the past 30 years, the epidemic of COPD has been largely fueled by the rise in COPD burden in women. For instance, between 1971–1975 and 1988–1994, the number of female adults with COPD ($FEV_1/FVC < 70\%$ and $FEV_1 < 80\%$ of predicted) in the United States increased by 141%; whereas in men, the increase has been much more modest at 44% (19). In 2000, the number of self-reported cases of COPD was 77% higher in women than in men. The number of office visits, emergency admissions, hospitalizations, and deaths from COPD were also 2%, 38%, 25%, and 1%, respectively, higher in women than in men. The number of female patients dying from COPD in the United States surpassed the number of men in 2000 and continues to rise disproportionately (Fig. 3) (32). Compared to female nonsmokers, female smokers are 13 times more likely to die from COPD. Whether women are more susceptible to cigarette smoking is still controversial. However, there is a growing body of evidence that supports this notion.

Maternal cigarette smoking during pregnancy is associated with decreased lung function in infancy and childhood (64–66). This adverse effect is more significant for female than for male infants (67,68). During adolescence, girls are more vulnerable to the adverse effects of cigarette smoking compared to boys (111). Gold and colleagues showed that compared with never smokers, smoking five or more cigarettes per day was associated with a 1.09% annual reduction in the growth rate of FEV_1 in girls, while in boys, the corresponding annual reduction was only 0.20% per year (111). Consistent with these data, exposure to cigarette smoke during childhood has been shown to be an independent risk factor for the development of obstructive airways disease in women but not in men (112).

In adults, the Danish longitudinal population study reported that female smokers had a faster decline in lung function compared with male smokers. The estimated excess loss in FEV_1 was 7.4 per pack-year for female current smokers and 6.3 mL per pack-year for male current smokers (113). More importantly, compared with male smokers, female smokers had a significantly higher risk of hospitalization for COPD after adjustments for daily tobacco consumption and years of smoking (113). Furthermore, compared with men, women with impaired lung function ($FEV_1 < 40\%$ of predicted) had a higher risk of death from all causes and from obstructive lung diseases (114). The Beijing Respiratory Health Study reported that female current smokers had significantly lower lung function compared with male smokers although female never smokers had better lung function than did male never smokers (115). A genetic study of early onset COPD found that female first-degree current or ex-smoking relatives of the probands were almost two times more likely to demonstrate mild airflow limitation ($FEV_1 < 80\%$ of predicted) and over three times more likely to have severe airflow limitation ($FEV_1 < 40\%$ of predicted) than did male relatives (110). A recent systematic review and meta-analysis synthesized 11 large population-based cohort studies. The results indicated that female smokers after age 45 to 50 years experience an accelerated decline in lung function compared with male smokers (116). On the other hand, smoking cessation appears to have a more beneficial effect for female than male smokers. The Lung Health Study reported that after the first year of smoking cessation, the average FEV_1 increased by 3.7% of predicted for female sustained quitters, whereas it increased by only 1.6% of predicted for male sustained quitters ($p < 0.001$). The larger gain in lung function for female sustained quitters persisted across the five-year of follow-up (46).

XI. Summary

COPD is a debilitating disease affecting one in every 10 adults in the western world and accounting for up to 5 million deaths worldwide. The physiologic hallmark of COPD is progressive and irreversible airflow obstruction, which is defined as FEV_1 to FVC ratio of less than 0.7 after bronchodilation. A large majority of COPD patients do not know they have the disease and most COPD patients are undertreated. Although COPD is currently the 13th leading cause of morbidity and the 4th leading cause of death, by the year 2020 it will be the 5th leading cause of disability and the 3rd leading cause of death worldwide. The economic burden from COPD will also increase by 90% to 140% at constant prices over the next decade. Cigarette smoking is the single most important risk factor for COPD, responsible for about 60% of the incident cases. Other environmental risk factors include passive smoking, outdoor air pollution such as suspended PM and sulfur dioxide, indoor air pollution from combustion of biomass fuel for heating and cooking, occupational exposure, and genetic factors such as α_1-antitrypsin deficiency. The burden of disease is growing disproportionately in the female population.

XII. Conclusions

COPD is one of the leading causes of morbidity and mortality worldwide. Owing to the aging population and increased prevalence of cigarette smoking especially in developing countries, COPD is one of the few chronic diseases for which the morbidity and mortality are expected to increase over the next two decades. COPD is not just a risk factor for respiratory failure but also contributes substantially to ischemic heart disease and lung cancer even in the milder stages of the disease. Remarkably, a large majority of COPD patients do not know they have the disease and many remained untreated because spirometry is underutilized in most parts of the world. Accordingly, COPD remains a silent worldwide epidemic. On the positive side, COPD is a preventable and treatable disease. Smoking cessation, improvements in indoor ventilation, and reductions in air pollution are some of the ways to decelerate disease progression and improve health outcomes of COPD patients. The first step is to increase awareness about this disease among health professionals and the general public.

Acknowledgments

This work is supported in part by the Canadian Institutes of Health Research and the GlaxoSmithKline/St. Paul's Hospital Foundation Professorship in COPD.

References

1. Murray CJ, Lopez AD. Regional patterns of disability-free life expectancy and disability-adjusted life expectancy: global Burden of Disease Study. Lancet 1997; 349(9062):1347–52.
2. Pauwels RA, Rabe KF. Burden and clinical features of chronic obstructive pulmonary disease (COPD). Lancet 2004; 364(9434):613–20.
3. Ferrer M, Alonso J, Morera J, et al. Chronic obstructive pulmonary disease stage and health-related quality of life. The Quality of Life of Chronic Obstructive Pulmonary Disease Study Group. Ann Intern Med 1997; 127(12):1072–9.
4. Sullivan SD, Ramsey SD, Lee TA. The economic burden of COPD. Chest 2000; 117(Suppl. 2):5S–9.
5. Jemal A, Ward E, Hao Y, Thun M. Trends in the leading causes of death in the United States, 1970–2002. J Am Med Assoc 2005; 294(10):1255–9.
6. Feenstra TL, van Genugten ML, Hoogenveen RT, Wouters EF, Rutten-van Molken MP. The impact of aging and smoking on the future burden of chronic obstructive pulmonary disease: a model analysis in the Netherlands. Am J Respir Crit Care Med 2001; 164(4):590–6.
7. Chronic Obstructive Pulmonary Disease. (http://www.who.int/respiratory/copd/en/)
8. Sin DD, Wu L, Man SF. The relationship between reduced lung function and cardiovascular mortality: a population-based study and a systematic review of the literature. Chest 2005; 127(6):1952–9.
9. Wasswa-Kintu S, Gan WQ, Man SF, Pare PD, Sin DD. Relationship between reduced forced expiratory volume in one second and the risk of lung cancer: a systematic review and meta-analysis. Thorax 2005; 60(7):570–5.
10. Wouters EF. Chronic obstructive pulmonary disease. 5: systemic effects of COPD. Thorax 2002; 57(12):1067–70.
11. Global Strategy for the Diagnosis, Management, and Prevention of Chronic Obstructive Pulmonary Disease. (http://www.goldcopd.com)
12. American Thoracic Society. Standards for the diagnosis and care of patients with chronic obstructive pulmonary disease. American Thoracic Society. Am J Respir Crit Care Med 1995; 152(5 Pt 2):S77–121.

13. Celli BR, MacNee W. Standards for the diagnosis and treatment of patients with COPD: a summary of the ATS/ERS position paper. Eur Respir J 2004; 23(6):932–46.

14. O'Donnell DE, Aaron S, Bourbeau J, Hernandez P, Marciniuk D, Balter M, Ford G, Gervais A, Goldstein R, Hodder R, et al. State of the Art Compendium: Canadian Thoracic Society recommendations for the management of chronic obstructive pulmonary disease. Can Respir J 2004; 11(Suppl. B):7B–59.

15. National Collaborating Centre for Chronic Conditions. Chronic obstructive pulmonary disease. National clinical guideline on management of chronic obstructive pulmonary disease in adults in primary and secondary care. Thorax 2004; 59(Suppl. 1):1–232.

16. Halbert RJ, Natoli JL, Gano A, Badamgarav E, Buist AS, Mannino DM. Global burden of COPD: systematic review and meta-analysis. Eur Respir J 2006; 28:523–32.

17. Siafakas NM, Vermeire P, Pride NB, Paoletti P, Gibson J, Howard P, Yernault JC, Decramer M, Higenbottam T, Postma DS, et al. Optimal assessment and management of chronic obstructive pulmonary disease (COPD). The European Respiratory Society Task Force. Eur Respir J 1995; 8(8):1398–420.

18. Lundback B, Lindberg A, Lindstrom M, et al. Not 15 but 50% of smokers develop COPD? Report from the Obstructive Lung Disease in Northern Sweden Studies. Respir Med 2003; 97(2):115–22.

19. Mannino DM, Homa DM, Akinbami LJ, Ford ES, Redd SC. Chronic obstructive pulmonary disease surveillance—United States, 1971–2000. MMWR Surveill Summ 2002; 51(6):1–16.

20. Kim DS, Kim YS, Jung KS, et al. Prevalence of chronic obstructive pulmonary disease in Korea: a population-based spirometry survey. Am J Respir Crit Care Med 2005; 172(7):842–7.

21. Pena VS, Miravitlles M, Gabriel R, et al. Geographic variations in prevalence and underdiagnosis of COPD: results of the IBERPOC multicentre epidemiological study. Chest 2000; 118(4):981–9.

22. Menezes AM, Perez-Padilla R, Jardim JR, et al. Chronic obstructive pulmonary disease in five Latin American cities (the PLATINO study): a prevalence study. Lancet 2005; 366(9500):1875–81.

23. Chapman KR, Mannino DM, Soriano JB, Vermeire PA, Buist AS, Thun MJ, Connell C, Jemal A, Lee TA, Miravitlles M, et al. Epidemiology and costs of chronic obstructive pulmonary disease. Eur Respir J 2006; 27(1):188–207.

24. Rennard S, Decramer M, Calverley PM, et al. Impact of COPD in North America and Europe in 2000: subjects' perspective of Confronting COPD International Survey. Eur Respir J 2002; 20(4):799–805.

25. Sin DD, Jones RL, Mannino DM, Paul Man SF. Forced expiratory volume in 1 second and physical activity in the general population. Am J Med 2004; 117(4):270–3.

26. Lacasse Y, Brooks D, Goldstein RS. Trends in the epidemiology of COPD in Canada, 1980 to 1995. COPD and Rehabilitation Committee of the Canadian Thoracic Society. Chest 1999; 116(2):306–13.

27. Facts and figures—Chronic Obstructive Pulmonary Disease. (http://www.phac-aspc.gc.ca/ccdpc-cpcmc/crd-mrc/facts_copd_e.html)

28. Clearing the air. (http://www.healthcare commission.org.uk/_db_/documents/COPD_report1.pdf)

29. Sin DD, Johnson M, Gan WQ, Man SF. Combination therapy of inhaled corticosteroids and long-acting beta2-adrenergics in management of patients with chronic obstructive pulmonary disease. Curr Pharm Des 2004; 10(28):3547–60.

30. Anderson RN, Smith BL. Deaths: leading causes for 2002. Natl Vital Stat Rep 2005; 53(17):1–89.

31. Dal Negro R, Rossi A, Cerveri I. The burden of COPD in Italy: results from the Confronting COPD survey. Respir Med 2003; 97(Suppl. C):S43–50.

32. Nishimura S, Zaher C. Cost impact of COPD in Japan: opportunities and challenges? Respirology 2004; 9(4):466–73.

33. Sin DD, Stafinski T, Ng YC, Bell NR, Jacobs P. The impact of chronic obstructive pulmonary disease on work loss in the United States. Am J Respir Crit Care Med 2002; 165(5):704–7.

34. Wouters EF. Economic analysis of the Confronting COPD survey: an overview of results. Respir Med 2003; 97(Suppl. C):S3–14.

35. Jansson SA, Andersson F, Borg S, Ericsson A, Jonsson E, Lundback B. Costs of COPD in Sweden according to disease severity. Chest 2002; 122(6):1994–2002.

36. Miravitlles M, Murio C, Guerrero T, Gisbert R. Costs of chronic bronchitis and COPD: a 1-year follow-up study. Chest 2003; 123(3):784–91.

37. Fletcher C, Peto R. The natural history of chronic airflow obstruction. Br Med J 1977; 1(6077):1645–8.

38. Anthonisen NR, Connett JE, Murray RP. Smoking and lung function of Lung Health Study participants after 11 years. Am J Respir Crit Care Med 2002; 166(5):675–9.

39. Rutgers SR, Postma DS, ten Hacken NH, et al. Ongoing airway inflammation in patients with COPD who do not currently smoke. Thorax 2000; 55(1):12–8.

40. Vestbo J, Prescott E, Lange P. Association of chronic mucus hypersecretion with FEV1 decline and chronic obstructive pulmonary disease morbidity. Copenhagen City Heart Study Group. Am J Respir Crit Care Med 1996; 153(5):1530–5.

41. Annesi I, Kauffmann F. Is respiratory mucus hypersecretion really an innocent disorder? A 22-year mortality survey of 1,061 working men. Am Rev Respir Dis 1986; 134(4):688–93.

42. de Marco R, Accordini S, Cerveri I, Corsico A, Anto JM, Kunzli N, Janson C, Sunyer J, Jarvis D, Chinn S, et al. Incidence of chronic obstructive pulmonary disease in a cohort of young adults according to the presence of chronic cough and phlegm. Am J Respir Crit Care Med 2007; 175(1):32–9.

43. Vestbo J, Lange P. Can GOLD Stage 0 provide information of prognostic value in chronic obstructive pulmonary disease? Am J Respir Crit Care Med 2002; 166(3):329–32.

44. Lindberg A, Eriksson B, Larsson LG, Ronmark E, Sandstrom T, Lundback B. Seven-year cumulative incidence of COPD in an age-stratified general population sample. Chest 2006; 129(4):879–85.

45. Chinn S, Jarvis D, Melotti R, Luczynska C, Ackermann-Liebrich U, Anto JM, Cerveri I, de Marco R, Gislason T, Heinrich J, et al. Smoking cessation, lung function, and weight gain: a follow-up study. Lancet 2005; 365(9471):1629–35 (discussion 1600–21).

46. Connett JE, Murray RP, Buist AS, et al. Changes in smoking status affect women more than men: results of the Lung Health Study. Am J Epidemiol 2003; 157(11):973–9.

47. James AL, Palmer LJ, Kicic E, et al. Decline in lung function in the Busselton Health Study: the effects of asthma and cigarette smoking. Am J Respir Crit Care Med 2005; 171(2):109–14.

48. Tashkin DP, Clark VA, Coulson AH, et al. The UCLA population studies of chronic obstructive respiratory disease. VIII. Effects of smoking cessation on lung function: a prospective study of a free-living population. Am Rev Respir Dis 1984; 130(5):707–15.

49. Xu X, Dockery DW, Ware JH, Speizer FE, Ferris BG, Jr. Effects of cigarette smoking on rate of loss of pulmonary function in adults: a longitudinal assessment. Am Rev Respir Dis 1992; 146(5 Pt 1):1345–8.

50. Wilson D, Adams R, Appleton S, Ruffin R. Difficulties identifying and targeting COPD and population-attributable risk of smoking for COPD: a population study. Chest 2005; 128(4):2035–42.

51. Niewoehner DE, Kleinerman J, Rice DB. Pathologic changes in the peripheral airways of young cigarette smokers. N Engl J Med 1974; 291(15):755–8.

52. Rennard SI, Vestbo J. COPD: the dangerous underestimate of 15%. Lancet 2006; 367(9518):1216–9.

53. Sin DD, McAlister FA, Man SF, Anthonisen NR. Contemporary management of chronic obstructive pulmonary disease: scientific review. J Am Med Assoc 2003; 290(17):2301–12.

54. Scanlon PD, Connett JE, Waller LA, Altose MD, Bailey WC, Buist AS. Smoking cessation and lung function in mild-to-moderate chronic obstructive pulmonary disease. The Lung Health Study. Am J Respir Crit Care Med 2000; 161(2 Pt 1):381–90.

55. Kanner RE, Connett JE, Williams DE, Buist AS. Effects of randomized assignment to a smoking cessation intervention and changes in smoking habits on respiratory symptoms in smokers with early chronic obstructive pulmonary disease: the Lung Health Study. Am J Med 1999; 106(4):410–6.

56. Sherrill DL, Enright P, Cline M, Burrows B, Lebowitz MD. Rates of decline in lung function among subjects who restart cigarette smoking. Chest 1996; 109(4):1001–5.

57. Anthonisen NR, Skeans MA, Wise RA, Manfreda J, Kanner RE, Connett JE. The effects of a smoking cessation intervention on 14.5-year mortality: a randomized clinical trial. Ann Intern Med 2005; 142(4):233–9.

58. Iribarren C, Tekawa IS, Sidney S, Friedman GD. Effect of cigar smoking on the risk of cardiovascular disease, chronic obstructive pulmonary disease, and cancer in men. N Engl J Med 1999; 340(23):1773–80.

59. Henley SJ, Thun MJ, Chao A, Calle EE. Association between exclusive pipe smoking and mortality from cancer and other diseases. J Natl Cancer Inst 2004; 96(11):853–61.

60. Wald NJ, Watt HC. Prospective study of effect of switching from cigarettes to pipes or cigars on mortality from three smoking related diseases. Br Med J 1997; 314(7098):1860–3.

61. Roth MD, Arora A, Barsky SH, Kleerup EC, Simmons M, Tashkin DP. Airway inflammation in young marijuana and tobacco smokers. Am J Respir Crit Care Med 1998; 157(3 Pt 1):928–37.

62. Fligiel SE, Roth MD, Kleerup EC, Barsky SH, Simmons MS, Tashkin DP. Tracheobronchial histopathology in habitual smokers of cocaine, marijuana, and/or tobacco. Chest 1997; 112(2):319–26.

63. Van Hoozen BE, Cross CE. Marijuana. Respiratory tract effects. Clin Rev Allergy Immunol 1997; 15(3):243–69.

64. Hanrahan JP, Tager IB, Segal MR, et al. The effect of maternal smoking during pregnancy on early infant lung function. Am Rev Respir Dis 1992; 145(5):1129–35.

65. Gilliland FD, Berhane K, McConnell R, et al. Maternal smoking during pregnancy, environmental tobacco smoke exposure and childhood lung function. Thorax 2000; 55(4):271–6.

66. Stick SM, Burton PR, Gurrin L, Sly PD, LeSouef PN. Effects of maternal smoking during pregnancy and a family history of asthma on respiratory function in newborn infants. Lancet 1996; 348(9034): 1060–4.

67. Lodrup Carlsen KC, Jaakkola JJ, Nafstad P, Carlsen KH. In utero exposure to cigarette smoking influences lung function at birth. Eur Respir J 1997; 10(8):1774–9.

68. Kerstjens HA, Rijcken B, Schouten JP, Postma DS. Decline of FEV1 by age and smoking status: facts, figures, and fallacies. Thorax 1997; 52(9):820–7.

69. Coultas DB. Health effects of passive smoking. 8. Passive smoking and risk of adult asthma and COPD: an update. Thorax 1998; 53(5):381–7.

70. Leaderer BP, Samet JM. Passive smoking and adults: new evidence for adverse effects. Am J Respir Crit Care Med 1994; 150(5 Pt 1):1216–8.

71. Sandler DP, Comstock GW, Helsing KJ, Shore DL. Deaths from all causes in non-smokers who lived with smokers. Am J Public Health 1989; 79(2):163–7.

72. Helsing KJ, Sandler DP, Comstock GW, Chee E. Heart disease mortality in nonsmokers living with smokers. Am J Epidemiol 1988; 127(5):915–22.

73. Enstrom JE, Kabat GC. Environmental tobacco smoke and tobacco related mortality in a prospective study of Californians, 1960–98. Br Med J 2003; 326(7398):1057.

74. Lebowitz MD. Epidemiological studies of the respiratory effects of air pollution. Eur Respir J 1996; 9(5):1029–54.

75. Sunyer J, Anto JM, Murillo C, Saez M. Effects of urban air pollution on emergency room admissions for chronic obstructive pulmonary disease. Am J Epidemiol 1991; 134(3):277–86 (discussion 287–9).

76. Sunyer J, Saez M, Murillo C, Castellsague J, Martinez F, Anto JM. Air pollution and emergency room admissions for chronic obstructive pulmonary disease: a 5-year study. Am J Epidemiol 1993; 137(7):701–5.

77. Anderson HR, Spix C, Medina S, Schouten JP, Castellsague J, Rossi G, Zmirou D, Touloumi G, Wojtyniak B, Ponka A, et al. Air pollution and daily admissions for chronic obstructive pulmonary disease in 6 European cities: results from the APHEA project. Eur Respir J 1997; 10(5):1064–71.

78. Burnett RT, Dales R, Krewski D, Vincent R, Dann T, Brook JR. Associations between ambient particulate sulfate and admissions to Ontario hospitals for cardiac and respiratory diseases. Am J Epidemiol 1995; 142(1):15–22.

79. Schwartz J, Dockery DW. Increased mortality in Philadelphia associated with daily air pollution concentrations. Am Rev Respir Dis 1992; 145(3):600–4.

80. Kelsall JE, Samet JM, Zeger SL, Xu J. Air pollution and mortality in Philadelphia, 1974–1988. Am J Epidemiol 1997; 146(9):750–62.

81. Xu X, Gao J, Dockery DW, Chen Y. Air pollution and daily mortality in residential areas of Beijing, China. Arch Environ Health 1994; 49(4):216–22.

82. Sunyer J, Schwartz J, Tobias A, Macfarlane D, Garcia J, Anto JM. Patients with chronic obstructive pulmonary disease are at increased risk of death associated with urban particle air pollution: a case-crossover analysis. Am J Epidemiol 2000; 151(1):50–6.

83. Braun-Fahrlander C, Vuille JC, Sennhauser FH, Neu U, Kunzle T, Grize L, Gassner M, Minder C, Schindler C, Varonier HS, et al. Respiratory health and long-term exposure to air pollutants in Swiss schoolchildren. SCARPOL Team. Swiss Study on Childhood Allergy and Respiratory Symptoms with Respect to Air Pollution, Climate and Pollen. Am J Respir Crit Care Med 1997; 155(3):1042–9.

84. Zemp E, Elsasser S, Schindler C, Kunzli N, Perruchoud AP, Domenighetti G, Medici T, Ackermann-Liebrich U, Leuenberger P, Monn C, et al. Long-term ambient air pollution and respiratory symptoms in adults (SAPALDIA study). The SAPALDIA Team. Am J Respir Crit Care Med 1999; 159(4 Pt 1):1257–66.

85. Euler GL, Abbey DE, Magie AR, Hodgkin JE. Chronic obstructive pulmonary disease symptom effects of long-term cumulative exposure to ambient levels of total suspended particulates and sulfur dioxide in California Seventh-Day Adventist residents. Arch Environ Health 1987; 42(4):213–22.

86. Chhabra SK, Chhabra P, Rajpal S, Gupta RK. Ambient air pollution and chronic respiratory morbidity in Delhi. Arch Environ Health 2001; 56(1):58–64.

87. Gauderman WJ, Avol E, Gilliland F, Vora H, Thomas D, Berhane K, McConnell R, Kuenzli N, Lurmann F, Rappaport E, et al. The effect of air pollution on lung development from 10 to 18 years of age. N Engl J Med 2004; 351(11):1057–67.

88. Tashkin DP, Detels R, Simmons M, et al. The UCLA population studies of chronic obstructive respiratory disease: XI. Impact of air pollution and smoking on annual change in forced expiratory volume in one second. Am J Respir Crit Care Med 1994; 149(5):1209–17.

89. Abbey DE, Burchette RJ, Knutsen SF, McDonnell WF, Lebowitz MD, Enright PL. Long-term particulate and other air pollutants and lung function in nonsmokers. Am J Respir Crit Care Med 1998; 158(1):289–98.

90. Balakrishnan K, Sankar S, Parikh J, et al. Daily average exposures to respirable particulate matter from combustion of biomass fuels in rural households of southern India. Environ Health Perspect 2002; 110(11):1069–75.

91. Ekici A, Ekici M, Kurtipek E, et al. Obstructive airway diseases in women exposed to biomass smoke. Environ Res 2005; 99(1):93–8.

92. Kiraz K, Kart L, Demir R, et al. Chronic pulmonary disease in rural women exposed to biomass fumes. Clin Invest Med 2003; 26(5):243–8.

93. Shrestha IL, Shrestha SL. Indoor air pollution from biomass fuels and respiratory health of the exposed population in Nepalese households. Int J Occup Environ Health 2005; 11(2):150–60.

94. Dennis RJ, Maldonado D, Norman S, Baena E, Martinez G. Woodsmoke exposure and risk for obstructive airways disease among women. Chest 1996; 109(1):115–9.

95. Chapman RS, He X, Blair AE, Lan Q. Improvement in household stoves and risk of chronic obstructive pulmonary disease in Xuanwei, China: retrospective cohort study. Br Med J 2005; 331(7524):1050.

96. Perez-Padilla R, Regalado J, Vedal S, et al. Exposure to biomass smoke and chronic airway disease in Mexican women. A case-control study. Am J Respir Crit Care Med 1996; 154(3 Pt 1):701–6.

97. Balmes J, Becklake M, Blanc P, et al. American Thoracic Society Statement: occupational contribution to the burden of airway disease. Am J Respir Crit Care Med 2003; 167(5):787–97.

98. Hendrick DJ. Occupational and chronic obstructive pulmonary disease (COPD). Thorax 1996; 51(9):947–55.

99. Humerfelt S, Gulsvik A, Skjaerven R, et al. Decline in FEV1 and airflow limitation related to occupational exposures in men of an urban community. Eur Respir J 1993; 6(8):1095–103.

100. Kauffmann F, Drouet D, Lellouch J, Brille D. Occupational exposure and 12-year spirometric changes among Paris area workers. Br J Ind Med 1982; 39(3):221–32.

101. Krzyzanowski M, Jedrychowski W, Wysocki M. Occupational exposures and changes in pulmonary function over 13 years among residents of Cracow. Br J Ind Med 1988; 45(11):747–54.

102. Sunyer J, Zock JP, Kromhout H, Garcia-Esteban R, Radon K, Jarvis D, Toren K, Kunzli N, Norback D, d'Errico A, et al. Lung function decline, chronic bronchitis, and occupational exposures in young adults. Am J Respir Crit Care Med 2005; 172(9):1139–45.

103. Post WK, Heederik D, Kromhout H, Kromhout D. Occupational exposures estimated by a population specific job exposure matrix and 25 years incidence rate of chronic nonspecific lung disease (CNSLD): the Zutphen Study. Eur Respir J 1994; 7(6):1048–55.

104. Hnizdo E, Sullivan PA, Bang KM, Wagner G. Association between chronic obstructive pulmonary disease and employment by industry and occupation in the U.S. population: a study of data from the Third National Health and Nutrition Examination Survey. Am J Epidemiol 2002; 156(8):738–46.

105. Dowson LJ, Guest PJ, Stockley RA. Longitudinal changes in physiological, radiological, and health status measurements in alpha(1)-antitrypsin deficiency and factors associated with decline. Am J Respir Crit Care Med 2001; 164(10 Pt 1):1805–9.

106. Sandford AJ, Silverman EK. Chronic obstructive pulmonary disease. 1: Susceptibility factors for COPD the genotype–environment interaction. Thorax 2002; 57(8):736–41.

107. Stoller JK. Clinical features and natural history of severe alpha 1-antitrypsin deficiency. Roger S. Mitchell Lecture. Chest 1997; 111(Suppl. 6):123S–8.

108. Kurzius-Spencer M, Sherrill DL, Holberg CJ, Martinez FD, Lebowitz MD. Familial correlation in the decline of forced expiratory volume in one second. Am J Respir Crit Care Med 2001; 164(7):1261–5.

109. McCloskey SC, Patel BD, Hinchliffe SJ, Reid ED, Wareham NJ, Lomas DA. Siblings of patients with severe chronic obstructive pulmonary disease have a significant risk of airflow obstruction. Am J Respir Crit Care Med 2001; 164(8 Pt 1):1419–24.

110. Silverman EK, Chapman HA, Drazen JM, Weiss ST, Rosner B, Campbell EJ, O'Donnell WJ, Reilly JJ, Ginns L, Mentzer S, et al. Genetic epidemiology of severe, early-onset chronic obstructive pulmonary disease. Risk to relatives for airflow obstruction and chronic bronchitis. Am J Respir Crit Care Med 1998; 157(6 Pt 1):1770–8.

111. Gold DR, Wang X, Wypij D, Speizer FE, Ware JH, Dockery DW. Effects of cigarette smoking on lung function in adolescent boys and girls. N Engl J Med 1996; 335(13):931–7.

112. Patel BD, Luben RN, Welch AA, et al. Childhood smoking is an independent risk factor for obstructive airways disease in women. Thorax 2004; 59(8):682–6.
113. Prescott E, Bjerg AM, Andersen PK, Lange P, Vestbo J. Gender difference in smoking effects on lung function and risk of hospitalization for COPD: results from a Danish longitudinal population study. Eur Respir J 1997; 10(4):822–7.
114. Lange P, Nyboe J, Appleyard M, Jensen G, Schnohr P. Relation of ventilatory impairment and of chronic mucus hypersecretion to mortality from obstructive lung disease and from all causes. Thorax 1990; 45(8):579–85.
115. Xu X, Li B, Wang L. Gender difference in smoking effects on adult pulmonary function. Eur Respir J 1994; 7(3):477–83.
116. Gan WQ, Man SF, Postma DS, Camp P, Sin DD. Female smokers beyond the perimenopausal period are at increased risk of chronic obstructive pulmonary disease: a systematic review and meta-analysis. Respir Res 2006; 7:52.

2

Smoking Cessation

STEPHEN I. RENNARD and LISA M. HEPP
Department of Internal Medicine, University of Nebraska, Nebraska Medical Center,
Omaha, Nebraska, U.S.A.

I. Introduction

Cigarette smoking is the most important cause of chronic obstructive pulmonary disease (COPD). In the United States, approximately 80% of individuals with low lung function who would qualify as COPD (1) and a similar percentage who die from COPD are current or former smokers (2). Cigarette smoking may also contribute to COPD among 20% of the nonsmokers with the disease, as passive smoke exposure is also a risk factor (3). Cigarette smoking can lead to COPD through a number of interacting mechanisms (4,5). These include direct damage to the lung, initiation of inflammation in the lung that leads to secondary lung damage and impairment of lung repair processes that can exacerbate lung damage. In addition, smoking by children who are still growing can compromise lung growth (6), which is a risk factor for subsequent development of COPD (7,8). Finally, infants born to mothers who were smoking during pregnancy are also at risk for the development of COPD (9,10), perhaps due to effects on lung development. Targeting smoking, therefore, is the most important strategy to address the etiology of COPD. The best strategy, of course, would be to prevent smoking initiation. The second best strategy, once smoking has been initiated, is to quit, the sooner the better. The current chapter will provide an overview of smoking cessation, particularly as it relates to the patient with COPD. A further strategy, which may be appropriate for individuals who cannot or will not quit, sometimes termed harm reduction (11), will be addressed only briefly as evidence supporting the utility of this approach is limited.

II. Cigarette Smoking

A. Cigarette Smoking as a Disease

Cigarette smoking has been regarded as a "lifestyle choice." While the decision to smoke or not to smoke is a matter of choice, at least to some extent, this oversimplification has confounded the perception of cigarette smoking in the general population and has compromised the approach to the problem by the medical community. For the majority of smokers, cigarette smoking is an addiction. Nicotine is recognized as the most important addictive substance in cigarette smoke (12,13). Smoke, however, contains other psychoactive compounds that may contribute to addiction.

Like most addictions, cigarette smoking should be regarded as a chronic, relapsing disorder (13). Cigarette smoking is, in addition, a heterogeneous condition. Most smokers begin smoking a few cigarettes on occasion and gradually progress to smoking regularly. The number of cigarettes usually increases over a period of about 10 years until a "mature" smoking behavior is established (14,15). Smoking behavior then remains remarkably constant. However, the rate of uptake and the final smoking behavior can vary tremendously. Most individuals who quit smoking will develop a well-defined withdrawal syndrome upon cessation of smoking (see below). A minority, perhaps 15% in the United States, may not be addicted (16). These individuals, sometimes termed "chippers," may smoke in certain social settings, for example on weekends, but will not smoke at other times. They experience no signs of withdrawal and no unwanted urges to smoke.

Regarding smoking simply as a "lifestyle choice" dramatically oversimplifies the physiologic effects of smoking and the consequent medical problem of smoking cessation. In this context, cigarette smoke has a number of potent psychological effects in the central nervous systems. These effects are mediated by virtue of the interaction of nicotine with nicotinic acetylcholine receptors. These receptors, which are hetero- or homo-pentameric ion channels are a large family of receptors widely distributed in the central nervous system as well as peripherally (17,18). In the central nervous system, nicotinic receptors can modulate the release of other neurotransmitters. Their signaling pathways also have pleotropic effects on many other cell types, and modulation of inflammatory mediator release (19–21) and cell survival (22) have also been described. With regard to addiction, actions on the $\alpha 4\beta 2$ receptor are believed to play a particularly important role (23–25). The $\alpha 4\beta 2$ receptor modulates release of dopamine in the mesolymbic system, a pathway believed important in endogenous reward and in consolidating behavioral memory. This pathway appears to be co-opted by most drugs of addiction.

The cellular mechanisms that lead to addiction are not fully understood. However, nicotine can upregulate its own receptors (26,27). As a result, when nicotine levels fall, unoccupied receptors are believed to mediate the initial features of the withdrawal syndrome, which are readily alleviated by readministration of nicotine. The symptoms of nicotine withdrawal are well recognized (Table 1). These symptoms, which develop rapidly and are usually the most intense within the first three days, gradually decrease over the next few weeks (13,28). Cravings for smoking, however, may persist for many years following cessation. These cravings may be precipitated by situational cues. While they decrease following cessation, the decrease in frequency is more prominent than the decrease in intensity, a feature that resembles a grief response.

Like most complex disorders, cigarette smoking shows important gene-by-environment interactions. In this context, societies that prevent individuals from smoking through strong social prohibitions have low prevalences of smoking. Conversely, societies that encourage smoking have high prevalences. Within a population, however, genetic factors can influence both smoking initiation and smoking persistence (29–32). The specific genes that control smoking behavior remain to be fully defined. However, several candidate genes in the dopamine signaling pathway have been suggested to play a role (33). In addition, genes that affect nicotine metabolism may also be involved. Pianezza and colleagues (34), for example, describe polymorphisms in the enzyme CYP2A6, which metabolizes nicotine to cotinine. Individuals with low enzyme activity are less likely to become smokers, perhaps

Table 1 Nicotine Withdrawal Symptoms (DSM-IV)

Dysphoric or depressed mood
Insomnia
Irritability, frustration, or anger
Anxiety
Difficulty concentrating
Decreased heart rate
Increased appetite or weight gain
Craving to smoke[a]

[a] Not included in the DSM-IV, as it was regarded as a tautology; craving to smoke is most predictive of relapse.
Abbreviation: DSM-IV, Diagnostic and Statistical Manual of Mental Disorders, Fourth Edition.

because they "overdose" when attempting to smoke. Individuals who learn to smoke despite their poor nicotine metabolism, interestingly, smoke fewer cigarettes than do individuals with more robust nicotine metabolism.

Polymorphisms in the CYP2A6 system that are associated with reduced nicotine metabolism are also associated with reduced risk for the development of COPD (35) and lung cancer (36). This is consistent with these individuals smoking less to maintain their addition and, therefore, having a reduced exposure to smoke toxins. Other genetic factors likely also modify the intensity of smoking (37).

Taken together, the available evidence supports a "medical" model for smoking cessation (13). Like most complex disorders, there are strong gene-by-environment interactions that account for heterogeneity in individuals' susceptibility to smoking. There are, moreover, genetic variations that account for heterogeneity in behavior among smokers. While this is no different than many complex multifactorial problems faced by the clinician, failure to recognize these features can compromise clinical care.

B. Conditioned Responses

While addiction plays a major role in driving persistent smoking, behavioral aspects do as well. In this context, smokers will frequently, habitually smoke during certain common situations; for example, when driving, after eating, while socializing, following stressful conversations or with many other activities. Since these events occur extremely often, this can lead to classic conditioning, i.e., "Pavlovian" responses associating smoking with specific cues. Animal models can clearly demonstrate the development and strength of these "Pavlovian" conditioned responses. The acquisition and strength of the responses, moreover, can be modified by the exogenous administration of psychoactive compounds. In this regard, nicotine greatly potentiates the development of conditioned responses (38).

The smoker, therefore, faces at least two mechanisms that tend to drive persistent smoking behavior (Fig. 1). The first is addiction with the well-developed withdrawal response. The second is the conditioned response, which may be particularly intense due to the reinforcing actions of nicotine. Both drivers of persistent smoking must be successfully addressed for a smoker to achieve abstinence. This conceptual model is consistent with the evidence that the most effective regimes combine behavioral and pharmacologic support (13).

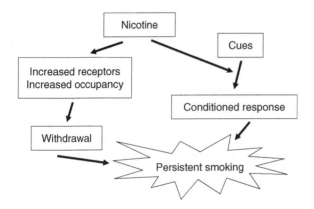

Figure 1 The multiple components leading to persistent smoking.

Finally like most addictions, smoking should be regarded as a chronic, relapsing disorder. A smoker who achieves abstinence should not be regarded as "cured" but as having achieved a remission. Relapse, in fact, is likely. Relapse should not be regarded as a failure, but rather as an event that needs to be addressed as part of the management program. Interventions that may help prevent relapse should be initiated. If relapse occurs, reinduction of remission at the earliest possible occasion should be planned.

III. Smoking Cessation: Behavioral Intervention

The first component in a smoking cessation intervention is assessing whether a smoker is interested in quitting. A useful model is the "stages of change" model (39). Smokers can be regarded as "precontemplators," who are not thinking of quitting, as "contemplators" who are considering quitting and who may benefit from specific information, and as individuals who are preparing for or are ready to begin a quit attempt. Behavioral interventions should be tailored to a patient's stage of change.

Individuals who are not ready to quit can, at times, be moved along the motivational scale. Providing patient-relevant information in a non-confrontational manner can be incorporated into a brief clinical encounter. The "5 Rs" can help guide this process (Table 2). Considerable evidence supports the concept that acute illness in both the inpatient (40) and outpatient setting (41), whether related to smoking or not, is a time when smokers are more likely to be motivated to quit. Clinicians should be aware of these "windows of opportunity" and should use them to initiate quit attempts.

Table 2 The 5 Rs for the Smoker Not Willing to Quit at the Present Time

RELEVANCE: Tailor advice and discussion to each patient
RISKS: Outline risks of continued smoking
REWARDS: Outline the benefits of quitting
ROADBLOCKS: Identify barriers to quitting
REPETITION: Reinforce the motivational message at every visit

For individuals willing to make a quit attempt, the best possible chance for achieving a remission should be given to each subject. In general, this means that the most intensive cessation regimen available should be used.

A large number of specific behavioral strategies have been developed and evaluated (42). In general, quit rates increase with the intensity of intervention (13). Many smokers, however, are unwilling to participate in more intensive programs; for example, group sessions. As a result, the majority of patients are likely to receive their behavioral support in the setting of the clinician's office. In addition to physician advice, participation of other healthcare personnel increases quit rates (13). Quit rates also increase with the number of sessions. Thus, follow-up evaluations should be part of all serious quit attempts. Behavioral interventions should help prepare the smoker for the initial withdrawal period, should anticipate problems associated with cessation and may help the smoker prevent relapse. Much of the advice given smokers may fit in the category of "common sense." A large number of specific suggestions have been reviewed elsewhere (13,43). Key issues should include: (*i*) informing others of the quit attempt and eliciting support from them, (*ii*) avoiding smoking in sites where much time is spent, and (*iii*) avoiding situations that are likely to be "high risk." In addition, previous quit attempts should be reviewed, and problems, particularly reasons for relapse, identified. The assessment should also include an evaluation of the intensity of the addiction and identification of factors that can guide pharmacologic support (see below). All of these should be noted systematically in the medical record and incorporated into the long-term management plan.

IV. Smoking Cessation: Pharmacotherapy

Every smoker willing to make a serious quit attempt should, in addition to behavioral support, be offered pharmacologic support, unless contraindicated. While up to 20% of highly motivated smokers may be able to quit with a behavioral intervention alone, pharmacologic support can increase quit rates two- to threefold. Because of the increased efficacy, more intense interventions that include pharmacologic support have been demonstrated to be more cost effective (44–46). Three categories of pharmacologic support for smoking cessation are currently approved by the Food and Drug Administration (FDA). Two off-label interventions are supported by a number of studies and are included in the Department of Health and Human Services guidelines (13). In addition, novel interventions are under investigation.

Detailed reviews of clinical trials of smoking cessation medications are available (13) as are other discussions of therapeutic approach (47,48). Prior to choosing a specific intervention, however, a careful assessment of the patient should be made. The presence of comorbid psychiatric disorders, especially depression should be evaluated. If present, depression can be a confounding factor (see below). In particular, the severity of addiction to nicotine should be gauged. Experience with past quit attempts and the severity of withdrawal will be helpful. In addition, the Fagerström's Test for Nicotine Dependence (FTND) (Table 3) has been widely used as a quick measure of nicotine dependence (49). A score of 7 or greater suggests strong nicotine dependence and a likely benefit of nicotine replacement therapy (NRT). Of the questions in the FTND, the time to first cigarette is believed to be the most important.

Table 3 Items and Scoring for Fagerström's Test for Nicotine Dependence

Questions	Answers	Points
1. How soon after you wake up do you smoke your first cigarette?	Within 5 minutes	3
	6–30 minutes	2
	31–60 minutes	1
	After 60 minutes	0
2. Do you find it difficult to refrain from smoking in places where it is forbidden, e.g., in church, at the library, in cinema, etc.?	Yes	1
	No	0
3. Which cigarette would you hate most to give up?	The first one in the morning	1
	All others	0
4. How many cigarettes per day do you smoke?	10 or less	0
	11–20	1
	21–30	2
	31 or more	3
5. Do you smoke more frequently during the first hours after waking than during the rest of the day?	Yes	1
	No	0
6. Do you smoke if you are so ill that you are in bed most of the day?	Yes	1
	No	0

Source: From Ref. 49.

Individuals who do not smoke until many hours after arising are unlikely to be heavily addicted.

Biochemical measures can also be used to assess smoking status (50,51). Exhaled breath carbon monoxide (CO) can be easily measured. Although not specific as endogenous CO production can result in levels of 1 to 3 parts per million (PPM), environmental exposures can result in much higher levels. Levels above 8 PPM are strongly indicative of active smoking in the absence of an environmental exposure. As CO has a half-life of two to four hours, however, and as one cigarette "bumps" the CO about 1 to 2 PPM, low levels do not exclude smoking. Nevertheless, this test is widely used in clinical trials to provide biochemical validation of self-reported abstinence. It has been used in clinical practice, where it may improve accuracy of diagnosis. Cotinine, which has a half-life of 26 hours, is also widely used to confirm smoking abstinence in clinical trials. While a "dipstick" test is available, there is little published experience of its use in clinical practice.

A. Nicotine Replacement Therapy

It may seem paradoxical that NRT can be used to facilitate smoking cessation since smoking, in large part, represents an addiction to nicotine. Like most addicting drugs, the psychoactive effects of nicotine depend on the pharmacokinetics of its delivery to the brain (Fig. 2) (52–54). A cigarette is a particularly effective delivery device, allowing relatively large amounts of nicotine to pass directly from the inhaled air into the pulmonary capillary blood and thence through the arterial circulation to the brain.

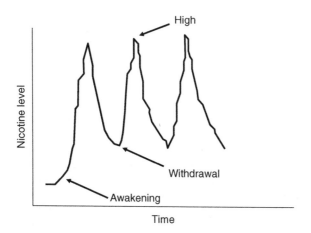

Figure 2 Nicotine levels in a smoker. When a smoker awakens, nicotine levels are low, due to overnight clearance. The first cigarette results in a rapid rise that is associated with the "hit." Many addicted smokers will smoke their first cigarette within minutes of awakening. Most will report this to be the most "satisfying" cigarette of the day, perhaps because the difference in level from baseline is greatest and perhaps because of alleviation of mild withdrawal. Nicotine levels then fall due to redistribution and metabolism. Withdrawal is believed to begin when levels fall below a threshold.

This results in a rapid "hit," which contributes both to the euphoric effects of nicotine as well as to its addictive potential. Current concepts suggest that, as nicotine levels decrease, initially through redistribution into other body pools and more slowly by metabolism, levels fall sufficiently low that craving to smoke and other withdrawal symptoms develop. The concept behind NRT, therefore, is to provide a relative steady state of nicotine that can mitigate craving and symptoms of nicotine withdrawal while, at the same time, not providing the reinforcing effects of bolus nicotine. Currently available formulations for NRT have a range of kinetics, but all deliver nicotine more slowly than does a cigarette (Table 4). The differences among the formulations, however, may have advantages for specific individual patients. In addition, the

Table 4 Nicotine Replacement Therapy Formulations

	Polacrilex	Patch	Inhaler	Nasal spray
Route	Oral	Skin	Oral	Nasal
Dosing	2, 4 mg gum	7–21 mg	2–5 mg/device	0.5 mg/actuation
	2, 4 mg lozenge ad lib	Continuous (patches changed daily)	Ad lib	Ad lib
Adverse effects	Local irritation	Local irritation	Local irritation	Local irritation
	Gastric irritation	Sleep disturbance		
	Dental and jaw problems (gum)			
Potential advantages	Variable dosing	Constant dosing	Variable dosing	Variable dosing
	Ease of use (lozenge)		Oral rituals	

combination of a transdermal system, which provides steady state nicotine levels, with a formulation that permits additional dosing as needed, may have added benefits. All forms of NRT are designed to reduce the severity of withdrawal, and all should be started on the intended quit day.

Nicotine Polacrilex

Nicotine polacrilex ("gum") was the first nicotine formulation approved for use in the United States by the FDA. It is available in 2 and 4 mg dosages. Proper use of this formulation requires considerable instruction. The nicotine is bound to the polacrilex resin and is released by act of chewing. Smokers, therefore, must be instructed to chew the gum in order to release the nicotine. The nicotine, which is released into solution in saliva, must be absorbed across the buccal mucosa, hence the smoker must not swallow. In addition, if the pH of the mouth is acidic, e.g., if the individual has been drinking an acidic beverage, the nicotine will become ionized and will not be absorbed transmucosally. If swallowed, the nicotine may cause local irritation in the stomach, resulting in gastrointestinal (GI) distress and hiccups. Swallowed nicotine will be absorbed from the GI tract, but high first-pass metabolism by the liver results in ineffective blood levels. Nicotine administered by polacrilex resin results in lower peak and sustained levels than are usually present in smokers. As a result, "gum" is thought to have a low addiction potential. However, the pharmacokinetics of nicotine derived from polacrilex gum appear to be sufficient to sustain addiction, as many smokers will have completely abstained from smoking, but remain chronic gum users. This is not a recommended indication. Nevertheless, because nicotine polacrilex gum is available over the counter and because the risks of chronic nicotine use are generally accepted as much less than that of chronic smoking, many individuals are chronic gum users. While the use of the gum has been found to approximately double quit rates in clinical trials, much lower results have been observed in clinical practice and in general use (13,55). This reduced effectiveness may be related to the instruction required to use this formulation properly.

Nicotine Lozenge

A nicotine polacrilex sublingual lozenge that slowly dissolves acts much like nicotine polacrilex gum releasing nicotine that is absorbed through the oral mucosa. Tablets containing 2 and 4 mg are available. The recommended dose is approximately one tablet per hour, although heavily dependent smokers have been reported to use more tablets effectively. Quit rates of 16% (vs. 7% on placebo) were achieved (56). The lozenge may offer advantages over the gum because of its simplicity of use and because the smoker can more readily use more pieces (and thus achieve more effective dosing).

Transdermal Nicotine Systems ("The Patch")

These systems administer nicotine topically through the skin resulting in a very slow rise in nicotine levels. While several formulations of patch are available, levels approximating one-half the blood nicotine levels of a 30-cigarette (one and a half packs per day) smoker are achieved (57). The patch may be worn at night, which may prevent nocturnal symptoms and may prevent strong cravings for smoking in the early morning. Alternatively, by delivering nicotine at night, the patch may be associated with disturbed sleep, particularly vivid dreams. In general, transdermal nicotine replacement achieves quit rates about twice that of placebo (13). It is most effective when combined with an intensive behavioral program. However, because of its ease of use, it is effective in a general practice setting (41), which contrasts with nicotine gum. Treatment with the patch is generally recommended at "full dose" (approximately 21 mg delivered dose/patch per day) for four to six weeks. A tapering regimen over four to six weeks is possible and is often recommended as intermediate (14 mg) and low (7 mg) dose patches are available. A very high dose patch (44 mg) has been tested and was found to have modest increased efficacy for heavy smokers (58). While titrating the dose of nicotine patch to smoking behavior is appealing, current evidence does not strongly support such a strategy.

Nicotine Inhaler

The nicotine inhaler consists of a plastic holder containing a nicotine-soaked pledget that contains about 10 mg of nicotine. Air is sucked through the inhaler entraining nicotine into the air stream. Approximately 4 to 5 mg of nicotine can be delivered, but this may require as many as 100 inhalations. Importantly, the nicotine is deposited in the mouth where it is readily absorbed through the oral mucosa and pharynx and is not very effectively delivered to the lower respiratory tract. As a result of the slow delivery from the device, the pharmacokinetics is relatively slow. Like other NRT products, quit rates about twice that of placebo have been reported (13). The mechanics of using the inhaler, which reproduces many of the actions of smoking, may be a benefit for selected smokers.

Nicotine Nasal Spray

Nicotine is available as aqueous solution that can be sprayed nasally. Each actuation delivers 0.5 mg as a 10 mg/mL solution. Of all the nicotine formulations, this delivers nicotine with the most rapid kinetics, achieving peak levels in approximately 10 minutes. Absorption, however, is into the venous circulation of the nasal mucosa. This differs considerably from that of a cigarette, although it is possible that nicotine via the nasal spray may have a greater addiction potential than nicotine delivered by formulations with slower rates of delivery. Local side effects due to irritation of the nasal mucosa are common. The nasal spray is currently available only by prescription.

In general, all forms of NRT approximately double quit rates when compared to placebo (13). As noted above, there is some rationale for the combination of nicotine formulations to provide a steady state nicotine level supplemented by increased dosing as needed. While this is an off-label indication, several studies suggest that there may be added benefits in selected individuals.

B. Psychotropic Agents

Bupropion

Bupropion was initially approved as an antidepressant. It was subsequently observed empirically to decrease craving for smoking. Its utility as an aid to smoking cessation was confirmed in randomized, prospective, placebo-controlled trials, and it was approved by the FDA for this indication (59,60). Many subsequent studies have confirmed the efficacy of bupropion for smoking cessation, including one study conducted specifically in COPD patients (61). Bupropion is administered 150 mg once daily for a week followed by 150 mg twice daily. Therapy should be started approximately one week prior to the quit date in order to establish adequate levels. Therapy is generally continued for 7 to 12 weeks. The major adverse effects are insomnia and dry mouth. Because bupropion can lower seizure threshold, it is contraindicated in individuals with increased seizure risk; the reported incidence of seizures is approximately 0.1%. Bupropion combined with NRT administered by a transdermal system has been reported to further increase the quit rate (59).

Varenicline

Varenicline is the most recently approved pharmacologic aid for smoking cessation. This agent, which was specifically developed to assist with smoking cessation, is a partial agonist at the $\alpha 4\beta 2$ nicotinic receptor. Because of its partial agonist activity, it results in some activation of the nicotinic receptor. This is believed to prevent nicotine withdrawal symptoms much as nicotine replacement products do. In addition, because varenicline occupies the receptor but is only a partial agonist, it prevents nicotine, if present, from fully activating the receptor (Fig. 3). As a result, should a smoker "slip" and inhale a cigarette, varenicline may prevent the fully reinforcing effects of nicotine. By this mechanism, varenicline has the potential for preventing relapse. In clinical trials, varenicline was found to increase quit rates more than threefold compared to placebo and was significantly better than was bupropion, although bupropion also was effective compared to placebo (62,63). The major adverse side effect associated with varenicline has been nausea, which appears to be reduced with a dose titration. For this reason, dosing is usually started with 0.5 mg once daily for three days followed by 1 mg once daily for three days and then "full " dosing at 1 mg twice daily. Dosing should be started one week before the quit day so that the smoker is on the full dose. Treatment

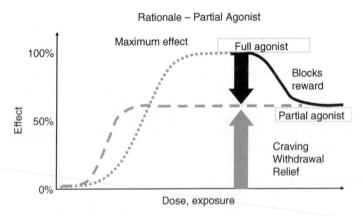

Figure 3 Rationale for a partial agonist to treat nicotine dependence. In contrast to a full agonist (dotted line) a partial agonist (dashed line) results in a reduced biological response. This reduced response may alleviate withdrawal without being fully reinforcing. In addition, by blocking the receptor, a partial agonist will block the activity of a full agonist (solid black line), reducing its biological effect.

is recommended for 12 weeks. Increased quit rates, however, were observed when treatment was extended to 24 weeks, perhaps because of prevention of relapse consequent to slips (64).

Other Agents

The tricyclic antidepressant nortriptyline has been demonstrated in several studies to have efficacy as an aid to smoking cessation. This appears to be the case both when used alone and when used in combination with NRT (65). While not specifically approved by the FDA, current guidelines suggest that clinicians who are comfortable with the use of nortriptyline, which is approved for other indications, should consider its use as an aid for smoking cessation (13).

Clonidine

Clonidine is approved as an antihypertensive. It acts centrally by modulating neurotransmission. Several studies support its use as an aid to smoking cessation. Although not consistently observed in all trials, these studies have been confirmed by a meta-analysis (66). While not approved specifically for smoking cessation, current guidelines also support clinicians comfortable in the use of clonidine who wish to consider it as an aid for smoking cessation (13). The major side effect of concern is postural hypotension.

Agents that do not Help

A large number of additional agents have been assessed as aids for smoking cessation (13,47). Because bupropion and nortriptyline, both antidepressants, were useful in this regard, a number of other antidepressants have been assessed. It is noteworthy that the selective serotonin reuptake inhibitors (SSRIs) have no effect whatsoever as aids for smoking cessation. The use of SSRIs for this purpose, therefore, is not supported (13,65).

C. Investigational Drugs

A number of additional compounds are under investigation as potential aids to smoking cessation (47). These include rimonabant, a canabinoid receptor antagonist, selegiline, a monoamine oxidase inhibitor and topimarate, an antiseizure agent with several mechanisms of action. Whether any of these agents will reach clinical practice remains to be seen, but additional pharmacological approaches to smoking cessation are likely.

In addition, several formulations of a nicotine vaccine have entered clinical trials. The concept behind the vaccine is that antibodies to nicotine bind nicotine in the peripheral blood. This prevents nicotine from rapidly diffusing from the blood into the brain since the antibodies will not cross the blood brain barrier. As a result, the presence of antibodies alters the pharmacokinetics of nicotine delivery by a cigarette, decreasing its reinforcing potential and making it potentially similar to NRT. One trial of a nicotine vaccine in a limited number of subjects suggests this approach may have utility as an aid to smoking cessation (67). Such an approach may also be useful for primary prevention and relapse prevention.

V. Special Considerations for the COPD Patient

A. Therapeutic Approaches

Although relatively few studies have been conducted regarding smoking cessation in the COPD patient, available evidence suggests that the same approaches used generally should be used in patients with COPD (68,69). Some reports have suggested that COPD patients may be "hard core" smokers who have not become abstinent despite having developed a major disease. In a Spanish study of 4000 subjects, smokers with COPD were found to be more addicted (Fagerström's Tolerance Questionnaire 4.7 vs. 3.3), to have higher exhaled CO (19.7 vs. 15.4), to smoke more and to have smoked longer. In addition, COPD subjects had lower social economic status and less completed education, all predictors of less success with cessation (70). Finally, the presence of comorbidities can influence motivation to quit. Data from the National Health Interview Survey suggest that quit attempts increase with medical comorbidities. In contrast, the number of quit attempts decrease with heavy alcohol use (71). Moreover, patients with COPD have an increased prevalence of depression (72) which can complicate smoking cessation attempts (see below) (73).

B. The Myth of the "Refractory Smoker with COPD"

While some studies have reported poor success with behavioral strategies for cessation in COPD patients, in general, cessation rates of 5% or so have been achieved (74–78). This compares with the effectiveness of physician advice in the general population and refutes the concept that COPD patients are "refractory" to cessation. Importantly, the addition of pharmacological support can significantly improve quit rates in COPD patients. In the Lung Health Study, long-term quit rates of more than 20% were achieved with counseling and NRT (79). The high quit rates achieved may have reflected a selection bias, because subjects entering a clinical trial may be more motivated to quit (80). Nevertheless, the available evidence suggests that pharma-cotherapy with NRT, bupropion and, perhaps nortritpyline, at least doubles quit rates compared to placebo in COPD patients, making them just as effective in COPD as in the general population (61,78,81). A study of varenicline in COPD patients is currently in progress (82). Taken together, the available data support smoking cessation invervention in COPD, but clearly indicate that pharmacological support is needed for optimal results.

A major question has been whether asymptomatic patients with COPD should be identified by spirometry. While this question has a number of implications, several studies have addressed whether spirometric diagnosis of reduced lung function affects cessation rate. In contrast to the concept that COPD patients are "refractory," several studies have shown higher quit rates among individuals with lower lung function (83–85). A study among Veterans Administration patients is also consistent with the utility of diagnosis of COPD to facilitate smoking cessation. Patients with COPD reported being advised to quit more often than smokers without COPD, although more than 20% reported no advice to quit in the preceding year (86). In addition, a number of studies have demonstrated the feasibility of spirometric screening coupled with cessation counseling in a general practice setting (87–90). Thus, the available data would support an aggressive COPD case identification program that should be coupled to smoking cessation intervention. To be most effective, the intervention should combine behavioral support and pharmacotherapy.

C. Psychiatric Comorbidities

One issue that can confound smoking cessation attempts is the concurrence of other psychopathology. Depression and alcohol dependency are major problems (91,92). Smoking has a modest antidepressant effect, and there is a higher prevalence of smoking among depressed individuals than in the general population. This has been suggested to be a form of self-medication; that is, individuals with depression discover smoking as a means of self-medication that partially addresses their dysphoric mood. Depression is also common among COPD patients (73,93), particularly as the disease progresses. This appears to be a specific relationship as depression is more prevalent among COPD patients than it is among similarly aged patients with other conditions of similar morbidity. Since smoking cessation may make depression worse (94), this is a problem that should be anticipated in the COPD patient. This is particularly important as psychiatric dysfunction, even if mild, can adversely affect exercise performance and morbidity in COPD (95,96).

Depressed individuals are less likely to succeed at a smoking cessation attempt than are individuals without depression (91,97,98). Interestingly, bupropion, which is an effective antidepressant, is equally effective among individuals with a past history of depression as it is among individuals without (59). This contrasts with NRT, which is less effective in individuals with a past history of depression and suggests that bupropion should be considered for smokers with a history of depression.

Concurrent alcohol use also complicates smoking cessation (92,99) and is often associated with relapse in smokers who have successfully quit (100). This may be because both alcohol and its related behaviors represent conditioned cues for smoking and because alcohol use reduces "resolve" to resist urges (101). While currently available strategies are limited efforts to prevent relapse, some success can be achieved (102), and the smoker should be counseled about the hazards of alcohol for relapse to smoking. Among those with alcohol abuse, current evidence suggests that smoking cessation interventions can be effective (103,104) and do not compromise attempts to treat the alcohol abuse (104,105).

VI. Harm Reduction

For smokers with COPD, who are unable or unwilling to quit, there are few options. Currently available therapies, other than smoking cessation, do little to alter the progressive nature of the disease. A number of anti-inflammatory and tissue modifying treatments are under investigation, but the efficacy of such approaches remains untested. "Harm reduction" is an approach to mitigate the consequences of smoking without the individual achieving abstinence. This strategy was the subject of a comprehensive review by the Institute of Medicine, which supported the concept as part of a comprehensive tobacco control program that includes primary prevention and cessation (11).

There are several strategies that might achieve harm reduction. Simple reduction of smoking is unlikely to be successful, as smokers generally alter smoking behavior to maintain nicotine intake (106–108). As a result, it is likely that a smoker who reduces, but continues to absorb the same amount of nicotine will not reduce the other associated toxins. Similarly, switching to low tar, low-nicotine cigarettes are unlikely to be of benefit.

Nicotine, which is the major addicting substance in cigarettes, is much less toxic than other components of smoke. This suggests the concept that pharmacologic replacement of part of the nicotine dose may reduce toxin exposure. Consistent with this, partial nicotine replacement with nicotine gum has been associated with reduced lower respiratory tract inflammation in normal volunteers (109). However, while smoking cessation is associated with reduced inflammation in normal smokers (110,111), similar effects have not been observed in COPD patients, in whom inflammation may no longer be dependent on continued smoking (111), although reduced sputum neutrophils and improved health status have been reported (112,113). Thus, while there is some potential for the harm reduction approach, the benefits, if any, among COPD patients remain to be defined.

In addition to use of pharmacological nicotine, tobacco products may have the potential for harm reduction (11,114,115). It is likely that tobacco products will have greater toxin burdens than pharmacologic nicotine, so demonstration of benefits for harm reduction will be more difficult. In addition, these products, which will be marketed by tobacco companies, raise a number of complex issues related to their regulation, promotion and use. The increasingly widespread availability of nonsmoked products, which have been associated with reduced disease prevalence in Sweden (116), is precipitating an active debate of these issues (116–118).

VII. Conclusion

Cigarette smoking is the major risk factor for the development and progression of COPD. Currently available strategies to smoking cessation can achieve considerable success in both the general population and in the COPD patient. The approach should be multicomponent. Both behavioral support and pharmacologic support are required to achieve optimal success and each smoker should be given the best chance of success with each quit attempt. Smoking, moreover, should be regarded as a chronic relapsing disorder. In this context, smoking cessation intervention needs to be regarded as a long-term therapeutic program. Success is induction of a remission. Relapse should not be regarded as failure, but as an event that can, in part, be prevented and, if it occurs, should lead to prompt retreatment. While COPD patients may have comorbidities such as depression that require special consideration, in general the same approaches that are used in the general population are applicable to the COPD population.

Finally, one must never forget that brief counseling (which takes a few minutes only) is an effective measure: if applied systematically to all smokers, it could double the number of subjects quitting smoking in the population (119). For those who are willing to make a quit attempt, the best chance of success should be assured, which means providing appropriate pharmacotherapy. This means that doctors must ask about smoking at each and every visit, even if the motive of the visit has nothing to do with complications of smoking, and be prepared to act appropriately.

References

1. Mannino DM, Gagnon RC, Petty TL, Lydick E. Obstructive lung disease and low lung function in adults in the United States: data from the National Health and Nutrition Examination Survey, 1988–1994. Arch Intern Med 2000; 160:1683–9.

2. Mannino DM, Buist AS, Petty TL, Enright PL, Redd SC. Lung function and mortality in the United States: data from the First National Health and Nutrition Examination Survey follow up study. Thorax 2003; 58:388–93.
3. Buist AS. Smoking and other risk factors. In: Murray JF, Nadel JA, eds. Textbook of Respirtory Therapy. Philadelphia, PA: W.B. Saunders Company, 1988:1001–29.
4. Rennard SI, Barnes PJ. Pathogenesis of COPD. In: Barnes P, Drazen J, Rennard S, Thomson N, eds. Asthma and COPD. Amsterdam: Academic Press, 2002:361–79.
5. Spurzem JR, Rennard SI. Pathogenesis of COPD. Semin Respir Crit Care Med 2005; 26:142–53.
6. Gold DR, Wang X, Wypij D, Speizer FE, Ware JH, Dockery DW. Effects of cigarette smoking on lung function in adolescent boys and girls. N Engl J Med 1996; 335:931–7.
7. Tager I, Segal M, Speizer F, Weiss S. The natural history of forced expiratory volumes. Am Rev Respir Dis 1988; 138:837–49.
8. Wang X, Mensinga TT, Schouten JP, Rijcken B, Weiss ST. Determinants of maximally attained level of pulmonary function. Am J Respir Crit Care Med 2004; 169:941–9.
9. Gilliland FD, Berhane K, McConnell R, et al. Maternal smoking during pregnancy, environmental tobacco smoke exposure and childhood lung function. Thorax 2000; 55:271–6.
10. DiFranza JR, Aligne CA, Weitzman M. Prenatal and postnatal environmental tobacco smoke exposure and children's health. Pediatrics 2004; 113:1007–15.
11. Stratton H, Shetty P, Wallace R, eds. Clearing the Smoke. Washington, DC: National Academy Press, 2001.
12. U.S. Department of Health and Human Services. The Health Consequences of Smoking: A Report of the Surgeon General. U.S. Department of Health and Human Services, Centers for Disease Control and Prevention, National Center for Chronic Disease Prevention and Health Promotion, Office on Smoking and Health, Washington, DC, 2004.
13. Fiore M, Bailey W, Cohen S, Dorfman S, Goldstein M, Gritz E, Heyman R, Jaen C, Kottke T, Lando H, et al. Treating Tobacco Use and Dependence. Rockville, MD: U.S. Department of Health and Human Services, 2000.
14. Gilpin EA, Lee L, Evans N, Pierce JP. Smoking initiation rates in adults and minors: United States, 1944–1988. Am J Epidemiol 1994; 140:535–43.
15. Pierce JP, Lee L, Gilpin EA. Smoking initiation by adolescent girls, 1944 through 1988. J Am Med Assoc 1994; 271:608–11.
16. Shiffman S. Tobacco "chippers"–individual differences in tobacco dependence. Psychopharmacology 1989; 97:539–47.
17. Dani JA, Bertrand D. Nicotinic acetylcholine receptors and nicotinic cholinergic mechanisms of the central nervous system. Annu Rev Pharmacol Toxicol 2007; 47:699–729.
18. Gotti C, Clementi F. Neuronal nicotinic receptors: from structure to pathology. Prog Neurobiol 2004; 74:363–96.
19. Lau PP, Li L, Merched AJ, Zhang AL, Ko KW, Chan L. Nicotine induces proinflammatory responses in macrophages and the aorta leading to acceleration of atherosclerosis in low-density lipoprotein receptor($-/-$) mice. Arterioscler Thromb Vasc Biol 2006; 26:143–9.
20. Yoshikawa H, Kurokawa M, Ozaki N, et al. Nicotine inhibits the production of proinflammatory mediators in human monocytes by suppression of I-kappaB phosphorylation and nuclear factor-kappaB transcriptional activity through nicotinic acetylcholine receptor alpha7. Clin Exp Immunol 2006; 146:116–23.
21. Takahashi HK, Iwagaki H, Hamano R, Yoshino T, Tanaka N, Nishibori M. Effect of nicotine on IL-18-initiated immune response in human monocytes. J Leukoc Biol 2006; 80:1388–94.
22. Nakayama H, Numakawa T, Ikeuchi T. Nicotine-induced phosphorylation of Akt through epidermal growth factor receptor and Src in PC12h cells. J Neurochem 2002; 83:1372–9.
23. Picciotto MR, Zoli M, Rimondini R, et al. Acetylcholine receptors containing the beta2 subunit are involved in the reinforcing properties of nicotine. Nature 1998; 391:173–7.
24. Tapper AR, McKinney SL, Nashmi R, et al. Nicotine activation of alpha4* receptors: sufficient for reward, tolerance, and sensitization. Science 2004; 306:1029–32.
25. Smith AD, Dar MS. Involvement of the alpha4beta2 nicotinic receptor subtype in nicotine-induced attenuation of delta9-THC cerebellar ataxia: role of cerebellar nitric oxide. Pharmacol Biochem Behav 2007; 86:103–12.
26. Buisson B, Bertrand D. Nicotine addiction: the possible role of functional upregulation. Trends Pharmacol Sci 2002; 23:130–6.

27. Wonnacott S. The paradox of nicotinic acetylcholine receptor upregulation by nicotine. Trends Pharmacol Sci 1990; 11:216–9.
28. Daughton DM, Rennard SI. The tobacco withdrawal syndrome: recognition of the physiological rebound phenomenon and treatment implications. Monaldi Arch Chest Dis 1993; 48:574–5.
29. Hardie TL, Moss HB, Lynch KG. Genetic correlations between smoking initiation and smoking behaviors in a twin sample. Addict Behav 2006; 31:2030–7.
30. Madden PA, Heath AC, Pedersen NL, Kaprio J, Koskenvuo MJ, Martin NG. The genetics of smoking persistence in men and women: a multicultural study. Behav Genet 1999; 29:423–31.
31. Madden PA, Pedersen NL, Kaprio J, Koskenvuo MJ, Martin NG. The epidemiology and genetics of smoking initiation and persistence: crosscultural comparisons of twin study results. Twin Res 2004; 7:82–97.
32. Morley KI, Medland SE, Ferreira MA, et al. A possible smoking susceptibility locus on chromosome 11p12: evidence from sex-limitation linkage analyses in a sample of Australian twin families. Behav Genet 2006; 36:87–99.
33. Arinami T, Ishiguro H, Onaivi ES. Polymorphisms in genes involved in neurotransmission in relation to smoking. Eur J Pharmacol 2000; 410:215–26.
34. Pianezza ML, Sellers EM, Tyndale RF. Nicotine metabolism defect reduces smoking. Nature 1998; 393:750.
35. Minematsu N, Nakamura H, Iwata M, et al. Association of CYP2A6 deletion polymorphism with smoking habit and development of pulmonary emphysema. Thorax 2003; 58:623–8.
36. Ariyoshi N, Miyamoto M, Umetsu Y, et al. Genetic polymorphism of CYP2A6 gene and tobacco-induced lung cancer risk in male smokers. Cancer Epidemiol Biomarkers Prev 2002; 11:890–4.
37. Saccone SF, Pergadia ML, Loukola A, Broms U, Montgomery GW, Wang JC, Agrawal A, Dick DM, Heath AC, Todorov AA, et al. Genetic linkage to chromosome 22q12 for a heavy-smoking quantitative trait in two independent samples. Am J Hum Genet 2007; 80:856–66.
38. Chaudhri N, Caggiula AR, Donny EC, et al. Operant responding for conditioned and unconditioned reinforcers in rats is differentially enhanced by the primary reinforcing and reinforcement-enhancing effects of nicotine. Psychopharmacology (Berl) 2006; 189:27–36.
39. DiClemente CC, Prochaska JO, Fairhurst SK, Velicer WF, Velasquez MM, Rossi JS. The process of smoking cessation: an analysis of precontemplation, contemplation, and preparation stages of change. J Consult Clin Psychol 1991; 59:295–304.
40. Rigotti NA, Munafo MR, Murphy MF, Stead LF. Interventions for smoking cessation in hospitalised patients. Cochrane Database Syst Rev 2003; (1):CD001837.
41. Daughton DM, Heatley SA, Prendergast JJ, et al. Effect of transdermal nicotine delivery as an adjunct to low-intervention smoking cessation therapy. Arch Intern Med 1991; 151:749–52.
42. Schwartz JL. Review and evaluation of smoking cessation methods: the United States and Canada, 1978–1985. NIH publication No. 87-2940. 1987:1125–56.
43. Sackey J. Behavioral Approach to Smoking Cessation (UpToDate). www.uptodate.com (last accessed January 1, 2007).
44. Godfrey C, Fowler G. Pharmacoeconomic considerations in the management of smoking cessation. Drugs 2002; 62(Suppl. 2):63–70.
45. Curry SJ, Grothaus LC, McAfee T, Painiak C. Use and cost effectiveness of smoking cessation services under four insurance plans in a health maintenance organization. N Engl J Med 1998; 339:673–9.
46. Cromwell J, Bartosch WJ, Barendregt JJ, Bonneux L. AHCPR guidelines on smoking cessation found cost-effective—more intensive interventions cost less per quitter. Am J Health Syst Pharm 1998; 55:211–2.
47. Rennard SI, Daughton DM. Overview of Smoking Cessation (UpToDate). www.uptodate.com (last accessed January 1, 2007).
48. Tonnesen P. Smoking cessation. In: Stockley RA, Rennard SI, Rabe K, Celli B, eds. Chronic Obstructive Pulmonary Disease. Malden: Blackwell, 2007:608–21.
49. Fagerstrom KO, Schneider NG. Measuring nicotine dependence: a review of the Fagerstrom tolerance questionnaire. J Behav Med 1989; 12:159–82.
50. Glasgow RE, Mullooly JP, Vogt TM, et al. Biochemical validation of smoking status: pros, cons, and data from four low-intensity intervention trials. Addict Behav 1993; 18:511–27.
51. Glynn SM, Gruder CL, Jegerski JA. Effects of biochemical validation of self-reported cigarette smoking on treatment success and on misreporting abstinence. Health Psychol 1986; 5:125–36.
52. Benowitz NL. Pharmacokinetic considerations in understanding nicotine dependence. Ciba Found Symp 1990; 152:186–200.

53. Benowitz NL. Pharmacodynamics of nicotine: implications for rational treatment of nicotine addiction. Br J Addict 1991; 86:495–9.

54. Le Houezec J. Role of nicotine pharmacokinetics in nicotine addiction and nicotine replacement therapy: a review. Int J Tuberc Lung Dis 2003; 7:811–9.

55. Lam W, Sze PC, Sacks HS, Chalmers TC. Meta-analysis of randomised controlled trials of nicotine chewing-gum. Lancet 1987; 2:27–30.

56. Shiffman S, Dresler CM, Hajek P, Gilburt SJ, Targett DA, Strahs KR. Efficacy of a nicotine lozenge for smoking cessation. Arch Intern Med 2002; 162:1267–76.

57. Lawson GM, Hurt RD, Dale LC, et al. Application of serum nicotine and plasma cotinine concentrations to assessment of nicotine replacement in light, moderate, and heavy smokers undergoing transdermal therapy. J Clin Pharmacol 1998; 38:502–9.

58. Hughes JR, Lesmes GR, Hatsukami DK, et al. Are higher doses of nicotine replacement more effective for smoking cessation? Nicotine Tob Res 1999; 1:169–74.

59. Jorenby DE, Leischow SJ, Nides MA, et al. A controlled trial of sustained-release bupropion, a nicotine patch, or both for smoking cessation. N Engl J Med 1999; 340:685–91.

60. Hurt RD, Sachs DP, Glover ED, et al. A comparison of sustained-release bupropion and placebo for smoking cessation. N Engl J Med 1997; 337:1195–202.

61. Tashkin D, Kanner R, Bailey W, et al. Smoking cessation in patients with chronic obstructive pulmonary disease: a double-blind, placebo-controlled, randomised trial. Lancet 2001; 357:1571–5.

62. Gonzales D, Rennard SI, Nides M, et al. Varenicline, an alpha4beta2 nicotinic acetylcholine receptor partial agonist, vs sustained-release bupropion and placebo for smoking cessation: a randomized controlled trial. J Am Med Assoc 2006; 296:47–55.

63. Jorenby DE, Hays JT, Rigotti NA, et al. Efficacy of varenicline, an alpha4beta2 nicotinic acetylcholine receptor partial agonist, vs placebo or sustained-release bupropion for smoking cessation: a randomized controlled trial. J Am Med Assoc 2006; 296:56–63.

64. Tonstad S, Tonnesen P, Hajek P, Williams KE, Billing CB, Reeves KR. Effect of maintenance therapy with varenicline on smoking cessation: a randomized controlled trial. J Am Med Assoc 2006; 296:64–71.

65. Hughes J, Stead L, Lancaster T. Antidepressants for smoking cessation. Cochrane Database Syst Rev 2004; (4):CD000031.

66. Gourlay SG, Stead LF, Benowitz NL. Clonidine for smoking cessation. Cochrane Database Syst Rev 2000; (2):CD000058.

67. Hatsukami DK, Rennard S, Jorenby D, et al. Safety and immunogenicity of a nicotine conjugate vaccine in current smokers. Clin Pharmacol Ther 2005; 78:456–67.

68. Wagena EJ, van der Meer RM, Ostelo RJ, Jacobs JE, van Schayck CP. The efficacy of smoking cessation strategies in people with chronic obstructive pulmonary disease: results from a systematic review. Respir Med 2004; 98:805–15.

69. Wagena EJ, Zeegers MP, van Schayck CP, Wouters EF. Benefits and risks of pharmacological smoking cessation therapies in chronic obstructive pulmonary disease. Drug Saf 2003; 26:381–403.

70. Jimenez-Ruiz CA, Masa F, Miravitlles M, et al. Smoking characteristics: differences in attitudes and dependence between healthy smokers and smokers with COPD. Chest 2001; 119:1365–70.

71. Schiller JS, Ni H. Cigarette smoking and smoking cessation among persons with chronic obstructive pulmonary disease. Am J Health Promot 2006; 20:319–23.

72. Wagena EJ, Kant I, van Amelsvoort LG, Wouters EF, van Schayck CP, Swaen GM. Risk of depression and anxiety in employees with chronic bronchitis: the modifying effect of cigarette smoking. Psychosom Med 2004; 66:729–34.

73. Wilhelm K, Arnold K, Niven H, Richmond R. Grey lungs and blue moods: smoking cessation in the context of lifetime depression history. Aust NZ J Psychiatry 2004; 38:896–905.

74. Taylor SJ, Candy B, Bryar RM, et al. Effectiveness of innovations in nurse led chronic disease management for patients with chronic obstructive pulmonary disease: systematic review of evidence. Br Med J 2005; 331:485.

75. Wilson JS, Fitzsimons D, Bradbury I, Stuart Elborn J. Does additional support by nurses enhance the effect of a brief smoking cessation intervention in people with moderate to severe chronic obstructive pulmonary disease? A randomised controlled trial Int J Nurs Stud 2006. [Epub ahead of print.]

76. Comparison of four methods of smoking withdrawal in patients with smoking related diseases. Report by a subcommittee of the Research Committee of the British Thoracic Society. Br Med J (Clin Res Ed) 1983; 286:595–7.

77. Research Committee of the British Thoracic Society. Smoking cessation in patients: two further studies by the British Thoracic Society. Thorax 1990; 45:835–40.

78. Tonnesen P, Mikkelsen K, Bremann L. Nurse-conducted smoking cessation in patients with COPD using nicotine sublingual tablets and behavioral support. Chest 2006; 130:334–42.

79. Anthonisen NR, Connett JE, Kiley JP, et al. Effects of smoking intervention and the use of an inhaled anticholinergic bronchodilator on the rate of decline of FEV_1. J Am Med Assoc 1994; 272:1497–505.

80. Willemse B, Lesman-Leegte I, Timens W, Postma D, ten Hacken N. High cessation rates of cigarette smoking in subjects with and without COPD. Chest 2005; 128:3685–7.

81. Wagena EJ, Knipschild PG, Huibers MJ, Wouters EF, van Schayck CP. Efficacy of bupropion and nortriptyline for smoking cessation among people at risk for or with chronic obstructive pulmonary disease. Arch Intern Med 2005; 165:2286–92.

82. Smoking Cessation in Subjects With Mild-to-Moderate Chronic Obstructive Pulmonary Disease (COPD). www.clinicaltrials.gov (last accessed February 1, 2007).

83. Bednarek M, Gorecka D, Wielgomas J, et al. Smokers with airway obstruction are more likely to quit smoking. Thorax 2006; 61:869–73.

84. Gorecka D, Bednarek M, Nowinski A, Puscinska E, Goljan-Geremek A, Zielinski J. Diagnosis of airflow limitation combined with smoking cessation advice increases stop-smoking rate. Chest 2003; 123:1916–23.

85. Stratelis G, Molstad S, Jakobsson P, Zetterstrom O. The impact of repeated spirometry and smoking cessation advice on smokers with mild COPD. Scand J Prim Health Care 2006; 24:133–9.

86. Sherman SE, Lanto AB, Nield M, Yano EM. Smoking cessation care received by veterans with chronic obstructive pulmonary disease. J Rehabil Res Dev 2003; 40:1–12.

87. Hilberink SR, Jacobs JE, Bottema BJ, de Vries H, Grol RP. Smoking cessation in patients with COPD in daily general practice (SMOCC): six months' results. Prev Med 2005; 41:822–7.

88. Hilberink SR, Jacobs JE, Schlosser M, Grol RP, de Vries H. Characteristics of patients with COPD in three motivational stages related to smoking cessation. Patient Educ Couns 2006; 61:449–57.

89. Giannopoulos D, Panagiotakopoulos T, Voulioti S, et al. ABS96: effectiveness of smoking cessation on COPD outpatients in three different settings in Greece. Prim Care Respir J 2006; 15(3):213.

90. DeJong SR, Veltman RH. The effectiveness of a CNS-led community-based COPD screening and intervention program. Clin Nurse Spec 2004; 18:72–9.

91. Hughes JR. Comorbidity and smoking. Nicotine Tob Res 1999; 1(Suppl. 2):S149–52 (discussion S165–6).

92. Hughes JR. Treating smokers with current or past alcohol dependence. Am J Health Behav 1996; 20:286–90.

93. Pentel P, Malin D. A vaccine for nicotine dependence: targeting the drug rather than the brain. Respiration 2002; 69:193–7.

94. Hughes JR. Depression during tobacco abstinence. Nicotine Tob Res 2007; 9:443–6.

95. Borak J, Chodosowska E, Matuszewski A, Zielinski J. Emotional status does not alter exercise tolerance in patients with chronic obstructive pulmonary disease. Eur Respir J 1998; 12:370–3.

96. Yohannes AM, Baldwin RC, Connolly MJ. Prevalence of sub-threshold depression in elderly patients with chronic obstructive pulmonary disease. Int J Geriatr Psychiatry 2003; 18:412–6.

97. Wilhelm K, Wedgwood L, Niven H, Kay-Lambkin F. Smoking cessation and depression: current knowledge and future directions. Drug Alcohol Rev 2006; 25:97–107.

98. Paperwalla KN, Levin TT, Weiner J, Saravay SM. Smoking and depression. Med Clin North Am 2004; 88:1483–94 (see also x–xi).

99. Hays JT, Schroeder DR, Offord KP, et al. Response to nicotine dependence treatment in smokers with current and past alcohol problems. Ann Behav Med 1999; 21:244–50.

100. Krall EA, Garvey AJ, Garcia RI. Smoking relapse after 2 years of abstinence: findings from the VA Normative Aging Study. Nicotine Tob Res 2002; 4:95–100.

101. McKee SA, Krishnan-Sarin S, Shi J, Mase T, O'Malley SS. Modeling the effect of alcohol on smoking lapse behavior. Psychopharmacology (Berl) 2006; 189:201–10.

102. Irvin JE, Bowers CA, Dunn ME, Wang MC. Efficacy of relapse prevention: a meta-analytic review. J Consult Clin Psychol 1999; 67:563–70.

103. Ait-Daoud N, Lynch WJ, Penberthy JK, Breland AB, Marzani-Nissen GR, Johnson BA. Treating smoking dependence in depressed alcoholics. Alcohol Res Health 2006; 29:213–20.

104. Hurt RD, Eberman KM, Croghan IT, et al. Nicotine dependence treatment during inpatient treatment for other addcitions: a prospective intervention trial. Alcohol Clin Exp Res 1994; 18:867–72.

105. Gulliver SB, Kamholz BW, Helstrom AW. Smoking cessation and alcohol abstinence: what do the data tell us? Alcohol Res Health 2006; 29:208–12.

106. Russell MAH, Sutton SR, Feyerabend C, Saloojee Y. Smokers' response to shortened cigarettes: dose reduction without dilution of tobacco smoke. Clin Pharmacol Ther 1980; 27:210–8.

107. Russell MAH, Wilson C, Patel VA. Plasma nicotine levels after smoking cigarettes with high, medium and low nicotine yields. Br Med J 1975; 2:414–6.

108. Scherer G. Smoking behaviour and compensation: a review of the literature. Psychopharmacology (Berl) 1999; 145:1–20.

109. Rennard SI, Daughton D, Fujita J, et al. Short-term smoking reduction is associated with reduction in measures of lower respiratory tract inflammation in heavy smokers. Eur Respir J 1990; 3:752–9.

110. Skold CM, Hed J, Eklund A. Smoking cessation rapidly reduces cell recovery in bronchoalveolar lavage, while alveolar macrophage fluorescence remains high. Chest 1992; 101:989–95.

111. Willemse BW, ten Hacken NH, Rutgers B, Lesman-Leegte IG, Postma DS, Timens W. Effect of 1-year smoking cessation on airway inflammation in COPD and asymptomatic smokers. Eur Respir J 2005; 26:835–45.

112. Swan GE, Hodgkin JE, Roby T, Mittman C, Jacobo N, Peters J. Reversibility of airways injury over a 12-month period following smoking cessation. Chest 1992; 101:607–12.

113. Romberger DJ, Spurzem JR, Von Essen SG, et al. Impact of smoking cessation on quality of life measures in COPD. PATS 2006; 3:A811.

114. Russell MA. Letter: safer cigarettes. Br Med J 1975; 3:41.

115. Company RJRT. New Cigarette Prototypes that Heat Instead of Burn Tobacco. Winston-Salem, NC: RJ Reynolds Tobacco Company, 1988.

116. Gray N. Mixed feelings on snus. Lancet 2005; 366:966–7.

117. Kozlowski LT. Harm reduction, public health, and human rights: smokers have a right to be informed of significant harm reduction options. Nicotine Tob Res 2002; 4(Suppl. 2):S55–60.

118. Henningfield JE, Fagerstrom KO. Swedish Match Company, Swedish snus and public health: a harm reduction experiment in progress? Tob Control 2001; 10:253–7.

119. West R, McNeill A, Raw M. Smoking cessation guidelines for health professionals: an update. Thorax 2000; 55:987–99.

3

The Relationship of Tobacco Smoking to COPD: Histopathogenesis

JAMES C. HOGG

Department of Pathology and Laboratory Medicine, University of British Columbia, McDonald Research Laboratories, St. Paul's Hospital, Vancouver, British Columbia, Canada

I. Introduction

The lungs of a 60-year-old person with a 40-pack-year smoking history starting at age 20 will have inhaled the smoke generated from approximately 290,000 cigarettes. The dose of inhaled toxic particles and gases received from each of these cigarettes varies with the nature of the tobacco, the size, and number of puffs of smoke drawn from the cigarette. The amount of air added as the smoke is inhaled and local conditions within the lung that determine the diffusion of toxic gases and deposition of particles. Tobacco smoking interferes with the innate defenses of the lung, which includes mucus production and clearance, epithelial barrier, and infiltrating inflammatory immune cells (1,2). This interference increases the opportunity for infection by both increasing the production of mucus and decreasing its clearance from the airways lumen (2,3); disruption of the tight junctions that form the epithelial barrier allows foreign material to enter the sub-epithelium (4,5). This stimulates the infiltration of the damaged tissue by polymorphonuclear and mononuclear phagocytes as well as natural killer (NK) cells, CD-4, CD-8, and B-cell lymphocytes (6–17). The organization of the lymphocytes into follicles with germinal centers can be demonstrated in about 5% of the smaller airways of smokers with the normal lung function (15) and this rises to 20% to 30% of airways in the later stages of chronic obstructive pulmonary disease (COPD) (15–17). The formation of these follicles provides anatomic evidence for the presence of an adaptive immune response to foreign antigen, but the source of antigen that drives this sharp increase in the adaptive immune response in GOLD-3 and GOLD-4 COPD is unknown. It could be related to either the colonization or infection of the lower airways by a variety of microbes in the later stages of the disease or to auto-antigens that develop in the damaged tissue. Interestingly this inflammatory immune process persists following smoking cessation (18,19), even though discontinuing the habit slows the rate of decline in the lung function and delays death in those who successfully quit (20,21). Most importantly the repetitive tissue injury caused in the lung tissues by smoking is associated with a repair and remodeling process that attempts to restore damaged tissue. The primary objective of this chapter is to briefly review the nature of the inflammatory immune process in relation to concurrent repair and remodeling of the lung tissue damaged by tobacco smoke and to discuss the contribution of these processes to the pathogenesis of the lesions that define COPD.

II. The Inflammatory Immune Response

The epithelial cells that cover the lung surface and the alveolar macrophages (AMs) that protect it are the first to come in contact with inhaled gases and particulates. Both of these cell types produce an impressive array of pro-inflammatory chemokines and cytokines when stimulated by tobacco smoke that can be measured in induced sputum (22) and bronchoalveolar lavage fluid from patients with COPD (23). Similarly, cytokines are released into supernates of cultured cells exposed to particles and gases under controlled in vitro conditions (24–29). A group more than 50 different types of chemokine ligands (L) spread over four different families determined by the position of the cysteine residue and designated CC, CXC, C, and CX_3C interact with more than 20 different chemokine receptors (R) to direct leukocyte traffic in the inflammatory immune response (30,31). Many chemokines interact with more than one receptor. IL-8 (CXCL8), for example, binds to CXCR1 and CXCR2 to control the infiltration of PMN into damaged the lung tissue. This chemokine is markedly increased in sputum from patients with COPD (32,33) and can readily be measured in the supernates of cultured human bronchial epithelial cells (HBEC) as they take up toxic particles (28,29). CXCL1 (GRO-α) is also secreted by airway epithelial cells and alveolar macrophages and activates PMN, monocytes, basophils, and T lymphocytes via the CXCR2 receptor (30,31). The migration of T lymphocytes is controlled by the expression CXCR3 that is expressed in human peripheral airways (34) interacts with a variety of chemokines that include CXCL9 (Mig), CXCL10 (IP10), and CXCL11 (I-TAC) (35). More complete reviews of this subject are available and the identification of the roles played by these ligand–receptor interactions provide hope that safe and effective inhibitors of individual chemokines might benefit those who suffer from COPD (30,31).

Reports of coculture experiments of AMs and HBECs indicate that paracrine stimulation between these cell types enhance production of chemokines and cytokines capable of controlling the recruitment and activation of leukocytes (TNF-α, IL-1β, IL-8, and MIP-1α), enhancing phagocytosis (IFN-γ), stimulating NK and T-cell function (IL-12), and initiating the repair process (granulocyte macrophage colony-stimulating factor) (36,37). Furthermore, the instillation of the supernatants from AMs and/or HBECs challenged with particles in vitro produces a systemic response similar to that achieved by instilling the same number of particles directly into the lungs of animals (36). Importantly, the magnitude of this systemic response correlates with the number of particles that have been phagocytosed by the macrophages (37). More limited studies of living subjects following inhalation exposure during natural forest fires indicate that cytokines produced in the lungs enter the blood (TNF-α, IL-1β, and IL-6) and stimulate the liver to produce acute-phase proteins and the bone marrow to increase their production of leukocytes and release them into the circulation (38,39). Other studies in humans have shown that there is a relationship between the level of the circulating leukocyte count, the decline in the lung function, and the early death from COPD (40,41). These and other reports indicate that the inhalation of toxic particles and gases sets up a local innate inflammatory immune response in the lung that initiates an adaptive immune response.

III. The Adaptive Immune Response

The transition from the innate response to the much more sophisticated adaptive immune response takes place in lymphoid follicles with germinal centers (Fig. 1) that are found either in regional lymph nodes or in lymphoid collections within the lung tissue (Fig. 2). Those found in the lung tissue are similar to the lymphoid collections observed in tonsils and adenoids in the nasopharynx, Peyers patches in the small bowel, and the appendix of the large bowel (15–17,42). All of these structures are part of the mucosal immune system and differ from true lymph nodes in that they have no capsule

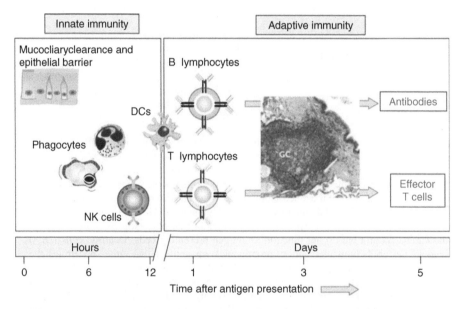

Figure 1 A diagram of the innate and adaptive immune system that includes the mucus production and clearance apparatus, the epithelial barrier, and the inflammatory immune response. Chronic stimulation of this system by tobacco smoke exposure results in both increased production and decreased clearance of mucus from the airways lumen, disruption of the tight junctions that form the epithelial barrier, and infiltration of the damaged tissue by polymorphonuclear and mononuclear phagocytes as well as NK cells, CD-4, CD-8, and B-cell lymphocytes. The adaptive immune response requires antigen presentation primarily by dendritic cells and the organization of the lymphocytes into follicles with GC. This type of response is rarely found in healthy non-smokers but has been documented in about 5% of peripheral lung units of smokers with normal lung function, increasing to about 20% to 30% of airways in the later stages of COPD. The source of antigen that drives this sharp increase in the adaptive immune response is unknown and may be related to either the colonization or infection of the lower airways by a variety of microbes in the later stages of the disease or to auto-antigens that develop in the damaged tissue. *Abbreviations*: DCs, dentritic cells; GCs, germinal centers; NK, natural killer.

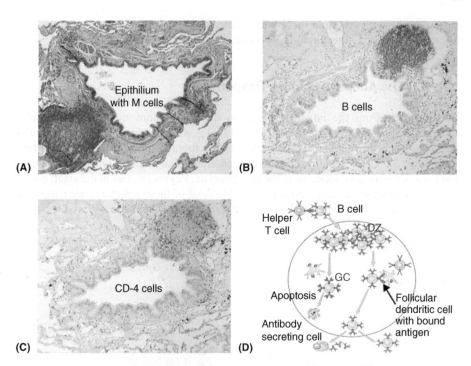

Figure 2 (**A**) A lymphoid follicle in an airway from a person with COPD. (**B**) The concentration of B cells in the center of this follicle. (**C**) The distribution of CD-4 cells around the edge of the follicle. These lymphoid collections are similar to those observed in tonsils and adenoids in the nasopharynx, Peyers patches in the small bowel, and the appendix of the large bowel. They are part of the mucosal immune system and differ from true lymph nodes in that they have no capsule and do not receive afferent lymphatics. The epithelium covering the surface of the follicles contains specialized M cells that transport antigens from the lumen to the lamina propria but do not function as antigen presenting cells. Dentritic cells (DCs) located in the epithelium and lamina propria pick up antigen that either penetrates the epithelial barrier or is transported by the M cells and carries it to these mucosal lymphatic collections. Lymphocytes enter these collections from the blood by attaching to specialized high endothelial cells lining the micro-vessels that supply mucosal lymphoid follicles. B cells concentrate in the GCs, and the CD-4 and CD-8 T cells concentrate in the dark zone surrounding the GC and in the space between the follicles. This separation and concentration of B and T lymphocytes increase the opportunity for the migrating DCs to present antigen to immature T and B lymphocytes as they make their way through the lymphoid collections to the efferent lymph. The diagram (**D**) illustrates that immature T and B cells activated by antigen presentation migrate to the edge or dark zone surrounding the GC where they enrich the numbers of CD-4 T helper cells as well as B and T lymphocytes that have recognized the same antigens. The B cells activated by the CD-4 T helper cells that have recognized the same antigen then mature to antibody secreting B cells and memory cells by a process termed affinity maturation where cells that produce high-affinity antibodies are able to interact with antigen presented by follicular dendritic cells and those producing low-affinity antibodies undergo apoptosis (see text for further explanation). *Abbreviation*: GC, germinal center. *Source*: From Ref. 15.

and do not receive afferent lymphatics (15,17). The epithelium that covers the follicles contained in bronchial associated lymphoid tissue contains specialized M cells (Fig. 2) that transport antigens from the lumen to the lamina propria but do not function as antigen presenting cells. Dentritic cells (DCs) located in the epithelium and lamina propria (7) pick up the antigen that either penetrates the epithelial barrier or is transported by the M cells and carries it either the mucosal lymphatic collections or regional lymph nodes. Lymphocytes enter these collections from the blood by attaching to specialized high endothelial cells lining the micro-vessels that supply mucosal lymphoid follicles (43,44). The B cells concentrate in B lymphocyte rich germinal centers and the CD-4 and CD-8 T cells concentrate at the edge of the follicles and in the space between them (15). This separation and concentration of B and T lymphocytes (Fig. 2) greatly increases the opportunity for the migrating DCs to present antigen to immature T and B lymphocytes as they make their way through the lymphoid collections to the efferent lymph. The T and B cells that are activated by the antigen presented to them migrate to the edge or dark zone surrounding the germinal center (Fig. 2) and enrich this zone with CD-4 T helper cells and B and T lymphocytes that have recognized similar antigens. This greatly increases the opportunity for CD-4 T helper cells, B cells, and T cells that have recognized the same antigen to interact with each other to initiate an adaptive response. The primary stimulus for antibody production is provided by the interaction between CD-4 T helper cell receptors and the MHC class II antigen complex on the B cell (44). Secondary co-stimulatory signals delivered by interaction between B-7 on the dendritic cell and its ligand CD-28 on the B cell as well as between CD-40 on CD-4 T helper cells and the CD-40 ligand on the B cells stimulate clonal proliferation of the B cell and antibody production (43,44).

The rich diversity of antigen receptors expressed on mature T and B lymphocytes is made possible by a somatic recombination of a limited number of gene segments encoded in spatially segregated regions of the germ line. The specificity of the antibodies that are produced is further enhanced by an affinity maturation process that depends upon the presentation of antigen to maturing B cells by a network of follicular dendritic cells located in the germinal center (44). The B cells that express high-affinity antibody to the antigen presented to them bind tightly to it and receive signals that allow them to survive and develop into either memory cells or antibody-producing plasma cells (Fig. 2). In contrast, those that produce low-affinity antibody fail to make this tight connection and subsequently undergo apoptosis (44). The antigens that drive antibody production in the lungs of cigarette smokers in either the early or the late stages of COPD are poorly understood at present. But the marked increase in the adaptive immune response that occurs in the later stages of the disease has been attributed to antigens introduced by colonization and infection of the lung with microorganisms (15,45,46) as well as auto-antigens arising from within damaged the lung tissue (47,48).

A persistent innate and adaptive immune inflammatory response that has been briefly described above is present in the lungs of all chronic smokers and appears to be amplified in those smokers that develop severe COPD (14,15,33) (Fig. 3). However, a multivariate analysis of the overall tissue response indicates that the remodeling of the small airway wall tissue explains more of the variance in the association between changes in airway histology and the decline in forced expiratory volume (FEV_1) than the infiltration of the tissue by any particular type of inflammatory cell (15).

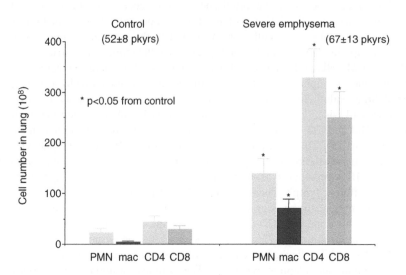

Figure 3 The innate and adaptive immune inflammatory response is presented in the lungs of chronic smokers with normal lung function (control subjects, *left*) and is amplified in those smokers that develop severe emphysema (*right*). Interestingly, this response persists many years after the smoking habit has stopped. *Abbreviations*: mac, macrophages; pkyrs, pack-years; PMN, polymorphonuclear neutrophil. *Source*: From Ref. 14.

IV. Tissue Remodeling

Tissue remodeling is an intrinsic property of the wound healing process that has been most carefully studied in tissue damaged by a single isolated injury (Fig. 4) (49,50). Activation of the coagulation and inflammatory cascades by this injury results in the formation of a clot that seals the wound and forms a primitive granulation tissue. The subsequent organization by the processes of angiogenesis and fibrogenesis produces a more mature granulation tissue that leads to the formation of provisional matrix and ultimately develops into a mature scar (49). Angiogenesis is a process that leads to the formation of new blood vessels within the granulation tissue by both budding from existing vessels at the edge of the wound and by deposition of bone marrow-derived angioblast-like endothelial progenitor cells (EPCs) in the provisional matrix (51–54). Vascular endothelial growth factor (VEGF) and one of its receptors (VEGFR2) enhance vascular permeability and encourage the proliferation of EPCs both in the bone marrow and at the site of injury. They also control the differentiation of the EPCs within the granulation tissue as they form fragile endothelial tubes. These early vascular structures are stabilized by the interaction of angiopoietin 1 with Tie-2 receptors on endothelial cells. Platelet-derived growth factor (PDGF) and transforming growth factor (TGF)-β control the recruitment of smooth muscle to the outer surface of the developing vessels and enhance the production of the extracellular matrix that stabilizes these newly formed structures (49,55). The migration of endothelial cells formed from EPCs is controlled by integrins especially $\alpha_v\beta_3$ and extracellular proteins that include thrombospondin, secreted proteins acidic and rich in cysteine (SPARCs), and tenacin C (49,55).

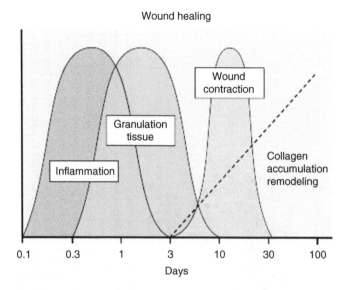

Figure 4   The remodeling process that follows a single clean surgical wound. This type of injury initiates an acute inflammatory response that lasts for about three days and is associated with an increase in microvascular permeability that allows large molecules like fibrinogen to leak out of the vessels and participate in the formation of primitive granulation tissue. This granulation tissue is subsequently organized by the processes of angiogenesis and fibrogenesis leading to the formation of a mature scar. A major difference between this process and that observed in the lung tissue of tobacco smokers is that persistent tissue damage by tobacco smoke results in chronic infiltration of the tissue by inflammatory immune cells that create a chemokine and cytokine milieu that drives the repair and remodeling process that is responsible for the lesions observed in chronic obstructive pulmonary disease. *Source*: Reproduced from Ref. 49.

The fibrogenic process is initiated by the activation of resting interstitial fibroblasts at the edge of the wound that migrate into the primitive granulation tissue (49). These resting fibroblasts have a stellate shape with octopus-like projections that form a network that connects the epithelial to the endothelial boundaries of the interstitial compartment (56–58). These projections send small short extensions through tiny preformed holes in both the endothelial and epithelial basement membranes. Walker and associates (56–58) have used very elegant three-dimensional reconstructions of serial electron micrographs of the interstitial space of the alveolar wall to show that the migrating inflammatory immune cells use both the preformed holes in the basement membrane and the surface of the fibroblast extensions to navigate through the interstitial space. They found (Fig. 5) that the migrating inflammatory cells exit the micro-vessels in the alveolar wall without disrupting the tight junctions by seeking out corners where three endothelial cells meet. Upon exit, the migrating cells come into contact with the endothelial basement membrane and follow its surface until they contact one of the preformed holes that normally accommodate a fibroblast extension and crawl through it to enter the interstitial space. This brings them in contact with the surface of a fibroblast which they use to guide their movement through the interstitial compartment and bring them into contact with the preformed holes in the epithelial basement membrane. After they crawl through the hole in the epithelial basement membrane and seek out the junctions between alveolar type 1

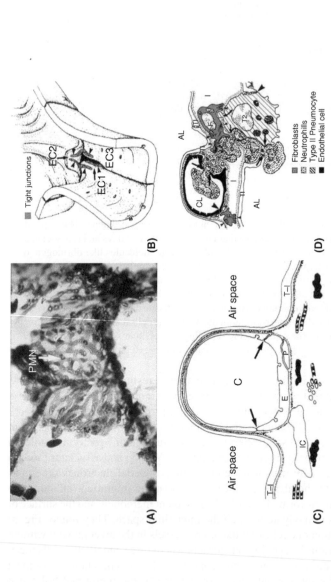

Figure 5 Migratory pathways for inflammatory cells in alveolar tissue. (**A**) Low-power view showing interconnected network of short capillary segments in the alveolar wall, with a PMN within one of the segments (*arrow*). (**B**) Diagram of a tight junction between endothelial cells lining capillaries. Two cells in the same plane (EC1 and EC3) are joined by the flap of a third cell (EC2) that is fastened to the other two, leaving an open pore that migrating cells use to penetrate the endothelial barrier. (**C**) Diagram of a cross section of a single capillary segment, showing that the capillary has a thin side that bulges into the alveolar lumen and a thick side that is in the plane of the alveolar wall. The pores shown in (**B**) are located near the thick side of the capillary (*arrows*). (**D**) Diagram of the migratory pathway used by PMNs as they leave the capillary through the pore in the endothelium shown in (**B**) and (**C**), using the surface of the fibroblast as a guide to cross the interstitial space and exit into the airspace between the type 1 and type-2 epithelial cells. Abbreviations: AL, alveolar airspace lumen; CL, capillary lumen; E, endothelium; F, fibroblast; I, interstitial space; IC, interstitial cell; PMN, polymorphonuclear neutrophil; P, pneumocyte; T1, type 1 epithelial cell; T2, type 2 epithelial cell. Source: Modified from Refs. 57,58, courtesy of Dr. David Walker.

and 2 epithelial cells to reach the alveolar surface (57,58). Similar but less well-studied pathways are used by migrating inflammatory cells to move from the bronchial microvasculature to the surface of the conducting airways.

Activation of the resting fibroblasts at the edge of a wound initiates their migration into the primitive granulation tissue with differentiation of the fibroblasts into proto-myofibroblasts that contain microfilament bundles termed stress fibers (59,60). These proto-myofibroblasts mature into myofibroblasts that contain both stress fibers and α-SM actin (49). The myofibroblasts generate contractile force within the granulation tissue in response to agonists such as endothelin and the increase in force that they generate correlates with the level of expression of α-SM actin. The forces generated by the myofibroblast as well as the reorganization of the extracellular matrix secreted by these cells combine to reduce the size of the damaged area (49,60,61). Recent reports indicate that precursors of the myofibroblasts also circulate in the blood and exhibit a mesenchymal stem cell phenotype with multilineage differentiation potential capable of directing specific types of tissue repair (62). The role of these cells in wound healing is currently under active investigation.

The lung tissues that are repetitively damaged by tobacco smoke are persistently infiltrated by inflammatory cells that create the chemokine and cytokine milieu that drives a repair and remodeling process where a balance between synthesis and degradation controls the deposition of collagen (fibrosis) within the damaged tissue. Synthesis is controlled by a wide variety of cytokines and growth factors and degradation is controlled by proteolytic enzymes such as the matrix metalloproteinases (MMPs) that are activated both by enzymes such as plasmin that are generated from the coagulation cascade and by serine proteases such as the elastase released from infiltrating neutrophils (49). This repair processes is known to be deregulated by the persistent injury that underlies chronic diseases such as rheumatoid arthritis, hepatic cirrhosis, and idiopathic pulmonary fibrosis (49) and we speculate that the deregulation of this process also underlies the pathogenesis of the lesions that develop in the lungs of smokers with COPD.

V. Chronic Bronchitis

In the 1950s, the British medical research council suggested that a diagnosis of chronic bronchitis was warranted when the symptoms of chronic cough and sputum production were present on most days of the month for at least three months in two consecutive years without any other underlying explanation (64). Reid used the size of the mucous gland layer as a yardstick for the postmortem diagnosis of this condition and subsequent studies of the lung tissue that had been surgically removed for cancer (Fig. 6) have shown that the symptoms of chronic bronchitis are associated with an inflammatory response involving the mucosal surface, sub-mucosal glands, and gland ducts, particularly in the smaller bronchi between 2 and 4 mm in diameter (66,67). Longitudinal studies of chronic bronchitis in persons with the normal lung function indicate that its presence does not predict future progression to more severe obstructive lung disease (20,68). However, when present in persons that already have severe airflow limitation chronic bronchitis appears to predict a more rapid decline in the lung function with higher risk of hospitalization compared with persons with a similar level of airflow limitation who do not have chronic bronchitis (68).

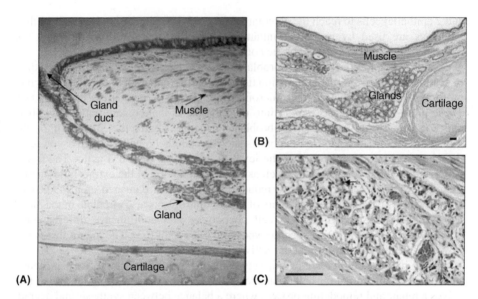

Figure 6 Compares a normal bronchial gland (**A**) to the enlarged bronchial glands (**B** and **C**) from a patient with chronic bronchitis. Several studies of human lungs have shown that the symptoms of chronic bronchitis are associated with an inflammatory response involving the mucosal surface, sub-mucosal glands, and gland ducts, particularly in the smaller bronchi between 2 and 4 mm in diameter. *Source*: Reproduced from Ref. 64.

The inflammatory immune cells that infiltrate the epithelium, sub-epithelium, and glandular tissue in chronic bronchitis include the PMN, macrophages, CD-8 positive and CD-4 positive T lymphocytes, and B cells that are part of the innate inflammatory immune process (9,13,67). This chronic inflammation, enlargement of the mucus glands, and remodeling of the walls of both large and small bronchi reflect a deregulated healing process taking place in tissue that is persistently damaged by the inhalation of toxic particles and gases. The loss of function associated with this process includes the development of a chronic cough and the accumulation of excess mucus in the airways lumen. However, these changes do not influence maximum expiratory flow unless they extend to the smaller conducting airways that are the major site of increased airway resistance in COPD (64).

Studies reported from Snider's laboratory (69) were the first to show that polymorphonuclear neutrophil (PMN) elastase was an important secretogogue for mucus secretion by epithelial goblet cells. Nadel and colleagues (70–76) extended these observations by linking PMN-induced mucin production to stimulation of the epidermal growth factor receptor (EGFR). This group showed that PMN elastase triggered the cleavage of membrane tethered TGF-α, allowing it to attach to the external binding site of EGFR. This step is followed by phosphorylation of the intracellular component of this receptor and stimulation of downstream signaling pathways that activate the expression of MUC5AC and lead to the production of mucus (70). This type of experiment established that EGFR and its ligands provide a regulatory axis for mucin production that involves several membrane bound ligands of EGFR, such as TGF-α and heparin-binding epidermal growth factor. The Nadel group has also shown that reactive oxygen species can bypass this regulatory axis and activate the EGFR intracellular domain directly (71,72).

Recent work in transgenic mice indicates that over expression of epithelial Na^+ channels results in excess epithelial sodium re-absorption and periciliary fluid volume depletion (77). This interferes with ciliary beat frequency resulting in decreased clearance and adherence of mucus to the airway surface. Depletion of the periciliary fluid in these animals was associated with the accumulation of mucus in both large and small airways with greater susceptibility to lower respiratory tract infection and early death.

VI. Chronic Airflow Limitation

Maximum expiratory flow is determined by the product of resistance to flow in the small conducting airways (cm $H_2O/L/sec$) and the elastic recoil of the lung parenchyma that drives expiratory flow (L/cm H_2O). The product of these two variables has the units of time and controls the way in which the lung fills and empties during respiration. Surprisingly the time constant of the lung remains constant over a wide range of breathing frequencies in the normal lungs, but if disease increases either the compliance (emphysema) or the resistance (small airway obstruction) the time required to empty the lung is prolonged (78). A person's ability to empty their lungs can be diagnosed by measuring the volume of air that they can forcibly expire from their lungs in one second (FEV_1) and its ratio to forced vital capacity (FEV_1/FVC). Fletcher et al.'s classic study of the natural history of chronic bronchitis and emphysema used this type of measurement to test the hypothesis that there is a natural progression from the tobacco smoking habit to symptoms of chronic bronchitis, recurrent chest infections, and chronic airflow limitation (18,63). Figure 7 shows the diagram of the natural history of the decline in forced expiratory flow that Fletcher and his associates to summarize their longitudinal study of a group of men working in West London over a period of about six years (18). The horizontal lines added to their diagram indicate the boundaries of the five-stage global initiative on obstructive lung disease (GOLD) classification of COPD severity introduced by the GOLD based on measurements (FEV_1) and its ratio to forced vital capacity (FEV_1/FVC) (79,80). According to this classification, GOLD-0 defines persons with a normal FEV_1 and FEV_1/FVC with symptoms attributable to significant tobacco smoke exposure as being at risk for developing COPD. The importance of Stage 0 in predicting subsequent decline has been questioned and this stage ("at risk") has been deleted from the most recent version of the guidelines (80). Individuals with mild, moderate, severe, and very severe COPD are included as GOLD classes 1 to 4, respectively (76).

Fletcher et al. made the important observations that only 15% to 25% of the smokers developed sufficient airflow limitation to be diagnosed with COPD and showed that stopping smoking slowed the rate of decline in the FEV_1 in those that were able to quit (18). However, they rejected the hypothesis that there is a continuum from smoking to obstructive bronchitis because the majority of subjects that developed airflow limitation during their study had no evidence of chronic bronchitis. Subsequent studies confirmed that the presence of chronic bronchitis in persons with the normal lung function (GOLD-0) does not predict disease progression (68). But others have shown that the symptoms of chronic bronchitis in persons with severe (GOLD-3) COPD are associated with an accelerated decline in FEV_1 (81).

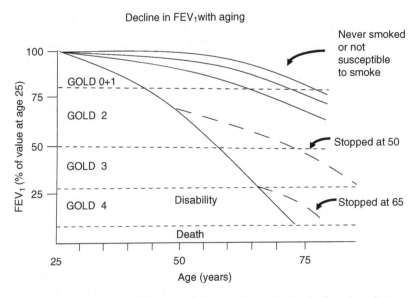

Figure 7 The diagram of the natural history of the decline in forced expiratory volume (FEV$_1$) from Fletcher and associates based on measurements in a group of working men in West London over a period of about six years. The horizontal lines that have been added to their diagram indicate the approximate boundaries of the global initiative on obstructive lung disease (GOLD) classification of chronic obstructive pulmonary disease severity, which is based on age-adjusted lung function. *Source*: Reproduced from Refs. 20, 64.

Acute exacerbations are a major problem in COPD that are attributed to viral (82–84) and bacterial infection, occupational and environmental air pollution with an important residual of cases where there is no obvious cause (80,81). Latent viral infection might explain some of the currently unexplained exacerbations of COPD because this can amplify the inflammatory response associated with colonization and infection of the lower respiratory tract (85,86). Although Fletcher et al. found that exacerbations had no effect on the rate of decline of FEV (18), the U.S. Lung Health Study showed that exacerbations were associated with a more rapid decline in FEV$_1$ in subjects with mild disease that continued to smoke (87). Others reports indicate that frequent exacerbations in patients with more severe COPD, especially those associated with an increased bacterial load, are followed by a more accelerated decline in FEV$_1$ (88,89). Collectively these data suggest that when the lung defenses become compromised in the later stages of COPD chronic infection might have a more important role in the pathogenesis of the airflow limitation in COPD.

VII. Small Airway Obstruction

Although the measurements of FEV$_1$ and the FEV$_1$/FVC provide a reliable way of diagnosing airflow limitation and of classifying its severity they cannot determine the precise contribution of either small airway obstruction or emphysematous destruction to the airflow limitation in individuals with COPD. Direct measurements of pressures and flows within the lung have shown that the smaller bronchi and bronchioles <2 mm

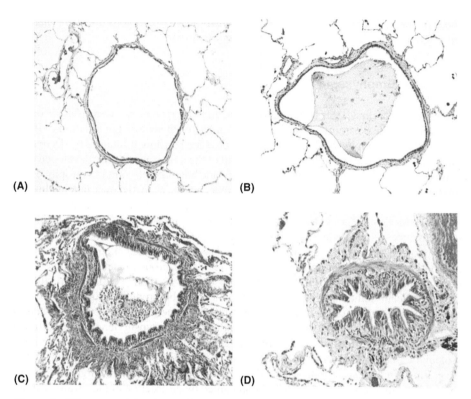

Figure 8 The nature of the obstruction in the small conducting airways <2 mm in diameter where an airway with an empty lumen (**A**) is compared to another airway where the lumen is partially filled with a bland mucus plug containing a few epithelial cells (**B**). An airway where the wall contains an active inflammatory process that also extends into and partially fills the lumen with inflammatory exudates containing mucus is shown in (**C**) and an airway that has been narrowed by collagen deposition in the peribronchiolar space is shown in (**D**). *Source*: Reproduced from Ref. 64.

in diameter are the major site of airway obstruction in COPD (90–92). Figure 8 shows that this obstruction is related to an inflammatory process that thickens the airway wall, fills the lumen with mucus containing exudates, and narrows the airway by depositing connective tissue in the airway wall. Both McLean (92) and Leopold and Gough (93) recognized that an inflammatory process was present in the smaller bronchi and bronchioles of the lungs affected by centrilobular (CLE) emphysema and the latter thought that CLE emphysema resulted from an extension of this process from the small conducting airways into the respiratory bronchioles (93). Matsuba and Thurlbeck (95) demonstrated an excess deposition of connective tissue in the adventitia of the small conducting airways in advanced emphysema and suggested that this peribronchiolar fibrosis narrowed the airway lumen. Cross-sectional studies of the pathology of COPD have shown that the peripheral lung inflammatory immune process found in all smokers is amplified in severe (GOLD-3) and very severe (GOLD-4) COPD (15,20). But the thickening of the airways and occlusion of the lumen by inflammatory exudates explain more of the variance in the relationship of small airway pathology to FEV_1 than the infiltration of the airways by any inflammatory cell type.

VIII. Emphysema

Emphysema was first described by Laennec in 1834 based on observations made on the cut surface of the postmortem human lungs that had been air-dried in inflation (96), but the concept that emphysematous destruction produced airflow limitation by decreasing the elastic recoil forces required to drive air out of the lung was not fully developed until 1967 (97). The major text books of Pathology attributed emphysema to atrophy of the lung tissue as a result of compression of the lung capillaries by the over inflated lung as late as 1940 (98). A major step forward in our understanding of this disease came with the studies of McLean (93) and Leopold and Gough (94) who were the first to implicate the inflammatory response in the pathogenesis of alveolar destruction in their early descriptions of CLE emphysema. However, there was persistent skepticism about this association because of the possibility that preterminal bronchopneumonia may have been responsible for the inflammation observed in their postmortem studies. The subsequent demonstration that emphysema could be produced experimentally by depositing the enzyme papain in the lung (99), combined with observational studies showing the association between emphysema and α_1-antitrypsin deficiency (100), led naturally to the hypothesis that the pathogenesis of emphysema was based on a functional proteolytic imbalance within the tobacco smoke-induced inflammatory response (101).

Emphysema is currently defined as "abnormal permanent enlargement of air spaces distal to terminal bronchioles, accompanied by destruction of their walls without obvious fibrosis" (102,103) and although it can now be diagnosed and quantified during life by several techniques its prevalence has not been measured in a truly representative sample of any population. Postmortem examinations have provided indirect information on the prevalence of emphysema (104,105) and an important study from the United Kingdom (105) showed that it was present in 62% (219/353) of consecutive postmortem examinations and that on average it occupied 12.6% (range 0.5–95%) of total lung volume in cases where it was present. In 179 of these cases where a smoking history could be confidently established, emphysema was present in 75% (80/106) of the smokers and the mean proportion of total lung volume occupied by emphysema was 10.8% (range 0–90%). Interestingly emphysema was also present in 28% (21/73) of non-smokers but the mean proportion of the lung taken up by emphysema was only 1.7% (range 0–40%). This study also showed that the non-smokers lived longer than the smokers (64.8 vs. 60.2 years $p < 0.05$) and that their emphysema appeared in the older age groups (105). A study from our laboratory (69) based on a series of over 400 lungs removed from patients being treated for the lung cancer confirmed that small amounts of emphysema are present in the lungs of non-smokers and that there is a rough dose response between the amount smoked and emphysema severity that achieved a plateau when about 40% of the heavy smokers showed evidence of emphysema (Fig. 9). Although the introduction of the computed tomography scan confirmed that emphysema can be found in persons who have a normal FEV_1, there are neither population-based studies of its prevalence in those with the normal lung function nor studies that address the question as to whether the appearance of emphysema in this group is a risk factor for the later development of severe COPD.

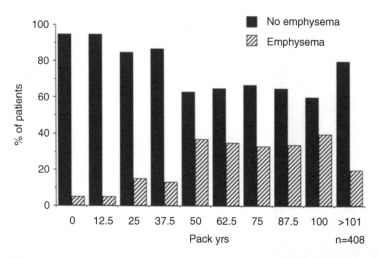

Figure 9 A rough dose response curve between the one smoking history and the percent of patients with morphologic evidence of significant emphysema in their lungs. This reaches a plateau with about 40% of the heavy smokers having emphysema. *Source*: Reproduced from Ref. 64.

IX. The CLE and Panacinar Forms of Emphysema

Figure 10 shows a postmortem bronchogram from a patient with CLE emphysema where the lesions can be seen a low power. The nature of these lesions is shown to better advantage in Figure 11 where several normal terminal bronchioles within a secondary lung lobule (A) and the histology of a normal acinus beyond a single terminal bronchiole (B) can be compared to a line drawing from Leopold and Gough's original description of CLE emphysema (C) and a postmortem radiograph showing the destruction of the respiratory bronchioles in (D). These CLE lesions affect the upper regions of the lung more commonly than the lower (Fig. 12) and are also larger and more numerous in the upper lung (101,102). Heppleston and Leopold (106) used the term focal emphysema to describe a less severe form of CLE but Dunnill has argued that this separation was unhelpful and suggested that both forms had similar origin with focal emphysema being more widely distributed and less severe than the classic CLE form (107). Dunnill also preferred the term centriacinar to CLE, which is logical, based on the fact that each secondary lobule contains several acini (Fig. 11A) and not all of them need be involved in emphysematous destruction.

Wyatt et al. (108) provided the first detailed account of the panacinar (PLE) form of emphysema (PLE) where there is more uniform destruction of all of the entire acinus in 1962. Thurlbeck (104) showed that, in its mildest forms, it can be difficult to separate the normal lung from mild forms of PLE unless fully inflated specimens are carefully examined using a dissecting microscope. In contrast to the CLE emphysema, the PLE form tends to be more severe in the lower compared with the upper lobe (Fig. 12) but this difference only becomes statistically significant in severe disease (104). PLE emphysema is the type of lesion commonly associated with α_1-antitrypsin deficiency but is also found in cases where no genetic abnormality has been identified (104).

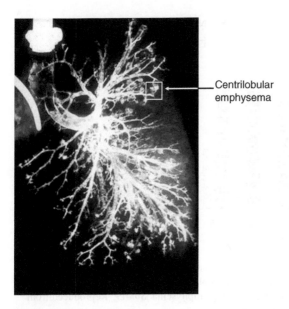

Centrilobular
emphysema

Figure 10 A postmortem bronchogram performed on the lungs of a person with centrilobular emphysema. The lesions hang from the distal airways like "Christmas tree balls" (*arrow*).

X.   Other Forms of Emphysema

Distal acinar, mantle, or paraseptal emphysema are terms used to describe lesions that occur in the periphery of the lobule. This type of lesion is found along the lobular septae particularly in the subpleural region. It also occurs in isolation and it has been associated with spontaneous pneumothorax in young adults (109) and bullous lung disease in older individuals where the removal of large individual cysts has been shown to improve the lung function (110). Unilateral emphysema (McLeod's syndrome) that occurs as a complication of severe childhood viral infection by rubella or adenovirus, congenital lobar emphysema which is a developmental abnormality in newborn children and paracicatricial emphysema that forms around scars and lacks any special distribution within the acinus are much less frequently seen than the other forms (104,107).

XI.   Pulmonary Hypertension

The invasive nature of right heart catheterization in elderly patients with comorbid disease has made it difficult to study the prevalence of pulmonary hypertension in COPD. One study (111) conducted over six years in a group of 131 patients ranging from moderate (GOLD-2) to very severe (GOLD-4) COPD has been reported. None of the subjects had pulmonary hypertension at the start of this study but by the end of the six-year follow-up it was present in 25% of the subjects at rest and in over half of the subjects during exercise. These data suggest that prevalence of pulmonary hypertension increases with COPD progression appearing first during exercise and later at rest.

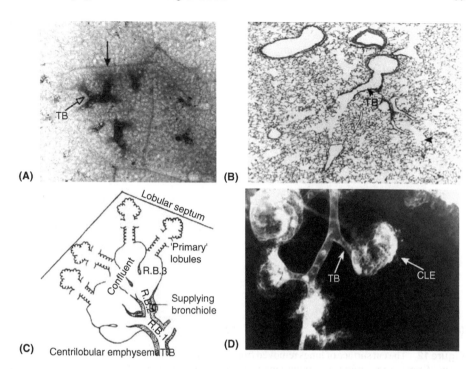

Figure 11 (**A**) Several normal TB within a secondary lung lobule defined by its surrounding connective tissue septa (*solid arrow*). This compares to the histology of a normal acinus beyond a single (**B**) in which the RB and the AD can be recognized. A line drawing from Leopold and Gough's original description of centrilobular emphysema (CLE) showing the destruction of the RBs is shown in (**C**) and a postmortem radiograph of the dilatation and destruction of the RBs in (**D**). *Abbreviations*: AD, alveolar duct; RB, respiratory bronchiole; TBs, terminal bronchioles. *Source*: Reproduced from Ref. 64.

When pulmonary hypertension is absent at rest but present during exercise some of the increase in pulmonary vascular pressures can be attributed to the mechanical events associated with dynamic hyperinflation of the lung in persons with airflow limitation. When the time required to exhale becomes longer than the time between breaths, lung volume tends to increase, first as the breathing rate increases during exercise and later at rest. This increase in intra-thoracic pressure produced by lung inflation is transmitted to all the vessels within the thorax. As a result both pulmonary artery and left atrial pressures are increased when referenced to the atmosphere but not when referenced to intra-thoracic pressure. Treatment with oxygen at this stage of the disease lowers both pulmonary artery pressure and left atrial pressures by slowing the breathing rate which relieves the dynamic hyperinflation and lowers intra-thoracic pressure (112–115). However, when lung emptying is more severely prolonged and alveolar pressure rises above intra-thoracic pressure, there is a shift from zone 3 to zone 2 conditions in the pulmonary circulation produces a true increase in pulmonary artery pressure (112). Hypoxic vasoconstriction of the muscular pulmonary arteries and emphysematous destruction of the pulmonary vascular bed are more likely to contribute to pulmonary hypertension in severe (GOLD-3) and very severe (GOLD-4)

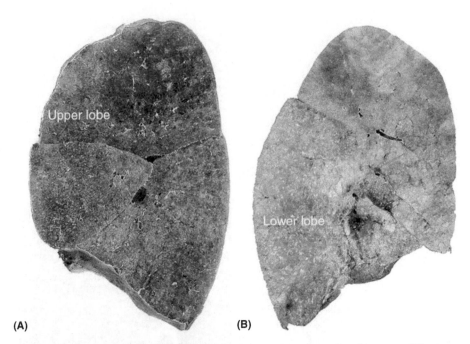

(A)   **(B)**

Figure 12   The cut surface of lungs removed from two patients that suffered from two different forms of emphysema prior to receiving a lung transplant. The lung labeled (**A**) is affected by the centrilobular form of emphysema, which involves the upper more severely than the lower lobe. The lung labeled (**B**) is from a person that suffered from α_1-antitrypsin deficiency, where lower lobes are affected to a greater degree than the upper lobes. *Source*: Courtesy of Dr. Joel Cooper.

COPD when patients more commonly experience chronic hypoxia and there is extensive destruction of the pulmonary capillary bed.

Studies of the lung micro-vessels in mild (GOLD-1) and moderate (GOLD-2) COPD show consistent changes in the intima whereas more severe (GOLD-3) and very severe (GOLD-4) COPD are more likely to be accompanied by fibroelastic thickening of the vessel wall, smooth muscle proliferation, and extension of the muscle into smaller vessels that do not normally contain muscle. Although the contribution of smooth muscle to vessel wall thickness is reported to increase steadily from non-smokers to smokers with normal lung function and smokers whose lung function is impaired (115). In patients who have very severe emphysema, the overall wall thickness of vessels of 100 to 200 µm in external diameter correlate with both the rise in pulmonary arterial pressure during exercise and the difference between the pulmonary artery pressures measured between rest and exercise (116,117). The increase in muscle in the pulmonary arteries is variable and probably dependent on the level of COPD severity. An increase in the amount of muscle has been observed in the pulmonary vessels of smokers compared with non-smokers (115) but in those with mild COPD little if any increase in muscle has been observed (112,118). Muscular medial thickening (119) as apposed to overall wall thickening (116,117) does not appear to have any clear relationship with the severity of the pulmonary hypertension or the vascular response to oxygen in patients with COPD (120).

Reports from Barbera and his associates indicate that this vascular remodeling process is also associated with, and possibly preceded by an inflammatory process where the vessels become infiltrated with a population of cells that is very similar to that found around the small conducting airways. The precise meaning of this finding and its role in the pathogenesis of the peripheral lung lesions observed in COPD is currently under investigation.

XII. Summary

The healing of wounds inflicted by stimuli that recur repetitively as healing takes place provides a model that could lead to useful insights into the pathogenesis of lesions found in the lungs of chronic smokers. According to this model, the amount of collagen that accumulates as fibrosis within the damaged tissue is determined by the net result of both collagen synthesis and degradation. This suggests the working hypothesis that deregulation of this process might result in both accumulation of the tissue in the airway walls and the destruction of the gas exchanging tissue in emphysema.

References

1. Abbas AK, Lichtman AH, Pober JS. Innate immunity. Cellular and Molecular Immunology. Philadelphia, PA: W.B. Saunders, 2000:270–90.
2. Knowles MR, Boucher RC. Mucus clearance as a primary innate defense mechanism for mammalian airways. J Clin Invest 2002; 109:571–7.
3. Drannic AG, Pouladi MA, Robbins CS, et al. Impact of cigarette smoke on clearance and inflammation after Pseudomonas aeruginosa infection. Am J Respir Crit Care Med 2004; 170:1164–71.
4. Hulbert WC, Walker DC, Jackson A, Hogg JC. Airway permeability to horseradish peroxidase in guinea pigs: the repair phase after injury by cigarette smoke. Am Rev Respir Dis 1981; 123(3):320–6.
5. Jones JG, Minty BD, Lawler P, Hulands G, Crawley JC, Veall N. Increased alveolar epithelial permeability in cigarette smokers. Lancet 1980; 1:66–8.
6. Niewoehner DE, Kleinerman J, Rice DP. Pathologic changes in the peripheral airways of young cigarette smokers. N Engl J Med 1974; 291:755–8.
7. Buzatu L, Chu F, Javadifard A, et al. The accumulation of dendritic and natural killer cells in the small airways at different levels of COPD severity. Proc Am Thorac Soc 2005; 2:A135.
8. Cosio MG, Majo J. Inflammation of the airways and lung parenchyma in COPD: role of T cells. Chest 2002; 121:160S–5.
9. O'Shaughnessy TC, Ansari TW, Barnes NC, Jeffery PK. Inflammation in bronchial biopsies of subjects with chronic bronchitis: inverse relationship of CD8+ T lymphocytes with FEV1. Am J Respir Crit Care Med 1997; 155:852–7.
10. Ekberg-Jansson A, Bake B, Andersson B, Skoogh BE, Lofdahl CG. Respiratory symptoms relate to physiological changes and inflammatory markers reflecting central but not peripheral airways. A study in 60-year-old 'healthy' smokers and never-smokers. Respir Med 2001; 95:40–7.
11. Aoshiba K, Koinuma M, Yokohori N, Nagai A. Differences in the distribution of CD4+ and CD8+ T cells in emphysematous lungs. Respiration 2004; 71:184–90.
12. Bosken CH, Hards J, Gatter K, Hogg JC. Characterization of the inflammatory reaction in the peripheral airways of cigarette smokers using immunocytochemistry. Am Rev Respir Dis 1992; 145:911–7.
13. Di Stefano A, Turato G, Maestrelli P, et al. Airflow limitation in chronic bronchitis is associated with T-lymphocyte and macrophage infiltration in the bronchial mucosa. Am J Respir Crit Care Med 1996; 153:629–32.
14. Retamales I, Elliott M, Meshi B, et al. Amplification of inflammation in emphysema and its association with latent adenoviral infection. Am J Respir Crit Care Med 2001; 164:469–73.
15. Hogg JC, Chu F, Utokaparch S, Woods R, Elliott WM, Buzatu L, Cherniack RM, Rogers RM, Sciurba FC, Coxson HO, et al. The nature of small-airway obstruction in chronic obstructive pulmonary disease. N Engl J Med 2004; 350:2645–53.

16. Richmond I, Prichard GE, Ashcroft PA, Walters EH. Bronchial associated lymphoid tissue. Thorax 1993; 48:1130–4.

17. Niagashi C. The lymphoid tissue of the lunga. Functional Anatomy and Physiology of the Lung. Baltimore and London: University Park Press, 1972:102–79.

18. Wright JL, Lawson LM, Pare PD, et al. Morphology of peripheral airways in current smokers and ex-smokers. Am Rev Respir Dis 1983; 127:474–7.

19. Rutgers SR, Postma DS, ten Haken NH, et al. Ongoing airway inflammation in patients with COPD who do not currently smoke. Thorax 2000; 55:12–8.

20. Fletcher C, Peto R, Tinker C, Speizer FE. The Natural History of Chronic Bronchitis and Emphysema. New York: Oxford University Press, 1976:93.

21. Anthonisen NR, Skeanes MA, Wise RA, et al. The effect of smoking cessation intervention on 14.5-year mortality. Ann Intern Med 2005; 142:233–8.

22. Traves SL, Culpitt S, Russell REK, Barnes PJ, Donnelly LE. Elevated levels of the chemokines GRO-α and MCP-1 in sputum samples from COPD patients. Thorax 2002; 57:590–5.

23. Morrison D, Strieter RM, Donnelly SC, Burdick MD, Kunkel SL, MacNee W. Neutrophil chemokines in bronchoalveolar lavage fluid and leukocyte-conditioned medium from nonsmokers and smokers. Eur Respir J 1998; 12:1067–72.

24. Becker S, Soukup JM, Gilmour MI, Devlin RB. Stimulation of human and rat alveolar macrophages by urban air particulates: effects on oxidant radical generation and cytokine production. Toxicol Appl Pharmacol 1996; 141(2):637–48.

25. Quay JL, Reed W, Samet J, Devlin RB. Air pollution particles induce IL-6 gene expression in human airway epithelial cells via NF-kappaB activation. Am J Respir Cell Mol Biol 1998; 19(1):98–106.

26. van Eeden SF, Tan WC, Suwa T, et al. Cytokines involved in the systemic inflammatory response induced by exposure to particulate matter air pollutants (PM_{10}). Am J Respir Crit Care Med 2001; 164:826–30.

27. Mukae H, Hogg JC, English D, Vincent R, van Eeden SF. Phagocytosis of particulate matter air pollutants (PM_{10}) by human alveolar macrophages stimulates the bone marrow. Am J Physiol (Lung Mol Biol) 2000; 279:L924–31.

28. Fujii T, Hayashi S, Hogg JC, Vincent R, van Eeden SF. Particulate matter induces cytokine expression in human bronchial epithelial cells. Am J Respir Cell Biol Med 2001; 25:1–7.

29. Fujii T, Hayashi S, Hogg JC, et al. Interaction of alveolar macrophages and airway epithelial cells following exposure to particulate matter produces mediators that stimulate the bone marrow. Am J Respir Cell Mol Biol 2002; 27:34–41.

30. Proudfoot AE. Chemokine receptors. Nat Rev Immunol 2002; 2:106–15.

31. Lukacs NW. Chemokines and their receptors in chronic pulmonary disease. Curr Drug Targets inflamm Allergy 2004; 4:313–7.

32. Yamamoto C, Yoneda C, Yoshikawa M, et al. Airway inflammation in COPD assessed by sputum levels of interlukin-8. Chest 1997; 112:505–10.

33. Keatings VM, Collins PD, Scott DM, Barnes PJ. Differences in interleukin-8 and tumour necrosis factor-alpha in induced sputum from patients with chronic obstructive pulmonary disease or asthma. Am J Respir Crit Care Med 1996; 153:530–4.

34. Seatta M. Increased expression of CXCR3 and its ligand CXCL-10 in peripheral airways of smokers with chronic obstructive pulmonary disease. Am J Respir Crit Care Med 2002; 165:1404–9.

35. Clark-Lewis I, Mattioli I, Gong JH, Loetscher P. Structure and function relationships between the human chemokine receptor CXCR3 and its ligands. J Biol Chem 2003; 278:289–95.

36. Goto Y, Hogg JC, Shih CH, Ishii H, Vincent R, van Eeden SF. Exposure to ambient particles accelerates monocyte release from the bone marrow in atherosclerotic rabbits. Am J Physiol Lung Cell Mol Physiol 2004; 287:L79–85.

37. Mukae H, Vincent R, Quinlan K, et al. The effect of repeated exposure to particulate air pollution (PM_{10}) on the bone marrow. Am J Respir Crit Care Med 2001; 163:201–9.

38. Tan WC, Qui D, Liam BL, et al. The human bone marrow response to fine particulate air pollution. Am J Respir Crit Care Med 2000; 161:1213–7.

39. van Eeden SF, Hogg JC. The response of human bone marrow to chronic cigarette smoking. Eur Respir J 2000; 15:915–21.

40. Weiss ST, Segal MR. Relationship of FEV1 and peripheral blood leukocyte counts to total mortality. Am J Epidemiol 1995; 142:493–8.

41. Chan-Yeung M, Abboud R, Buncio AD, Vidal S. Periheral leukocyte count and longitudinal decline in lung function. Thorax 1988; 43:462–6.

42. Pabst RG, Gehrke I. Is the bronchus associated lympoid tissue (BALT) an integral structure in the lungs of normal mammals, including humans? Am J Respir Cell Mol Biol 1990; 3:131–5.
43. Abbas AK, Lichtman AH, Pober JS. Activation of T lymphocytes. Cellular and Molecular Immunology. Philadelphia, PA: W.B. Saunders, 2000:161–81.
44. Abbas AK, Lichtman AH, Pober JS. B cell activation and antibody production. Cellular and Molecular Immunology. Philadelphia, PA: W.B. Saunders, 2000:182–207.
45. Sethi S, Evans N, Grant BJB, Murphy TF. New strains of bacteria and exacerbations of chronic obstructive pulmonary disease. N Engl J Med 2002; 347:465–71.
46. Murphy TF, Kirkham C, Sethi S, Lesse AJ. Moraxella catarrhalis in chronic obstructive pulmonary disease: burden of disease and immune response. Am J Respir Crit Care Med 2005; 172(2):195–9.
47. Agusti A, MacNee W, Donaldson K, Cosio M. Hypothesis: does COPD have an autoimmune component? Thorax 2003; 58:832–4.
48. Voelkel N, Taraseviciene-Stewart L. Emphysema: an autoimmune disease? Proc Am Thorac Soc 2005; 2:23–5.
49. Robbins AH, Cotran RS. Tissue renewal and repair: regeneration, healing and fibrosis. In: Kumar V, Abbas A, Fausto N, eds. Pathologic Basis of Disease. Philadelphia, PA: Elsevier, 2005:87–118 (chap. 3).
50. Clark RAF. Wound repair. In: Clark RAF, ed. The Molecular and Cellular Biology of Wound Repair. 2nd ed. New York: Plenum Press, 1996:3–50.
51. Kubo H, Alitalo K. The bloody fate of endothelial stem cells. Genes Dev 2003; 17:322.
52. Rafii S, Meeus S, Dias S, et al. Contribution of marrow-derived progenitors to vascular and cardiac regeneration. Semin Cell Dev Biol 2002; 13:61.
53. Reyes M, Dudek A, Jahagirdar B, Koodie L, Marker PH, Verfaillie CM. Origin of endothelial progenitors in human postnatal bone marrow. J Clin Invest 2002; 109:337.
54. Hill JM, Zalos G, Halcox JP, et al. Circulating endothelial progenitor cells, vascular function, and cardiovascular risk. N Engl J Med 2003; 348:593.
55. Conway EM, Collen D, Carmeliet P. Molecular mechanisms of blood vessel growth. Cardiovasc Res 2001; 49:507.
56. Behzad A, Chu F, Walker DC. Fibroblasts are in a position to provide directional information to migrating neutrophils during pneumonia in rabbit lungs. Microvasc Res 1996; 51(3):303–16.
57. Walker DC, Behzad A, Chu F. Neutrophil migration through preexisting holes in the basal laminae of alveolar capillaries and epithelium during streptococcal pneumonia. Microvasc Res 1995; 50(3):397–416.
58. Burns AR, Smith CW, Walker DC. Unique structural features that influence neutrophil emigration into the lung. Physiol Rev 2003; 83:309–36.
59. Werner S, Grose R. Regulation of wound healing by growth factors and cytokines. Physiol Rev 2003; 83:835–70.
60. Cross KJ, Mustoe TA. Growth factors in wound healing. Surg Clin North Am 2003; 83:531–45.
61. Tomasek JJ, Gabbiani G, Chaponnier C, Hinz B, Brown RA. Myofibroblasts and mechano-regulation of connective tissue remodelling. Nat Rev Mol Cell Biol 2002; 3:349.
62. Sabbatinni F, Petecchia L, Tavian M, dE Villerosche VJ, Rossi GA, Boutre Boi D. Human bronchial fibroblasts exhibit a stem cell phenotype and multi lineage differentiating potentialities. Lab Invest 2005; 85:962–71.
63. Medical Research Council. Definition and classification of chronic bronchitis for clinical and epidemiological purposes. Lancet 1965; i:775–9.
64. Hogg JC. Pathophysiology of airflow limitation in chronic obstructive pulmonary disease. Lancet 2004; 364(9435):709–21.
65. Reid L. Measurement of the bronchial mucous gland layer: a diagnostic yardstick in chronic bronchitis. Thorax 1960; 15:132–41.
66. Mullen JBM, Wright JL, Wiggs BR, Paré PD, Hogg JC. Reassessment of inflammation of airways in chronic bronchitis. Br Med J 1985; 291:1235–9.
67. Saetta M, Turato G, Facchini FM, et al. Inflammatory cells in the bronchial glands of smokers with chronic bronchitis. Am J Respir Crit Care Med 1997; 156:1633–9.
68. Vestbo J, Lange P. Can GOLD Stage 0 provide information of prognostic value in chronic obstructive pulmonary disease? Am J Respir Crit Care Med 2002; 166:329–32.
69. Breuer R, Christensen TG, Lucey EC, Bolbochan G, Stone PJ, Snider GL. Elastase causes secretory discharge in bronchi of hampsters with elastase-induced secretory cell metaplasia. Exp Lung Res 1993; 19(2):273–82.

70. Takeyama K, Dabbagh K, Lee HM, et al. Epidermal growth factor system regulates mucin production in airways. Proc Natl Acad Sci USA 1999; 96(6):3081–6.
71. Takeyama K, Dabbagh K, Jeong Shim J, Dao-Pick T, Ueki IF, Nadel JA. Oxidative stress causes mucin synthesis via transactivation of epidermal growth factor receptor: role of neutrophils. J Immunol 2000; 164(3):1546–52.
72. Kohri K, Ueki IF, Nadel JA. Neutrophil elastase induces mucin production by ligand dependent epidermal growth factor receptor activation. Am J Lung Cell Mol Physiol 2002; 283:L531–40.
73. Burgel PR, Escudier E, Coste A, et al. Relation of epidermal growth factor receptor expression to goblet cell hyperplasia in nasal polyps. J Allergy Clin Immunol 2000; 106(4):705–12.
74. Lee HM, Takeyama K, Dabbagh K, Lausier JA, Ueki IF, Nadel JA. Agarose plug instillation causes goblet cell metaplasia by activating EGF receptors in rat airways. Am J Physiol Lung Cell Mol Physiol 2000; 278(1):L185–92.
75. Takeyama K, Fahy JV, Nadel JA. Relationship of epidermal growth factor receptors to goblet cell production in human bronchi. Am J Respir Crit Care Med 2001; 163:511–6.
76. Takeyama K, Jung B, Shim JJ, et al. Activation of epidermal growth factor receptors is responsible for mucin synthesis induced by cigarette smoke. Am J Physiol Lung Cell Mol Physiol 2001; 280:L165–72.
77. Mall M, Grubb BR, Harkema JR, O'Neal WK, Boucher RC. Increased airway Na+ absorption produces cystic fibrosis-like lung disease in mice. Nat Med 2004; 10:487–93.
78. Otis AB, McKerrow CB, Bartlett RA, et al. Mechanical factors in the distribution of pulmonary ventilation. J Appl Physiol 1956; 8:427–43.
79. Pauwels R, Buist A, Calverley P, Jenkins C, Hurd S. Global strategy for the diagnosis, management and prevention of chronic obstructive pulmonary disease. NHLBI/WHO global initiative for chronic obstructive lung disease (GOLD) workshop summary. Am J Respir Crit Care Med 2001; 163:1256–76.
80. Gold website: www.goldcopd.com, November 2006.
81. Vestbo J, Prescott E, Lange P, The Copenhagen City Heart Study Group. Association of chronic mucus hypersecretion with FEV_1 decline and COPD morbidity. Am J Respir Crit Care Med 1996; 153:1530–5.
82. Seemungle TS, Harper-Owen R, Bhowmic A, et al. Symptoms, inflammatory markers and respiratory viruses in acute exacerbations and stable COPD. Am J Respir Crit Care Med 2001; 164:1618–23.
83. Monto AS, Higgins MW, Ross HW. The Tecumseh Study of Respiratory Illness. VIII. Acute infection in chronic respiratory disease and comparison groups. Am Rev Respir Dis 1975; 111:27–36.
84. Smith CB, Golden CA, Canner RE, Renzetti AD. Association of viral and mycoplasmal pneumonia infections with acute respiratory illness in patients with COPD. Am Rev Respir Dis 1980; 121:225–32.
85. Gonzales S, Hards J, van Eeden SF, Hogg JC. The expression of adhesion molecules in cigarette smoke-induced airways obstruction. Eur Respir J 1996; 9:1995–2001.
86. Kiecho N, Elliott W, Hogg JC, Hayashi S. Adenovirus E1A gene dysregulates ICAM-1 expression in transformed pulmonary epithelial cells. Am J Respir Cell Mol Biol 1997; 16:23–30.
87. Kanner RE, Anthonisen NR, Lung Health Study Research Group. Lower respiratory illnesses promote FEV1 decline in current smokers but not ex-smokers with mild chronic obstructive pulmonary disease. Am J Respir Crit Care Med 2001; 164:358–64.
88. Donaldson GC, Seemungal TAR, Bhomik A, Wedzicha JA. Relationship between exacerbation frequency and lung function decline in chronic obstructive pulmonarydisease. Thorax 2002; 57:847–52.
89. Wilkinson TMA, Patel IS, Wilks M, Donaldson GC, Wedzicha JA. Airway bacterial load and FEV_1 decline in patients with chronic obstructive lung disease. Am J Respir Crit Care Med 2003; 167:1090–5.
90. Hogg JC, Macklem PT, Thurlbeck WM. Site and nature of airways obstruction in chronic obstructive lung disease. N Engl J Med 1968; 278:1355–60.
91. van Brabandt H, Cauberghs M, Verbeken E, Moerman P, Lauweryns JM, Van de Woestijne KP. Partitioning of pulmonary impedance in excised human and canine lungs. J Appl Physiol 1983; 55:1733–42.
92. Yanai M, Sekizawa K, Ohrui T, Sasaki H, Takishima T. Site of airway obstruction in pulmonary disease: direct measurement of intrabronchial pressure. J Appl Physiol 1992; 72:1016–23.
93. McLean KH. Microscopic anatomy of pulmonary emphysema. Aust Ann Intern Med 1956; 5:73–88.
94. Leopold JG, Gough J. Centrilobular form of hypertrophic emphysema and its relation to chronic bronchitis. Thorax 1957; 12:219–35.

95. Matsuba K, Thurlbeck WM. The number and dimensions of small airways in emphysematous lungs. Am J Pathol 1972; 67:265–75.
96. Laennec RTH. A Treatise on Diseases of the Chest and on Mediate Auscultations. 4th ed. London: Longmans, 1834 (translation by Forbes J).
97. Mead J, Turner JM, Macklem PT, Little J. Significance of the relationship between lung recoil and maximum expiratory flow. J Appl Physiol 1967; 22:951–8.
98. McCallum WG. Types of Injury—Destruction of the Respiratory Tract. A Textbook of Pathology. 7th ed. Philadelphia, PA: W.B. Saunders, 1940:419.
99. Gross P, Babyuk MA, Toller E, Kashak M. Enzymatically produced pulmonary emphysema. J Occup Med 1964; 6:481–4.
100. Laurel CB, Erickson S. The electrophoretic alpha-1 globulin pattern of serum α-1 anti-trypsin deficiency. Scand J Clin Lab Invest 1963; 15:132–40.
101. Gadek JE, Fells JA, Crystal RG. Cigarette smoke induces a functional anti-protease deficiency in the lower respiratory tract. Science 1979; 206:315–6.
102. Ciba Guest Symposium. Terminology, definitions and classifications of chronic pulmonary emphysema and related conditions. Thorax 1959; 14:286–99.
103. Snider GL, Kleinerman JL, Thurlbeck WM, Bengally ZH. Definition of emphysema. Report of a National Heart, Lung and Blood Institute, Division of Lung Diseases. Am Rev Respir Dis 1985; 132:182–5.
104. Thurlbeck WM. The incidence of pulmonary emphysema with observations on the relative incidence and spatial distribution of various types of emphysema. Am Rev Respir Dis 1963; 87:207–15.
105. Ryder RC, Dunnill MS, Anderson JA. A quantitative study of bronchial mucus gland volume, emphysema and smoking in a necropsy population. J Pathol 1971; 104:481–7.
106. Heppleston AG, Leopold JG. Chronic pulmonary emphysema: anatomy and pathogenesis. Am J Med 1961; 31:279–91.
107. Dunnill MS. Emphysema in Pulmonary Pathology. Edinburgh, London/New York: Churchill Livingston/Longman Group limited, 1982:81–112 (chap. 6).
108. Wyatt JP, Fischer VW, Sweet AC. Panlobular emphysema: anatomy and pathogenesis. Dis Chest 1962; 41:239–59.
109. Ohtaka M, Suzuki H. Pathogenesis of spontaneous pneumothorax with special reference to the ultrastructure of emphysematous bullae. Chest 1980; 77:771–6.
110. Morgan L. Bullous lung disease. In: Calverly P, Pride N, eds. Obstructive Pulmonary Disease. London: Chapman and Hall, 1995:548–60 (chap. 22).
111. Kessler R, Faller M, Weitzenblum E, et al. "Natural history" of pulmonary hypertension in a series of 131 patients with chronic obstructive pulmonary disease. Am J Respir Crit Care Med 2001; 164:219–24.
112. Weitzenblum E, Hirth C, Ducolone A, et al. Prognostic value of pulmonary artery pressure in chronic obstructive pulmonary disease. Thorax 1981; 36:752–8.
113. Wright JL, Lawson L, Pare PD, et al. The structure and function of the pulmonary vasculature in mild chronic obstructive pulmonary disease. Am Rev Respir Dis 1983; 128:702–7.
114. Jezek V, Schrijen F, Sadoul P. Right ventricular function and pulmonary hemodynamics during exercise in patients with chronic obstructive pulmonary disease. Cardiology 1973; 58:20–31.
115. Horsefield K, Segel M, Bishop JM. Pulmonary circulation in chronic bronchitis at rest and during exercise breathing air and 80% oxygen. Clin Sci 1968; 43:473–83.
116. Hale KA, Ewing SL, Goxnell BA, et al. Lung disease in long-term cigarette smokers with and without chronic air-flow obstruction. Am Rev Respir Dis 1984; 130:716–21.
117. Kubo K, Ge R-L, Koizumi T, et al. Pulmonary artery remodelling modifies pulmonary hypertension during exercise in severe emphysema. Respir Physiol 2000; 120:71–9.
118. Haniuda M, Kubo K, Fujimoto K, et al. Effects of pulmonary artery remodeling on the pulmonary circulation following lung volume reduction surgery. Thorac Cardiovasc Surg 2003; 51:154–8.
119. Barbera JA, Peinado VI, Santos S. Pulmonary hypertension in chronic obstructive pulmonary disease. Eur Respir J 2003; 21:892–905.
120. Wright JL, Petty TL, Thurlbeck WM. Analysis of the structure of the muscular pulmonary arteries in patients with pulmonary hypertension and COPD: National Institutes of Health Nocturnal Oxygen Therapy Trial. Lung 1992; 170:109–24.

4

COPD as a Systemic Disease

ALVAR AGUSTI

Hospital Universitario Son Dureta and Fundació Caubet-CIMERA, Palma, Mallorca, Spain

I. Introduction

Chronic obstructive pulmonary disease (COPD) is a multi-component disease with pulmonary and extra-pulmonary manifestations (Fig. 1) (1). The latter (so-called, systemic effects of COPD) is currently an area of intense research. This chapter describes the systemic effects of COPD identified to date, and discusses their pathogenesis and potential clinical implications (2,3). Given that systemic inflammation is thought to be a key pathogenic mechanism of these systemic effects (albeit probably not the only one) it is discussed first.

II. Systemic Inflammation

COPD is characterized by an abnormal inflammatory response of the lungs to a variety of noxious inhaled gases or particles (mostly cigarette smoking) (4). This inflammatory response is characterized by: (*i*) increased number of neutrophils, macrophages, and T-lymphocytes with a CD8+ predominance; (*ii*) augmented concentration of proinflammatory cytokines, such as leukotriene B-4, interleukin-8, and tumor necrosis factor α (TNFα) among others; and (*iii*) evidence of oxidative stress caused directly by the inhalation of oxidant substances (tobacco smoke) and/or by the activated inflammatory cells mentioned above (4).

Similar inflammatory changes can be also detected in the systemic circulation of these patients, including evidence of oxidative stress (5,6), presence of activated inflammatory cells (7–11) and increased plasma levels of several proinflammatory cytokines, such as TNFα and its soluble receptors (TNF-R55 and TNF-R75), IL-6, IL-8, C-reactive protein (CRP), lipopolysaccharide binding protein, Fas and, Fas-L (12–15). These observations have been recently summarized in the form of a meta-analysis (16). Systemic inflammation can be detected in patients considered clinically stable but it increases during the episodes of exacerbation of the disease (17).

The origin of systemic inflammation in COPD is unclear. Several potential and not mutually exclusive mechanisms can be conceived. Tobacco smoke (and other inhaled pollutants) cause systemic inflammation (18,19). However, it is unlikely that tobacco smoking is the only mechanism explaining systemic inflammation in COPD because patients who had quit smoking years ago still present systemic inflammation (16).

Lung inflammation can also be the source of the systemic inflammation because, in theory, it can either "spill over" into the systemic circulation and/or contribute to

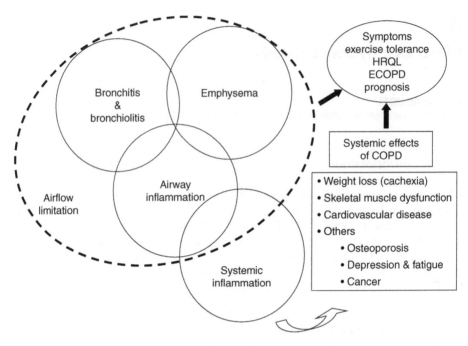

Figure 1 Multi-component nature of COPD. *Abbreviation*: COPD, chronic obstructive pulmonary disease. *Source*: Modified from Ref. 1.

prime and activate different inflammatory cells in their transit through the pulmonary circulation (3). If this was the case, however, one should expect some correlation between the type and intensity of inflammation in the lung and in the systemic circulation. Vernooy et al. could not find such a relationship when investigating the levels of different inflammatory cytokines in the lung (sputum) and in blood (20). There is however, another mechanistic possibility that involves the diseased lungs of these patients as a potential source of systemic inflammation. This is related to lung hyperinflation, which is frequent in patients with moderate to severe disease and has been shown to be a potent stimulus for the production of lung cytokines (21). In this context, it is worth noting the observation by Casanova et al. that lung hyperinflation influences prognosis in COPD very significantly (22).

Tissue hypoxia can also contribute to systemic inflammation in COPD, as shown by Takabatake and colleagues who reported a relationship between the severity of arterial hypoxemia and the circulating levels of TNFα, sTNF-R55, and sTNF-R75 in patients with COPD patients (23). Likewise, other potential sites of origin of systemic inflammation in COPD are skeletal muscle (24–26) and the bone marrow, although the latter has not been systematically studied in these patients. Yet, several observations may point toward a role of the bone marrow response to smoking in patients with COPD. First, it is well established that smoking causes leukocytosis and induces a number of distinct phenotypic changes in circulating polymorphonuclear leukocytes, such as increased band cell counts with a higher content of myeloperoxidase and enhanced surface expression of L-selectin (27) as well as results in the sequestration of polymorphonuclear leukocytes in lung microvessels (28). Second, peripheral monocytes appear to be primed for the production of TNFα, particularly in patients with COPD and low body weight (29). Finally, the recent observation of an inverse relationship between forced expiratory volume in one second (FEV_1) and CRP in subjects with lung function values within the normal range (including never smokers) (30) suggests that systemic inflammation occurs with very mild perturbations of pulmonary function and questions whether it precedes or follows lung function changes.

When considering the origin of systemic inflammation in COPD, it should finally be taken into account that the normal ageing process is associated with low-grade systemic inflammation (31–33), and COPD is an age-related disease (34). Further, smoking has been shown to enhance telomeric loss (a marker of cell aging) (35), and evidence for cell senescence has been recently identified in the lung parenchyma of patients with emphysema (36,37). All in all, these observations identify a new area for research, namely the potential influence of lung ageing in the pathogenesis of COPD.

Finally, an intriguing possibility is that, irrespectively of its origin, systemic inflammation may "feed back" to the lungs and enhance the chronic destructive process that characterizes the disease (38).

III. Nutritional Abnormalities and Weight Loss

Patients with COPD often present a variety of nutritional abnormalities that include alterations in basal metabolic rate, intermediate metabolism, and body composition (12). The cause(s) of these nutritional abnormalities is unclear, although several mechanisms can contribute. These include the increased work of breathing that characterizes the disease (39), the use of β2 agonists to treat airflow obstruction (40), the presence of tissue hypoxia (41), and systemic inflammation (12).

The most obvious clinical expression of these nutritional abnormalities is unexplained weight loss. This is particularly prevalent in patients with severe COPD and chronic respiratory failure, occurring in about 50% of these patients, but it can be seen also in about 10% to 15% of patients with mild to moderate disease (42). Loss of skeletal muscle mass is the main cause of weight loss in COPD, while loss of fat mass contributes to a lesser extent (42). Importantly, however, alterations in body composition (detected by dual-energy X-ray absorption (DEXA-scan) or bio-electrical impedance) can occur in COPD in the absence of clinically significant weight loss (15). This seems particularly prevalent in patients with computed tomography diagnosed emphysema (43).

Unexplained weight loss is an important prognostic factor in COPD patients and importantly, its prognostic value is independent of that of other more traditional prognostic indicators, such as FEV_1 or PaO_2 (44,45). Low body weight, therefore, identifies a new systemic domain of COPD, not considered previously by the traditional measures of lung function, but recently incorporated in a multi-dimensional index (the BODE index) proposed by Celli and collaborators (46).

IV. Skeletal Muscle Dysfunction

Killian and co-workers were the first to indicate that skeletal muscle was abnormal in patients with COPD by showing that many patients stop exercise because of leg fatigue and not because of dyspnea (47). It is now well established that skeletal muscle dysfunction (SMD) is common in patients with COPD, and that it contributes significantly to limit their exercise capacity and quality of life (48,49). Interestingly, the respiratory muscles, particularly the diaphragm, appear to behave quite differently, both from the structural and functional points of view, probably due to the very different conditions under which both work in these patients, the skeletal muscles being generally under-used while the diaphragm is constantly working against an increased load (50,51).

SMD is characterized by two different, but possibly related, phenomena: (*i*) net loss of muscle mass coupled with a switch of fiber type, an intrinsic muscular phenomenon, and (*ii*) dysfunction or malfunction of the remaining muscle (48,49). Several mechanisms can contribute to SMD in patients with COPD (48,49). First, patients with COPD often adopt a sedentary lifestyle, and physical inactivity causes net loss of muscle mass, reduces the force generation capacity of the muscle and decreases its resistance to fatigue (52). Second, chronic hypoxia suppresses protein synthesis in muscle cells causes net loss of amino acids and reduces the expression of myosin heavy chain isoforms (53). Third, systemic inflammation can also influence skeletal muscle structure and function. For instance, TNFα activates the transcription nuclear factor-κB (NF-κB), degrades myosin heavy chains through the ubiquitin–proteasome complex, induces the expression of a variety of genes, such as the inducible form of the nitric oxide synthase (iNOS) (54) and can induce apoptosis (55). Interestingly, skeletal muscle of patients with COPD shows evidence of nuclear translocation of NF-κB, increased expression of iNOS (56) and evidence of enhanced apoptosis (57). Finally, other mechanisms that can also contribute to SMD in patients with COPD are oxidative stress (58), an abnormal regulation of several hormone pathways (59,60) and reduced plasma leptin levels (61,62).

SMD has two clinically relevant consequences in patients with COPD. First, it causes unexplained weight loss, which is a poor prognostic factor in these patients (44,45). Second, it is an important factor limiting exercise in these patients (thus, activities of daily living) (48,49). Appropriate treatment of SMD therefore should be a priority in the clinical management of COPD. Currently, this is based upon rehabilitation programs, nutritional support, and perhaps, oxygen therapy. More specific and effective, therapies need to be developed. Since TNFα might be a biological mediator of SMD in COPD, antibodies directed against TNFα may theoretically provide some benefit in these patients. Unfortunately, very recent data does not seem to support this hypothesis (63).

V. Cardiovascular Effects

Tobacco smoking is a well recognized risk factor for both COPD and cardiovascular diseases. It has been recently recognized, however, that the presence of COPD increases the risk of cardiovascular disease among smokers even further (64). The mechanism(s) for this synergy are still under investigation but, given that systemic inflammation is a well established factor in the pathogenesis of cardiovascular disease (65), the low-grade persistent systemic inflammation that characterizes COPD is likely to contribute significantly to the pathobiology of these cardiovascular abnormalities (64).

Endothelial cells are key controllers of vascular tone and tissue perfusion (66). In resected lung specimens studied in vitro Dihn-Xuan was the first to show that endothelial function is abnormal in COPD (67). The use of echo-Doppler technology has allowed the non-invasive study of endothelial function in other vascular territories in vivo (68–70). Using these techniques it has been shown that in patients with COPD the endothelial function of the renal circulation is also abnormal (71,72). Similar abnormalities were more recently identified in the bronchial circulation (part of the systemic circulation) in COPD (73).

Interestingly, the use of inhaled steroids to treat pulmonary inflammation may have unexpected systemic effects and contribute also to reduce systemic inflammation (74), and potentially, to reduce cardiovascular morbidity and mortality in patients with COPD (64,75,76).

VI. Nervous System Effects

Different aspects of the nervous system may be abnormal in patients with COPD. For instance, there is high prevalence of depression in these patients (77). Even though it is possible that this may simply represent a physiological response to a chronic debilitating disease, it is also possible that it may related to systemic inflammation in these patients, because TNFα and other cytokines and molecules such as nitric oxide have been implicated in the pathogenesis of depression (78–80). Likewise, the use of nuclear magnetic resonance spectroscopy has shown that the bio-energetic metabolism of the brain is altered in these patients (81). Finally, Takabatake et al. showed indirect evidence of abnormal control of the autonomic nervous system in patients with COPD, particularly those with low body weight, and a related deregulation of the normal circadian rhythm of leptin (82). Given that leptin has important effects on neuroendocine function, apetite regulation, body weight control, and thermogenesis in humans (82), and that previous studies have shown reduced plasma leptin concentration in patients with COPD (61,62), these findings may well be relevant also for the pathogenesis of SMD and weight loss in COPD.

VII. Osteoskeletal Effects

The prevalence of osteoporosis is increased in patients with COPD (83,84). Many of the same factors that are considered potential pathogenic factors of SMD in COPD, can theoretically contribute also to osteoporosis. These include: malnutrition, sedentarism, smoking, steroid treatment, and systemic inflammation (84–86). Similarly, excessive osteoporosis in relation to age could also be considered a systemic effect of COPD (43,83).

VIII. Conclusions

COPD can no longer be considered a disease affecting the lungs only. Available evidence indicates that COPD has an important systemic component, that the clinical assessment of COPD must take it into consideration, and that the treatment of these extra-pulmonary effects can be important in the clinical management of the disease.

References

1. Agusti AG. COPD, a multicomponent disease: implications for management. Respir Med 2005; 99:670–82.
2. Agusti A. Thomas A. Neff lecture. Chronic obstructive pulmonary disease: a systemic disease. Proc Am Thorac Soc 2006; 3:478–81.
3. Agusti AG, Noguera A, Sauleda J, Sala E, Pons J, Busquets X. Systemic effects of chronic obstructive pulmonary disease. Eur Respir J 2003; 21:347–60.
4. Celli BR, MacNee W, Agusti AG, Anzueto A, Berg BR, Buist AS, Calverley P, Chavannes N, Dillard T, Fahy B, et al. Standards for the diagnosis and treatment of patients with COPD: a summary of the ATS/ERS position paper. Eur Respir J 2004; 23:932–46.
5. Rahman I, Morrison D, Donaldson K, MacNee W. Systemic oxidative stress in asthma, COPD, and smokers. Am J Respir Crit Care Med 1996; 154:1055–60.
6. Praticò D, Basili S, Vieri M, Cordova C, Violi F, Fitzgerald GA. Chronic obstructive pulmonary disease is associated with an increase in urinary levels of isoprostane F_{2a}-III, an index of oxidant stress. Am J Respir Crit Care Med 1998; 158:1709–14.
7. Burnett D, Hill SL, Chamba A, Stockley RA. Neutrophils from subjects with chronic obstructive lung disease show enhanced chemotaxis and extracellular proteolysis. Lancet 1987; 2:1043–6.
8. Noguera A, Batle S, Miralles C, et al. Enhanced neutrophil response in chronic obstructive pulmonary disease. Thorax 2001; 56:432–7.
9. Noguera A, Busquets X, Sauleda J, Villaverde JM, MacNee W, Agustí AGN. Expression of adhesion molecules and G proteins in circulating neutrophils in chronic obstructive pulmonary disease. Am J Respir Crit Care Med 1998; 158:1664–8.
10. Sauleda J, Garcia-Palmer FJ, Gonzalez G, Palou A, Agusti AG. The activity of cytochrome oxidase is increased in circulating lymphocytes of patients with chronic obstructive pulmonary disease, asthma, and chronic arthritis. Am J Respir Crit Care Med 2000; 161:32–5.
11. Noguera A, Sala E, Pons AR, Iglesias J, MacNee W, Agusti AGN. Expression of adhesion molecules during apoptosis of circulating neutrophils in COPD. Chest 2004; 125:1837–42.
12. Schols AM, Buurman WA, Staal van den Brekel AJ, Dentener MA, Wouters EF. Evidence for a relation between metabolic derangements and increased levels of inflammatory mediators in a subgroup of patients with chronic obstructive pulmonary disease. Thorax 1996; 51:819–24.
13. Di Francia M, Barbier D, Mege JL, Orehek J. Tumor necrosis factor-alpha levels and weight loss in chronic obstructive pulmonary disease. Am J Respir Crit Care Med 1994; 150:1453–5.
14. Yasuda N, Gotoh K, Minatoguchi S, et al. An increase of soluble Fas, an inhibitor of apoptosis, associated with progression of COPD. Respir Med 1998; 92:993–9.
15. Eid AA, Ionescu AA, Nixon LS, et al. Inflammatory response and body composition in chronic obstructive pulmonary disease. Am J Respir Crit Care Med 2001; 164:1414–8.
16. Gan WQ, Man SF, Senthilselvan A, Sin DD. Association between chronic obstructive pulmonary disease and systemic inflammation: a systematic review and a meta-analysis. Thorax 2004; 59:574–80.
17. Pinto-Plata VM, Livnat G, Girish M, et al. Systemic cytokines, clinical and physiological changes in patients hospitalized for exacerbation of COPD. Chest 2007; 131:37–43.
18. van Eeden SF, Tan WC, Suwa T, et al. Cytokines involved in the systemic inflammatory response induced by exposure to particulate matter air pollutants (PM_{10}). Am J Respir Crit Care Med 2001; 164:826–30.
19. Morrow JD, Frei B, Longmire WA, et al. Increase in circulating products of lipid peroxidation (F_2-isoprostanes) in smokers. N Engl J Med 1995; 332:1198–203.
20. Vernooy JH, Kucukaycan M, Jacobs JA, et al. Local and systemic inflammation in patients with chronic obstructive pulmonary disease: soluble tumor necrosis factor receptors are increased in sputum. Am J Respir Crit Care Med 2002; 166:1218–24.
21. Vassilakopoulos T, Roussos C, Zakynthinos S. The immune response to resistive breathing. Eur Respir J 2004; 24:1033–43.
22. Casanova C, Cote C, de Torres JP, et al. Inspiratory-to-total lung capacity ratio predicts mortality in patients with chronic obstructive pulmonary disease. Am J Respir Crit Care Med 2005; 171:591–7.
23. Takabatake N, Nakamura H, Abe S, et al. The relationship between chronic hypoxemia and activation of the tumor necrosis factor-alpha system in patients with chronic obstructive pulmonary disease. Am J Respir Crit Care Med 2000; 161:1179–84.

24. Rabinovich RA, Figueras M, Ardite E, et al. Increased tumour necrosis factor-alpha plasma levels during moderate-intensity exercise in COPD patients. Eur Respir J 2003; 21:789–94.
25. Couillard A, Maltais F, Saey D, et al. Exercise-induced quadriceps oxidative stress and peripheral muscle dysfunction in patients with chronic obstructive pulmonary disease. Am J Respir Crit Care Med 2003; 167:1664–9.
26. Koechlin C, Couillard A, Cristol JP, et al. Does systemic inflammation trigger local exercise-induced oxidative stress in COPD? Eur Respir J 2004; 23:538–44.
27. van Eeden SF, Hogg JC. The response of human bone marrow to chronic cigarette smoking. Eur Respir J 2000; 15:915–21.
28. MacNee W, Wiggs B, Belzberg AS, Hogg JC. The effect of cigarette smoking on neutrophil kinetics in human lungs. N Engl J Med 1989; 321:924–8.
29. De Godoy I, Donahoe M, Calhoun WJ, Mancino J, Rogers RM. Elevated TNF-alpha production by peripheral blood monocytes of weight-losing COPD patients. Am J Respir Crit Care Med 1996; 153:633–7.
30. Aronson D, Roterman I, Yigla M, et al. Inverse association between pulmonary function and C-reactive protein in apparently healthy subjects. Am J Respir Crit Care Med 2006; 174:626–32.
31. De MM, Franceschi C, Monti D, Ginaldi L. Inflammation markers predicting frailty and mortality in the elderly. Exp Mol Pathol 2006; 80:219–27.
32. De MM, Franceschi C, Monti D, Ginaldi L. Inflamm-ageing and lifelong antigenic load as major determinants of ageing rate and longevity. FEBS Lett 2005; 579:2035–9.
33. Ginaldi L, De MM, Monti D, Franceschi C. Chronic antigenic load and apoptosis in immunosenescence. Trends Immunol 2005; 26:79–84.
34. Fabbri LM, Ferrari R. Chronic disease in the elderly: back to the future of internal medicine. Breathe 2006; 3:40–9.
35. Morla M, Busquets X, Pons J, Sauleda J, MacNee W, Agusti AG. Telomere shortening in smokers with and without COPD. Eur Respir J 2006; 27:525–8.
36. Muller KC, Welker L, Paasch K, et al. Lung fibroblasts from patients with emphysema show markers of senescence in vitro. Respir Res 2006; 7:32.
37. Tsuji T, Aoshiba K, Nagai A. Alveolar cell senescence in patients with pulmonary emphysema. Am J Respir Crit Care Med 2006; 174:886–93.
38. Agusti A, MacNee W, Donaldson K, Cosio M. Hypothesis: does COPD have an autoimmune component? Thorax 2003; 58:832–4.
39. Baarends EM, Schols AM, Slebos DJ, Mostert R, Janssen PP, Wouters EF. Metabolic and ventilatory response pattern to arm elevation in patients with COPD and healthy age-matched subjects. Eur Respir J 1995; 8:1345–51.
40. Amoroso P, Wilson SR, Moxham J, Ponte J. Acute effects of inhaled salbutamol on the metabolic rate of normal subjects. Thorax 1993; 48:882–5.
41. Sridhar MK. Why do patients with emphysema lose weight? Lancet 1995; 345:1190–1.
42. Schols AM, Soeters PB, Dingemans AM, Mostert R, Frantzen PJ, Wouters EF. Prevalence and characteristics of nutritional depletion in patients with stable COPD eligible for pulmonary rehabilitation. Am Rev Respir Dis 1993; 147:1151–6.
43. Engelen MP, Schols AM, Lamers RJ, Wouters EF. Different patterns of chronic tissue wasting among patients with chronic obstructive pulmonary disease. Clin Nutr 1999; 18:275–80.
44. Schols AM, Slangen J, Volovics L, Wouters EF. Weight loss is a reversible factor in the prognosis of chronic obstructive pulmonary disease. Am J Respir Crit Care Med 1998; 157:1791–7.
45. Landbo C, Prescott E, Lange P, Vestbo J, Almdal TP. Prognostic value of nutritional status in chronic obstructive pulmonary disease. Am J Respir Crit Care Med 1999; 160:1856–61.
46. Celli BR, Cote CG, Marin JM, et al. The body-mass index, airflow obstruction, dyspnea, and exercise capacity index in chronic obstructive pulmonary disease. N Engl J Med 2004; 350:1005–12.
47. Killian KJ, Leblanc P, Martin DH, Summers E, Jones NL, Campbell EJM. Exercise capacity and ventilatory, circulatory, and symptom limitation in patients with chronic airflow limitation. Am Rev Respir Dis 1992; 146:935–40.
48. American Thoracic Society/European Respiratory Society. Skeletal muscle dysfunction in chronic obstructive pulmonary disease. Am J Respir Crit Care Med 1999; 159:S2–40.
49. Gosker HR, Wouters EF, Van der Vusse GJ, Schols AM. Skeletal muscle dysfunction in chronic obstructive pulmonary disease and chronic heart failure: underlying mechanisms and therapy perspectives. Am J Clin Nutr 2000; 71:1033–47.

50. Levine S, Kaiser L, Leferovich J, Tikunov B. Cellular adaptations in the diaphragm in chronic obstructive pulmonary disease. N Engl J Med 1997; 337:1799–806.
51. Sauleda J, Gea J, Orozco-Levi M, et al. Structure and function relationships of the respiratory muscles. Eur Respir J 1998; 11:906–11.
52. Roca J, Whipp BJ, Agustí AGN, Anderson SD, Casaburi R, Cotes JE, Donner CF, Estenne M, Folgering H, Higenbottam T, et al. Clinical exercise testing with reference to lung diseases: indications, standardization and interpretation strategies. Eur Respir J 1997; 10:2662–89.
53. Bigard AX, Sanchez H, Birot O, Serrurier B. Myosin heavy chain composition of skeletal muscles in young rats growing under hypobaric hypoxia conditions. J Appl Physiol 2000; 88:479–86.
54. Li YP, Schwartz RJ, Waddell ID, Holloway BR, Reid MB. Skeletal muscle myocytes undergo protein loss and reactive oxygen-mediated NF-κB activation in response to tumor necrosis factor α. FASEB J 1998; 12:871–80.
55. Petrache I, Otterbein LE, Alam J, Wiegand GW, Choi AM. Heme oxygenase-1 inhibits TNF-alpha-induced apoptosis in cultured fibroblasts. Am J Physiol Lung Cell Mol Physiol 2000; 278:L312–9.
56. Agusti A, Morla M, Sauleda J, Saus C, Busquets X. NF-κB activation and iNOS upregulation in skeletal muscle of patients with COPD and low body weight. Thorax 2004; 59:483–7.
57. Agusti AGN, Sauleda J, Miralles C, et al. Skeletal muscle apoptosis and weight loss in chronic obstructive pulmonary disease. Am J Respir Crit Care Med 2002; 166:485–9.
58. Reid MB, Shoji T, Moody MR, Entman ML. Reactive oxygen in skeletal muscle. II. Extracellular release of free radicals. J Appl Physiol 1992; 73:1805–9.
59. Kamischke A, Kemper DE, Castel MA, et al. Testosterone levels in men with chronic obstructive pulmonary disease with or without glucocorticoid therapy. Eur Respir J 1998; 11:41–5.
60. Casaburi R. Rationale for anabolic therapy to facilitate rehabilitation in chronic obstructive pulmonary disease. Baillieres Clin Endocrinol Metab 1998; 12:407–18.
61. Creutzberg EC, Wouters EF, Vanderhoven-Augustin IM, Dentener MA, Schols AM. Disturbances in leptin metabolism are related to energy imbalance during acute exacerbations of chronic obstructive pulmonary disease. Am J Respir Crit Care Med 2000; 162:1239–45.
62. Takabatake N, Nadamura H, Abe S, et al. Circulating leptin in patients with chronic obstructive pulmonary disease. Am J Respir Crit Care Med 1999; 159:1215–9.
63. Rennard SI, Fogarty C, Kelsen S, Long W, Ramsdell J, Allison J, Mahler D, Saadeh C, Siler T, Snell P, et al. The safety and efficacy of infliximab in moderate-to-severe chronic obstructive pulmonary disease. Am J Respir Crit Care Med 2007; 175:926–34.
64. Sin DD, Man SF. Why are patients with chronic obstructive pulmonary disease at increased risk of cardiovascular diseases? The potential role of systemic inflammation in chronic obstructive pulmonary disease Circulation 2003; 107:1514–9.
65. Hansson GK. Inflammation, atherosclerosis, and coronary artery disease. N Engl J Med 2005; 352:1685–95.
66. Moncada S, Higgs A. The L-arginine–nitric oxide pathway. N Engl J Med 1993; 329:2002–12.
67. Dinh-Xuan AT, Higenbottam TW, Clelland CA, et al. Impairment of endothelium-dependent pulmonary-artery relaxation in chronic obstructive lung disease. N Engl J Med 1991; 324:1539–47.
68. Celermajer DS, Sorensen KE, Gooch VM, et al. Non-invasive detection of endothelial dysfunction in children and adults at risk of atherosclerosis. Lancet 1992; 340:1111–5.
69. Celermajer DS, Adams MR, Clarkson P, et al. Passive smoking and impaired endothelium-dependent arterial dilatation in healthy young adults. N Engl J Med 1996; 334:150–4.
70. Raitakari OT, Adams MR, McCredie RJ, Griffiths KA, Celermajer DS. Arterial endothelial dysfunction related to passive smoking is potentially reversible in healthy young adults. Ann Intern Med 1999; 130:578–81.
71. Howes TQ, Deane CR, Levin GE, Baudouin SV, Moxham J. The effects of oxygen and dopamine on renal and aortic blood flow in chronic obstructive pulmonary disease with hypoxemia and hypercapnia. Am J Respir Crit Care Med 1995; 151:378–83.
72. Baudouin SV, Bott J, Ward A, Deane C, Moxham J. Short term effect of oxygen on renal haemodynamics in patients with hypoxaemic chronic obstructive airways disease. Thorax 1992; 47:550–4.
73. Mendes ES, Campos MA, Wanner A. Airway blood flow reactivity in healthy smokers and in ex-smokers with or without COPD. Chest 2006; 129:893–8.
74. Sin DD, Lacy P, York E, Man SFP. Effects of fluticasone on systemic markers of inflammation in chronic obstructive pulmonary disease. Am J Respir Crit Care Med 2004; 170:760–5.

75. Huiart L, Ernst P, Ranouil X, Suissa S. Low-dose inhaled corticosteroids and the risk of acute myocardial infarction in COPD. Eur Respir J 2005; 25:634–9.
76. Vestbo J. The TORCH (toward a revolution in COPD health) survival study protocol. Eur Respir J 2004; 24:206–10.
77. Wagena EJ, Huibers MJ, Van Schayck CP. Antidepressants in the treatment of patients with COPD: possible associations between smoking cigarettes, COPD and depression. Thorax 2001; 56:587–8.
78. Tracey KJ, Cerami A. Tumor necrosis factor: a pleiotropic cytokine and therapeutic target. Annu Rev Med 1994; 45:491–503.
79. Holden RJ, Pakula IS, Mooney PA. An immunological model connecting the pathogenesis of stress, depression and carcinoma. Med Hypotheses 1998; 51:309–14.
80. Worrall NK, Chang K, Suau GM, et al. Inhibition of inducible nitric oxide synthase prevents myocardial and systemic vascular barrier dysfunction during early cardiac allograft rejection. Circ Res 1996; 78:769–79.
81. Mathur R, Cox IJ, Oatridge A, Shephard DT, Shaw RJ, Taylor-Robinson SD. Cerebral bioenergetics in stable chronic obstructive pulmonary disease. Am J Respir Crit Care Med 1999; 160:1994–9.
82. Takabatake N, Nakamura H, Minamihaba O, et al. A novel pathophysiologic phenomenon in cachexic patients with chronic obstructive pulmonary disease: the relationship between the circadian rhythm of circulating leptin and the very low-frequency component of heart rate variability. Am J Respir Crit Care Med 2001; 163:1314–9.
83. Incalzi RA, Caradonna P, Ranieri P, et al. Correlates of osteoporosis in chronic obstructive pulmonary disease. Respir Med 2000; 94:1079–84.
84. Gross NJ. Extrapulmonary effects of chronic obstructive pulmonary disease. Curr Opin Pulm Med 2001; 7:84–92.
85. Nishimura Y, Nakata H, Matsubara M, Maeda H, Yokoyama H. Bone mineral loss in patients with chronic obstructive pulmonary disease. Nihon Kyobu Shikkan Gakkai Zasshi 1993; 31:1548–52.
86. Goldstein MF, Fallon JJ, Jr, Harning R. Chronic glucocorticoid therapy-induced osteoporosis in patients with obstructive lung disease. Chest 1999; 116:1733–49.

5

Early Diagnosis of COPD: Usefulness, Tools, and Actors

DENNIS E. DOHERTY
Division of Pulmonary, Critical Care, and Sleep Medicine, Respiratory Care Services, Department of Medicine, University of Kentucky, Veterans Administration Medical Center, Lexington, Kentucky, U.S.A.

KETAN BUCH
Division of Pulmonary, Critical Care, and Sleep Medicine, Department of Medicine, University of Kentucky, Lexington, Kentucky, U.S.A.

I. Introduction

Chronic obstructive pulmonary disease (COPD), an umbrella term for chronic obstructive bronchitis and emphysema, has long been labeled as a disease that is "irreversible" with little to offer therapeutically to alter the course of the disease. Accordingly, little interest has existed to identify this disease, which may be debilitating, earlier in its course. But the tone in the 21st century is now changed to one of optimism! COPD is now defined by two major worldwide Clinical Practice Guidelines (CPGs) (1–3) as a "partially reversible" disease process with several therapeutic interventions available, non-pharmacologic and pharmacologic, which improve the quality of life and activities of daily living of our patients with this disease. In the past, COPD was usually not identified until it was in its advanced stages, when those afflicted finally acknowledged their symptoms and sought medical care, or when clinicians recognized COPD after patients presented with this disease's associated comorbidities: e.g., coronary disease, stroke, lung cancer, osteoporosis, depression, and anxiety.

A clinical–pathologic study of emphysema published in 1964 by Cole and Roberts, observed that emphysema was diagnosed antemortem in less than half of the patients in which it was found at autopsy, and they concluded that—"If timed vital capacity estimations (carried out at the bedside with a simple portable apparatus) were a part of every physical examination, early diagnosis of airway obstructive disease such as the chronic bronchitis–emphysema syndrome would be commonplace and differential diagnosis would be more accurate. Preventive treatment could then be instituted. Though leaving much to be desired, it could at least slow down the progress of the disease, especially the bronchitic element" (4). Since then we have come a long way, or have we?

This chapter examines the need for an earlier diagnosis of COPD, describes the tools available currently to accomplish this goal, and reviews some investigational modalities waiting in the wings for prime time. In light of the current state-of-the art management paradigms available for COPD, as well as our efforts to prevent progression of this chronic disease, it is imperative that COPD be detected as early as possible, perhaps even before it becomes clinically apparent.

II. Burden of COPD and the Need for Early Diagnosis

The exact prevalence of COPD can only be estimated due to variances in the collection and statistical analysis of epidemiologic studies to date. However, as reviewed in an earlier chapter, the third National Health and Nutrition Examination Survey (NHANES III) conducted in the U.S.A. between 1988 and 1994 (5) and the Proyecto Latinoamericano (PLATINO) study para la Investigacion de la Enfermedad Pulmonar Obstructiva Cronica conducted in five cities in Latin America between 2001 and 2004 (6) provide excellent epidemiological data on COPD. The NHANES III estimated the prevalence of COPD in those aged 25 to 75 years old was 16%. This study also reported that COPD (both mild and moderate) was more prevalent in males than in females and among white versus black subjects, and that the prevalence of COPD increased markedly with age (5). The PLATINO study estimated that the prevalence of COPD was 7.8% to 19.7% in subjects living in the five Latin American cities studied, based on post-bronchodilator forced expiratory volume in one second (FEV_1) measurements (6). If one were to utilize the most conservative estimates of prevalence, it could be estimated that there are over 280 million cases of COPD worldwide. In the United States, COPD is currently the fourth leading cause of death and it is estimated that by 2020, it will be the third cause of death not only in the U.S. but also worldwide (7). These numbers only represent the tip of an iceberg as COPD remains grossly under-recognized and under-diagnosed. In NHANES III, less than half of patients with airflow obstruction self-reported that they were diagnosed with COPD by a doctor; moreover, it was found by use of spirometry testing in a sub-cohort of these subjects that more than 45% of the patients documented to have advanced COPD (FEV_1 50% of predicted with an $FEV_1/FVC < 70\%$) [forced vital capacity (FVC)] were unaware of their condition (5).

The financial costs of COPD are also staggering. In 2002, the total economic cost of COPD was $32.1 billion ($14.1 billion in indirect cost in addition to $18 billion in direct medical costs). Annually, COPD accounts for approximately 119,000 deaths, 550,000 hospitalizations, 16 million health care office visits, 50 million days of disability, and 14 million days of restricted activity (3).

Taking these data together, the need to identify, diagnose, and to initiate appropriate and optimal management (assess and monitor disease, reduce risk factors, manage stable COPD, and manage exacerbations) for COPD in an earlier timely manner cannot be overemphasized (2,3,8). Although the medical environment is rapidly changing for the better, given the current awareness of COPD, the nonspecific clinical features of early COPD, and the low utilization of currently available diagnostic tests, the goal of making an early diagnosis of COPD, before clinical manifestations are present and/or recognized, is easier stated than done.

III. Currently Available Tools for Prevention and Early Diagnosis of COPD

The diagnosis of COPD is often elusive in its early stages. Thus, the various diagnostic modalities and tools available should be utilized in a complimentary fashion in order for the optimal identification and monitoring of management for this potentially deadly disease. It goes without saying that the majority of COPD could be prevented by the reduction of known risk factors (tobacco smoke, biomass fuels, and other occupational and environmental exposures), and a better understanding of genetic predisposition(s) for the disease (e.g., α_1 antitrypsin deficiency). These areas were reviewed earlier in this book; therefore the following discussion focuses on tools available to aid in the early diagnosis of COPD:

1. Education
2. Clinical features (history of symptoms, risk factors, and physical examination)
3. Pulmonary function testing—including office spirometry
4. Radiographic imaging and newer techniques (actors awaiting prime time)

A. Education

Traditionally COPD has been viewed as an irreversible disease with no treatment and a poor prognosis. It is of paramount importance that educational programs increase the awareness of COPD and ensure the implementation of current comprehensive CPGs for COPD; the Global Initiative for Chronic Obstructive Lung Disease (GOLD) (1,3) and the American Thoracic Society/European Respiratory Society (ATS/ERS) (2) guidelines. These guidelines define COPD more optimistically than previous guidelines. Specifically, COPD is no longer defined as an irreversible disease process but rather a potentially "partially" reversible process. This changes the paradigm of COPD management and signals justified optimism and hope for those who suffer from the disease.

The physiological impairment in COPD is characterized by airflow limitation, air trapping, and hyperinflation—depending on the severity of the disease. These abnormalities can lead to dyspnea, which is unpleasant, and often severely limits the activities patients can or want to undertake—prompting them to avoid situations that demand certain levels of physical activity. COPD patients slowly modify their lifestyle over years to decades and often avoid activities that lead to dyspnea; accordingly, they frequently do not present with respiratory complaints to clinicians until the disease is severe. The classic time course of COPD is a slow deterioration of lung function with a decrease in activity which leads to de-conditioning and which is often associated with an increase in the frequency and severity exacerbations. As COPD worsens, patients are more likely to experience a compromised quality of life, respiratory failure, cardiovascular disease, other comorbidities as described below, and ultimately death.

Misdiagnosis, "silent" unrecognized and/or unacknowledged early signs and symptoms of COPD, or coexistent conditions (comorbidities) are all believed to contribute to under-diagnosis of COPD—despite the availability of CPGs for earlier diagnosis and appropriate treatment of COPD. Educating patients and health care providers alike—about the risk factors, clinical features of COPD, and the usefulness of spirometry to establish airflow obstruction in patients at risk for COPD—is the cornerstone of National Lung Health Education Program (NLHEP) (9). The NLHEP recommends to identify individuals "at risk" for COPD, and then to determine if airflow obstruction is present or absent by use of spirometry testing. Several accurate, reliable, inexpensive handheld spirometers are now available worldwide. The NLHEP does not currently recommend "screening," but rather an approach of "case finding" or "selected early detection," i.e., only to perform spirometry on individuals older than 44 years of age who have smoked tobacco or recently quit smoking, as well as on anyone, regardless of age, who has one or more of the cardinal signs/symptoms of COPD— chronic cough with or without chronic sputum (mucus) production, shortness of breath on mild exertion out of proportion to the activity being performed, or wheeze (10). If the FEV_1/FVC is below the lower limit of normal (LLN), airflow obstruction is present (5,10–12). The degree of airflow obstruction, measured by the FEV_1 as a percent of predicted, can then be utilized to stratify the severity of COPD (2,3). Current CPGs (2,3) support the above NLHEP concepts and emphasize the need for identifying persons with airflow obstruction who have been chronically exposed to tobacco smoke or other environmental/occupational risk factors for COPD *before* their clinical symptoms are recognized and acknowledged by either the patient or their health care clinician. Increased public and clinician awareness of COPD and implementation of comprehensive educational programs about this disease will lead to better understanding of the clinical course of COPD and perhaps avoidance of risk factors and improved compliance with prescribed therapies.

B. Clinical Features

Clinical findings—symptoms as well as signs are nonspecific, especially in the early stages of the disease. By the time patients complain of dyspnea, their lung function is lower by 50% or more and the pathologic changes in lungs are no longer completely reversible. The majority of patients have an insidious onset of exertional dyspnea around which they slowly modify their lifestyle to do less strenuous activities that do not lead to dyspnea, and therefore they are not aware, or do not experience a sensation of dyspnea. Similarly, most patients and their physicians tend to ignore the early signs of COPD—cough and sputum production—but rather attribute these to smoking, e.g., "smoker's cough." Physical examination findings of hyper-expansion, hyperresonance, distant breath sounds, and prolonged expiratory phase with expiratory wheezes are not early signs but rather signs of advanced disease. Physicians should actively seek a history of chronic cough or sputum production and changes in lifestyle suggesting dyspnea with exertion from their patients at risk for developing COPD. A positive history should lead to appropriate diagnostic testing even in patients with a normal physical examination.

There appears to be a gender bias associated with the diagnosis of COPD, despite the recent speculation that women may be more susceptible than men to the harmful effects of tobacco smoke. Indeed, a study has suggested that women with clinical features and risk factors similar to their male counterparts are more likely to be diagnosed with asthma as opposed to the correct diagnosis of COPD (13). It was also noted in this study that female patients were less likely to be referred for pulmonary function testing to evaluate symptoms of cough, mucus production, or dyspnea versus men. All clinicians must be vigilant and avoid falling into this gender bias trap.

Similarly, one must be aware of the disparate risk of COPD in African American and other minorities. The mortality from COPD in African Americans is on the rise (14). Recent data suggest that African Americans, especially females, are more susceptible to the damaging effects of tobacco smoke—as assessed by the rate of decline in lung function (FEV_1) (15).

C. Pulmonary Function Testing and Office Spirometry

Documentation of airflow obstruction by spirometry is the cornerstone for the diagnosis of COPD. Spirometry is currently the most practical tool to document the diagnosis of COPD and to stratify its severity based on the degree of airflow obstruction. The Agency for Healthcare Research and Quality (AHRQ) recently stated that spirometry, in addition to clinical examination, improves COPD diagnostic accuracy (16). Spirometry is essential for establishing the diagnosis of COPD, but by itself is inadequate to optimally follow the course of the disease or the impact of therapies. Spirometry, in addition to the history and physical exam, improves diagnostic accuracy of COPD in adults with a history of risk factors (e.g., tobacco use) and respiratory symptoms—one should not make a diagnosis of COPD based on clinical manifestations alone. However, when monitoring the course of COPD, spirometry should be used in conjunction with other outcome measures, e.g., quality of life, health status, dyspnea, exacerbation rate, associated comorbidities, etc. It is important to note that spirometry is sensitive in detecting airflow obstruction, and measurable airflow obstruction may be present in certain individuals before the appearance or their acknowledgement of symptoms—the effects of their lung function impairment may not be seen in the very early stages of the disease—especially if they have modified their life style to perform less strenuous activity. In addition, repeated testing may be needed in persons at risk in order to establish the onset of airflow obstruction and to detect disease earlier.

A recent report by the AHRQ reviewed the use of spirometry for case finding, diagnosis, and management of COPD (16). This report concluded that: (*i*) spirometry, besides improving diagnostic accuracy also provides prognostic value for predicting respiratory and overall morbidity and mortality; (*ii*) spirometry is a useful tool in those whose symptoms suggest COPD (case finding); (*iii*) the primary benefit of spirometry is to identify those who might benefit from therapies to improve exacerbations; (*iv*) current evidence (randomized controlled studies—RCT) does not support widespread use of spirometry in the primary care setting for all adults with persistent respiratory symptoms or risk factor exposure for COPD, but states that more RCT research is needed to evaluate this approach; (*v*) spirometry may reduce the number of patients being labeled as having COPD—i.e., many have been diagnosed with COPD based only on clinical features, yet they have no airflow obstruction present when tested; and (*vi*) further RCT investigations should be conducted on the utility of spirometry in aiding smoking cessation and its impact on COPD therapy.

Spirometry is not a new invention; it has been around for centuries. The history of the spirometer dates back to 1846 when an English surgeon, John Hutchinson, invented the device and coined the term "vital capacity." Dr Hutchinson reported measurements on 2130 individuals and showed that vital capacity was directly proportional to height and inversely proportional to age (17). These data were deemed a monumental advancement by actuaries who used the information to predict patient longevity and mortality. Nonetheless, the spirometer was not widely appreciated nor implemented into day-to-day practice, and Dr Hutchinson retired to Fiji at the age of 40 and then died without appreciating the eventual impact his invention would have on medical practice worldwide. More than a century later, another surgeon, Edward A. Gaensler, further demonstrated the value of vital capacity and added a timing element to the measure (18). Thus, the concept of "forced expiratory volume as a function of time"—FEV_1 and FVC—was created in 1951. Nearly three decades later, the Framingham Study corroborated Hutchinson's observations by reporting that FEV_1 is a powerful prognostic indicator for both pulmonary disease and cardiac failure (19), suggesting that it may have utility for primary care practitioners, pulmonologists, and cardiologists alike.

Reference values, for the spirometric parameters an individual would be predicted to, have been established and found useful for decades (20). A limitation that has recently received some criticism is that these values are based upon studies of healthy people, as opposed to the health-compromised patients (e.g., COPD) typically seen in practice. Predicted values, like the percentage of predicted FEV_1, are normalized to airflow for height, age, gender, and, in some cases, race, but generally are not as accurate for African American and Hispanic populations (21). Further, weight is not a factor in estimating predicted value, even though extreme overweight can at times reduce lung function. Several sets of predicted values have been reported. The NHANES III conducted from 1988 to 1994, collected spirometry data on 20,627 survey participants, which included an over-sampling of African American and Mexican American populations allowing for valid comparisons among different race/ethnic groups. The NHANES III spirometry data have generated reference equations to describe normal pulmonary function for three major race/ethnic groups: Caucasians, African Americans, and Mexican Americans (22). Many experts agree that NHANES III reference equations are much better suited to COPD practice than most other predicted value standards.

Spirometry is not the end all test; it has its limitations like any diagnostic instrument or procedure. However, spirometry is probably the best practical test currently available to the majority of practicing clinicians to assist them in an earlier detection of COPD in those individuals at risk (23–25). As noted above, the NLHEP recommends widespread use of spirometry in the offices of primary care practitioners for establishing the diagnosis of COPD—in those patients at risk (smokers, patients 45 years or older, those with chronic cough in the presence of absence of mucus production, wheezing, or dyspnea) (10). This can be successfully accomplished in the primary care provider's office (26) with new generation handheld spirometers that are easy to use, accurate, and cost-effective. The NLHEP and NHANES III recommend the use of the LLN FEV_1/FVC to establish airflow obstruction, and also recommend the use of the FEV_6 as a surrogate measurement for FVC in the office setting (5,10,12). Airflow obstruction is established when both the FEV_1 and the FEV_1/FEV_6 ratio are below the LLN. The use of FEV_6 in diagnosing airflow obstruction and its predicted values have been reported and validated (27,28). This allows for relative ease and accuracy of performance in the office setting as it is less demanding on the patient and the test provider. Patients with abnormal test results can then be referred to a pulmonary function laboratory for more formal testing if clinically warranted.

The association between FEV_1 measures and prognosis was established more than 15 years ago when Burrows and colleagues revealed that 10-year mortality in COPD patients was directly related to the degree of airflow obstruction (29). These findings were further quantified by Hodgkin and colleagues, who reported that an

$FEV_1 > 1.00$ L resulted in a low mortality at 10 years, an $FEV_1 < 0.75$ L resulted in a one year mortality of 30% increase, and an $FEV_1 < 0.75$ L resulted in a 10-year mortality of as high as 95% (30). Marked reversibility of FEV_1 was shown to be a favorable prognostic factor in COPD, suggesting that elevation of FEV_1 may prompt other physiological changes to improve prognostic outlook. Based on this and other medical evidence, both ATS/ERS and GOLD guidelines recommend that post-bronchodilator FEV_1 readings be used to establish the severity of COPD to determine the patient's prognosis (2,3). The ATS/ERS guidelines stipulate, however, that patient activity level is a more significant prognostic factor than the FEV_1 measure (2). This suggests that a more active patient will have a better prognosis despite the level of FEV_1 and also suggests that spirometry alone is a suboptimal tool for assessing patient outcomes.

Within a broader framework, spirometry classification has proven useful in predicting health status (31), utilization of health-care resources (32), and development of acute exacerbations (33,34), as well as mortality (35). Thus, an abnormal FEV_1 reading is a highly useful clinical tool as it provides a signal for physicians to focus the clinical history and examination to probe not just for COPD, but also for a broad spectrum of diseases associated with tobacco use that are increased in prevalence in COPD patients.

While one parameter may serve as a useful predictor of outcome, often the combination of two or more parameters combined will result in better prediction. The Body-mass index, Obstruction, Dyspnea, and Exercise Capacity (BODE) index combines factors to predict mortality in COPD: *B*ody-mass index, *O*bstruction (Airflow-FEV_1), *D*yspnea (Medical Research Council scale), and *E*xercise limitation (6-minute walk) (36). This index is used to capture systemic manifestations that are not reflected by the FEV_1 alone in order to better categorize and predict the outcome of mortality. Adding the frequency of acute exacerbations to the BODE index assessment may help clinicians to better prognosticate, but in the original report, the addition of this parameter to the other four did not increase the predictive value for mortality.

Baseline and follow-up spirometry is also now recommended for patients being considered for, and placed on, inhaled medications such as inhaled insulin. Abnormal spirometry in "at risk" asymptomatic individuals may promote smoking cessation—the most important intervention to prevent the development and progression of airflow obstruction/COPD (37,38). Evidence from non-randomized studies indicates that markers of respiratory impairment, including spirometry, may be utilized as motivational tools, as a part of a multidisciplinary approach, in smoking cessation programs. However, evidence from randomized trials has yet to definitively prove that knowledge of abnormal spirometry values provides more than small improvements in smoking cessation rates. Indeed, if a smoker has normal spirometry, this should not be a reenforcement to continue smoking. Rather, the clinician should mention that airflow obstruction may occur down the road and that they will retest the patient—but they should still stop smoking in order to prevent the development of heart disease, cancer, and/or stroke. There are no large well-controlled studies to date that have evaluated the impact of obtaining spirometry on avoidance of other risk factors such as pollution and cooking-biomass fuels.

Several studies have suggested that spirometry should be an integral part of the primary care approach to COPD, but that it is of utmost importance that the staff performing the test is well trained and that there is oversight to ensure the quality of spirometry data (39–41). Airway disease and airflow obstruction is common but often not suspected in patients admitted to a general medicine service (42). Although more studies are needed to confirm this observation, one study suggested that spirometry not only aided clinicians in their diagnosis of COPD but also positively impacted upon their management plan in patients identified with significant airflow obstruction (43). Again, the ATS/ERS, GOLD, NLHEP, and others emphasize the important of a quality assurance program to ensure the quality and accuracy of spirometry obtained in the office (44), and for that matter, hospital settings (2,3,9,10,24,45).

The overall utility of spirometry for an earlier and accurate diagnosis of COPD and asthma has led the National Committee for Quality Assurance to establish a Health plan Employer Data and Information Set (HEDIS) measure specially for spirometry use to document airflow limitation when a diagnosis of COPD is considered (46). Spirometry has also been incorporated as a standard parameter in the pay-for-performance, or physician-reporting program, of the Centers for Medicare and Medicaid Services. The Joint Commission, formerly known as the Joint Commission on Accreditation of Healthcare Organizations is also developing accreditation programs for COPD, which will likely establish additional standards for use of spirometry in the inpatient, outpatient, and emergency department settings. These developments suggest that use of spirometry for a definitive diagnosis of COPD will soon be inexorably related to provider reimbursement in virtually every practice setting.

D. Radiographic Imaging and Newer Techniques (Actors Awaiting Prime Time)

Routine postero-anterior and lateral chest roentgenograms are insensitive in detecting early airflow obstruction. Changes of airflow obstruction characterized by increased antero-posterior diameter of the thorax, hyper-expansion of lung fields, flattening of diaphragms, and increase in retrosternal airspace are all signs indicating advanced disease.

Regional lung scintigraphy detects ventilation defects in patients with smoking-related lung disease but its routine use for detection of early lung disease in symptomatic or asymptomatic patients has not been established.

High resolution computed tomography scan (HRCT) of chest can show emphysematous changes prior to development of symptoms, however this test is not practical for every at risk patient. In one small study of 36 asymptomatic volunteers with normal pulmonary function, HRCT showed emphysema and air trapping in one-third of smokers and in none of the nonsmokers (47). HRCT may be used to identify lung lesions in asymptomatic smokers. However, clinical significance of such lesions and their progression to symptomatic disease has not been established. Also, cost effectiveness of such expensive modality for screening purposes is yet to be determined.

Apparent diffusion coefficient (ADC) measurements obtained from diffusion-weighted hyperpolarized helium 3 (^{3}He) magnetic resonance imaging (48) in asymptomatic smokers and healthy nonsmokers of similar age showed statistically significant correlation between mean ADC values and pulmonary function test measurements, especially carbon monoxide diffusing capacity. Mean ADC values also had a positive correlation with pack-years of smoking and age. These observations, however, need to be confirmed by studies involving more subjects.

IV. Actors Awaiting Prime Time

A. Pulmonary Biomarkers for COPD—Plasma, Tissue, and Exhaled Breath Condensates

COPD is a multisystem inflammatory disease that manifests itself primarily by respiratory dysfunction. Markers of inflammation are present in the plasma, tissue, alveolar lining cells—the epithelial lining fluid of pulmonary surfaces—and exhaled air (49–51). Sputum induction is not always easy to perform and bronchoalveolar lavage is invasive and hence these are not currently procedures of choice for routinely measuring inflammatory markers in respiratory secretions, although both are being used in the research setting. Collection of exhaled breath condensate (EBC) involves collection of exhaled air in cooled condensers and is likely to be of less risk and discomfort to the subject, and serial measurements may be more readily obtainable versus more invasive procedures (52). Studies have shown that levels of inflammatory markers such as interleukin-6 and leukotriene B_4 are increased in EBC of smokers and patients with COPD and may serve as early indication of smoking-induced lung damage (53). Although EBC analysis has not been standardized in COPD, and all studies of EBC in COPD involve small number of patients, this noninvasive evaluation of airway inflammation holds promise. It may help identify smokers at risk of developing clinical disease, and may help identify patients who are more likely to respond to broad spectrum anti-inflammatory treatments. It may also help us in developing new specific anti-inflammatory agents specifically targeting the markers of airway inflammation in defined clinical COPD phenotypes.

No blood tests are currently available in practice to routinely identify smokers at risk of developing COPD. A panel of protein biomarkers that can distinguish patients with COPD from closely matched controls was identified using plasma protein profiles from surface enhanced laser desorption/ionization time-of-flight mass spectrometry (54). In this pilot study involving 30 COPD subjects and 30 controls matched for age, gender, and smoking history researchers identified a panel of five biomarkers that could distinguish COPD patients from controls with sensitivity and specificity of 91.7% and 88%, respectively. This test needs to be validated in larger cohorts before it can be used routinely for clinical purposes.

V. Summary

COPD remains a formidable opponent in the 21st century. Significant advances have been made in diagnosing COPD and reversing some of its devastating effects on respiratory function and overall quality of life (health status). "Prevention is better than cure"—this adage cannot be truer for any other disease. Smoking cessation and avoiding other environmental and occupational risk factors before the development of clinical disease should be the foundation of managing all patients at risk for developing COPD. Educating clinicians and patients about the disease and the ease and utility of spirometry to make an earlier and accurate diagnosis of COPD needs to be emphasized. More studies are needed to validate the impact of spirometric values on the management plans and their outcomes for patients with COPD. Additional diagnostic modalities such as biomarkers (to identify specific clinical COPD phenotypes), or other techniques yet to be developed, will certainly advance the clinician's ability to make an even earlier, perhaps preclinical, diagnosis of COPD. Accordingly, clinicians will have the ability to initiate clinically proven management plans that will hopefully not only be disease modifying and alter the course of this chronic disease, but perhaps also lead to a cure for COPD.

References

1. Global Initiative on Obstructive Lung Disease. Global strategy for the diagnosis, management, and prevention of chronic obstructive pulmonary disease. Am J Respir Crit Care Med 2001; 163:1256–76.
2. The American Thoracic Society/European Respiratory Society (ATS/ERS). Standards for the diagnosis and management of patients with COPD. Eur Respir J 2004; 23:932–46.
3. Global strategy for the diagnosis, management, and prevention of chronic obstructive pulmonary disease: executive summary. 2006. www.goldcopd.com (last accessed August 29, 2007).
4. Cole MB, Roberts FE. A clinico-pathologic study of emphysema—the importance of early diagnosis. J Am Geriatr Soc 1964; 12:415–9.
5. National Center for Health Statistics. Plan and operation of the Third National Health and Nutrition Examination Survey: United States 1988–1994. U.S. Department of Health and Human Services, Public Heath Service, CDC, Hyattsville, MD, 1994.
6. Menezes A, Perez-Padilla R, Jardim J, et al. Chronic obstructive pulmonary disease in five Latin American cities: the PLATINO study. Lancet 2005; 366:1875–81.
7. Mannino DM, Homa DM, Akinbami LJ, Ford ES, Redd SC. Chronic obstructive pulmonary disease surveillance—United States, 1971–2000. MMWR Morb Mortal Wkly Rep 2002; 51(S506):1–16.
8. Ramsey SD, Sullivan SD. Chronic obstructive pulmonary disease: is there a case for early intervention? Am J Med 2004; 117(Suppl. 12A):3S–10.
9. Petty TL, Doherty DE. The National Lung Health Education Program: roots, mission, future directions. Respir Care 2004; 49(6):678–83.
10. Ferguson GT, Enright PL, Buist AS, Higgins MW. Office spirometry for lung health assessment in adults: a consensus statement from the National Lung Health Education Program. Respir Care 2000; 45(5):513–30.
11. Aggarwal A, Gupta D, Behera D, Jindal S. Comparison of fixed percentage method and lower confidence limits for defining limits of normality for interpretation of spirometry. Respir Care 2006; 51(7):737–43.
12. Hansen J, Sun X, Wasserman K. Spirometric criteria for airway obstruction: use percentage of FEV_1/FVC ratio below the fifth percential, not <70%. Chest 2007; 131(2):349–55.
13. Chapman KR, Tashkin DP, Pye DJ. Gender bias in the diagnosis of COPD. Chest 2001; 119(6):1691–5.
14. Chatila W, Hoffman E, Gaughan J, Robinswood G, Criner G, National Emphysema Treatment Trial Research Group. Advanced emphysema in African American and white patients. Chest 2006; 130:108–18.
15. Dransfield M, Bailey W. COPD: racial differences in susceptibility, treatment, and outcomes. Clin Chest Med 2006; 27:463–71.
16. Wilt TJ, Niewoehner D, Kim C, et al. Use of spirometry for case finding, diagnosis, and management of chronic obstructive pulmonary disease (COPD). Evidence Report/Technology Assessment No. 121. In: Agency for Healthcare Research and Quality (ed) (Prepared by the Minnesota Evidence-Based Practice Center under Contract No. 290-02-0009, September 2005 AHRQ Publication No. 05-E017-2).
17. Hutchinson J. On the capacity of the lungs and on the respiratory function with a view of establishing a precise and easy method of detecting disease by the spirometer. Med Chir Trans (Lond) 1846; 29:137.
18. Gaensler E. Analysis of the ventilatory defect by timed vital capacity. Am Rev Tuberc 1951; 69:256–78.
19. Kannel W, Lew E, Hubert H. The value of measuring vital capacity for prognostic purposes. Trans Assoc Life Insure Med Dir Am 1980; 64:66–83.
20. Brusasco V, Crapo R, Viegi G, et al. ATS/ERS Task Force: standardization of lung function testing. Eur Respir J 2005; 26:319–38.
21. Miller M. Standardization of spirometry. Eur Respir J 2005; 26:319–38.
22. Hankinson J, Odencrantz J, Fedan K. Spirometric reference values from a sample of the general U.S. population. Am Rev Resp Crit Care Med 1999; 159:179–87.
23. Doherty D. Detecting and managing COPD in the younger patient. J Respir Dis 2003; 24(12):S14–28.

24. Doherty DE. Early detection and management of COPD. What you can do to reduce the impact of this disabling disease. Postgrad Med 2002; 111(6):41–4 (see also 49, 50, 53 passim).

25. Doherty DE, Gross NJ, Briggs DD. Today's approach to the diagnosis and management of COPD. Clin Rev 2004; 14(1):97–105.

26. Buffels J, Degryse J, Heyrman J, Decramer M. Office spirometry significantly improves early detection of COPD in general practice: the DIDASCO study. Chest 2004; 125:1394–9.

27. Hankinson J, Crapo R, Jensen R. Spirometric reference values for the 6 second FVC maneuver. Chest 2003; 124(5):1805–11.

28. Jensen R, Crapo R, Enright P, Others from the Family Heart Study. A statistical rationale for the use of forced expiratory volume in 6 seconds. Chest 2006; 130(6):1650–6.

29. Burrows B. Airways obstructive diseases: pathogenetic mechanisms and natural histories of the disorders. Med Clin North Am 1990; 74(3):547–59.

30. Hodgkin JE. Prognosis in chronic obstructive pulmonary disease. Clin Chest Med 1990; 11(3):555–69.

31. Ferrer M, Alonso J, Morera J, et al. Chronic obstructive pulmonary disease stage and health-related quality of life. Ann Intern Med 1997; 127(12):1072–9.

32. Friedman M, Serby CW, Menjoge SS, Wilson JD, Hilleman DE, Witek TJ, Jr. Pharmacoeconomic evaluation of a combination of ipratropium plus albuterol compared with ipratropium alone and albuterol alone in COPD. Chest 1999; 115(3):635–41.

33. Burge PS, Calverley PM, Jones PW, Spencer S, Anderson JA, Maslen TK. Randomised, double blind, placebo controlled study of fluticasone propionate in patients with moderate to severe chronic obstructive pulmonary disease: the ISOLDE trial. Br Med J 2000; 320(7245):1297–303.

34. Dewan NA, Rafique S, Kanwar B, et al. Acute exacerbation of COPD: factors associated with poor treatment outcome. Chest 2000; 117(3):662–71.

35. Anthonisen N, Connett J, Murray R. Smoking and lung function of Lung Health Study participants after 11 years. Am J Respir Crit Care Med 2002; 166:675–9.

36. Celli B, Cote CG, Marin JM. The body-mass index, airflow obstruction, dyspnea, and exercise capacity index in chronic obstructive pulmonary disease. N Engl J Med 2004; 350:1005–12.

37. Gorecka D. Diagnosis of airflow limitation combined with smoking cessation advise increases stop-smoking rates. Chest 2003; 123:1916–23.

38. Zielinski J, Bednarek M. Early detection of COPD in high-risk population using spirometric screening. Chest 2001; 119:731–6.

39. Enright P, Beck K, Sherrill D. Repeatability of spirometry in 18,000 adult patients. Am J Respir Crit Care Med 2004; 169:235–8.

40. Kaminsky D, Marcy T, Bachand M, Irvin C. Knowledge and use of office spirometry for the detection of chronic obstructive pulmonary disease by primary care physicians. Respir Care 2005; 50:1639–48.

41. Schermer T, Jacobs J, Chavannes N, Hartman J, Folgering H, van Weel C. Validity of spirometric testing in a general practice population of patients with chronic obstructive pulmonary disease (COPD). Thorax 2003; 58:861–6.

42. Zas D, Wise R, Wiener C, Longcope Spirometry Investigation Team. Airway obstruction is common but unsuspected in patients admitted to a general medicine service. Chest 2004; 125:106–11.

43. Dales R, Vandemheen K, Clinch J, Aaron S. Spirometry in the primary care setting: influence on clinical diagnosis and management of airflow obstruction. Chest 2005; 128:2443–7.

44. Eaton T, Withy S, Garret J, Mercer J, Whitlock R, Rea H. Spirometry in primary care: the importance of quality assurance and the impact of spirometry workshops. Chest 1999; 116:416–23.

45. Doherty DE. Identification and assessment of chronic obstructive pulmonary disease in the elderly. J Am Med Dir Assoc 2003; 4(Suppl. 5):S116–20.

46. NCQA. NCQA releases HEDIS 2006: New measures address overuse, followup, 2006. www.ncqa.org/communications/news/hedis_2006.htm (last accessed September 10, 2007).

47. Spaggaiari E, Zompatori M, Verduri A, et al. Early smoking-induced lesions in asymptomatic subjects. Correlation between high resolution dynamic CT and pulmonary function testing. Radiol Med 2005; 109:27–39.

48. Fain SB, Panth SR, Evans MD, et al. Early emphysematous changes in asymptomatic smokers: detection with ^{3}He MR imaging. Radiology 2006; 239(3):875–83.

49. Barnes P, Chowdhury B, Kharitonov S, et al. Pulmonary biomarkers in chronic obstructive pulmonary disease. Am J Respir Crit Care Med 2006; 174:6–14.

50. Hurst J, Donaldson G, Perera W, et al. Use of plasma biomarkers at exacerbation of chronic obstructive pulmonary disease. Am J Respir Crit Care Med 2006; 174:867–74.

51. American Thoracic Society. ATS workshop proceedings: exhaled nitric oxide and nitric oxide oxidative metabolism in exhaled breath condensate: executive summary. Am J Respir Crit Care Med 2006; 173:811–3.

52. Effros RM, Dunning MB, III, Biller J, Shaker R. The promise and perils of exhaled breath condensates. Am J Physiol Lung Cell Mol Physiol 2004; 287(6):L1073–80.

53. Carpagnano GE, Kharitonov SA, Foschino-Barbaro MP, Resta O, Gramiccioni E, Barnes PJ. Increased inflammatory markers in the exhaled breath condensate of cigarette smokers. Eur Respir J 2003; 21(4):589–93.

54. Bowler RP, Canham ME, Ellison MC. Surface enhanced laser desorption/ionization (SELDI) time-of-flight mass spectrometry to identify patients with chronic obstructive pulmonary disease. J Chronic Obstructive Pulm Dis 2006; 3:41–50.

6

Assessment of Symptoms and Quality of Life in the COPD Patient

CARME SANTIVERI
Department of Respiratory Medicine, St. George's, University of London, London, U.K., and Dos de maig Hospital, Consorci Sanitari Integral, Barcelona, Spain

PAUL W. JONES
Department of Respiratory Medicine, St. George's, University of London, London, U.K.

I. Introduction

This chapter is about the quantification of symptoms and health status in chronic obstructive pulmonary disease (COPD), which now are integrated in a group of measurements termed patient-reported outcomes (PROs). It addresses some conceptual and methodological issues, describes the importance of the evaluation of symptoms and health status and approaches to their assessment.

II. Why Make Measurements of Symptoms and Quality of Life?

COPD is a chronic condition with multiple respiratory and systemic effects. Current treatment is directed toward management of symptoms. The aim is not to cure but improve patient's living condition. In this context, the patient's perception of their disease and its impact on their life is an important clinical and research endpoint.

In clinical practice, the assessment of symptoms—their presence and severity—is needed to assist diagnosis, monitor disease activity, and evaluate therapy. All these assessments aim ultimately at improving the patient health-related quality of life (HRQL) by decreasing the symptom burden. However a standardized evaluation with health status instruments is not a routine clinical practice. Clinicians usually approach the assessment of HRQL through a clinical interview with unstructured nonquantifiable global questions, which is a valid approach with individual patients in the clinical setting.

In the research field, symptoms, and health status are important PROs that need to be quantified and measured in a standardized manner. They measure what the patient experiences and what it is important to them. They contribute to evaluation of disease severity and can measure changes in clinical status due to exacerbations, disease progression, or the response to clinical interventions such as drugs, surgery, or rehabilitation programs. Since these measures are reported by patients, their changes are more relevant to them than physiological measurements and might provide better and more comprehensive information about the actual impact of clinical interventions. They complement traditional data such physiological measures which correlate only poor to moderately with health status and survival (1,2).

Symptoms and health status measurement are important in health care planning policies. Symptoms drive the patient to seek medical attention and an individual's rating of overall health is among the best predictors of mortality and future use of health services (3). In this respect, health utilities are being increasingly used in cost-effectiveness analysis.

The Food and Drug Administration and the European Agency for the Evaluation of Medicinal products recognize the importance and contribution of PROs such as symptoms and health status questionnaires and have published guidelines for their use in clinical trials, respectively (4,5). These will set the requirements of the clinical outcomes used in clinical trials to quantify the effects of treatment and may have important implications for their design, execution, and analysis (4,5).

III. Symptoms and Health Status

Symptoms and HRQL are subjective, multifaceted experiences reported by the patients and modulated by physical, psychological, and social factors which might be perceived and expressed in different ways depending on the individual and their cultural setting. There are complex relationships between biological/physiological variables and symptom reports, and between symptoms and HRQL (6).

A. The Relationship Between Symptoms and Health Status

Symptoms and their impact on the patient's life constitute a significant component of health status assessment. Many instruments that evaluate health status have items pertaining to symptoms; however, the definition and the choice of relevant symptoms may differ (7).

Symptoms are more tied to health status than to lung function (8) and their management influences patient's quality of life. It has been demonstrated, in a variety of symptoms, that people with more numerous or more severe symptoms tend to have lower functional health status, less effective role performance, lower cognitive functioning, lower quality of life, and lower physical performance capabilities (9). A symptom-based chronic lung disease index severity that summarizes frequency and intensity of coughing, sputum, wheezing, and dyspnea has been shown to relate more strongly to general health status measured using the short form 36 Item (SF-36) than peak expiratory flow rates (PEFRs) (8).

Symptoms, such as cough and dyspnea, are in themselves distressing and the resultant limitation in functioning and the importance attributed to them by the patient are related to their HRQL. Restrictions on daily living due to disease of airflow obstruction may cause more distress than the symptoms themselves (10). An assessment of the patient's limitations and perceptions, together with their physiological parameters might help determine the choice of treatment better than reliance on lung function tests alone.

B. Symptoms

A symptom is a "feature which indicates a condition of disease, in particular one apparent to the patient" as stated in the Compact Oxford English dictionary (11). Several alternative definitions could be applied to this term; all of them stress the concept of individual's perception. Symptoms are subjective experiences that can only be measured from the patient's perspective as they are the most reliable witness of their disease.

Some symptoms can be observed and measured but some are not observable and are only known by the patient. They can be classified as: (*i*) externally verifiable such as cough and sputum; (*ii*) both directly and indirectly verifiable such as breathlessness which can be assessed directly by the patient during an exercise test or indirectly through its impact on daily basis through the use of dyspnea questionnaires; and (*iii*) cannot be verified externally, such as mood or fatigue. These have to be evaluated in a similar way to health status, through questionnaires.

The patient's subjective report of symptoms may not correlate well with objective measures. Some biological parameters can be altered with no symptoms and symptoms can be experienced with no evidence of abnormal biological parameters (6). In COPD, dyspnea intensity has a low to moderate correlation with exercise tolerance and low correlation with pulmonary function (7,12). Although all these measures are related to the physical limitations that patients experience, the low concordance might be attributed to the fact that they reflect different aspects of the disease.

C. Factors that Influence Symptom Perception

Symptoms are the result of the interaction of different physiopathological mechanisms and patient specific characteristics. The relative importance of the different components may shift as disease progresses. For instance, shortness of breath and repeated exacerbations have major adverse effects on health status as COPD severity increases (13).

People differ in the way they perceive, report, and interpret their symptoms. The selection of words for describing symptoms and the variability in expression is related to the characteristics of the subject such as educational background, language skill, and any perceptual disorders together with environmental and sociocultural factors (14).

Even within the same patient, the choice of question to the patient about symptoms may influence the response. One study showed that a diary card question phrased to address the level of asthma symptoms produced a more severe mean score over 14 days than a similar question in the same diary that addressed the effect of asthma on daily life (15).

The meanings of words may vary between different languages and cultural settings and the endpoints of scales for a given symptom domain may also have very different meanings across cultures or socioeconomic groups (16). This highlights the need for cross-cultural validated instruments for symptom assessment and research (16).

Similarly, simply because a tool has been validated in one culture does not mean that it is equally valid with individuals from another, either within in the same society or in different societies with a common language (16). Furthermore, patients might not report symptoms unless asked directly. A prospective study using diary cards, revealed that moderate to severe COPD patients only reported 50% of their exacerbations (17). Patients might under-assess both the number and severity of symptoms and assume that they are just part of their illness or the normal aging process. They might also avoid their expression in accordance to what is socially acceptable in order not to be seen as a burden. Cultural factors may lead to either exaggeration or denial of symptoms.

Psychological state may influence attention to, interpretation of, and response to symptoms (14). Psychiatric comorbidity is common in patients with COPD and psychological factors such as depression and anxiety have been linked to the reporting of respiratory symptoms in cross-sectional studies (18). In a recent longitudinal study over a nine-year-period, the risk of developing dyspnea was increased in subjects who developed symptoms of anxiety and depression during the follow-up (19).

The social environment such as employment, marital and family status, social support, annual income, availability of and access to health care resources may affect the individual's experience and reporting of symptoms (14).

Common symptoms experienced by COPD patients include dyspnea, cough, sputum, fatigue, sleep difficulties, and emotional symptoms. Dyspnea and fatigue are the most prevalent ones and are closely related one to each other (20). Fatigue comes second to dyspnea in its influence on health status (20). Other symptoms, such as dry mouth and itching, have been reported by COPD patients. Apart from symptoms secondary to COPD, patients often have associated comorbidities, each with their own symptoms. In a study that included 104 severe COPD patients, an average of nine symptoms were reported by each patient using a generic symptom questionnaire, the Memorial Symptom Assessment Scale-Short Form (MSAS-SF) (21).

D. Health Status

Quality of Life, HRQL, and Health Status are subjective, multidimensional, abstract concepts, perceived, and reported by the patient. They encompass a broad range of physical, psychological, and social factors that impact on the patient's life. These interrelated domains are summarized in Figure 1. Various definitions have been used and although they are not equivalent, they are often applied interchangeably in the literature (22–24).

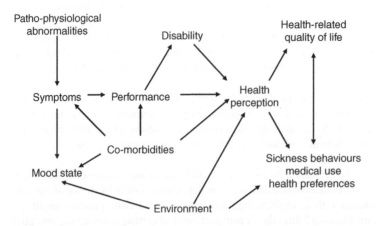

Figure 1 Conceptual scheme of the complex relationship between symptoms, health-related quality of life, and other factors in chronic obstructive pulmonary disease.

Quality of Life may be defined as a subjective evaluation of a *person's situation* in terms of their satisfaction with life in domains that each individual considers important. It includes concepts unrelated to health, such as education, occupation, freedom of action, social, and intellectual fulfillment, among others.

The HRQL refers to the *individual's satisfaction* with multiple domains of life that are affected by health conditions, its treatment, or health services (25). It is an individual concept, unique to every individual.

Health status refers to *common*, i.e., *not individualized effects/consequences* of the disease in the domains that constitute the patient's HRQL. It is a standardized, population-based concept tailored to fit into a specific disease or a generic idea of health, but not tailored to the individual patient's perspective (26). It attempts to measure how different variables of health/disease relate to different domains of life such as physical, social, and psychological functioning. It is an attempt to quantify and turn into numbers, for measurement purposes, the abstract and individual concept of HRQL. In this respects, health status is a surrogate marker of HRQL.

E. Methods of Measurement

An instrument provides a means by which to capture data (symptom or health status) using a standard format for data collection, methods for scoring, analysis, and interpretation of results (4). The key objectives in measuring symptoms and health status are to collect data that are valid, reliable, unbiased, discriminating, and responsive to change and interpretable (27).

Instruments are designed with a specific purpose: diagnostic—to provide a dichotomous answer—present or absent; discriminative—to distinguish different levels of disease between patients; or evaluative—to detect response to intervention or changes over time. Some instruments have both discriminate and evaluative properties as well as having predictive power. A number of different formats are used: semi-structured and structured interviews, checklists, diaries, and questionnaires (self- or interviewer-administered). Diaries are used when measuring a small number of symptoms frequently. Questionnaires are the most widely instruments. They consist of items that are often grouped in domains; every domain representing a different aspect or construct of the patient's experience of the disease.

The current instruments have different item response scales, which basically can be classified into dichotomous and multiple category responses. The dichotomous responses are mostly phrased in terms of yes or no and the responses can be either weighted [e.g., sickness impact profile (SIP), St. George's Respiratory Questionnaire (SGRQ)] or unweighted Airways Questionnaire 20 (AQ20). The multiple category responses adopt a modified type Likert scale [e.g., Chronic Respiratory Questionnaire (CRQ)]. Most of the instruments use a four to seven-point modified Likert scale and assume that the distance between each pair of points is the same along all the scale and the scores are given the same weight and then aggregated into a simple sum. Rasch modeling should be used to test whether they act as true interval scales (28).

The selection of appropriate and clinically meaningful outcome measures is a complex issue. When selecting the measurement instrument, different factors have to be taken into account. Some of them relate to the characteristics of the instrument itself, such as the purpose for which the instrument was designed, and its psychometric properties. It should be used for the patient's population for which it was designed.

Under some circumstances, the method of administration and the recall period may become very important. Other factors include its understandability, the burden it imposes on the patients and possible cultural and language barriers that might influence the responses. Other factors are the investigator's experience with the instrument and issues of copyright (29). Once all the properties of a specific instrument have been taken into account, the selection of the appropriate measure will depends on the aspect of the disease being addressed and the purpose of the study being conducted. Neither the American Thoracic Society (ATS) nor the European Respiratory Society have recommended any specific assessments as standards.

Ideally an assessment tool should provide a simple, interpretable, and well-standardized scoring system, which should quantify both the degree of severity and the change over time.

Finally, using more than one method of assessment may be helpful as no one method is free of error or is likely to meet all demands. Instruments measuring the same construct may differ since the developers' concept of the construct may vary. Indeed, the identification of the items to form a construct is one of the challenges that the researcher has to face. Defining symptoms and health status might prove a difficult task and consensus agreement for symptoms such as fatigue that might be interpreted as sleepiness, muscle weakness, tiredness, among others, is lacking.

F.   Methods of Administration

Different administration methods can be used: self-administered, interview, via telephone or computerized. One randomized trial has evaluated the measurement properties of the CRQ while being self- or interviewer-administered (30). Validity and responsiveness were maintained in both forms; the self-administered questionnaire proved to be more responsive, although as the authors suggested this enhanced responsiveness appeared largely due to lower baseline scores on the self-administered group. The increase in responsiveness may be related to patients being more willing to acknowledge severe dysfunction in the absence of an interviewer (30). No differences have been found in internal consistency between self- and interview-administered SGRQ (31).

G.   Validation Principles

All instruments used for clinical research should have accepted psychometric properties, which include validity, reliability, and responsiveness.

Validity is the most fundamental property as it refers to whether the instrument is measuring what it intends to measure. Specific types of validity include: Face validity (Does the test appear to measure what it is supposed to measure to a nonexpert?); Content validity (Do the items cover the relevant aspects of the domain?); Construct validity (Does the test correlate with other objective tools such as other questionnaires or physiological measures related to the construct being measured?).

Reliability refers to the ability of the instrument to produce a consistent and reproducible result in response to the same clinical state on different occasions. In the absence of intervening variables such as drug therapy or rehabilitation, scores should remain stable even when administered by different assessors.

The reliability of responses to questions can be improved by asking about a specific time period (27). Determination of the correct time frame is a balance between reducing recall bias and maximizing the amount of time for which data are available (32). Recall of minor symptoms is likely to be poor when the reference period exceeds one week (27). One month is the maximum over which patients could provide reliable data on frequency of symptoms of asthma or diabetes and on the impact of those symptoms (32). The time frame should be clearly stated in any tool.

Responsiveness tests whether the questionnaire is capable of detecting changes in a condition over time or in response to treatment. The range of variation over which the instrument operates might differ depending on the population studied and its disease severity. In these respects, Ceiling (best possible score) and Floor (worst possible score) effects must be considered in making the proper choice of a measurement instrument (7).

IV. Instruments for Symptoms

COPD patients usually present with more than one symptom due to COPD and often have associated comorbidities. For these reasons, consideration must be given to the number of symptoms to be measured, whether multiple items are needed to measure each symptom and whether it is appropriate to produce an overall assessment. The issue of how many symptoms to assess will depend on the purpose of assessment (27).

In collecting self-report data on symptoms, the two main methods are diaries and questionnaires. Diaries allow data to be recorded contemporaneously, reducing the risk of recall bias. They can capture day-to-day fluctuation in symptoms, the coincidence of symptoms, potential exacerbating factors, and symptom free days (27). However, the number of symptom-free days calculated from diary cards will depend on the questions used and standardization is required before symptom-free days can be used as a reliable measure of treatment efficacy (15). Diaries place a considerable respondent burden and carry the risk of "hoarding" (retrospective completion of diary entries) although this can be avoided through the use of electronic devices (Table 1) (27).

A. Generic Symptoms

The MSAS-SF is a widely used generic symptom questionnaire developed to provide multidimensional information about a diverse group of common symptoms and has been validated in a population of patients with cancer (33). It rates the frequency, intensity, and distress of 32 physical and psychological symptoms during the week prior to filling in the questionnaire. It has been used in COPD (21) where the report of physical symptoms was related to fatigue. When analyzed by gender, fatigue in women had a stronger correlation with the amount of physical symptoms than with dyspnea.

B. Respiratory Specific Symptoms

Among the respiratory specific symptoms questionnaires, some of them were designed for epidemiological studies such as the Medical Research Council (MRC) questionnaire (34) and the ATS Inventory (35). Few instruments have been designed to assess symptomatic outcomes in COPD for use within the context of a clinical trial. Recently developed questionnaires include the chronic lung disease severity index (8), which uses a three-month recall period. Another three-item scale, the breathlessness, cough, and sputum scale, has been developed for diary card use (36). This instrument

Table 1 Summary of Symptom Instruments

	(Number) and item scale	Symptoms	Traits evaluated	Recall period	Reliability validity
Generic					
MSAS-SF	(32 items) Dichotomous 4- and 5-point Likert type scale	32 symptoms; physical symptom subscale; psychologic symptom subscale; global distress index	Frequency Intensity Distress	Past week	Validated in cancer patients
COPD-specific					
Multiple symptoms					
CLDSI	(6 items) 4- and 5-point Likert type scale	Dyspnea; wheezing; cough	Severity	3 months	Low to moderate correlation with SF-36
BCSS	(3 items) 5-point Likert type scale	Breathlessness; cough; sputum	Severity	Daily (part of a diary card)	Moderate to good correlations with SF-36 and SGRQ
One symptom: dyspnea					
MRC dyspnea scale	(5 items) yes/no	Severity		Daily life	Moderate correlation with FEV_1 and other dyspnea measures
Modified Borg dyspnea scale	0 to 10 rating scale	Intensity during activity		Now	High correlation with FEV_1
OCD	Visual analogue scale	Exercise tolerance		Daily life	Good correlation with 6-MWT
SAC BDI		Functional impairment; magnitude of task; magnitude of effort		At a single point in time	High correlation with interview administered BDI
SAC TDI		Functional impairment; magnitude of task; magnitude of effort		Changes from the baseline state	High correlation with interview administered TDI

Abbreviations: BCSS, breathlessness, cough, and sputum scale; CLDSI, chronic lung disease severity index; MRC, Medical Research Council; MSAS-SF, Memorial Symptom Assessment Scale–Short Form; OCD, oxygen cost diagram; SAC BDI, self-administered computerized baseline dyspnea index; SAC TDI, self-administered computerized transition dyspnea index; 6-MWT, 6-minute walking test.

evaluates the severity of symptoms day-to-day and provides guidelines for clinical interpretation of score changes.

C. Dyspnea

Dyspnea is the subjective perception of respiratory discomfort. It is the primary symptom experienced by COPD patients and is a major determinant of HRQL but it correlates only modestly with measures of lung function (37). Measures of dyspnea are used commonly in evaluating outcomes in COPD (38).

A number of instruments are available to assess dyspnea in daily life. One-dimensional scales include the Borg scale (39), a 0 to 10 rating scale for intensity of breathlessness during activity, and the modified MRC dyspnea scale (34), which is a five-point scale which ranges from patients getting breathless only with strenuous exercise to severe dyspnea that prevents the patient from leaving the house or getting dressed comfortably. One-dimensional scales are easy to administer and score, but cannot provide an accurate assessment of the type of tasks which are likely to cause dyspnea and do not take into account the variation of effort which patients may exert in completing certain activities (40).

Multidimensional scales cover information on more components of dyspnea. Examples include the baseline dyspnea index and transition dyspnea index (BDI–TDI) (41), oxygen cost diagram (OCD) (42). The BDI/TDI have three components: functional impairment, magnitude of task, and effort needed to evoke dyspnea (41). A 1 U change in the TDI total score has been demonstrated to be clinically relevant (40). Evidence of the validity of the different dyspnea questionnaires has been made through different criterion including comparisons with six-minute walking test (six-MWT), PEFR, forced expiratory volume in one second (FEV_1) and other dyspnea measures.

It is difficult to determine which method is the most reliable and valid measure for any given setting (38). There are no methods of converting between them so it is not possible to make direct comparisons of breathlessness measurements made using different scales and units (43). Hajiro carried out a cross-sectional study to clarify relationships between different dyspnea ratings and health status questionnaires in mild to severe COPD. Factor analysis demonstrated that the MRC, BDI, OCD, and the component Activity of the SGRQ, and Dyspnea component of the CRQ, both disease-specific health status measures, were grouped into the same factor. The Borg scale at the end of maximum exercise was found to be a different factor. The MRC, BDI, OCD, and activity in the SGRQ and Dyspnea in the CRQ demonstrated the same pattern of correlation with physiologic data, and maximal oxygen uptake (44).

D. Fatigue

The most widely used questionnaires in COPD include in their assessment dyspnea, other symptoms such as sputum, cough, and wheezing, but few of them address fatigue, which comes second to dyspnea in prevalence and impact on health status (20). There are several fatigue questionnaires in the literature; most of them validated in cancer, multiple sclerosis, and chronic fatigue syndrome populations (45). Four of them have been used in COPD; however none has been fully validated in COPD population (46–49).

V. Instruments for Health Status

The simplest measures of health status are global questions such as "how would you rate your health overall?" Although these simple and quick measures have proven to be predictive of mortality and use of health resources (3), they do not provide a detailed picture of the different factors contributing to the answer.

Health status questionnaires provide a means of quantifying the overall impact of the disease or response to therapy on patient's daily life in a standardized manner. They aggregate into a single score the effect of multiple pathophysiological processes. For this reason, they are useful for detecting a change when a treatment acts through different mechanisms, but they cannot identify the underlying mechanisms. There are two basic approaches to health status measurement: generic and specific instruments (Table 2).

A. Generic

Generic instruments describe outcomes for people with a range of conditions in a comprehensive manner and are useful for population surveys and to compare different populations and conditions (3). Due to their comprehensiveness and inclusion of generic terms, they might detect only large improvements and may not be very sensitive to treatment effects in specific diseases. However for the same reason, they might detect unanticipated side effects.

The Medical Outcomes Study SF-36 is one of the most widely used generic questionnaires (50). It includes eight health concepts: physical functioning, role-physical, bodily-pain, general health perceptions, vitality, social functioning, role-emotional, and mental health. Two summary components (Physical and Mental) can be calculated. The SF-36 scales are scored as a percentage of impairment with zero representing worst health and 100 indicating best health. When compared with other health status measures, the SF-36 has been found to discriminate better among individuals with varying levels of self-reported general health status and comorbidity (51). It has been validated and widely used in COPD and has shown responsiveness in pulmonary rehabilitation (52). Other widely used generic health status questionnaires include the SIP (53) and the Nottingham Health Profile (54).

B. Specific

Disease-specific questionnaires provide a standardized method of measuring the impact of disease and treatment on the patient's well being in a specific condition. They can summarize the effects of the disease into one overall score and are able to distinguish between different degrees of severity (1). Since they focus on specific problems, they may be more acceptable from the patient's perspective and they should be more responsive to changes in health status than generic measures.

There are a number of disease-specific questionnaires in COPD: the CRQ (55), the SGRQ (56), the breathing problems questionnaire (BPQ) (57), and the AQ20 (58). The CRQ is a 20-item questionnaire that evaluates four domains: dyspnea (five items), fatigue (four items), emotional function (seven items), and mastery (four items). On all questions, patient rate their experience on a seven-point Likert scale ranging from one (maximum impairment) to seven (no impairment). The SGRQ contains 50 items divided into three domains: symptoms (eight items), activity (16 items), and impacts

Table 2 Summary of Generic and Airways-Specific Health Status Questionnaires

Questionnaires	Items	Item response scale	Domains	MID	Reliability validity	Recall period[a]	Administration method
Generic							
SIP	136	Dichotomous, weighted	12 and 2 overall domains		Yes		Self, face-to-face or telephone interview
MOS SF-36	36	Dichotomous and 5-point Likert scale	8 and 2 summary scores	5 points	Yes	1 or 4 weeks	Self, face-to-face or telephone interview, computerized
NHP	38	Dichotomous, items weighted	6 No total score		Yes	Usual health	Self
HUI2		Standard gamble 3 to 5 levels	7		Yes	1, 2, or 4 weeks and usual health	Self, interview
QWB	50	Weighted	4		Yes	3 or 6 previous days	Self, interview
COPD-specific							
SGRQ	50	Dichotomous and 5-point Likert scale	3 and a total score	4 for all domains	Yes	4 weeks	Self, face-to-face or telephone interview
CRQ	20	7-point Likert scale Items weighted	4	0.5 per question for all domains	Yes	2 weeks	Self, interview
AQ20		Dichotomous, unweighted	4 and a total score		Yes		Self
SOLQ	29	5- and 7-point Likert type scales	4	6 for physical function domain	Yes		Self

[a] Some questionnaires are available with different recall periods.

Abbreviations: AQ20, Airways Questionnaire 20; CRQ, chronic respiratory questionnaire; HUI2, Health Utilities Index 2; MID, minimally important difference; MOS-SF36, Medical Outcomes Study–Short Form; NHP, Nottingham Health Profile; QWB, quality of well-being scale; SGRQ, St. George's Respiratory Questionnaire; SIP, sickness impact profile; SOLQ, Seattle Obstructive Lung Disease Questionnaire.

(26 items). Each item response has an empirically derived weight. Demographic and disease factors seem to have little influence on the importance that individual patients attach to each item in the questionnaire (59). A total score can be calculated. Scores range from 0 to 100, zero indicating no impairment of health status. A shorter version has recently been developed specifically for COPD, the SGRQ-C.

Few studies have compared the performance of different questionnaires. The SGRQ, the BPQ, and the CRQ have been compared in patients with mild to severe COPD with no substantial differences in the correlations with physiologic parameters, although the BPQ was less discriminatory than both the SGRQ and the CRQ in evaluating health status cross sectionally (44). Moderate to high correlations of the CRQ domains with dimensions of the SF-36 and the SGRQ have been observed in a wide range of COPD patients while comparing the discriminative and evaluative properties of both questionnaires (30).

Two generic questionnaires, the SF-36 and the Euroqol Classification of Health (EQ-5D), and two disease-specific instruments, the CRQ and SGRQ, have been compared for their psychometric, discriminative and evaluative properties in COPD patients at baseline, at 6 and 12 months. All instruments proved to be valid and reliable over time. The SF-36 was superior to the EQ-5D and the CRQ performed slightly better than the SGRQ (60).

C. Utility Measures

Utility measures are generic instruments that are designed from a health-economic perspective. They measure individuals' preferences for certain health states in the decision-making process associated with treatments, diagnostic strategies, and health spending (61). Health utilities allow calculation of the quality adjusted life year and are being applied increasingly in cost-utility and cost-effectiveness analyses. They place outcomes for trials of COPD treatments in the context of all treatments in healthcare (62).

Using a utility instrument, a single number rates the value of health states on a continuum scale ranging from zero to one (or 100), where zero usually represents death and one (100) represents perfect health (63). Health utilities can be measured either directly (using techniques such as the standard gamble or time trade-off) or indirectly (using multidimensional HRQL questionnaires developed using multi-attribute utility theory) (61). They may have discriminative properties in COPD, but might be weak at evaluating changes (26).

The EQ-5D, the Health Utilities Index 2 and 3 (HUI2, HUI3), the SF-6D, and the quality of well-being scale are among the most widely used generic utility measures (61). Recently, a disease-specific utility measure has been developed for its use in COPD: the Health States-COPD. A comprehensive review is available elsewhere (64,65).

D. Interpretation

Although physicians might be able to make reasonable judgments of overall treatment efficacy (Fig. 2), they may not be still familiar with the meaning and clinical relevance of the health status scores and its changes. Different approaches have been made to provide an understandable interpretation, chief of which has been the concept of the "minimal clinically important difference" (MCID). The concept as first defined by

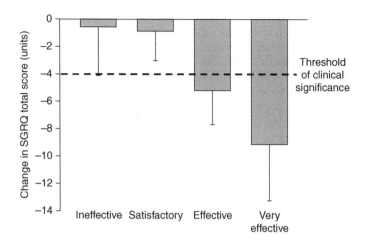

Figure 2 Change in SGRQ score after 16 weeks in chronic obstructive pulmonary disease patients recruited to a trial of salmeterol versus placebo, categorized by the physicians' retrospective judgment of treatment efficacy. The error bars are 95% confidence intervals. *Abbreviation*: SGRQ, St. George's Respiratory Questionnaire. *Source*: Reproduced from Ref. 66.

Jaeschke is "the smallest difference in score in the domain of interest which patients perceive as beneficial and which would mandate, in the absence of troublesome side effects and excessive cost, a change in the patient's management" (67). A number of different approaches have been used to establish the MCID, which include distribution-based methods, opinion-based methods (expert and patient preference-based estimates), and anchor-based methods (using anchors such as results in clinical trials, other clinical parameters such as dyspnea or prediction of future events such as hospital admission). Value judgments are always required at some stage in the establishment of threshold for a MCID (62).

The MCID is specific to each instrument. A minimum clinically significant change has been established for some health status instruments; for example a change of 4 U in the overall score for the SGRQ (1) and a change of at least 0.5 on the seven-point scale for the CRQ (55). One study which compared the MICD for the SGRQ and the CRQ showed that a change of 0.5 on the CRQ dyspnea domain was associated with a change of 3.1 on the SGRQ total score (68).

Since all MCID estimates are made in populations of patients and have both sampling and measurement error, they should be used as indicatives values. For the same reason, different approaches to its estimation rather than a single one should be used (69). It remains unclear whether the MCID has the same value along the whole scaling range of the instrument.

The MCID of a health status score is a population-based estimate and cannot be used in the medical decision-making process in individual patients. Although the repeatability of the SGRQ as measured by the intraclass correlation is high (0.92), this still means that approximately half of the patients with stable COPD may have a change in SGRQ greater than 4 U in repeated testing (26).

Once the MCID has been defined, data on the proportion of patients achieving a threshold for clinically important change, and the number needed to treat, can be calculated. This type of responder analysis provides a different, but equally valid perspective about the change in health status with treatment. These estimates may be quite reliable because they supply relevant information that cannot be obtained from group mean change assessments. However there is still no agreement on the proportion of patients that constitutes a clinically significant change. One advantage of this approach however is the observation, made with both the CRQ and SGRQ, that the proportion of responders appears to be relatively independent of the precise threshold chosen (69,70). Indeed, the proportion of patients who will benefit from treatment can be estimated from the effect size, a distribution-based approach method of interpretation, since the effect size and the proportion benefiting from treatment and the number needed to be treated have shown a linear relationship (70).

VI. Factors that Are Related to Health Status in COPD

Health status in stable COPD patients is affected by many factors. Variables that affect the physical health component of HRQL include breathlessness, physical impairment, reduced daily activities, and variables that affect the mental health component such as hopelessness, anxiety, and a negative affective trait (71).

A. Psychological Status

Psychological status has an impact on the health status of COPD patients. Hospital anxiety and depression scale scores have been related to most aspects of HRQL, with anxiety and depression consistently correlating with impaired health. Emotional wellbeing has been reported to be significantly related to symptoms, especially fatigue, and to coping pattern (72).

Besides improving health status, pulmonary rehabilitation may decrease psychosocial morbidity in COPD patients even when no specific psychological intervention is performed (73).

B. Dyspnea

There is a significant association between the MRC dyspnea grade and the SGRQ scores (Fig. 3). COPD patients who report more severe dyspnea and exhibit more impaired lung function have, in general, lower health status scores (74). The SGRQ scores, together with depression and exercise performance, is one of the determinants of patient's disability between MRC Grades 3 and 4 (74).

Categorization of patients with COPD on the basis of the level of dyspnea is useful in the prediction of health status (75). Improvements in exercise performance and health status in patients with COPD after pulmonary rehabilitation has been reported to depend on the initial degree of dyspnea, even at similar degree of airflow obstruction (76).

C. Lung Function

Lower FEV_1 is associated with worse health, but the correlation between spirometry and health status is weak (1,31). Different stages of COPD, based on the FEV_1, separate

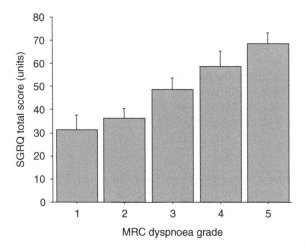

Figure 3 SGRQ score in chronic obstructive pulmonary disease patients categorized by MRC grade. The error bars are 95% confidence intervals. *Abbreviations*: MRC, Medical Research Council; SGRQ, St. George's Respiratory Questionnaire. *Source*: From Ref. 1.

groups of patients with varying degrees of impairment in health status using the SGRQ (77), but within each stage there is a very wide variation in SGRQ scores between patients (Fig. 4). Even patients with pre-bronchodilator $FEV_1 \geq 50\%$ predicted have impaired health status compared with a normal population (77,79).

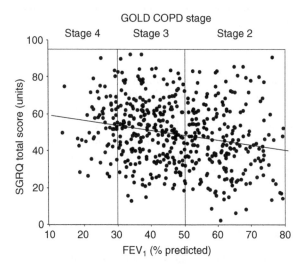

Figure 4 SGRQ score plotted against post-bronchodilator FEV_1, with the superimposition of the Global Initiative for Chronic Obstructive Lung Disease (GOLD COPD) stages. *Abbreviations*: FEV_1, forced expiratory volume in one second; SGRQ, St. George's Respiratory Questionnaire. *Source*: From Ref. 78.

Long-term changes in health status have been evaluated in patients with COPD, in comparison to the changes in FEV_1. A significant but weak correlation has been reported between the decline in FEV_1 and the decline in health status using the SGRQ (80). No significant relationships have been shown between change in health status measured by the CRQ and the change in pulmonary function (81).

In contrast, correlations between health status and other physiological measures such as exercise performance and PaO_2 may be stronger. HRQL has been related to the severity of hypoxemia in patients with severe COPD (82).

D. Exercise Tests

Health status tends to correlate better with exercise performance than with FEV_1 (78). Exercise capacity as measured by the six-MWT, progressive cycle ergometry, and the cycle endurance test correlates significantly with the activity and total scores of the SGRQ (83).

Walk test results show a moderate correlation with functional status questionnaires that focus on dyspnea in daily living, suggesting that they may reflect patients' HRQL quite well (84,85). The results of maximal exercise tests correlate poorly with quality of life measures (84,85).

E. Body Weight

Low body mass index (BMI ≤ 20) in patients with COPD has been related to worsening of dyspnea and deterioration of both generic and disease-specific health status. Underweight patients compared with normal weight patients show significantly worse total, and subscales scores of the SGRQ, and in the physical functioning, role emotional, bodily pain, and general health scores of the SF-36 (86). Low lean body mass has been associated with greater impairment in symptoms, activity and impact scores, and the total SGRQ scores (87).

F. Comorbidity

Comorbidity may modify health status scores and be a prognostic marker in patients with COPD. Up to 84% of COPD patients report coexisting chronic conditions (77). Comorbidities such as chronic renal failure or electrocardiogram signs of myocardial ischemia are associated with mortality in COPD (88). Patients with pre-bronchodilator $FEV_1 > 50\%$ predicted and comorbidities have a significant more impaired health status than patients with the same level of airways obstruction and no comorbidities. However, this difference is smaller in patients with more severe obstruction (77). The association between COPD disease stage and health status is stronger for patients without comorbid conditions (77).

G. Socioeconomic Factors

The associations between employment and health status in COPD patient have been examined in a study that included 210 COPD patients. Patients with COPD who were disabled for work showed equal severity of airflow limitation but worse health status measured by the CRQ, as compared with paid workers. Within the group of paid workers, patients with many work-related clinical symptoms and susceptible to various work-related irritants experienced poorer health status than those who had no symptoms, or were not susceptible to the irritants (89).

H. Imaging of the Lungs

The degree of HRCT scan abnormality is related to patients disability and impairment in alpha1-antitrypsin deficiency, when assessed using the SGRQ ($r = -0.38$ to 0.50) and the SF-36 (physical functioning score $r = -0.39$ to 0.54) (90).

I. Inflammatory Markers

Patients with raised C-reactive protein (CRP) levels have been reported to have high and worse-SGRQ total scores. Compared with those with normal CRP levels the differences exceeded the MCID (91).

J. Health Status and Smoking

Health status is improved by smoking cessation in non-COPD populations, especially on dimensions related to mental health, as assessed by the SF-36 (51,92). Improvement in health status has been identified as an outcome criterion for the effectiveness of treatment for addictions (51).

Current COPD smokers have worse health than COPD ex-smokers as measured by the SGRQ and the SF-36. The SGRQ symptoms and Impacts scores and the SF-36 psychosocial scales are most affected by smoking status; neither the physical scales of the SF-36 nor the Activity component of the SGRQ seem to be related to smoking. Nevertheless, health status declines at the same rate in smokers and ex-smokers (93).

K. Health Status and Exacerbations

Exacerbations are frequent events in the natural history of the disease. The presence of daily symptoms and a high exacerbation frequency contribute to impaired health status in COPD (17).

L. Acute Impact on Health Status

A recent review of the use of health status instruments to evaluate COPD exacerbations found that most measures, both generic and disease-specific, perform adequately when used during COPD exacerbations and indicate impaired health status during an exacerbation, which improves on its resolution (94). Relationships are evident between health status during an exacerbation and various outcomes, including post-exacerbation functional status, hospital readmission for exacerbation, and mortality (94).

Changes in health status scores 10 days after presentation with an exacerbation have shown moderate–high correlations with changes in FEV_1 and in the Transitional Dyspnea Index (95). Patients who suffered a clinical relapse within 10 days of the previous exacerbation did not show further impairment, possibly due to a floor effect phenomenon (95).

Although the greatest improvement takes place during the first month after an infective exacerbation, the effect of the exacerbations on health status may persist for many months (96). A second episode within six months limits recovery (96).

M. Long-Term Impact on Health Status

In a two-year observational study that included 336 patients, exacerbations had a negative long-term effect on health status in patients with moderate COPD (97). The change in SGRQ total score of moderate patients with ≥ 3 exacerbations was almost two points per year greater (worse) than those with < 3 exacerbations during the follow up (97). The greatest difference between frequent and infrequent exacerbators was observed in the symptoms scale. The SF-12, a generic instrument, did not detect any significant change during the follow-up period. At the end of the study, moderate patients with frequent exacerbations had worse health status scores than severe patients with infrequent exacerbations, which highlights the impact of exacerbations on health status. Indeed, the frequency of exacerbations is a separate factor from decline in FEV_1 on the impacts on health status (80).

Health status declines progressively in COPD whether measured by the SF-36 or using the SGRQ by a clinically significant amount every 15 months in patients just receiving short-acting bronchodilators (93). The rate of deterioration over three years is linked to the rate of exacerbations, which suggests a cumulative effect of exacerbations on health status. Preventing exacerbation by means of therapy may reduce health status decline (80,93).

N. Predictive Validity of Health Status Scores

Generic and specific health status measures, such as the SF-36 and the SGRQ have been useful in predicting health resource utilization (3) and both have been proved to be independent predictors of mortality (88).

Poor health status is associated with increased use of resources and rehospitalization/death rate in moderate to severe COPD patients (98).

Patients with poor health status are at greater risk of hospital readmission, are more likely to be provided with home nebulizers and are also more likely to be referred to respiratory specialists (98). In patients with COPD, those with greater distress and poorer coping are more likely to be readmitted to hospital following an admission for a COPD exacerbation (98). When health status improves, even though lung function does not, consultations and hospital admissions decrease (99).

Both generic and specific health status questionnaires have been shown to predict the survival of patients with COPD, independently of airflow limitation and age (100). Health status measured, by the SF-36 and the SGRQ has been associated with all-cause and respiratory mortality. This association is stronger with respiratory than with non-respiratory mortality (88). There is an estimate of 3.3% to 4% increased risk of mortality at one year associated with a 4-U difference in the SGRQ scores (69).

Different disease-specific health status questionnaires have shown different abilities to predict mortality. The total scores of the SGRQ and the BPQ have been significantly correlated with mortality; but the CRQ has not (100). Possible explanations for these differences could be that CRQ does not examine activity restrictions, has lower correlations with pulmonary function and exercise capacity and is more influenced by psychological status (100).

These findings should not mislead clinicians into assuming that HRQL might be a good indicator of a patient's life-sustaining treatment preferences. Health status scores have not shown to predict treatment preferences and should not influence clinicians' views. In one study of 101 COPD patients on oxygen-therapy, health status measured by the SGRQ was not associated with preferences for either resuscitation or mechanical ventilation. Depression was significantly associated with preferences for resuscitation, but not with preferences for mechanical ventilation (101). These findings highlight the individuality of life values, expectancies and hopes, which can only be captured partially by any of the current health status instruments.

O. Health Status Measurements in Clinical Trials

The importance of measuring health status in clinical trials can be appreciated in studies where no other measurements are able to document the effects of health care interventions on patient outcomes. Possibly, the most important contribution of health status questionnaires in effectiveness measurement is to assess the overall effect of the treatment; however the beneficial effects of treatment on health status may be mediated through different mechanisms, each with a different time course (80).

When using health status questionnaires in clinical trials, some potential bias have to be taken into account. One is the use of relatively short run-in periods; the implications of which emerged with the observation that SGRQ scores continued to recover for many months after an exacerbation (26). Another factor is the analysis of the dropout patients; the common "last observation carried forward" approach may underestimate the size of the difference between the active treatment and placebo groups. Health status declines progressively and patients who drop out of trials are not only more severe but also their health status declines faster (26,102).

Improvements in health status have been found in clinical trials with a variety of inhaled agents, rehabilitation programs and after COPD-specific surgery (103–106). It is possible to calculate the annual rate of deterioration in health for some health status questionnaires and show that this changes with treatment (93).

VII. Bronchodilators

A. Short-Acting β₂-Agonists

Short-acting bronchodilators provide symptomatic relief and improve exercise tolerance. Short-acting β_2-agonists improve the dyspnea and fatigue scores of the CRQ and ipratropium improved the symptoms domain of the SGRQ (107).

B. Long-Acting β₂-Agonists

The long-acting β_2-agonists (LABA) improve symptoms, and health status in patients with COPD (108,109). In one study that measured the efficacy of a LABA, changes in the SGRQ and the SF-36 were evaluated in patients with COPD following treatment with placebo, salmeterol 50 µg twice a day, or 100 µg twice a day at baseline and after 16 weeks of treatment. Compared with placebo, salmeterol 50 µg twice a day was associated with significant improvements in SGRQ Total and Impacts scores that exceeded the threshold for a clinically significant change. This was not seen with salmeterol 100 µg twice a day, which might have been related to side effects such as tremor. Although both doses showed similar change in FEV_1, health status measured by SGRQ improved only in the group in which a lower dose was given (66).

Similar findings have been reported with formoterol compared with placebo. After 12 weeks of treatment, formoterol showed clinically significant improvement on all domains of the SGRQ. The lower formoterol dose seemed to perform better than the higher dose (105). The same study showed some advantage of formoterol over regular four times daily ipratropium (105) and a similar advantage of salmeterol over ipratropium four times a day has been shown using the CRQ (110).

One study has used the CRQ to test the effect of adding theophylline to salmeterol and found a higher proportion of patients who had a clinically significant improvement with the combination than with either agent used alone (111).

C. Tiotropium

Tiotropium reduces COPD exacerbations and related hospitalizations compared with placebo and ipratropium (112). It has been shown to produce significant health status benefits compared with both placebo and regular ipratropium (104,113) and a small advantage compared with salmeterol, but that was not clinically significant (114).

There are not yet convincing data to date to show whether this drug is superior or inferior to LABA in improving health status in patients with moderate to severe COPD (109).

D. Inhaled Corticosteroids

Inhaled Corticosteroids

Most pharmacological studies to test health status benefits have been one year or less, and the test of treatment effect has been a direct comparison between the drug under test, and the comparator. The three-year inhaled steroids in obstructive lung disease in Europe study of fluticasone versus placebo required a different method of analysis, since this was the first study to show that health status declined at a measurable rate, whether measured using a disease-specific questionnaire (SGRQ) or a generic instrument (SF-36) (93). In the placebo limb, the SGRQ score worsened at 3.2 U/yr compared with 2.0 U/yr with fluticasone (103). This was an important observation since it showed that the effect of treatment increased over time, which is evidence for a possible overall disease-modifying effect of therapy.

Combination Therapy with LABA

There have been three large one year trials of combination therapy, comparing inhaled corticosteroid (ICS) and LABA, i.e., ICS+LABA with the monocomponents and placebo. Two of the studies (115,116) suggest only modest health status benefits compared with the single agents, however a third (117) showed a clear advantage over the single agents alone. The major difference between that study and the other two was that, instead of a traditional treatment withdrawal run-in period, the patients received two weeks of treatment intensification with prednisolone plus formoterol. That produced an improvement over two weeks which exceeded the minimum clinically important difference for the SGRQ; thereafter the ICS+LABA combination appears to have maintained that benefit and produced a small additional improvement over the next year. It is not known whether this was due to the design of the run-in period. This important study design needs to be tested again.

E. Rehabilitation

Improvements in health status following pulmonary rehabilitation have been shown with both generic (SF-36) and disease-specific measures (SGRQ, CRQ) (118).

In the pulmonary rehabilitation component of the National Emphysema Treatment Trial (NETT) study with 1218 patients there was a significant improvement in two disease-specific questionnaires, one generic and one utility measures after 6 to 10 weeks of a rehabilitation program. Changes in health status correlated with changes in the six-MWT (119). In another randomized controlled trial that included 200 patients assigned to a six week multidisciplinary program or to standard therapy, there was improvement in all domains of two disease-specific questionnaires and in all dimensions except pain of the SF-36. The differences between the groups for many of the health status measures, although smaller, remained significant after one year. At one year there was a lack of significant benefit in the mental component score of the SF-36 and the emotion domain in the CRQ, suggesting that the emotionally-based benefits of rehabilitation might be less robust than the physical ones (52).

On average, pulmonary rehabilitation improves CRQ dyspnea domain scores by 4.1 CRQ units and SGRQ total scores by 4.4 SGRQ units, both clinically and statistically significant. Two trials have reported long-term gains on the dyspnea domain of the CRQ of 1.11 CRQ units and two more trials have reported long-term gains on SGRQ, -5.6 SGRQ units (109). The relative improvements in patients' health status have been maintained to some extent during 18 months of follow-up in some studies (109).

F. Oxygen Therapy

Studies measuring health status have been performed in patients on long-term oxygen therapy or supplemental oxygen during exercise (120,121), but there have been no randomized control trials so it is not possible to state whether or not there is a definite health status benefit. It has been reported that the mode of oxygen delivery may be influential (122). Ambulatory oxygen from liquid source or lightweight cylinders seems to improve health status in selected patients who partake in regular outdoor activity. Whether continuous oxygen therapy from oxygen concentrators might be beneficial in improving quality of life is less clear (122). Withdrawal of oxygen therapy in patients who do not longer accomplish oxygen prescription criteria does not appear to affect their health status (123).

G. Surgery

Improvement in dyspnea, exercise tolerance and health status after lung volume reduction surgery has been documented in patients with an FEV_1 less than 30% of predicted. Improvement in health status appears to be better preserved over longer-term follow-up than physiological improvement (124). Bronchoscopic lung volume reduction with one-way valves might be an alternative to the surgical approach to improve HRQL. Health status has been measured as a secondary outcome in the Endobronchial Valve for Emphysema Palliation Trial, whose results have not been published yet (125).

Five prospective studies (125 patients) have examined health status in transplant recipients. Patients report significantly better physical functioning, with fewer restrictions in social and leisure activities, more favorable health impressions, more energy, and less pain and discomfort in comparison to their pre-transplant level of functioning (126).

VIII. Specific Issues about Symptoms and Health Status Assessment

A. Women

Sociocultural and biological factors are thought to play a role in the gender differences in the perception, reporting, and diagnostic interpretation of respiratory symptoms (127).

Shortness of breath is consistently reported more frequently by women than men (127). In a population study involving more than 20,000 adults, reporting rates for shortness of breath were lower with better levels of FEV_1 in a similar way in both men and women, but at all levels of FEV_1 reporting rates were higher in women than in men. These gender differences increased, after standardizing for potential confounders such as smoking, occupational exposure, educational level, obesity, and FEV_1 level (127). Similar findings have been reported in COPD patients in a primary care setting (128). In a population of patients with COPD attending a pulmonary clinic, for the same level of FEV_1, women had better oxygenation, better $PaCO_2$, and fewer comorbidities than men, however they performed poorer in walking distance, had higher symptoms score, a higher degree of dyspnea and worse health status scores (129). When analyzed longitudinally, however, differences in symptom reports between males and females seem to disappear (130).

Women are known to have a different attitude toward test taking and self-report assessments in general. Females perceive more impaired health status when compared with matched male subjects in sleep-breathing disorders and healthy populations (131,132). Males show a stronger association between symptoms and lung function and seem to have a risk of developing new symptoms of phlegm and wheeze caused by an increase in smoking, but not females (130).

When a group of 146 patients with chronic bronchitis and emphysema were asked to rate the frequency with which 89 symptoms and experiences occurred during breathlessness, women reported more anxiety and helplessness–hopelessness than men during their breathing difficulties (133).

The relationship between symptom indicators and functional performance may differ across gender. Several somatic symptoms, such as fatigue, provide the best indicator of overall, psychosocial and physical performance in women whereas dyspnea after the six-MWT served as the most accurate measurement of total and psychosocial performance in men (134).

Gender differences can also be observed in respect to the response to rehabilitation. In a randomized clinical trial of 3 months versus 18 months exercise therapy in COPD patients, there were significant improvements in all CRQ scores for men and women after three months of treatment. At 18 months, these effects were moderated by gender. Men in the long-term group reported significantly more favorable scores than the short-term group for all CRQ domains. The CRQ data on women demonstrated that long-term exercise therapy added little benefit for women compared with short-term exercise therapy (135).

B. Use of Proxies for Health Status Assessments

Symptoms and health status are measured best from the patient's perspective. However, patients unable to cooperate because of their advanced age, cognitive disorder, or impaired clinical condition might not provide reliable scores and surrogates such as proxies might be used instead. The use of assessments provided by relatives is common in clinical practice.

Attempts to measure symptoms and health status by observers such as relatives, caregivers or health professionals in a number of chronic diseases have shown a moderate to good level of agreement between patients and proxies' scores (40–75%) with a systematic bias showing underestimation of symptoms and overestimation of impairment of health status by proxies (136–138).

Proxies tend to overestimate the degree of patient health status impairment in all dimensions evaluated; physical domains correlate better than psychological aspects (139,140). Although a COPD-specific health status questionnaire, such as the SGRQ has proved to have adequate psychometric properties and the ability to discriminate across disease stages when answered by proxies, they systematically over-report impairment in health status (141). For research purposes, the patients should be the information source.

C. Use and Application of Health Status Data

It is clear that health status and symptom measurement form important outcomes that may be more important for making to clinical decisions and allocation of health resources than differences in traditional measures of pulmonary function.

The interest, use, and application of the various symptoms and health status questionnaires may differ according to the type of user: patient, clinicians, researchers, medical societies, and pharmaceutical companies, agencies responsible for drug registration or health authorities.

From the perspective of the patient, health status questionnaires are accessible and understandable tools that are close to their experience, especially disease-specific instruments. This gives them an opportunity to express what is important to them.

From the clinician's point of view, health status questionnaires include relevant information to the patient that might be missed in an unstructured clinical interview and provide a more comprehensive understanding of the disease and its effects and a wider perspective than the biologic pathways.

For the researcher, symptoms and health status measurements are important clinical outcomes that provide an overall measure of efficacy which may be particularly important when assessing therapies with more than one beneficial effects.

Health status instruments provide standardized assessments and treat each patient as is they were typical. Much has been learnt from their use, but there is a need for methods of assessment that address more individual aspects of HRQL.

D. Future Directions

Current COPD staging for guiding treatment decisions, such as suggested by Global Initiative for Chronic Obstructive Lung Disease is based upon FEV_1 (142). However, current treatment is largely directed toward improving symptoms, so it makes sense to develop staging processes that are more symptoms based. As health status and symptoms, such as dyspnea, have proved to influence patient outcomes and mortality, their assessment should play a role in addition to current staging to improve prognostic classification (37).

Future developments in health status measurements include establishing cross-cultural equivalence of questionnaires, defining clinical significant intraindividual changes, establishing equivalence scoring of different between questionnaires, simplifying existing instruments, and optimizing computerized versions (25,42).

References

1. Jones PW, Quirk FH, Baveystock CM, Littlejohns P. A self-complete measure of health status for chronic airflow limitation: the St. George's Respiratory Questionnaire. Am Rev Respir Dis 1992; 145:1321–7.
2. Curtis JR, Deyo RA, Hudson LD. Health-related quality of life among patients with chronic obstructive pulmonary disease. Thorax 1994; 49:162–70.
3. Clancy CM, Eisenberg JM. Outcomes research: measuring the end results of health care. Science 1998; 282:245–6.
4. U.S. Food and drug administration. Center for Drug Evaluation and Research. Guidance Documents. Patient-Reported Outcome Measures: use in Medical Product Development to Support Labelling Claims. [draft document updated 2006 February 2; cited 2006 July 20]. (Available from: http://www.fda.gov/cder/guidance/index.htm)
5. Chassany O, Sagnier P, Marquis P, Fulleton S, Aaronson N. Patient reported outcomes and regulatory issues: the example of health-related quality of life—a European Guidance Document for the improved integration of HRQL assessment in the drug regulatory process. Drug Inf J 2002; 36:209–38.
6. Wilson IB, Cleary PD. Linking clinical variables with health-related quality of life. J Am Med Assoc 1995; 273:59–65.
7. American Thoracic Society [homepage on the Internet]. Research. Quality of Life Resources. [updated 2006; cited 2006 July 20]. (Available from: http://www.atsqol.org/)
8. Selim AJ, Ren XS, Fincke G, et al. A symptom-based measure for the severity of chronic lung disease: results from the Veterans Health Study. Chest 1997; 111:1607–14.
9. Graydon JE, Ross E, Webster PM, Goldstein RS, Avendano M. Predictors of functioning of patients with chronic obstructive pulmonary disease. Heart Lung 1995; 24(5):369–75.
10. Quirk FH, Baveystock CM, Wilson RC, Jones PW. Influence of demographic and disease related factors on the degree of distress associated with symptoms and restrictions on daily living due to asthma in six countries. Eur Respir J 1991; 4:167–71.
11. Compact Oxford English Dictionary [updated 2006; cited 2006 July 20]. (Available from: http://www.askoxford.com/concise_oed/symptom?view=uk)
12. Curtis JR. Assessing health-related quality of life in chronic pulmonary disease. In: Fishman AP, ed. Pulmonary Rehabilitation. New York: Marcel Dekker, 1996; p. 329–354.
13. Wouters EFM. Management of severe COPD. Lancet 2004; 364:883–95.
14. Lenz ER, Pugh LC, Milligan RA, Suppe F. The middle-range theory of unpleasant symptoms: an update. Adv Nurs Sci 1997; 19:14–27.
15. Barley EA, Jones PW. A comparison of global questions versus health status questionnaires as measures of the severity and impact of asthma. Eur Respir J 1999; 14:591–6.
16. Mathers CD, Sadana R, Salomon JA, Murray, Lopez AD. Estimates of DALE for 191 countries: methods and results. Global Programme on Evidence for Health Policy Working Paper No. 16, WHO, June 2000. [updated 2006 July 10; cited 2006 July 20]. (Available from: http://www.who.int/health-systems-performance/docs/articles/paper16.pdf)
17. Seemungal TA, Donaldson GC, Paul EA, Bestall JC, Jeffries DJ, Wedzicha JA. Effect of exacerbation on quality of life in patients with chronic obstructive pulmonary disease. Am J Respir Crit Care Med 1998; 157:1418–22.
18. Gudmundsson G, Gislason T, Janson C, et al. Risk factors for rehospitalisation in COPD: role of health status, anxiety and depression. Eur Respir J. 2005; 26:414–9.
19. Neuman A, Gunnbjornsdottir M, Tunsater A, et al. Dyspnea in relation to symptoms of anxiety and depression: a prospective population study. Respir Med 2006; 100:1843–9.
20. Guyatt G, Townsend M, Berman L, Pugsley S. Quality of life in patients with chronic airflow limitation. Br J Dis Chest 1987; 81:45–54.

21. Gift AG, Shepard CE. Fatigue and other symptoms in patients with chronic obstructive pulmonary disease: do women and men differ? J Obstet Gynecol Neonatal Nurs 1999; 28:201–8.
22. Bergner M. Quality of life, health status, and clinical research. Med Care 1989; 27:S148–56.
23. Gill TM, Feinstein AR. A critical appraisal of the quality of quality of life measurements. J Am Med Assoc 1994; 272:619–26.
24. Jones PW. Measurement of quality of life in chronic obstructive lung disease. Eur Respir Rev 1991; 1:445–53.
25. Patrick DL, Chiang YP. Measurement of health outcomes in treatment effectiveness evaluations: conceptual and methodological challenges. Med Care 2000; 38(9 Suppl.):II14–25.
26. Jones PW. Health status: what does it mean for payers and patients? Proc Am Thorac Soc 2006; 3:222–6.
27. McColl E. Best practice in symptom assessment: a review. Gut 2004; 53(IV):49–54.
28. Spencer S, Jones PW, Duprat-Lomon I, Sagnier PP. An acute bronchitis questionnaire (AECB-SS) discriminates between GOLD categories for COPD severity in patients screened for the MOSAIC study. Eur Respir J 2004; 24(Suppl. 48):239S.
29. Ingham JM, Farooqi M. Chapter 3: assessment of physical symptoms. In: O'Neil JF, Selwyn PA, Sehietinger H, eds. A Clinical Guide on Supportive and Palliative Care for People with HIV/AIDS. U.S. Department of Health and Human Services, Health Resources and Services Administration, HIV/AIDS Bureau, 2003.
30. Schunemann HJ, Goldstein R, Mador MJ, et al. A randomised trial to evaluate the self-administered standardised chronic respiratory questionnaire. Eur Respir J 2005; 25:31–40.
31. Ferrer M, Alonso J, Prieto L, et al. Validity and reliability of the St George's Respiratory Questionnaire after adaptation to a different language and culture: the Spanish example. Eur Respir J 1996; 9:1160–6.
32. Fraser A, Delaney B, Moayyedi P. Symptom-based outcome measures for dyspepsia and GERD trials: a systematic review. Am J Gastroenterol 2005; 100:442–52.
33. Portenoy RK, Thaler HT, Kornblith AB, Lepore JM, Friedlander-Klar H, Kiyasu E, Sobel K, Coyle N, Kemeny N, Norton L, et al. The memorial symptom assessment scale: an instrument for the evaluation of symptom prevalence, characteristics and distress. Eur J Cancer 1994; 30A(9):1326–36.
34. Medical Research Council. Standardized questionnaire on respiratory symptoms. Br Med J 1960; 2:1665.
35. American Thoracic Society. Evaluation of impairment/disability secondary to respiratory disease. Am Rev Respir Dis 1982; 126:945–51.
36. Leidy NK, Schmier JK, Jones MK, Lloyd J, Rocchiccioli K. Evaluating symptoms in chronic obstructive pulmonary disease: validation of the breathlessness, cough and sputum scale. Respir Med 2003; 97:S59–70.
37. Nishimura K, Izumi T, Tsukino M, Oga T. Dyspnea is a better predictor of 5-year survival than airway obstruction in patients with COPD. Chest 2002; 121(5):1434–40.
38. Kaplan RM, Ries AL. Quality of life as an outcome measure in pulmonary diseases. J Cardiopulm Rehabil 2005; 25:321–31.
39. Borg G. Psychological scaling with applications in physical work and the perception of exertion. Scand J Work Environ Health 1990; 16(Suppl. 1):55–8.
40. Jones PW, Lareau S, Mahler DA. Measuring the effects of COPD on the patient. Respir Med 2005; 99:S11–8.
41. Mahler DA, Weinberg DH, Wells CK, Feinstein AR. The measurement of dyspnea. Contents, interobserver agreement, and physiologic correlates of two new clinical indexes. Chest 1984; 85(6):751–8.
42. McGavin CR, Artvinli M, Nace H, McHardy GJ. Dyspnoea, disability and distance walked: comparison of estimates of exercise performance in respiratory disease. Int J Rehabil Res 1980; 3(2):235–6.
43. Jones PW, Agusti AGN. Outcomes and markers in the assessment of chronic obstructive pulmonary disease. Eur Respir J 2006; 27:822–32.
44. Hajiro T, Nishimura K, Tsukino M, Ikeda A, Koyama H, Izumi T. Comparison of discriminative properties among disease-specific questionnaires for measuring health-related quality of life in patients with chronic obstructive pulmonary disease. Crit Care Med 1998; 157:785–90.
45. Dittner AJ, Wessely SC, Brown RG. The assessment of fatigue. A practical guide for clinicians and researchers. J Psychosom Res 2004; 56:157–70.
46. Breslin E, van der Schams C, Breukink S, et al. Perception of fatigue and quality of life in patients with COPD. Chest 1998; 114:958–64.

47. Small SP, Lamb M. Measurement of fatigue in chronic obstructive pulmonary disease and in asthma. Int J Nurs Stud 2000; 37:127–33.
48. Breukink SO, Strijbos JH, Koorn M, Koeter GH, Breslin EH, Van der Schans CP. Relationship between subjective fatigue and physiological variables in patients with chronic obstructive pulmonary disease. Respir Med 1998; 92:676–82.
49. Eui-Geum O, Cho-ja K, Won-Hee L, So-sun K. Correlates of fatigue in Koreans with chronic lung disease. Heart Lung 2004; 33:13–20.
50. Ware JE, Jr., Sherbourne CD. The MOS 36-Items Short-form health survey (SF-36): I. Conceptual framework and item selection. Med Care 1992; 30:473–81.
51. Croghan IT, Schroeder DR, Hays JT, et al. Nicotine dependence treatment: perceived health status improvement with 1-year continuous smoking abstinence. Eur J Public Health 2005; 15(3):251–5.
52. Griffiths TL, Burr ML, Campbell IA, et al. Results at 1 year of outpatient multidisciplinary pulmonary rehabilitation: a randomised controlled trial. Lancet 2000; 355:362–8.
53. Bergner M, Bobbitt RA, Pollard WE, Martin DP, Gilson BS. The sickness impact profile: validation of a health status measure. Med Care 1976; 14(1):57–67.
54. Hunt SM, McEwen J, McEwen J, McKenna SP. Measuring health status: a new tool for clinicians and epidemiologists. J R Coll Gen Pract 1985; 35:185–8.
55. Guyatt GH, Berman LB, Townsend M, Pugsley SO, Chambers LW. A measure of quality of life for clinical trials in chronic lung disease. Thorax 1987; 42:773–8.
56. Jones PW, Quirk FH, Baveystock CM. The St George's Respiratory Questionnaire. Respir Med 1991; 85:25–31.
57. Hyland ME, Bott J, Singh S, Kenyon CA. Domains, constructs and the development of the breathing problems questionnaire. Qual Life Res 1994; 3(4):245–56.
58. Barley EA, Quirk FH, Jones PW. Asthma health status measurement in clinical practice: validity of a new short and simple instrument. Respir Med 1998; 92:1027–34.
59. Quirk FH, Jones PW. Patients' perception of distress due to symptoms and effects of asthma on daily living and an investigation of possible influential factors. Clin Sci 1990; 79:17–21.
60. Harper R, Brazier JE, Waterhouse JC, et al. Comparison of outcome measures for patients with chronic obstructive pulmonary disease (COPD) in an outpatient setting. Thorax 1997; 52:879–87.
61. Marra CA, Woolcott JC, Kopec JA, et al. A comparison of generic, indirect utility measures (the HUI2, HUI3, SF-6D, and the EQ-5D) and disease-specific instruments (the RAQoL and the HAQ) in rheumatoid arthritis. Soc Sci Med 2005; 60(7):1571–82.
62. Jones PW, Kaplan RM. Methodological issues in evaluating measures of health as outcomes for COPD. Eur Respir J 2003; 21:8s–13.
63. Weinstein MC, Siegel JE, Gold MR, Kamlet MS, Russell LB. Recommendations of the panel on cost-effectiveness in health and medicine. J Am Med Assoc 1996; 276:1253–8.
64. Kopec JA, Willison KD. A comparative review of four preference-weighted measures of health-related quality of life. J Clin Epidemiol 2003; 56:317–25.
65. Drummond M. Introducing economic and quality of life measurements in clinical studies. Ann Med 2001; 33:344–9.
66. Jones PW, Bosh TK. Quality of life changes in COPD patients treated with salmeterol. Am J Respir Crit Care Med 1997; 155(4):1283–9.
67. Jaeschke R, Singer J, Guyatt GH. Measurement of health status: ascertaining the minimal clinically important difference. Control Clin Trials 1989; 10:407–15.
68. Schunemann HJ, Griffith L, Jaeschke R, Goldstein R, Stubbing D, Guyatt GH. Evaluation of the minimal important difference for the feeling thermometer and the St. George's Respiratory Questionnaire in patients with chronic airflow obstruction. J Clin Epidemiol 2003; 56(12):1170–6.
69. Jones PW. St George's respiratory questionnaire: MCID. J Chronic Obstructive Pulmonary Dis 2005; 1:1–6.
70. Norman GR, Sridhar FG, Guyatt GH, Walter SD. Relation of distribution- and anchor-based approaches in interpretation of changes in health-related quality of life. Med Care 2001; 39:1039–47.
71. Hu J, Meek P. Health-related quality of life in individuals with chronic obstructive pulmonary disease. Heart Lung 2005; 34(6):415–22.
72. Engström CP, Persson LO, Larsson S, Sullivan M. Health-related quality of life in COPD: why both disease-specific and generic measures should be used. Eur Respir J 2001; 18:69–76.
73. Guell R, Resqueti V, Sangenis M, et al. Impact of pulmonary rehabilitation on psychosocial morbidity in patients with severe COPD. Chest 2006; 129(4):899–904.

74. Bestall JC, Paul EA, Garrod R, Garnham R, Jones PW, Wedzicha JA. Usefulness of the Medical Research Council (MRC) dyspnoea scale as a measure of disability in patients with chronic obstructive pulmonary disease. Thorax 1999; 54:581–6.

75. Hajiro T, Nishimura K, Tsukino M, et al. A comparison of the level of dyspnea vs disease severity in indicating the health-related quality of life of patients with COPD. Chest 1999; 116:1632–7.

76. Wedzicha JA, Bestall JC, Garrod R, Garnham R, Paul EA, Jones PW. Randomized controlled trial of pulmonary rehabilitation in severe chronic obstructive pulmonary disease patients, stratified with the MRC dyspnoea scale. Eur Respir J 1998; 12:363–9.

77. Ferrer M, Alonso J, Morera J, et al. Chronic obstructive Pulmonary Disease Stage and health-related quality of life. Ann Intern Med 1997; 127:1072–9.

78. Jones PW. Health status measurement in chronic obstructive pulmonary disease. Thorax 2001; 56:880–7.

79. Mahler DA. How should health-related quality of life be assessed in patients with COPD? Chest 2000; 117:54S–7.

80. Spencer S, Calverley PMA, Burge PS, Jones PW. Impact of preventing exacerbations on deterioration of health status in COPD. Eur Respir J 2004; 23:1–5.

81. Oga T, Nishimura K, Tsukino M, et al. Longitudinal changes in health status using the chronic respiratory disease questionnaire and pulmonary function in patients with stable chronic obstructive pulmonary disease. Qual Life Res 2004; 13(6):1109–16.

82. Okubadejo AA, Jones PW, Wedzicha JA. Quality of life in patients with chronic obstructive pulmonary disease and severe hypoxemia. Thorax 1996; 51:44–7.

83. Oga T, Nishimura K, Tsukino M, Hajiro T, Ikeda A, Mishima M. Relationship between different indices of exercise capacity and clinical measures in patients with chronic obstructive pulmonary disease. Heart Lung 2002; 31(5):374–81.

84. Guyatt GH, Thompson PJ, Berman LB, et al. How should we measure function in patients with chronic heart and lung disease? J Chronic Dis 1985; 38:517–24.

85. Wijkstra PJ, TenVergert EM, van der Mark TW, et al. Relation of lung function, maximal inspiratory pressure, dyspnoea, and quality of life with exercise capacity in patients with chronic obstructive pulmonary disease. Thorax 1994; 49:468–72.

86. Katsura H, Yamada K, Kida K. Both generic and disease specific health-related quality of life are deteriorated in patients with underweight COPD. Respir Med 2005; 99(5):624–30.

87. Shoup R, Dalsky G, Warner S, et al. Body composition and health-related quality of life in patients with obstructive airways disease. Eur Respir J 1997; 10(7):1576–80.

88. Domingo-Salvany A, Lamarca R, Ferrer M, et al. Health-related quality of life and mortality in male patients with chronic obstructive pulmonary disease. Am J Respir Crit Care Med 2002; 166(5):680–5.

89. Orbon KH, Schermer TR, van der Gulden JW, et al. Employment status and quality of life in patients with chronic obstructive pulmonary disease. Int Arch Occup Environ Health 2005; 78(6):467–74.

90. Dowson LJ, Guest PJ, Hill SL, Holder RL, Stockley RA. High-resolution computed tomography scanning in alpha1-antitrypsin deficiency: relationship to lung function and health status. Eur Respir J 2001; 17(6):1097–104.

91. Broekhuizen R, Wouters EFM, Creutzberg EC, Schols AMW. Raised CRP levels mark metabolic and functional impairment in advanced COPD. Thorax 2006; 61(1):17–22.

92. Wilson D, Parsons J, Wakefield M. The health-related quality of life of never-smokers, ex-smokers and light, moderate and heavy smokers. Prev Med 1999; 29:139–44.

93. Spencer S, Calverley PM, Sherwood Burge P, Jones PW, Inhaled Steroids in Obstructive Lung Disease (ISOLDE) Study Group. Health status deterioration in patients with chronic obstructive pulmonary disease. Am J Respir Crit Care Med 2001; 163(1):122–8.

94. Dolll H, Miravitlles M. Health-related QOL in acute exacerbations of chronic bronchitis and chronic obstructive pulmonary disease: a review of the literature. Pharmacoeconomics 2005; 23(4):345–63.

95. Aaron SD, Vandemheen KL, Clinch JJ, et al. Measurement of short-term changes in dyspnea and disease-specific quality of life following an acute COPD exacerbation. Chest 2002; 122:688–96.

96. Spencer S, Jones PW. Time course of recovery of health status following an infective exacerbation of chronic bronchitis. Thorax 2003; 58:589–93.

97. Miravitlles M, Ferrer M, Pont A, et al. Effect of exacerbations on quality of life in patients with chronic obstructive pulmonary disease: a 2 year follow up study. Thorax 2004; 59(5):387–95.

98. Osman IM, Godden DJ, Friend JA, Legge JS, Douglas JG. Quality of life and hospital readmission in patients with chronic pulmonary obstructive disease. Thorax 1997; 52(1):67–71.

99. Cox NJ, Hendricks JC, Binkhorst RA, van Herwaarden CL. A pulmonary rehabilitation program for patients with asthma and mild chronic obstructive pulmonary diseases (COPD). Lung 1993; 171:235–44.
100. Oga T, Nishimura K, Tsukino M, Sato S, Hajiro T. Analysis of the factors related to mortality in chronic obstructive pulmonary disease. Am J Respir Crit Care Med 2003; 167:544–9.
101. Stapleton RD, Nielsen EL, Engelberg RA, Patrick DL, Curtis JR. Association of depression and life-sustaining treatment preferences in patients with COPD. Chest 2005; 127(1):328–34.
102. Calverley PMA, Spencer S, Willits L, Burge PS, Jones PW. Withdrawal from treatment as an outcome in the ISOLDE study of COPD. Chest 2003; 124:1350–6.
103. Burge PS, Calverley PM, Jones PW, Spencer S, Anderson JA, Maslen TK. Randomised, double blind, placebo controlled study of fluticasone propionate in patients with moderate to severe chronic obstructive pulmonary disease: the ISOLDE trial. Br Med J 2000; 320:1297–303.
104. Vincken W, van Noord JA, Greefhorst AP, et al. Improved health outcomes in patients with COPD during 1 yr's treatment with tiotropium. Eur Respir J 2002; 19(2):209–16.
105. Dahl R, Greefhorst LA, Nowak D, et al. Inhaled formoterol dry powder versus ipratropium bromide in chronic obstructive pulmonary disease. Am J Respir Crit Care Med 2001; 164(5):778–84.
106. Lacasse Y, Goldstein R, Lasserson TJ, Martin S. Pulmonary rehabilitation for chronic obstructive pulmonary disease. Cochrane Database Syst Rev 2002; (4):CD003793.
107. Tomas LHS, Varkey B. Improving health-related quality of life in chronic obstructive pulmonary disease. Curr Opin Pulm Med 2004; 10(2):120–7.
108. Stockley RA, Chopra N, Rice L. Addition of salmeterol to existing treatment in patients with COPD: a 12 month study. Thorax 2006; 61(2):122–8.
109. Sinn DD, McAlister FA, Man SF, Anthonisen NR. Contemporary management of chronic obstructive pulmonary disease: scientific review. J Am Med Assoc 2003; 290(17):2301–12.
110. Mahler DA, Donohue JF, Barbee RA, et al. Efficacy of salmeterol xinafoate in the treatment of COPD. Chest 1999; 115:957–65.
111. ZuWallack RL, Mahler DA, Reilly D, et al. Salmeterol plus theophylline combination therapy in the treatment of COPD. Chest 2001; 119:1661–70.
112. Barr RG, Bourbeau J, Camargo CA, Ram FSF. Tiotropium for stable chronic obstructive pulmonary disease. Cochrane Database Syst Rev 2005; (2):CD002876.
113. Casaburi R, Mahler DA, Jones PW, et al. A long-term evaluation of once-daily inhaled tiotropium in chronic obstructive pulmonary disease. Eur Respir J 2002; 19:217–24.
114. Brusasco V, Hodder R, Miravitlles M, Korducki L, Towse L, Kesten S. Health outcomes following treatment for six months with once daily tiotropium compared with twice daily salmeterol in patients with COPD. Thorax 2003; 58:399–404.
115. Szafranski W, Cukier A, Ramirez A, et al. Efficacy and safety of budesonide/formoterol in the management of chronic obstructive pulmonary disease. Eur Respir J 2003; 21(5):912.
116. Calverley P, Pauwels R, Vestbo J, et al. Combined salmeterol and fluticasone in the treatment of Chronic Obstructive Pulmonary Disease: a randomised controlled trial. Lancet 2003; 361:449–56.
117. Calverley PM, Boonsawat W, Cseke Z, Zhong N, Peterson S, Olsson H. Maintenance therapy with budesonide and formoterol in chronic obstructive pulmonary disease. Eur Respir J 2003; 22:912–9.
118. Nici L, Donner C, Wouters E, Zuwallack R, Ambrosino N, Bourbeau J, Carone M, Celli B, Engelen M, Fahy B, et al. American Thoracic Society/European Respiratory Society statement on pulmonary rehabilitation. Am J Respir Crit Care Med 2006; 173:1390–413.
119. Kaplan RM, Ries AL, Reilly J, Mohsenifar Z. Measurement of health-related quality of life in the national emphysema treatment trial. Chest 2004; 126(3):781–9.
120. Eaton T, Lewis C, Young P, Kennedy Y, Garrett JE, Kolbe J. Long-term oxygen therapy improves health-related quality of life. Respir Med 2004; 98(4):285–93.
121. Eaton T, Garrett JE, Young P, et al. Ambulatory oxygen improves quality of life of COPD patients: a randomised controlled study. Eur Respir J 2002; 20(2):306–12.
122. Andersson A, Strom K, Brodin H, et al. Domiciliary liquid oxygen versus concentrator treatment in chronic hypoxaemia: a cost-utility analysis. Eur Respir J 1998; 12:1284–9.
123. Guyatt GH, Nonoyama M, Lacchetti C, et al. A randomized trial of strategies for assessing eligibility for long-term domiciliary oxygen therapy. Am J Respir Crit Care Med 2005; 172:573–80.
124. Martinez FJ, Chang A. Surgical therapy for chronic obstructive pulmonary disease. Semin Respir Crit Care Med 2005; 26(2):167–91.

125. Clinical trials.gov. Endobronchial Valve for Emphysema Palliation Trial (VENT) Cost-Effectiveness Sub-Study. [updated 2005 December 12; cited 2006 September 12]. (Available from: http://www.clinicaltrials.gov/ct/show/NCT00137956)
126. Rodriguez JR, Baz MA, Kanasky WF, Jr., MacNaughton KL. Does lung transplantation improve health-related quality of life? The University of Florida experience J Heart Lung Transplant 2005; 24(6):755–63.
127. Becklake MR. Gender differences in airway behaviour over the human life span. Thorax 1999; 54:1119–38.
128. Dales RE, Mehdizadeh A, Aaron SD, Vandemheen KL, Clinch J. Sex differences in the clinical presentation and management of airflow obstruction. Eur Respir J 2006; 28:319–22.
129. Torres JP, Casanova C, Hernández C, Abreu J, Aguirre-Jaime A, Celli BR. Gender and COPD in patients attending a pulmonary clinic. Chest 2005; 128(4):2012–6.
130. Watson L, Schouten JP, Lofdahl CG, Pride NB, Laitinen LA, Postma DS. Predictors of COPD symptoms: does the sex of patient matter? Eur Respir J 2006; 28:311–8.
131. Breugelmans JG, Ford DE, Smith PL, et al. Differences in patient and bed partner-assessed quality of life in sleep-disordered breathing. Am J Respir Crit Care Med 2004; 170:547–52.
132. Seculi E, Fuste J, Brugulat P. Health status and gender in Catalonia. An approach using the information sources available. Gac Sanit 2001; 15:54–60.
133. Kinsman RA, Yaroush RA, Fernandez E, Dirks JF, Schocket M, Fukuhara J. Symptoms and experiences in chronic bronchitis and emphysema. Chest 1983; 83(5):755–61.
134. Gift A, Shepard C, Pugh L. Fatigue and other symptoms in patients with chronic obstructive pulmonary disease: do women and men differ? J Obstet Gynecol Neonatal Nurs 1999; 28(2):201–8.
135. Foy CG, Rejeski WJ, Berry MJ, Zaccaro D, Woodard CM. Gender moderates the effects of exercise therapy on health-related quality of life among COPD patients. Chest 2001; 119(1):70–6.
136. Sneeuw KCA, Aaronson NK, Sprangers MAG, et al. Evaluating the quality of life of cancer patients: assessments by patients, significant others, physicians and nurses. Br J Cancer 1999; 81:87–94.
137. Sneeuw KCA, Albertsen PC, Aaronson NK. Comparison of patient and spouse assessments of health related quality of life in men with metastatic prostate cancer. J Urol 2001; 165:478–82.
138. Andressen EM, Vahle VJ, Lollar D. Proxy reliability: health-related quality of life measures for people with disability. Qual Life Res 2001; 10:609–19.
139. Pickard AS, Johnson JA, Feeny DH, et al. Agreement between patient and proxy assessments of health-related quality of life after stroke using the EQ-5D and health utilities index. Stroke 2004; 35:607–12.
140. Sneeuw KCA, Sprangers MAG, Aaronson NK. The role of health care providers and significant others in evaluating the quality of life of patients with chronic disease. J Clin Epidemiol 2002; 55:1130–43.
141. Santiveri C, Espinalt M, Diaz Carrasco FX, Marin A, Miguel E, Jones PW. Evaluation of male COPD patients' health status by proxies. Respir Med 2007; 101: 439–45.
142. Global Initiative for chronic obstructive lung disease. Executive Summary: Global Strategy for the Diagnosis, Management, and Prevention of COPD. http://www.goldcopd.org (last accessed on August 31, 2007).

7

Measuring Ventilatory and Respiratory Impairment in COPD

RIK GOSSELINK
Respiratory Rehabilitation and Respiratory Division, University Hospitals, and Faculty
of Kinesiology and Rehabilitation Sciences, Katholieke Universiteit Leuven, Leuven, Belgium

THIERRY TROOSTERS
Respiratory Rehabilitation and Respiratory Division, University Hospitals, and Faculty of Kinesiology
and Rehabilitation Sciences, Katholieke Universiteit Leuven, Leuven, Belgium, and Postdoctoral
Fellow of the Research Foundation–Flanders, Brussels, Belgium

MARC DECRAMER
Respiratory Rehabilitation and Respiratory Division, University Hospitals, and Faculty
of Kinesiology and Rehabilitation Sciences, Katholieke Universiteit Leuven, Leuven, Belgium

I. Introduction

Dyspnea, impaired exercise tolerance, and reduced quality of life are common complaints in patients with chronic respiratory disease. Several pieces of evidence point to the fact that the symptoms associated to chronic obstructive pulmonary disease (COPD) show only a weak relation to lung function impairment (1). Prediction of exercise performance based solely on resting pulmonary function tests is inaccurate (2–4). Other factors, such as peripheral and respiratory muscle weakness and deconditioning are now recognized as important contributors to reduced exercise tolerance (5–7). Respiratory muscle weakness contributes to hypercapnia (8), dyspnea (5,9), and nocturnal oxygen desaturation (10). Signs of inspiratory muscle fatigue during exercise were observed by several authors (11–13), while debated by others (14). Moreover, inspiratory muscle strength was significantly correlated to walking distance (6,15). A higher mortality rate was observed in patients with severe muscle weakness due to steroid-induced myopathy (16). These are important observations since peripheral and respiratory muscle training might thus be able to improve physical performance, symptoms, quality of life, and perhaps, survival in these patients. In many diseases including COPD, interstitial lung disease, primary pulmonary hypertension, chronic heart failure, and cystic fibrosis, exercise tolerance showed to be one of the most important predictors of mortality (17–25). Ergometry is performed to answer the question whether exercise capacity is impaired, which factors may contribute to the exercise limitation are and to investigate the safety or risks of exercise (26). Exercise testing is particularly important to quantify the gains after interventions such as medication, surgical procedures or rehabilitation. Depending on the specific question, clinicians will rely on more complex tests, accurately measuring pulmonary gas exchange, cardiocirculatory, and muscular system, or may prefer more simple, yet useful tests to answer clinical questions. In the former case, maximal incremental or constant work rate (endurance) exercise tests may be

119

required, in the latter, field walking tests may suffice. For some of these tests, however, the lack of reference values and the absence of physiological measures are important limitations of the test. Incremental exercise testing and field testing have complementary value in the assessment of exercise performance (27).

II. Exercise Testing

The gold standard in exercise testing is the incremental maximal exercise test. Incremental exercise testing is first choice to assess impaired exercise capacity, to investigate the factors limiting exercise performance, to assess prognosis, to identify risk factors to participate in exercise programs or to prescribe exercise training (26). For all these indications incremental exercise testing provides clinicians with key data that cannot be obtained from resting measures of pulmonary function, cardiac function, blood gases, or other field exercise tests. The introduction of computerized breath-by-breath equipment made the test available to most clinical settings (28). Therefore, standardized maximal exercise tests were developed (29–31).

Two types of ergometers can be selected: a treadmill or a cycle ergometer. In treadmill exercise, a larger amount of muscle mass is put at work, which results in 5% to 10% higher VO_{2peak}. On a bicycle ergometer the workload is better controlled, and the external work is less dependent on the body weight. Factors such as walking efficiency (depending on footwear, length of the lower limb, and training status on treadmills) and the use of arm support may have unpredictable influence on the VO_2 profile during treadmill testing. Walking is, compared to cycling, a more natural movement, and for iso-VO_2, less lactate is produced on a treadmill. It is no surprise that treadmill exercises are less fatiguing for the lower limb muscles. Hence, to evaluate the ventilatory impairment, treadmill walking may be particularly sensitive. For example, the effect of bronchodilators is best assessed using endurance walking, rather than cycling (32,33).

As mentioned above, prior to a respiratory rehabilitation program maximal exercise performance has to be investigated for diagnosis of impaired exercise capacity, identification of factors limiting exercise performance and prescription of exercise training.

III. Maximal Incremental Exercise Testing

An incremental exercise test consists of baseline measurements of at least two to three minutes, then a three minutes period of unloaded pedaling, followed by the incremental part of the exercise test. The choice of the adequate increment size is one of the important steps in the tailoring of the test to the individual patient. Ideally peak work rate is reached within 8 to 12 minutes. Standardization and technical procedures for reproducible exercise testing were described in an American Thoracic Society/ American College of Chest Physicians document (28). Over the last 15 years more extensive use of specially trained nonphysicians (physiologists, physiotherapists, technicians) conducting exercise tests with a physician immediately available for consultation or emergency situations, has been become routine in hospitals and medical centers (34).

A. Measurements

Ergometry provides an integrated view on the bodies' response to exercise. In clinical practice, work rate, 12-lead electrocardiography, blood pressure, and pulmonary gas exchange (VO_2 and VCO_2) measurements are performed. The ventilatory response to exercise is assessed by analyzing breath-by-breath ventilation, arterial blood gasses or transcutaneous oxygen saturation, and symptom scores. More recent technology allows further insight into the operating lung volumes during exercise by the assessment of inspiratory capacity (IC) during exercise. Flow limitation can be assessed by evaluation of the tidal flow-volume loops during exercise. This measurement has become important in the assessment of the development of dynamic hyperinflation (DH). DH is now recognized as an important constraint of ventilatory capacity during exercise (35) and parallels the onset of dyspnea during exercise (36,37). Typically IC measurements are performed at the end of every step in the incremental loading exercise protocol and have shown to be reliable in patients with COPD.

Symptom scores for dyspnea and exertion showed also to be valuable tools during exercise testing. Visual analog scales and Borg-scales cannot be interchanged, but both show good agreement (R^2 0.72) and hence are valid tools to evaluate symptoms of dyspnea and perceived exertion (38). These scales may be available in paper format or electronic format. For research purposes, symptoms may also be asked at specific time points during the tests, or patients can indicate any change in dyspnea on an electronic score.

IV. How to Interpret the Maximal Exercise Test

The main outcome of the maximal exercise test is maximal oxygen uptake, standardized per kilogram body weight. Comparison with reference values allows judging on the level of exercise impairment. The European Respiratory Society report on exercise impairment in patients with respiratory disease (39) reported on two equations for reference values to VO_{2max}. The equation of Jones et al. (40) seems useful in clinical practice for cycle ergometry. In physiological sense the exercise is maximal when one or more components related to oxygen transport or muscle force generation are maximally loaded. Pulmonary gas exchange, ventilation, circulation, and muscle function (including peripheral gas exchange) are considered the components of the oxygen transport chain. In addition, intolerable symptoms mostly terminate exercise performance. Killian et al. (41) found that Borg scores of 7 to 8 were perceived as an unacceptable symptoms.

Exercise performance will be limited by the weakest component of the physiological chain of ventilation, pulmonary gas exchange, muscle cell metabolism, muscle force, and perception of fatigue and dyspnea (42,43). More specific the following limitations might be identified (Table 1).

A cardio circulatory limitation is identified when cardiac output fails to increase in order to meet the required oxygen delivery. Heart rate assessment is used as a noninvasive indicator of cardiac output. Achievement of the age-specific maximal heart rate [220 age (± 10) beats/min] is indicative of the maximum cardiac output. This limitation is observed in healthy subjects and frequently in patients with an forced expiratory volume in one second (FEV_1) larger than 50% predicted (44). This exercise limitation is not a direct consequence of the pulmonary disease. In other conditions, like heart failure, or ischemia, the maximal heart rate may not be reached, but a low ratio of

Table 1 Causes of Exercise Limitation

	PaO_2	$PaCO_2$	(A–a)DO_2	HR	VE_{max}	$PIpl_{max}/PEpl_{max}$	Borg score (D/E)
Cardiocirculatory limitation	=	↓	<2 kPa	>HR_{max}	<MVV	Not reached	↑ E
V/Q mismatch	↓/=	=	↑/=	<HR_{max}	<MVV	Not reached	↑ D
Ventilatory limitation	↓/=	↑	<2 kPa	<HR_{max}	>70%MVV	Possibly reached	↑ D
Pulmonary gas exchange	↓	=/↓	>2 kPa	<HR_{max}	<MVV	Possibly reached	↑ D
Peripheral muscle weakness	=	=/↓	<2 kPa	<HR_{max}	<MVV	Not reached	↑↑ E
Psychogenic limitation	=	=	<2 kPa	<HR_{max}	<MVV	Not reached	↑↑ D

Abbreviations: (A–a)DO_2, alveolar–arterial oxygen difference; D, dyspnea sensation; E, exertion; HR, heart rate at maximal exercise; HR_{max}, 220 age (years) (predicted maximal heart rate); MVV, maximal voluntary ventilation; $PEpl_{max}$, maximal expiratory pleural pressure; $PIpl_{max}$, maximal inspiratory pleural pressure; VE_{max}, maximal minute ventilation; V/Q, ventilation–perfusion mismatch; =, no change; ↑, increase; ↓, decrease.

VO_2/HR and high submaximal heart rates, together with other findings (echocardiography, electrocardiogram changes) may help to interpret a cardio circulatory limitation.

A ventilatory limitation is reached when the ventilatory pump system fails to further adequately increase ventilation despite higher demands. Several factors may increase the load on the ventilatory pump: airway obstruction (dynamic) hyperinflation, reduced compliance, and increased ventilatory demand. The latter may be excessive at a given oxygen consumption due to early lactic acidosis (45–48), hypoxia, and increased dead space ventilation. The capacity of the ventilatory pump might be impaired due to expiratory or inspiratory flow limitation, respiratory muscle weakness (49) (see later) and/or reduced ventilatoire drive. A ventilatory limitation is frequently observed in patient with more advanced lung disease and airway obstruction, chest wall deformities, respiratory muscle weakness, and in patients with interstitial lung disease and neuromuscular disease. A ventilatory limitation can be identified in different ways. An increase in arterial PCO_2 during the exercise test can be observed, but this response might be influenced by the central drive. Secondly, minute ventilation that exceeds 70% to 80% of the maximal voluntary ventilation (MVV $\sim 37.5 \times FEV_1$) is considered a ventilatory limitation. More recently, the assessment of DH during exercise (reducing the capacity of the ventilatory pump), by measurements of IC, or flow-volume loops was found to be useful (50). The onset of DH parallels the onset of dyspnea during exercise (51,52). Finally, the application of negative mouth pressure (53) and abdominal compression (54) during exercise were introduced as assessment tools to identify ventilatory limitation. Both have been shown reliable. It is clear that besides the interpretation of the ventilatory limitation as such, an exercise test also may be helpful to identify whether, or to what extent, a patient is limited only by the boundaries of the ventilatory system (i.e., simply due to a low MVV). This could be called primary ventilatory limitation. Alternatively ventilation is larger than expected at a given work rate, leading to premature ventilatory limitation. In this case the ventilatory limitation is secondary to another factor leading to increased ventilatory drive. A high dead space ventilation (indicated by a high Vd/Vt ratio), an early "anaerobic threshold," or emerging hypoxia are factors that can be identified as factors leading to increased ventilatory demands and hence premature (secondary) ventilatory limitation. This is illustrated in Figure 1.

Pulmonary gas exchange limitation is identified by an isolated reduction in arterial PO_2, and/or an increase of the alveolar–arterial oxygen gradient of more than 2 kPa (43). It is unclear why these patients stop exercise. When patients are given oxygen supplements during exercise lactate levels are slightly reduced. In addition, when healthy subjects are exercised in hypoxia, quadriceps contractile fatigue at isotime is more pronounced (55). Hypoxia, hence may likely contribute to exercise termination indirectly by affecting skeletal muscle metabolism or by increasing the ventilatory response to exercise (see above). Some patients do not sense hypoxemia and continue exercise up to very low values of PaO_2, while other patients stop exercise already when PaO_2 has hardly decreased (56). For safety reasons, exercise tests will generally be terminated by the investigator when oxygen saturation drops below 80%. Resting pulmonary function is often a poor predictor of oxygen desaturation during exercise (57). Although a low $T_{L,co}$ has some prediction for exercise-induced hypoxemia (15,58,59). In the absence of significant airflow limitation, $T_{L,co}$ values below 50% predicted will cause hypoxemia in most patients. During exercise in more severe COPD ventilation–perfusion inhomogeneity will decrease, while diffusion will deteriorate. The net effect will be that PaO_2 and $(A–a)DO_2$ do not alter (60).

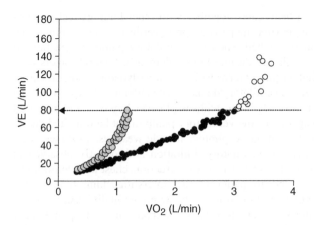

Figure 1 Two cases of ventilatory limitation are indicated in a subject with a predicted maximal voluntary ventilation (MVV) of 180 L/min (*solid line*) and a measured MVV of 80 L/min (*dashed line*). The black symbols indicate a primary ventilatory limitation. The ventilation at submaximal work VO_2 is essentially normal, the patient interrupts the test when the ventilatory ceiling is reached. The open symbols indicate how ventilation would have increased in the absence of a ventilatory limitation. In this patient the Vd/Vt is normal, there is no hypoxia and it is unlikely to see high levels of circulating lactate. A secondary ventilatory limitation is seen in the patient with grey symbols. Ventilation is elevated at submaximal work rate and the patient reaches prematurely the MVV. The ventilatory limitation is secondary to a high dead space ventilation (high Vd/Vt), hypoxia (reduced PaO_2), or deconditioning (early rise in lactate). *Abbreviation*: VE, minute ventilation.

In addition, peripheral muscle weakness might also contribute to reduced exercise capacity (6,7). Reduced cross sectional area (61), changes in fiber type composition resulting in a decrement of fatigue-resistant slow fibers (61–63) and a reduction in oxidative capacity due to a decrement in the presence of oxidative enzymes (48,64–66) are the main morphological and histochemical alterations found in lower limb skeletal muscles. Following morphological and histochemical studies, it may be hypothesized that lower limb muscle endurance is decreased. Indeed, several studies showed an early onset of lactic acidosis during exercise in COPD patients (45–48).

The contribution of muscle weakness to the exercise test can be objectified by repeated muscle strength measurement before and after exercise testing (67). The decline in force is associated to subjective rating of the level of exertion with the Borg score (67). Additional muscle strength measurements of leg and arm muscles are needed to further explore muscle weakness as the limiting factor of exercise performance.

Finally, psychological factors, such as fear, anxiety or lack of motivation can also contribute to low exercise performance. A psychological limitation is concluded when no other limitations of exercise performance can be identified as pointed out above.

V. Exercise Endurance Tests

In the follow-up of patients after respiratory rehabilitation and medication, constant work rate tests performed on a bicycle or treadmill showed to be sensitive (68,69).

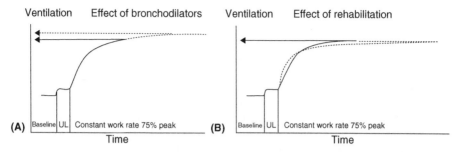

Figure 2 Effect of bronchodilators (**A**) and pulmonary rehabilitation (**B**) on pulmonary ventilation during constant work rate testing. Bronchodilators typically allow for somewhat more peak ventilation, which in a patient not suffering from leg fatigue allows for enhanced endurance time. Pulmonary rehabilitation leads to a lower ventilatory requirement, and a faster kinetic. Again it will take longer to reach an unchanged ventilatory ceiling. *Abbreviation*: UL, unloaded cycling.

After pulmonary rehabilitation the endurance time at isowork is on the average of 80% larger when compared to before training (70). After bronchodilator therapy endurance time is increased typically by 15% to 20% (71,72). Test–retest reliability is good (73). These tests, however, require at least one maximal incremental exercise test preceding the consecutive follow-up tests. The follow-up tests are made at a fixed work rate (mostly 75% of the peak work rate of the preceding incremental test). Nevertheless, the data obtained during a constant work rate test are of physiological relevance. These tests can vary in complexity from analysis of exercise time, ventilation, heart rate, and symptom scores to the analysis of the organ system responses at the onset of exercise. The measurement of ventilatory parameters (respiratory rate, tidal volume, and IC) yields unique insight in the mechanisms of action of interventions such as bronchodilators, oxygen, and pulmonary rehabilitation on respiratory mechanics. In general the effects of interventions are amplified since patients are studied at submaximum work rates high enough to elicit slowly increasing ventilation (slow phase). In contrast to incremental exercise testing this slow rise in ventilation yields a large time benefit when the ventilatory possibilities are slightly increased (as with bronchodilators in COPD) or when the ventilatory requirement is reduced (such as with pulmonary rehabilitation or oxygen therapy). This is schematically displayed in Figure 2. It also allows to study in detail the ventilatory response in terms of operating lung volumes (by studying IC), work of breathing (by studying the esophageal pressures during tidal breathing), and symptoms (by studying Borg symptom rates). After bronchodilator treatment, for example, changes in endurance time are best predicted by changes in IC (72). The response to bronchodilators on a bicycle endurance test may be blunted due to leg fatigue (7) this is much less seen after walking endurance exercise (32). Recently it has been suggested that the reduction in hyperinflation during exercise resulted in an improved cardiac function during exercise (74). Again it should be emphasized that exercise tests, particularly endurance exercises allow studying the complex interactions of different organ systems upon interventions.

Oxygen uptake, carbon dioxide production, ventilation, and heart rate responses are characterized by a time constant (τ). This is the time needed to reach 63% of the final steady state change (75). This last approach is mostly reserved for research and standardization is critical to obtain reliable results.

The power output that can be sustained (theoretically) forever, is called the critical power (76). No large studies have been performed to establish normal values, but the critical power in healthy subjects was found to be 65% of the peak work load, whereas in COPD patients it was slightly higher (77). Obviously the critical power expressed as a percentage of the peak work rate is biased by the incremental protocol used to achieve the peak exercise tolerance. Although not formally studied, it can be expected that the critical power as a percentage of peak work rate would be lower if the incremental protocol would be done with larger incremental work rates (i.e., peak work rate will be higher, whereas the critical work rate will not be influenced). This makes comparisons amongst studies particularly difficult.

VI. Respiratory Muscle Testing

Appropriate respiratory pump functioning is vital for the movement of air to the gas exchange part of the respiratory system. The respiratory muscles are the driving part of ventilation. Impairment of the respiratory pump will compromise ventilation, gas exchange and finally tissue respiration. Respiratory muscle weakness or inadequate neuromuscular coupling may be related to clinical consequences such as hypercapnia, dyspnea, impaired exercise performance, ineffective coughing, respiratory insufficiency, weaning failure and survival (78). Dysfunction of respiratory muscles is observed in several conditions, such as neuromuscular disease, spinal cord injury, congestive heart failure, critical illness, COPDs, asthma, and cystic fibrosis (78). Skeletal muscle function is an independent marker of disease severity (79). Muscle function assessment enables to diagnose muscle weakness and thus to state the indication for rehabilitation. Indeed, isometric muscle testing seems helpful in selecting candidates for exercise training in healthy subjects (80) and in COPD patients (81). COPD patients with muscle weakness seem to be better responders to rehabilitation (81). Assessment of respiratory muscle function will be discussed from the point of view of both strength and endurance capacity of the muscles.

A. Respiratory Muscle Strength Testing

In clinical routine, respiratory muscle strength is measured as maximal inspiratory and maximal expiratory mouth pressures (PI_{max} and PE_{max}, respectively). It is important to note upfront that the assessment hence does not provide a direct measure of muscle strength, but rather an assessment of the pressure generated during in and expiration. This pressure is the net result of the interplay of the respiratory muscle force, the mechanical properties, compliance of the lungs, and chest wall. These pressure measurements are often made by applying a small cylinder to the mouth with a circular mouthpiece. A small leak (2 mm diameter and 15 mm length) prevents artificially high pressures due to contraction of cheek muscles (82). An important part of the standardization is the lung volume from which the pressures are measured (83). In order to prevent the contribution of chest wall and lung recoil pressure to the pressure generation of the inspiratory muscles, measurements are preferably done at functional residual capacity. However, this lung volume is difficult to standardize. In clinical practice, PI_{max} is measured from residual volume whereas PE_{max} is taken from total lung capacity. At least five repetitions should be performed. A recent American Thoracic Society/European Respiratory Society statement describes respiratory muscle testing in more details (78).

Several groups developed normal values (82,84,85). Whatever normal values are used, there remains a large standard deviation. Since the technique is very much dependent on the standardization and the equipment, it is recommended to assess a series of healthy subjects to be able to choose the most appropriate reference values. Even then, it remains that weakness is not easy to define (86). Inspiratory weakness is accepted when PI_{max} is lower than 50% of the predicted value (87). Indeed, in studies investigating the effects of inspiratory muscle training, significant improvement in exercise performance or nocturnal desaturation time were observed in patients with a mean PI_{max} of less than 60% of the predicted value (10,44,88). Finally, respiratory muscle strength was a significant determinant of survival in patients with COPD (16).

Other techniques have also been developed to assess global respiratory muscle function, such as sniff maneuvers (89). The latter showed especially reliable in testing children with neuromuscular disease. To assess expiratory muscle function cough pressures, or more recently pressures obtained during sneezing have been used. In general these techniques can be considered as secondary techniques to confirm or reject a diagnosis of respiratory muscle weakness based on the assessment of mouth pressures. More invasive techniques such as electric or magnetic diaphragm stimulation have certainly more accurate information on isolated diaphragm function (90,91) and are useful in diagnosis of diaphragmatic paresis. However, for clinical application, assessment of inspiratory and expiratory mouth pressure is often sufficient. It needs to be said that given the large normal range, respiratory muscle assessment should always be interpreted in the context of other lung function assessment, e.g., static and dynamic lung volumes, vital capacity sitting, and supine, arterial blood gases, or other available tests (e.g., radiology) and proper anamnesis of the symptoms.

B. Respiratory Muscle Endurance Testing

Several tests for endurance capacity are described. The most frequently used are tests in which the patient breathes against a submaximal inspiratory load (60–75% PI_{max}) for as long as possible (88,92). This test has been shown to be sensitive to changes after inspiratory muscle training. Incremental threshold loading, breathing against an every two minutes incremental load (~ 5 cm H_2O) has also been shown reproducible (93). The highest load that can be sustained for two minutes is the "sustainable pressure," expressed as a percentage of the maximal load (93,94). Normal subjects were able to sustain 70% of the PI_{max} for two minutes (94). Johnson et al. (93) found that this percentage varied considerable among subjects and tended to decrease with age. The sustainable pressure has been shown to be more reduced than PI_{max} and PE_{max} in COPD (95). A third method (96–98) is repetitive maximal inspiratory or expiratory maneuvers against an occluded airway with a well-defined contraction duration (10 seconds) and relaxation time (five seconds). The relative decline in maximal pressure after 18 contractions is a measure of endurance capacity.

Tests for respiratory muscle function are helpful in detecting muscle weakness. All these tests have their limitations, such as motivation dependency, reproducibility, availability of reference values, and costs. However, these measurements have become more important in clinical practice, especially, when low values for muscle function are associated with clinical symptoms of weakness (fatigue, dyspnea). The addition of tests of muscle endurance needs further research to define its contribution to the diagnosis of muscle dysfunction.

In conclusion, several techniques can be used to gain insight in the ventilatory and respiratory impairment of patients. Exercise testing is clearly the most comprehensive assessment that has gained popularity in a variety of clinical conditions and specifically in respiratory disease, and rehabilitation. Maximal incremental exercise testing has its main emphasis on the diagnosis of exercise impairment and the mechanisms related to this impairment. Field exercise tests are mostly used in longitudinal assessment of exercise performance, such as evaluation of treatment. Endurance tests on a bicycle ergometer or on a treadmill have recently been used to gain insight in the mechanisms of improvement after interventions in ventilatory limited patients. More specific insight in respiratory and peripheral muscle function is obtained by specific assessment of muscle force and endurance. These tests may therefore complement routine exercise testing.

Acknowledgments

TT is a postdoctoral fellow of the FWO-Vlaanderen. This work is partially funded by FWO-Vlaanderen grant G 0523.06.

References

1. Wasserman K, Sue DY, Casaburi R, Moricca RB. Selection criteria for exercise training in pulmonary rehabilitation. Eur Respir J Suppl 1989; 7:604s–10.
2. McGavin CR, Gupta SP, McHardy GJR. Twelve-minute walking test for assessing disability in chronic bronchitis. Br Med J 1976; 1:822–3.
3. Morgan AD, Peck DF, Buchanan DR, McHardy GJR. Effect of attitudes and beliefs on exercise tolerance in chronic bronchitis. Br Med J 1983; 286:171–3.
4. Swinburn CR, Wakefield JM, Jones PW. Performance, ventilation, and oxygen consumption in three different types of exercise test in patients with chronic obstructive lung disease. Thorax 1985; 40:581–6.
5. Hamilton N, Killian KJ, Summers E, Jones NL. Muscle strength, symptom intensity, and exercise capacity in patients with cardiorespiratory disorders. Am J Respir Crit Care Med 1995; 152:2021–31.
6. Gosselink R, Troosters T, Decramer M. Peripheral muscle weakness contributes to exercise limitation in COPD. Am J Respir Crit Care Med 1996; 153:976–80.
7. Saey D, Debigare R, Leblanc P, et al. Contractile leg fatigue after cycle exercise: a factor limiting exercise in patients with chronic obstructive pulmonary disease. Am J Respir Crit Care Med 2003; 168:425–30.
8. Begin P, Grassino A. Inspiratory muscle dysfunction and chronic hypercapnia in chronic obstructive pulmonary disease. Am Rev Respir Dis 1991; 143:905–12.
9. Killian KJ, Jones NL. Respiratory muscles and dyspnea. Clin Chest Med 1988; 9:237–48.
10. Heijdra YF, Dekhuijzen PN, van Herwaarden CL, Folgering HT. Nocturnal saturation improves by target-flow inspiratory muscle training in patients with COPD. Am J Respir Crit Care Med 1996; 153:260–5.
11. Grassino A, Gross D, Macklem PT, Roussos C, Zagelbaum G. Inspiratory muscle fatigue as a factor limiting exercise. Bull Eur Physiopathol Respir 1979; 15:105–11.
12. Pardy RL, Rivington RN, Despas PJ, Macklem PT. The effects of inspiratory muscle training on exercise performance in chronic airflow limitation. Am Rev Respir Dis 1981; 123:426–33.
13. Fitting JW. Respiratory muscle fatigue limiting physical exercise? Eur Respir J 1991; 4:103–8.

14. Polkey MI, Kyroussis D, Keilty SE, et al. Exhaustive treadmill exercise does not reduce twitch transdiaphragmatic pressure in patients with COPD. Am J Respir Crit Care Med 1995; 152:959–64.
15. Wijkstra PJ, Ten Vergert EM, Van der Mark TW, et al. Relation of lung function, maximal inspiratory pressure, dyspnoea, and quality of life with exercise capacity in patients with chronic obstructive pulmonary disease. Thorax 1994; 49:468–72.
16. Decramer M, de Bock V, Dom R. Functional and histologic picture of steroid-induced myopathy in chronic obstructive pulmonary disease. Am J Respir Crit Care Med 1996; 153:1958–64.
17. Oga T, Nishimura K, Tsukino M, Sato S, Hajiro T. Analysis of the factors related to mortality in chronic obstructive pulmonary disease: role of exercise capacity and health status. Am J Respir Crit Care Med 2003; 167:544–9.
18. Pinto-Plata VM, Cote C, Cabral H, Taylor J, Celli BR. The 6-min walk distance: change over time and value as a predictor of survival in severe COPD. Eur Respir J 2004; 23:28–33.
19. Corra U, Mezzani A, Bosimini E, Giannuzzi P. Cardiopulmonary exercise testing and prognosis in chronic heart failure: a prognosticating algorithm for the individual patient. Chest 2004; 126:942–50.
20. Gibbons RJ, Balady GJ, Beasley JW, Bricker JT, Duvernoy WF, Froelicher VF, Mark DB, Marwick TH, McCallister BD, Thompson PD, Jr., et al. ACC/AHA Guidelines for Exercise Testing. A report of the American College of Cardiology/American Heart Association Task Force on Practice Guidelines (Committee on Exercise Testing). J Am Coll Cardiol 1997; 30:260–311.
21. Gerardi DA, Lovett L, Benoit-Connors ML, Reardon JZ, ZuWallack RL. Variables related to increased mortality following out-patient pulmonary rehabilitation. Eur Respir J 1996; 9:431–5.
22. Nixon PA, Orenstein DM, Kelsey SF, Doershuk CF. The prognostic value of exercise testing in patients with cystic fibrosis. N Engl J Med 1992; 327:1785–8.
23. King TE, Jr., Tooze JA, Schwarz MI, Brown KR, Cherniack RM. Predicting survival in idiopathic pulmonary fibrosis: scoring system and survival model. Am J Respir Crit Care Med 2001; 164:1171–81.
24. Miki K, Maekura R, Hiraga T, et al. Impairments and prognostic factors for survival in patients with idiopathic pulmonary fibrosis. Respir Med 2003; 97:482–90.
25. Wensel RCF, Opitz SD, Anker J, et al. Assessment of survival in patients with primary pulmonary hypertension: importance of cardiopulmonary exercise testing. Circulation 2002; 106:319–24.
26. Palange P, Ward SA, Carlsen KH, et al. Recommendations on the use of exercise testing in clinical practice. Eur Respir J 2007; 29:185–209.
27. Solway S, Brooks D, Lacasse Y, Thomas S. A qualitative systematic overview of the measurement properties of functional walk tests used in the cardiorespiratory domain. Chest 2001; 119:256–70.
28. American Thoracic Society/American College of Chest Physicians. ATS/ACCP Statement on cardiopulmonary exercise testing. Am J Respir Crit Care Med 2003; 167:211–77.
29. Hermansen L, Saltin B. Oxygen uptake during maximal treadmill and bicycle exercise. J Appl Physiol 1969; 25:31–7.
30. McArdle WD, Katch FI, Pechar GS. Comparison of continuous and discontinuous treadmill and bicycle tests for max VO$_2$. Med Sci Sports Exerc 1973; 5:156–60.
31. Astrand P-O, Saltin B. Maximal oxygen uptake and heart rate in various types of muscular activity. J Appl Physiol 1961; 16:977–81.
32. Pepin V, Saey D, Whittom F, Leblanc P, Maltais F. Walking versus cycling: sensitivity to bronchodilation in chronic obstructive pulmonary disease. Am J Respir Crit Care Med 2005; 172:1517–22.
33. Pepin V, Brodeur J, Lacasse Y, et al. Six-minute walking versus shuttle walking: responsiveness to bronchodilation in chronic obstructive pulmonary disease. Thorax 2007; 62:291–8.
34. Franklin BA, Gordon S, Timmis GC, O'Neill WW. Is direct physician supervision of exercise stress testing routinely necessary? Chest 1997; 111:262–5.
35. Diaz O, Villafranca C, Ghezzo H, et al. Role of inspiratory capacity on exercise tolerance in COPD patients with and without tidal expiratory flow limitation at rest. Eur Respir J 2000; 16:269–75.
36. Puente-Maestu L, Garcia dP, Martinez-Abad Y, Ruiz de Ona JM, Llorente D, Cubillo JM. Dyspnea, ventilatory pattern, and changes in dynamic hyperinflation related to the intensity of constant work rate exercise in COPD. Chest 2005; 128:651–6.
37. O'Donnell DE. Hyperinflation, dyspnea, and exercise intolerance in chronic obstructive pulmonary disease. Proc Am Thorac Soc 2006; 3:180–4.
38. Wilson RC, Jones PW. Differentiation between the intensity of breathlessness and the distress it evokes in normal subjects during exercise. Clin Sci (Lond) 1991; 80:65–70.
39. Cotes JE. Rating respiratory disability: a report on behalf of a working group of the European Society for Clinical Respiratory Physiology. Eur Respir J 1990; 3:1074–7.

40. Jones NL, Makrides L, Hitchcock C, Chypchar T, McCartney N. Normal standards for an incremental progressive cycle ergometer test. Am Rev Respir Dis 1985; 131:700–8.
41. Killian KJ, Leblanc P, Martin DH, Summers E, Jones NL, Campbell EJM. Exercise capacity and ventilatory, circulatory, and symptom limitation in patients with chronic airflow limitation. Am Rev Respir Dis 1992; 146:935–40.
42. Dempsey JA. Is the lung built for exercise? Med Sci Sports Exerc 1986; 2:143–55.
43. Wasserman K, Hansen JE, Sue DY, Whipp BJ, Casaburi R. Principles of Exercise Testing and Interpretation. 2nd ed. Philadelphia, PA: Lea and Febiger, 1994.
44. Dekhuijzen PN, Folgering HT, van Herwaarden CL. Target-flow inspiratory muscle training during pulmonary rehabilitation in patients with COPD. Chest 1991; 99:128–33.
45. Casaburi R, Wasserman K, Patessio A, Loli F, Zanaboni S, Donner CF. A new perspective in pulmonary rehabilitation: anaerobic threshold as a discriminant in training. Eur Respir J 1989; 2:618s–23.
46. Casaburi R, Patessio A, Ioli F, Zanaboni S, Donner CF, Wasserman K. Reductions in exercise lactic acidosis and ventilation as a result of exercise training in patients with obstructive lung disease. Am Rev Respir Dis 1991; 143:9–18.
47. Patessio A, Casaburi R, Carone M. Comparison of gas exchange, lactate, and lactic acidosis thresholds in patients with chronic obstructive pulmonary disease. Am Rev Respir Dis 1993; 148:622–6.
48. Maltais F, Simard AA, Simard C, Jobin J, Desgagnes P, Leblanc P. Oxidative capacity of the skeletal muscle and lactic acid kinetics during exercise in normal subjects and in patients with COPD. Am J Respir Crit Care Med 1996; 153:288–93.
49. Efthimiou J, Fleming J, Gomes C, Spiro SG. The effect of supplementary oral nutrition in poorly nourished patients with chronic obstructive pulmonary disease. Am Rev Respir Dis 1988; 137:1075–82.
50. O'Donnell DE. Exercise limitation and clinical exercise testing in chronic obstructive pulmonary disease. In: Weisman IM, Zeballos RJ, eds. Clinical Exercise Testing. Basel: Karger, 2002:138–58.
51. O'Donnell DE, Bertley JC, Chau LK, Webb KA. Qualitative aspects of exertional breathlessness in chronic airflow limitation: pathophysiologic mechanisms. Am J Respir Crit Care Med 1997; 155:109–15.
52. O'Donnell DE, Hamilton AL, Webb KA. Sensory-mechanical relationships during high intensity, constant work rate exercise in COPD. J Appl Physiol 2006; 101:1025–35.
53. Koulouris NG, Dimopoulou I, Valta P, Finkelstein R, Cosio MG, Milic-Emili J. Detection of expiratory flow limitation during exercise in COPD patients. J Appl Physiol 1997; 82:723–31.
54. Abdel KS, Serste T, Leduc D, Sergysels R, Ninane V. Expiratory flow limitation during exercise in COPD: detection by manual compression of the abdominal wall. Eur Respir J 2002; 19:919–27.
55. Romer LM, Miller JD, Haverkamp HC, Pegelow DF, Dempsey JA. Inspiratory muscles do not limit maximal incremental exercise performance in healthy subjects. Respir Physiol Neurobiol 2007; 156:353–61.
56. Mak VHF, Bugler JR, Roberts CM. Effect of arterial oxygen saturation on six-minute walking distance, perceived effort, and perceived breathlessness in patients with airflow limitation. Thorax 1993; 48:33–8.
57. Ries AL, Farrow JT, Clausen JL. Pulmonary function tests cannot predict exercise-induced hypoxaemia in chronic obstructive pulmonary disease. Chest 1988; 93:454–9.
58. D'Urzo AD, Mateika J, Bradley DT, Li D, Contreras MA, Goldstein RS. Correlates of arterial oxygenation during exercise in severe chronic obstructive pulmonary disease. Chest 1989; 95:13–7.
59. Kaminsky DA, Whitman T, Callas PW. DLCO versus DLCO/VA as predictors of pulmonary gas exchange. Respir Med 2007; 101:989–94.
60. Agusti ACN, Barbera JA, Roca J. Hypoxic pulmonary vasoconstriction and gas exchange during exercise in chronic obstructive pulmonary disease. Chest 1990; 97:268–75.
61. Whittom F, Jobin J, Simard P-M, et al. Histochemical and morphological characteristics of the vastus lateralis muscle in patients with chronic obstructive pulmonary disease. Med Sci Sports Exerc 1998; 30:1467–74.
62. Satta A, Migliori GB, Neri M, et al. Fibre types in skeletal muscles of chronic obstructive pulmonary disease patients related to respiratory function and exercise tolerance. Eur Respir J 1997; 10:2853–60.
63. Jakobsson P, Jorfeldt L, Brundin A. Skeletal muscle metabolites and fibre types in patients with advanced chronic obstructive pulmonary disease (COPD), with and without chronic respiratory failure. Eur Respir J 1990; 3:192–6.
64. Wuyam B, Payen JF, Levy P, et al. Metabolism and aerobic capacity of skeletal muscle in chronic respiratory failure related to chronic obstructive pulmonary disease. Eur Respir J 1992; 5:157–62.

65. Tada H, Kato H, Misawa T, et al. ^{31}P-nuclear magnetic resonance evidence of abnormal skeletal muscle metabolism in patients with chronic lung disease and congestive heart failure. Eur Respir J 1992; 5:163–9.

66. Maltais F, Jobin J, Sullivan MJ, et al. Metabolic and hemodynamic responses of lower limb during exercise in patients with COPD. J Appl Physiol 1998; 84:1573–80.

67. Mador MJ, Kufel TJ, Pineda L. Quadriceps fatigue after cycle exercise in patients with chronic obstructive pulmonary disease. Am J Respir Crit Care Med 2000; 161:447–53.

68. O'Donnell DE, McGuire MA, Samis L, Webb KA. General exercise training improves ventilatory and peripheral muscle strength and endurance in chronic airflow limitation. Am J Respir Crit Care Med 1998; 157:1489–97.

69. O'Donnell DE, Webb KA. Measurement of symptoms, lung hyperinflation, and endurance during exercise in chronic obstructive pulmonary disease. Am J Respir Crit Care Med 1998; 158:1557–65.

70. Troosters T, Casaburi R, Gosselink R, Decramer M. Pulmonary rehabilitation in chronic obstructive pulmonary disease. Am J Respir Crit Care Med 2005; 172:19–38.

71. Casaburi R, Kukafka D, Cooper CB, Witek TJ, Jr., Kesten S. Improvement in exercise tolerance with the combination of tiotropium and pulmonary rehabilitation in patients with COPD. Chest 2005; 127:809–17.

72. O'Donnell DE, Sciurba F, Celli B, et al. Effect of fluticasone propionate/salmeterol on lung hyperinflation and exercise endurance in COPD. Chest 2006; 130:647–56.

73. van't Hul AJ, Gosselink R, Kwakkel G. Constant-load cycle endurance performance: test-retest reliability and validity in patients with COPD. J Cardiopulm Rehabil 2003; 23:143–50.

74. Travers J, Laveneziana P, Webb KA, Kesten S, O'Donnell DE. Effect of tiotropium bromide on the cadiovascular response to exercise in COPD. Respir Med 2007; 101(9):2017–24.

75. Whipp BJ, Wagner PD, Agusti A. Factors determining the response to exercise in healthy subjects. In: Roca J, Whipp BJ, eds. Clinical Exercise Testing. Sheffield, U.K.: European Respiratory Journals Ltd, 1998:3–31.

76. Moritani T, Nagata A, Devries HA, Muro M. Critical power as a measure of physical work capacity and anaerobic threshold. Ergonomics 1981; 24:339–50.

77. Neder JA, Jones PW, Nery LE, Whipp BJ. Determinants of exercise endurance capacity in patients with chronic obstructive pulmonary disease. The power-duration relationship. Am J Respir Crit Care Med 2000; 162:497–504.

78. American Thoracic Society/European Respiratory Society. ATS/ERS Statement on respiratory muscle testing. Am J Respir Crit Care Med 2002; 166:518–624.

79. Marquis K, Debigare R, Lacasse Y, et al. Midthigh muscle cross-sectional area is a better predictor of mortality than body mass index in patients with chronic obstructive pulmonary disease. Am J Respir Crit Care Med 2002; 166:809–13.

80. Wilson GJ, Murphy AJ. Strength diagnosis: the use of test data to determine specific strength training. J Sports Sci 1996; 14:167–73.

81. Troosters T, Gosselink R, Decramer M. Exercise training: how to distinguish responders from non-responders. J Cardiopulm Rehabil 2001; 21:10–7.

82. Black LF, Hyatt RE. Maximal respiratory pressures: normal values and relationship to age and sex. Am Rev Respir Dis 1969; 99:696–702.

83. Coast JR, Weise SD. Lung volume changes and maximal inspiratory pressure. J Cardiopulm Rehabil 1990; 10:461–4.

84. Rochester D, Arora NS. Respiratory muscle failure. Med Clin North Am 1983; 67:573–98.

85. Wilson DO, Cooke NT, Edwards RHT, Spiro SG. Predicted normal values for maximal respiratory pressures in Caucasian adults and children. Thorax 1984; 39:535–8.

86. Polkey MI, Green M, Moxham J. Measurement of respiratory muscle strength. Thorax 1995; 50:1131–5.

87. DeVito E, Grassino A. Respiratory muscle fatigue. Rationale for diagnostic tests. In: Roussos C, ed. The Thorax. 2nd ed. New York/Basel/Hongkong: Marcel Dekker Inc., 1995:1857–79.

88. Wanke T, Formanek D, Lahrmann H, et al. The effects of combined inspiratory muscle and cycle ergometer training on exercise performance in patients with COPD. Eur Respir J 1994; 7:2205–11.

89. Koulouris N, Mulvey DA, Laroche CM, Sawicka EH, Green M, Moxham J. The measurement of inspiratory muscle strength by sniff esophageal, nasopharyngeal, and mouth pressures. Am Rev Respir Dis 1989; 139:641–6.

90. Yan S, Gauthier AP, Similowski T, Macklem PT, Bellemare F. Evaluation of human contractility using mouth pressure twitches. Am Rev Respir Dis 1992; 145:1064–9.

91. Similowski T, Fleury B, Launois S, Cathala HP, Bouche P, Derenne JP. Cervical magnetic stimulation: a new painless method for bilateral phrenic nerve stimulation in conscious humans. J Appl Physiol 1989; 67:1311–8.

92. Rochester DF. Tests of respiratory muscle function. Clin Chest Med 1988; 9:249–61.

93. Johnson PH, Cowley AJ, Kinnear W. Incremental threshold loading: a standard protocol and establishment of a reference range in naive normal subjects. Eur Respir J 1997; 10:2868–71.

94. Martyn JB, Moreno RH, Pare PD, Pardy RL. Measurement of inspiratory muscle performance with incremental threshold loading. Am Rev Respir Dis 1987; 135:919–23.

95. van't Hul AJ, Chadwick-Straver RVM, Wagenaar RC, Sol G, de Vries PMJM. Inspiratory muscle endurance is reduced more than maximal respiratory pressures in COPD patients. Eur Respir J 1997; 10:168s.

96. McKenzie DK, Gandevia SC. Strength and endurance of inspiratory, expiratory and limb muscles in asthma. Am Rev Respir Dis 1986; 134:999–1004.

97. McKenzie DK, Gandevia SC. Influence of muscle length on human inspiratory and limb muscle endurance. Respir Physiol 1987; 67:171–82.

98. Gandevia SC, McKenzie DK, Neering IR. Endurance capacity of respiratory and limb muscles. Respir Physiol 1983; 53:47–61.

8

Imaging of Lung Morphology and Function in COPD

PHILIPPE GRENIER, CATHERINE BEIGELMAN-AUBRY, and ANNE-LAURE BRUN
Department of Radiology, Pitié-Salpêtrière Hospital, Pierre and Marie Curie University,
Paris, France

PIERRE-YVES BRILLET
Department of Radiology, Avicenne Hospital, Bobigny Paris XIII University, Bobigny, France

I. Introduction

Chronic obstructive pulmonary disease (COPD) is a slowly progressive disorder characterized by airway obstruction resulting from some combination of pulmonary emphysema and small airways disease. Although it may induce some changes on radiographs, chronic bronchitis has a purely clinical definition and is not a radiological diagnosis. By contrast, emphysema is defined anatomically and is best detected by chest radiography and computed tomography (CT). The CT is not only the primary and most widely used imaging technique to assess the presence and extent of emphysema: it may also be useful in differentiating COPD patients who have emphysema-predominant disease from those having airway remodeling-predominant disease (1–4). As surgical and endoscopic treatment of emphysema progresses, it becomes necessary to characterize emphysema in an objective and reproducible manner. Besides, since pharmacological disease-modifying treatments may be soon available, it could be helpful to detect emphysema before symptoms or physiologic consequences have developed, and to quantify it to assess the progression of disease and the influence of treatments. A number of recent and evolving pulmonary imaging methods have the potential to provide quantitative methods for assessing extent and distribution of emphysema and dimensions of airways on CT. However, despite numerous and extensive studies, these methods have not yet been standardized (5). Single photon emission CT (SPECT) and magnetic resonance (MR) may provide functional displays of regional ventilation perfusion abnormalities (6). Diffusion-weighted MR images using hyperpolarized gas seem to be very promising to detect early emphysema in smokers before clinical, functional, and radiological abnormalities (7).

II. Chest Radiography

In spite of its obvious limitations when compared with CT, chest radiography remains the first-line imaging modality in patients with COPD. Because the normal respiratory bronchioles in the secondary pulmonary lobule cannot be visualized on chest radiography, the radiological diagnosis of COPD has been based on secondary manifestations such as alterations in the vascular pattern and the presence of hyper-inflation. Other manifestations may also be present including bullae, thickening of the bronchial walls, increased lung markings, and saber-sheath trachea.

A. Alterations of Lung Vessels

Vascular abnormalities related to COPD include arterial depletion (oligemia), decrease in caliber and number in peripheral vessels, and enlargement of the main pulmonary arteries. Local avascular areas, distortion of the vessels, and widened branching angles with loss of side branches suggest the presence of emphysematous regions (8–10). Diminution in the caliber of the pulmonary vessels with increased tapering toward the periphery has a relatively high specificity for the diagnosis of emphysema. However, it has a sensitivity of only 15% for the detection of mild to moderate disease and 40% for the detection of severe involvement (10). Peripheral arterial deficiency is often localized to certain areas of the lung, whereas vessels in other areas are of normal or even increased caliber (Fig. 1A) (11). In such cases, the hilar arteries are usually of normal size, suggesting that the relatively uninvolved portions of the lung are the sites of redistributed blood flow. In cases of general arterial deficiency, in which redistribution of blood flow to normal regions is impossible, the development of pulmonary hypertension is associated with an increased size of hilar arteries and a greater difference in caliber between central and peripheral vessels. A diameter of the

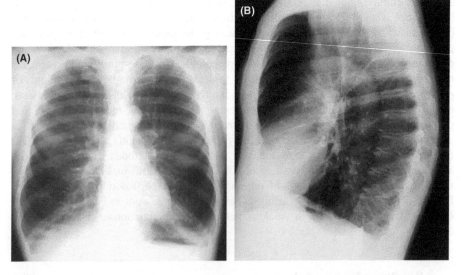

Figure 1 Posteroanterior (**A**) and lateral (**B**) chest radiographs in a patient with severe chronic obstructive pulmonary disease. Pulmonary vessels within the mid- and lower-lung zones appear diminished in caliber with increased tapering toward distal areas. Hyperinflation is present with flattening of the diaphragm. The costal attaches of the diaphragm are abnormally visible. On the lateral view, the dimension of the retrosternal space is increased and the diaphragm is flattened. Lung is visible beneath the heart due to the depression of the diaphragm.

right interlobar artery and the descending left pulmonary artery exceeding 16 and 18 mm, respectively, should be regarded as convincing evidence of pulmonary arterial hypertension (12). Although localized avascular areas, narrowing of mid-lung vessels, and an enlarged interlobar pulmonary artery have proven to be associated with the extent of emphysema observed pathologically, the diagnostic value of these parameters is inferior to that of hyperinflation (13).

B. Hyperinflation

Hyperinflation reflects ballooning of emphysematous spaces because of reduced elastic recoil as well as air trapping caused by obstruction of small airways. The most reliable sign of hyperinflation is flattening of the diaphragmatic domes (14–16). In general, a right hemidiaphragm that is at or below the anterior end of the seventh rib on the mid-clavicular line can be considered low (10,17). However, large lung volume can also be found in some healthy normal patients. In addition, this finding has low sensitivity (18) and is less of less diagnostic value than a change of contour of the diaphragmatic dome. Flattening of a hemidiaphragm can be assessed subjectively or objectively by drawing a line from costophrenic to cardiophrenic angles and measuring the largest perpendicular to the diaphragm silhouette. A value of <1.5 cm indicates flattening of the diaphragm (Fig. 1A) (15,16,19). Other helpful signs of hyperinflation include increases in the retrosternal space and in lung height, and depression (lowering) of the diaphragm. A large retrosternal space is defined by a distance between the sternum and the most anterior margin of the ascending aorta measuring >2.5 cm (Fig. 1B) (15,16). The lung height is considered to be increased when it measures 30 cm or more from the dome of the right hemidiaphragm to the tubercle of the first rib (Fig. 1A) (20). A narrow cardiac diameter <11.5 cm with a vertical heart and visible lung beneath the heart reflects the depression of the diaphragm (Fig. 1A). When the configuration of the diaphragm is concave superiorly, the presence of emphysema is virtually certain in adults. Nicklaus et al. found that a flat diaphragm on the postero-anterior chest radiograph detected 94% of patients with severe, 76% with moderate, and 21% with mild emphysema, with a low false-positive rate of only 4% (14).

The combination of hyperinflation and vascular alterations probably increases the accuracy of chest radiography for the diagnosis of emphysema. Thurlbeck et al. (21), using this combination, correctly diagnosed emphysema in 29 of 30 autopsy-proven and symptomatic cases and 8 of 17 autopsy-proven but asymptomatic cases. On the other hand, as mentioned above the arterial deficiency pattern alone identified only 41% of cases of moderate or severe emphysema (10). Although detecting alteration in lung vessels on radiographs is more subjective and less reproducible than detecting hyperinflation, the information provided by the vascular pattern is important and can help the diagnosis when hyperinflation is not present (14).

Hyperinflation with oligemia may occur in the absence of emphysema, as a consequence of conditions such as chronic obstructive bronchitis, asthma, and obliterative (constrictive) bronchiolitis that cause obstruction of small airways. Hyper-inflation reflects air trapping, and lung vessels are markedly attenuated, reflecting reflex vasoconstriction. In all these conditions, however, the vessels are often thin, but their branching pattern is not distorted. By contrast, in emphysema vessels are often sparse and their branching pattern is distorted by the patchy lung destruction and bullae.

C. Bullae

A bulla produces an avascular transradiant area usually separated from the remaining lung by a thin curvilinear wall of very variable extent (Fig. 2) (22). Sometimes the wall is only visible on short segments and it may even be completely absent, making the bulla difficult to detect. It is well admitted that chest radiographs markedly underestimate the number of bullae. The wall is usually of hairline thickness. Sometimes segments of the wall are thicker, due to redundant pleura or collapsed adjacent lung (23). Bullae due to paraseptal emphysema or centrilobular emphysema are much more common in the upper zones, but when associated with widespread panlobular emphysema, there is a much more even distribution. Bullae vary in diameter from 1 cm to the whole hemithorax, causing marked relaxation collapse of the adjacent lung. They can even extend across into the opposite hemithorax, particularly through the anterior junctional area. Large bullae observed pathologically can be invisible on the chest radiograph even in retrospect (8). Such bullae are usually situated anteriorly or posteriorly, their presence being masked by normal lung parenchyma. In subpleural zones, bullae are also difficult to detect since the absence of visible blood vessels prevents appreciation of vascular distortion (8).

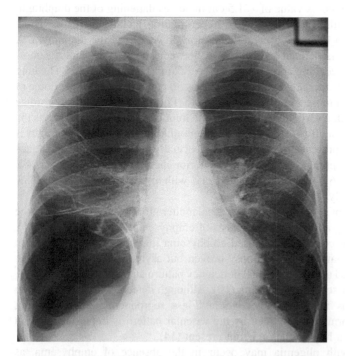

Figure 2 Posteroanterior chest radiograph in a patient with bullous emphysema. Voluminous bullae are visible in the upper lobes and in the lower third of the right hemithorax. They are seen as avascular areas apparently separated from the remaining lung by curvilinear opacities. Hyperinflation is present with flattening of the diaphragm. The right and left hilar areas are in an abnormally low position, reflecting the predominant extent of emphysema in the upper lobes. Increased lung markings are seen in the right paracardiac area, mainly due to relaxation atelectasis of the lung in the parenchyma adjacent to the compressive bullae.

D. Thickening of the Bronchial Walls

Bronchial wall thickening causes ring shadows when seen end-on and parallel linear shadows (tubular shadows), when seen en face (24,25). In roughly 80% of subjects, airways identified on chest radiographs are visualized end-on in the parahilar zones and represent branches of the anterior or posterior segmental bronchi of the upper lobes, or the superior segmental bronchi of the lower lobes. On the basis of a subjective assessment of bronchial wall thickness, 67% of 81 patients who had chronic bronchitis were interpreted as having increased wall thickness, compared with 42% of 81 normal individuals (25). On the basis of this information, the presence of thickening cannot be used as absolute criteria for the presence of chronic bronchitis, nor can its absence be used as evidence against that diagnosis. Tubular shadows are seldom seen on the chest radiographs of normal individuals, but the value of this finding for the diagnosis of chronic bronchitis remains extremely controversial.

E. Increased Lung Markings

This term is widely used in patients with COPD to describe a loss a clarity of lung vessels on chest radiographs; it should not be confused with extra shadowing related to the walls of bullae or thickened bronchial walls (Fig. 3) (19). The mechanisms underlying the loss of clarity of vessels remain controversial. Accumulation of inflammatory cells and fibrous tissue in the airway walls may raise the density of the lungs,

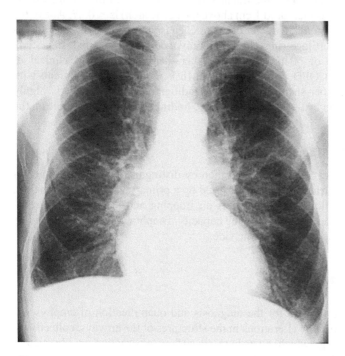

Figure 3 Posteroanterior chest radiography in a patient with chronic obstructive pulmonary disease and chronic bronchitis. Hyperinflation is mild. Increased lung markings are visible in the lung bases, particularly on the right side. Notice the slight enlargement of the proximal pulmonary arteries and right atrium and ventricle, related to pulmonary artery hypertension.

making vessels stand out less distinctly. Thickening of the walls of bronchi could also add to background density. Blood flow redistribution from emphysematous areas of reflex vasoconstriction result from decreased ventilation and may also contribute to the increase in lung density. In addition, patchy hyperinflation of some parts of the lung causes relaxation atelectasis and underinflation of other parts. Underinflated tissue is dense, and vessels within it are indistinct. As emphasized by Takasagi and Godwin, relaxation atelectasis and the consequent underinflation are major factors in the increased marking pattern of emphysema in cigarette smokers (19). In these cases, emphysema is mainly distributed in the apices, and the increased markings are found in the bases. In the apices, the emphysema destroys tissue and decreases elastic recoil, causing local hyperinflation. In the bases, where emphysema is less severe, elastic recoil is relatively preserved and relaxation atelectasis occurs, causing underinflation, crowding of vessels, and increased density, which render vessels indistinct. However "increased lung markings," also called "dirty chest," is a nonspecific radiographic feature, as it may be seen not only in patients with COPD but also in patients with interstitial lung disease such as viral pneumonia and lymphangitic carcinomatosis.

F. Saber-Sheath Trachea

This deformity is defined as a flattening from side to side of the intrathoracic part of the trachea, such that the coronal diameter is two-third or less of the sagittal diameter at the same level (26). In other words, the tracheal index (the ratio of the coronal to the sagittal tracheal diameter, as measured 1 cm above the aortic arch) is <0.67. Above the thoracic inlet the normal coronal diameter of the trachea is preserved. This deformity is fixed and rigid, and the cartilage rings are commonly calcified or ossified. In a study from Greene et al., 95% of 60 patients with saber-sheath trachea had clinical or physiological evidence of COPD, as compared with 18% of the 60 control patients with normal diameter (27). Saber-sheath trachea is a radiographic finding that is highly suggestive of COPD. It can be the only radiographic finding of COPD depictable on the chest radiograph.

G. Expiratory Air Trapping

Expiratory films can detect air trapping and thereby distinguish pulmonary oligemia caused by reflex vasoconstriction from that caused by a primary vascular abnormality. Reduction in diaphragmatic excursion reflects air trapping and increased lung compliance with consequent increase in total lung capacity. Diaphragmatic motion may be asymmetric if emphysema is worse on one side.

III. Computed Tomography

CT is the major imaging method for the diagnosis and quantification of emphysema in vivo. CT is also able to show alterations in the structures of the airways, collectively termed airway remodeling, which contribute to airflow obstruction in obstructive lung disease. CT may also contribute to separate COPD patients according to their predominant phenotype (emphysema or airway remodeling), and this may prove useful in applying specific therapies designed to prevent and ameliorate the airway remodeling of parenchymal destruction.

A. Technique

The original CT scans designed to assess airways and lung parenchyma involved thin slice images (typically 1–2 mm axial) which were acquired using a "stop and shoot" protocol and were reconstructed using an edge-enhancing algorithm known as the high resolution CT (HRCT) protocol. Usually there was a gap of 10 mm or more between the images because of radiation concerns and the limitations in obtaining truly sequential images using the axial technique. Even the advent of spiral CT scanner, where images can be acquired while the table moves continuously, did not change this approach significantly. However, multidetector row CT scanners have completely changed the approach to CT image acquisition. It is now possible to acquire the entire lung volume during a single breath hold (8–15 seconds). Contiguous or overlapped axial images are reconstructed with 0.6- to 1-mm thickness. According to this thin collimation and volumetric acquisition, these scanners produce true isotropic voxels, which allow image reconstructions in which the Z dimension (slice thickness) is the same as the X and Y (in plane) resolution (28). The isotropic voxels make it possible to measure airways in true cross section at any location using retrospective reconstruction of the images to achieve a cross-sectional image of the airways. They also allow multi-planar reformations of high quality along the long axis of the airways (Fig. 4A) (29).

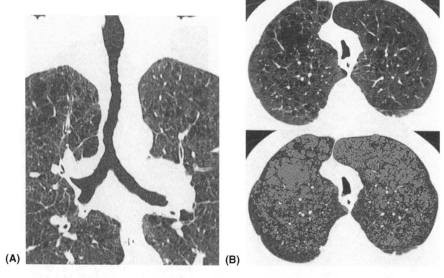

(A)   (B)

Figure 4 High resolution helical multidetector computed tomography in a patient with severe chronic obstructive pulmonary disease. (**A**) Coronal oblique reconstruction along the long axis of the trachea. The coronal diameter of the intrathoracic portion of the trachea is significantly reduced due to saber-sheath deformation. (**B**) (*Top*): Axial thin section scan across the upper lobes showing the reduction of the coronal diameter of the trachea and the presence of bilateral large clusters of emphysema. (*Bottom*): The application of a lung attenuation threshold (−960 HU) allows the segmentation and highlighting of the pixels that have an attenuation value lower than the threshold.

Maximum intensity projection (i.e., projecting the pixels that have the highest attenuation value) is used to increase the detection of small nodular opacities due to inflammatory or infectious changes in the small airways. Minimum intensity projection (i.e., projecting the pixels that have the lowest attenuation value) is applied on 3- to 7-mm thick slabs containing the trachea and proximal airways. This results in blurring the pulmonary vessels and increasing the visualization of airway lumens, ground glass opacities, emphysematous spaces, and lung cysts (Fig. 5) (29).

Volume rendering techniques applied at the level of central airways allow reconstruction of three-dimensional (3D) images of the airways visualized in semi-transparent mode (CT bronchography) similar to conventional bronchograms. Virtual bronchoscopy provides an internal rendering of the tracheobronchial walls and lumens. Owing to perspective-rendering algorithms, this simulates an endoscopist's view of the inner surface of the airways (29).

Images acquired for analysis of airways and lung parenchyma are usually obtained during suspended inspiration. Complementary acquisition during a forced expiratory maneuver is often requested, particularly to assess the degree of tracheobronchomalacia and the extent of air trapping.

Some investigators have proposed the use of spirometric gating, particularly for measurements of airways dimensions, since airways dilate with increases in lung volume (29–31).

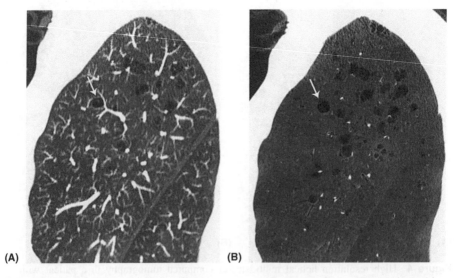

(A)   (B)

Figure 5 High resolution helical multidetector computed tomography scan in a patient with centrilobular emphysema. (**A**) Sagittal 5-mm thick slab reformatted with maximum intensity projection. The visibility of centrilobular artery in the mid part of the small hypoattenuated area (*arrow*) characterizes centrilobular emphysema. (**B**) Sagittal 5-mm thick slab reformatted with minimum intensity projection. The pulmonary vessels are not visible anymore. Many small emphysematous spaces, not depicted on the maximum intensity projection image, are now well visible.

B. Emphysema

Findings

CT is much more sensitive than chest radiography in assessing the presence and extent of emphysema. A significant number of asymptomatic and clinically undiagnosed smokers tend to have some degree of emphysema (32).

CT scans and particularly HRCT scans are the most accurate means of detecting emphysema and determining its type and extent in vivo. On CT scans, emphysema is characterized by the presence of areas of abnormally low attenuation, which can be easily contrasted by surrounding normal lung parenchyma (Fig. 5) (33–36). Usually, areas of emphysema lack distinct walls, but occasionally walls of 1 mm or less may be seen. On HRCT scans, vessels can be seen within the areas of low attenuation. Strong correlations have been found between HRCT findings and pathological grading of sections of inflated-fixed lung, except when emphysema is very mild (34,37–43). Although emphysema is more clearly defined on HRCT than on conventional CT, the extent of emphysema as compared with pathological grading is underestimated by both techniques. In addition, mild emphysematous disease can be missed by CT (34).

Visualization of small, subtle areas of emphysema on HRCT scans can be improved by the use of sufficiently low window levels [−800 to −1000 Hounsfield Units (HU)] and narrow window widths (−1000 HU or less) (35,37,40), or by the use of minimum intensity projection after helical CT acquisition using 1 mm collimation through a volume of lung of several mm in thickness. The images are reconstructed as a single slab based on the lowest attenuation values present within the slab. This technique suppresses the visualization of pulmonary vessels and optimizes visualization of low attenuation areas (Fig. 5) (44).

In many patients, it is possible to classify the type of emphysema on the basis of its HRCT appearance, although the different types are often present in association in the same patient, together with bullae.

Centrilobular emphysema, which predominantly affects the central portion of the lobule, is characterized on HRCT scans by the presence of multiple localized small areas of low attenuation, which measure <1 cm in diameter (Fig. 5).

Although emphysema can be distributed diffusely throughout the lungs, it commonly involves mainly the upper lobes (Fig. 4). When small, the emphysematous spaces often appear to be grouped near the center of the secondary lobules surrounding the centrilobular arterial branches (37,40,45). Severe centrilobular emphysema may be indistinguishable from panlobular emphysema on HRCT.

Panlobular emphysema is characterized on HRCT by widespread areas of abnormally low attenuation expressing the uniform destruction of the pulmonary lobule. Pulmonary vessels in the affected lung appear fewer and smaller than normal (36). Panlobular emphysema is often most severe in the lower lobes (Fig. 6). If the characteristic appearances of extensive lung destruction and the associated paucity of vascular markings are easily recognized, mild and even moderately severe panlobular emphysema can be very subtle and difficult to detect radiologically (43,46). Expiratory CT showing diffuse air trapping confirms the presence of small airways obstruction, but this does not allow a specific diagnosis. Even more, if air trapping is the most prominent finding, panlobular emphysema can be misdiagnosed as obliterative bronchiolitis (Fig. 7). Both conditions are characterized by bronchial wall thickening and, particularly in advanced stages, by bronchial enlargement and a generalized decrease

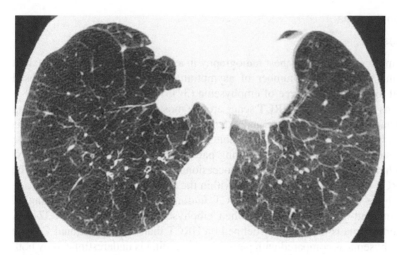

Figure 6 High resolution computed tomography scan in a patient with α_1-antitrypsin deficiency and panlobular emphysema. Decreased lung attenuation areas with pulmonary vessels in decreased number and caliber are present, mainly at the lung bases. The long lines visible through the lower lungs reflect the thickening of the remaining interlobular septa by mild fibrosis.

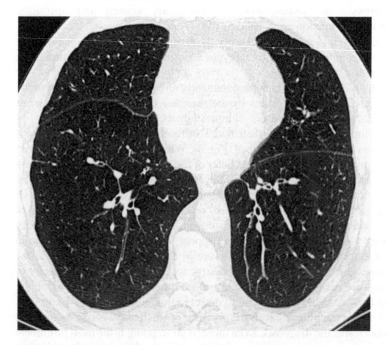

Figure 7 High resolution helical multidetector computed tomography scan in a severe chronic obstructive pulmonary disease patient. Diffuse hypoattenuation of lung parenchyma and paucity of peripheral pulmonary vessels associated with bronchial wall thickening.

in attenuation of the lung parenchyma. However, panlobular emphysema is characterized by a greater extent of parenchymal destruction and high prevalence and extent of long lines, particularly in the lower lobes, that may represent linked and thickened interlobular septa (Fig. 6) (47).

Paraseptal emphysema predominantly involves the airspaces located in the distal part of the secondary pulmonary lobule and is therefore often marginated by interlobular septa and is more striking in a subpleural location (35). On HRCT scans, paraseptal emphysema is characterized by areas of low attenuation in the subpleural area, along the peripheral or mediastinal pleura, mainly in the upper lobes, and along the fissures (36). The emphysematous spaces often have very thin and incomplete but visible walls, mostly corresponding to interlobular septa thickened by associated mild fibrosis (Fig. 8). In case of markedly visible walls, paraseptal emphysema can be mistaken for honeycomb cysts in lung fibrosis. In such cases, looking for vessels of residual lung tissue within the emphysematous spaces can be helpful for the recognition of emphysema, as they are absent in honeycomb cysts or in lung cysts such as those in histiocytosis X. In addition, honeycomb cysts of lung fibrosis are arranged commonly in multiple layers along the visceral pleura, whereas the paraseptal emphysematous spaces are typically confined to a single layer and are present along the fissures.

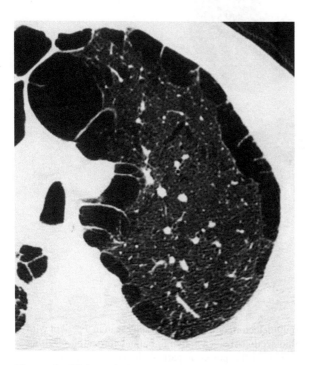

Figure 8 High resolution computed tomography scan targeted on the left lung in a patient with paraseptal emphysema. Numerous spaces of paraseptal emphysema are present along the peripheral and mediastinal pleura. Many of these spaces are marginated by thickened interlobular septa. Some of these emphysematous spaces reflect subpleural bullae.

Bullae, defined by emphysematous spaces larger than 1 cm, are generally seen in patients with centrilobular and/or paraseptal emphysema. They present as avascular, low attenuation areas that are larger than 1 cm and can have a thin but perceptible wall. CT allows greatly improved visibility of bullae identified on the radiograph and may reveal unsuspected bullae. It is also particularly valuable for defining the morphology of bullae and determining the extent of emphysema (22,23). CT scans can reveal whether hyperlucent regions seen on chest radiographs represent true bullae or areas of severe diffuse emphysema; it can also be used to determine whether the adjacent compressed lung tissue is normal or emphysematous (Fig. 9) (22,48). In bullous emphysema, compressed lung parenchyma often manifests as areas of ground glass attenuation due to relaxation atelectasis, and the vessels within them are crowded together (19,23,49). Occasionally, compression can result in atelectasis of sufficient volume to appear as a mass-like opacity (49). Although significant ventilation of large

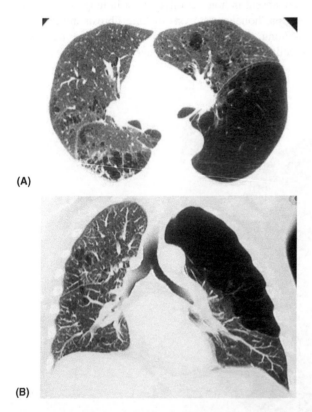

(A)

(B)

Figure 9 High resolution helical multidetector computed tomography scan in a patient with bullous emphysema. On the axial thin section slice (**A**), a large bullous formation resulting from parenchymal destruction is visible in the posterior part of the culmen and superior segment of the left lower lobe. This bulla displaces the left hilum anteriorly and downwards, the anterior mediastinum toward the right hemithorax, and the left fissure anteriorly. Centrilobular emphysematous spaces are also present in the right lung. Coronal (**B**) 8-mm thick slabs provide a good assessment of the extent and distribution of disease.

bullae is rare, this can be assessed by comparison of inspiratory and expiratory CT scans (50). The majority of bullae decrease in size at expiration. Occasionally, they may remain unchanged in size.

Extent, Distribution, and Quantification

Clinical applications. With the recent development of surgical, bronchoscopic interventional and pharmacological methods for treating patients with emphysema, accurate quantification of lung destruction in this disease is becoming increasingly relevant (50–59). Besides, in patients with giant bullous disease, CT remains the most important preoperative evaluation because it is useful assessing the extent of bullous disease and the quality of the surrounding lung tissue (60).

CT in the context of LRVS. Lung volume reduction surgery (LVRS) is being performed more frequently to improve pulmonary function, exercise tolerance and quality of life in patients with severe emphysema (55), even if the improvement usually vanishes about three years after surgery (56). An upper lobe predominance of emphysema (Fig. 4), a greater degree of parenchymal compression, a higher amount of regional heterogeneity, and a larger percentage of normal or mildly emphysematous lung showed the highest association with improvement following surgery (57). Heterogeneity of emphysema between lungs was directly correlated with the improvement at 36 months in forced expiratory volume in one second (FEV_1) in a series of 97 patients who underwent interventional unilateral LVRS (58). Morphologic scoring systems grading the degree of hyperinflation, impairment in diaphragmatic mechanics, heterogeneity, and extent in parenchymal destruction may help defining different patient groups before LVRS (59).

Although there is no difference between HRCT and spiral CT in assessing the degree of emphysema in candidates for LVRS, spiral CT is superior to HRCT for visual determination of the heterogeneity of emphysema. They should be included in a preoperative CT evaluation of LVRS candidates (61,62).

Some investigators have played attention to the core-rind in distribution of emphysema as a determinant of gas transfer (63–65). An increase in the percentage of emphysema within the core-rind is associated with lower diffusion capacity, whereas uniformity of emphysematous changes correlates with the severity of airway obstruction (63). Assessing the distribution of emphysematous destruction within the lungs using CT has become of great importance in establishing clinical indications for LVRS. Nakano et al. demonstrated that the greater extent of severe emphysema in the rind of the upper lung predicts increased benefit from LVRS, because it identifies the lesions most accessible to removal by LVRS (66). The assessment of heterogeneity of lung destruction may also be provided by the analysis of lung texture with the aim of identifying individuals with a pattern of emphysema that is not diffuse but clustered with admixed islands of normal lung. Size and number of clusters have to be taken into account (63,67).

The CT quantification of emphysema has been used to evaluate or predict surgical outcome in these patients. Gierada et al. have shown that, in patients undergoing bilateral LVRS for emphysema, many quantitative CT measures correlate with outcome measures (68). Significant differences were found among groups stratified by quantitative CT. Thus, standardized quantitative methods should improve in the preoperative imaging evaluation. Quantification of emphysema may be done at a regional level in different parts of each lung and illustrated in a diagram indicating the position of measurements in the lung (from cranial to caudal and on the axial plane). The slope of the fitted line may be used as a method for classification of emphysema heterogeneity (69). Determining the area of emphysema by quantitative CT has proven to be useful in predicting early postoperative recovery after lung lobectomy for cancer (70). Quantitative CT was also used to develop an objective model to improve clinical decision regarding LVRS (71).

Assessment of disease progression. Quantitative assessment of emphysema using CT has proven to be a sensitive indicator of disease progression in cohorts of patients with emphysema. Dowson et al., in a series of 111 patients with α_1-antitrypsin deficiency, confirmed the relationship between HRCT and lung physiology, and suggested that this relationship is even stronger in patients with predominantly lower lobes panlobular emphysema. The extent of emphysema on CT also was related to the patient's disability and impairment, as defined by health status questionnaires (72).

Methods of quantitative image analysis. CT and particularly HRCT may provide both subjective evaluation and objective quantitative measurement of CT attenuation values in the lung. Subjective (visual) CT scoring has been accomplished by (*i*) estimating the percentage of lung affected by emphysema (37,73), (*ii*) comparing CT scan images with anatomic standards for pathologic grading of emphysema (40,41), and (*iii*) placing a grid over the CT scan image and analyzing the severity and extent of emphysema in each square centimeter (34). These types of scoring have shown very good correlation with pulmonary function tests and pathology scores. However, they provide a systematic overestimation of emphysema and exhibit only moderate interobserver agreement. Bankier et al. compared subjective visual grading of emphysema with macroscopic morphometry and CT densitometry in 62 consecutive patients who underwent HRCT before surgical lung resection (74). Subjective grading of emphysema showed less agreement with the macroscopic reference standard results than with objective CT densitometric results (74). Objective quantitative methods are based on evaluation of lung attenuation as an index of emphysema. Densitometric methods include histograms and thresholding techniques. The histogram-based approach provides a density value below which a given percent of the pixels fall (75). Extent of emphysema is defined by the relative surface of lung occupied by attenuation values lower than a predetermined percentile. Dirksen et al. analyzed the attenuation histograms at various thresholds as well as at various percentiles and found percentiles of 10% to 30% to be the most appropriate for assessment of the extent of emphysema (51). Parr et al. recently showed that the 15th percentile point is a consistent measure of lung density loss for monitoring emphysema in patients with α_1-antitrypsin deficiency (76). However, this technique suffers from low CT–microscopic correlation, and the results are biased in case of coexisting interstitial lung disease that shifts the density pike toward the right of the curve.

The threshold techniques consist in quantifying the lung area that has abnormally low attenuation values (42,77,78). The pixels included within the lungs and having attenuation below a given threshold are highlighted and automatically counted (Fig. 4). This pixel index represents the relative area (RA) of lung parenchyma that has an attenuation value lower than the threshold in both lungs on a single scan. The optimal threshold for assessing the presence and extent of emphysema depends on the depth of inspiration and on the slice thickness. A threshold of -910 HU is optimal on conventional CT using 5- to 10-mm slice thickness (42). Using 1-mm thick spirometrically triggered HRCT with 10 mm intervals acquired at 90% of vital capacity, Gevenois et al. measured the RAs having attenuation values lower than eight different thresholds ranging from −900 to −970 HU prior to surgery in 63 patients (39). They compared the results with those obtained from the corresponding pathological specimen cut in the same plane at that used for the HRCT scans. The optimal threshold value for quantification of emphysema on HRCT scan was −950 HU, providing no significant difference between the extent of emphysema as assessed by HRCT or morphometry. This threshold also provided the best correlation with the macroscopic extent of emphysema. Recently, Madani et al. from the same group demonstrated that the best threshold attenuation value to quantify emphysema is −960 to −970 HU when using multidetector CT (MDCT) (79).

The threshold techniques, which are simple and available with current CT scanners, can be applied to both two-dimensional (2D) axial images as well as 3D volumetric reconstruction (Fig. 10) (77,80). Helical CT allows rapid quantification of the volume of lung involved with emphysema. The predetermined threshold attenuation value enables displays of the distribution of emphysema in multiple planes and in 3D, with good correlations between densitometric quantification from 3D CT analysis compared with 2D analysis and visual scoring (81). Using this technique, emphysema distribution can be quantified by reconstructing the upper and lower halves of the lungs separately on 3D. CT also allows measurement of overall lung volumes (82–85). This is appreciated in the assessment of the volume of lung involved with emphysema and regional changes in lung volume after LVRS (82,86,87).

Minimizing variability. Although lung attenuation, as measured by CT, is affected by many variables, including not only patient size, depth of inspiration, and location of areas of emphysema, but also the type of scanner, collimation, kilovoltage, and reconstruction algorithms (88–90), objective assessment of emphysema using

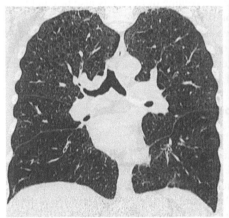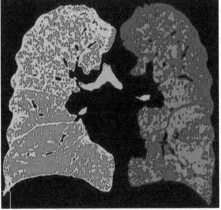

Figure 10 High resolution helical multidetector computed tomography scan in a chronic obstructive pulmonary disease patient. Regional distribution and quantitative assessment of emphysema. Coronal reformation before (*left*) and after (*right*) applying a thresholding technique to segment the emphysematous voxels having an attenuation value lower than −960 HU.

a threshold CT attenuation value has been shown to correlate closely with the visual assessment of emphysema and pathological extent of emphysema (42). On a given CT scanner, lung density is reproducible if correction for poor air calibration has been made (88). Parr et al. recommend incorporating a correction factor after air calibration (91). Repeatability of quantitative CT index of emphysema is high, but a little lower than in spirometric gating study. The variation in quantitative CT results in ungated CT is mainly relative to differences in lung volume (92,93). According to Gierada et al., repeatability of quantitative CT test results in LVRS candidates is unlikely to improve by spirometric gating. Volume adjustment of lung density may be applied to limit the variation in RA of emphysema and percentile density, due to variation in total lung volume at acquisition (94).

In follow-up studies, both dose and section thickness must be kept constant. Tube current-time product can be reduced to 16 or 20 mA (95), although Zaporozhan et al. recommend not decreasing below 50 mA (96). Because of a greater sensitivity of MDCT compared with conventional CT for the assessment of emphysema progression, Stoel et al. advocate the use of MDCT scanners in clinical multicentre trials (97).

Expiratory CT. CT evaluation of lung attenuation at expiration can also be helpful. Spirometric control of expiration scans may enhance the difference between normal lung and emphysema. Gevenois et al. demonstrated that HRCT scans obtained at the end of maximum expiration (10% of vital capacity) and analyzed with a threshold attenuation value of -910 HU provide better correlation with airflow obstruction than HRCT scans obtained at full inspiration (90% of vital capacity) and analyzed using a -950 HU threshold (98). This finding probably reflects air trapping due to airway disease, more than reduction of the alveolar wall surface.

CT measurement of lung air and tissue volumes. The volume of air and tissue present in the lung may be derived from CT lung attenuation values, given the volume of the voxels and the lung surface area. This approach allows calculation of plethysmographic lung volumes with excellent correlations, particularly for total lung capacity. The amount of parenchymal tissue per volume of lung may also be calculated as a very sensitive index of lung destruction (99).

Texture analysis. In addition to measures of attenuation values to quantify emphysema, preliminary data indicate that quantitative texture analysis using adaptive multiple features holds promise for the objective evaluation of emphysema below the direct spatial resolution of the CT scan (84,100,101).

C. Airway Inflammation and Remodeling

Findings

Bronchial wall thickening is commonly present on thin-section CT scans of patients with COPD (Fig. 7). It may also be present in smokers before the development of COPD (102). Abnormal thickening of bronchial wall in COPD is the main pathologic change described in proximal airways of these patients and is related to hypertrophy and hyperplasia of the bronchial glands, chronic inflammatory cell infiltration of the bronchial mucosa, and hypertrophy of the bronchial wall smooth muscle. After CT acquisition using helical thin-section MDCT protocol, the application of minimum intensity projection technique on 3- to 7-mm thick slabs including proximal airways allows the visualization of small air collections in the wall of the main and lobar bronchi. These air-filled outpouchings or diverticula may be numerous enough to give rise to the accordion-like (or comb-wide teeth) appearance previously described using bronchography (Fig. 11) (103). The virtual endoscopic view shows the irregular inner surface with the presence of small pits corresponding to the outpouchings and diverticula. These radiologic abnormalities may be related to the pathological changes previously described. Depression and dilation of the bronchial gland ducts are present on the mucosal surface; when multiple depressions and dilations fuse, they form a diverticulum which herniates between and through the smooth muscle cellular bundles; this diverticulum may enlarge in case of rupture of these bundles.

Cartilage abnormalities are also frequent in COPD, associating atrophy and scaring. This deficiency of bronchial cartilage induces alternated narrowing and dilation of the airways in advanced disease, explaining why bronchiectasis may be depicted on thin section CT scans in COPD patients. Bilateral bronchiectasis, affecting the upper lobes most commonly, is particularly frequent in patients with panlobular emphysema associated with antitrypsin deficiency (46,104–106). Cartilage deficiency is also responsible for prominent collapse of airway lumen occurring at maximum forced expiratory maneuver. On expiratory CT scans, the lumen of segmental or subsegmental bronchi may collapse exaggeratedly, particularly in the lower lobes where the cartilage deficiency is the most apparent. In some COPD patients, the cartilage deficiency involves the trachea and the main bronchi. The diagnosis of tracheobronchomalacia on CT is based on a >70% expiratory decrease in the cross-sectional area of the tracheal lumen (Fig. 12). Dynamic expiratory multislice CT may offer a feasible alternative to bronchoscopy in patients with suspected tracheomalacia (107,108). The reduction of airway may have an oval or crescentic shape. The crescentic form is due to the bowing of the posterior membranous trachea (109).

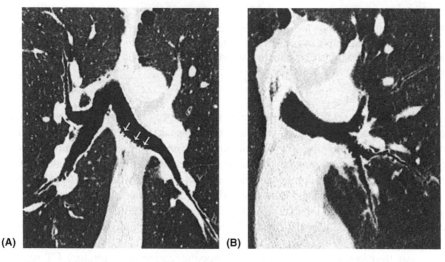

(A) (B)

Figure 11 High resolution helical multidetector computed tomography scan in a chronic obstructive pulmonary disease patient. (**A**) Coronal reformation with 5-mm thickness and minimum intensity projection technique showing multiple outpouchings and diverticula along the wall of the main bronchi, and to a lesser extent the lobar bronchi. (**B**) Oblique reformation targeted on the left bronchial tree with minimum intensity projection technique showing irregularities of the inner contours of the bronchial lumens (comb-wide teeth appearance).

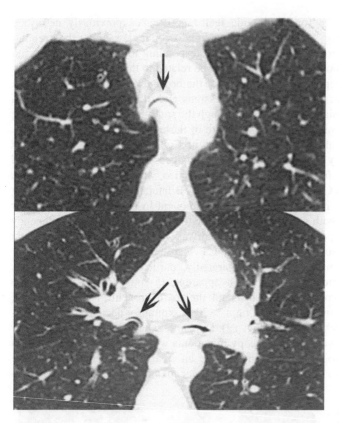

Figure 12 High resolution helical multidetector computed tomography scan during the last phase of a forced expiratory maneuver in a chronic obstructive pulmonary disease patient. The lumens of the trachea (*top*), right intermediate bronchus, and left main bronchus are collapsed, expressing tracheobronchomalacia (*bottom*).

Small airways abnormalities may also be present on CT scans of COPD patients: in particular, small nodular centrilobular opacities may reflect either reversible (mucus plugging and inflammation) or irreversible (peribronchiolar fibrosis) pathologic changes and may be present in smokers before the development of COPD (Fig. 13) (102). In the group of persistent current smokers with small nodules on the initial CT scan, Rémy-Jardin et al. noticed, after a minimal follow-up period of four years, no change in one-third of subjects, an increase in the number of small nodules in one-third of patients and replacement of small nodules by emphysema in the remaining third (110).

Air trapping, reflected by areas of hypoattenuation on expiratory CT scans in COPD patients, probably reflects fibrosis and stenosis of small airways, as well as smooth muscle hyperplasia rather than a reduction of the alveolar wall surface (98,111). However, expiratory air trapping in these patients may also be the result of airway obstruction caused by loss of alveolar attachments to the airways, which is directly related to emphysema (112).

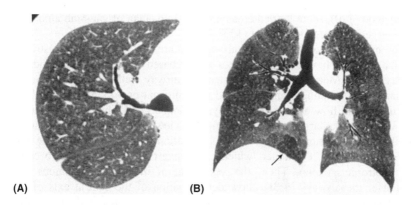

(A) **(B)**

Figure 13 High resolution helical multidetector computed tomography scan in a heavy smoker suffering from mild airflow obstruction. (**A**) Axial thin slice. (**B**) 5-mm thick coronal slab with minimum intensity projection. Presence of multiple ill-defined centrilobular nodular opacities reflecting respiratory bronchiolitis. Notice the presence of paraseptal emphysematous spaces along the mediastinal pleura in the apex of the left lung. Also notice the presence of lobular areas of decreased attenuation in the right lower lobe (*arrow*) corresponding to air trapping due to obstruction of the small airways.

Quantification of Airway Dimensions

Technical advances in CT allow the assessment of airway dimensions, and are ideally suited for the noninvasive evaluation of the pathogenesis of airway wall remodeling and the evaluation of new therapeutic interventions. Orlandi et al. showed that bronchial wall measurements using CT differ between patients who have COPD with chronic bronchitis and those who have COPD without chronic bronchitis (113). They concluded that the correlation between airway dimension and indexes of airway obstruction in patients with COPD and chronic bronchitis indicates that the bronchial tree is the site of anatomic-functional alterations in this patient group. Deveci et al., in a series of subjects including COPD patients with different levels of severity, healthy current smokers and healthy non smokers, found that airway wall thickening is inversely related to the degree of airflow obstruction and positively related to cumulative smoking history (114). Aziz et al., using stepwise regression analysis on a series of 101 patients with emphysema, revealed that bronchial wall thickness and the extent of emphysema on CT were the strongest independent determinants of FEV_1 (63).

A number of investigators have reported techniques to measure airway diameter using CT. An increasing number of quantitative methods have been developed.

In initial studies, investigators relied on manual tracing of the inner and outer contours of the airway cross section on axial CT images (115–118). These techniques are extremely time-consuming and suffer from large intra and interobserver variability. Therefore, computer aided and automated techniques have been developed to measure airway dimensions, with different types of algorithms to segment the inner and outer contours of airway cross section. Full width at half maximum (FNHM) has been widely used (119). Although this method provides a standardized and unbiased measurement, it has limitations since the CT scan constantly overestimates airway area and underestimates lumen area (119). Other techniques have been developed including maximum likelihood method (120), score guided erosion (121), Laplacian of gaussian algorithm (122), and energetic aggregation model (123).

Measurements of airway lumen and airway wall area (WA) have to be restricted to airways that appear to have been cut in cross section based on the apparent roundness of the airway lumen. Measuring airway lumen and airway walls when they are not perpendicular to the scanning plane may lead to significant errors, the magnitude of which will depend on how acutely the airways are angled and what the collimation and field of view are. The larger the angle and field of view and thicker the collimation, the greater the overestimation airway WA. This limitation is surmounted with the new generation of multislice CT scanner, which can convert the CT voxels into cubic dimension (isotropic voxels). Then, the segmentation of bronchial lumens and reconstruction of the airways in 3D allow determination of the central axis of the airways and reconstruction of the airway cross section in a plane perpendicular to this axis (Fig. 14) (124). These new algorithm softwares have been validated on phantom studies and excised animal lungs or by developing a realistic modeling of airways and pulmonary arteries included in CT scans of animal lungs obtained in vivo. Their accuracy in measuring the airways lumen and WAs is very good only for bronchi measuring at least 2 mm in diameter. Looking for differences in the dimensions of a given bronchus between two different CT examinations requires comparing measurements of bronchial cross sections performed at the same level. Thus, the lung volume needs to be very close from one acquisition to another. Since even in normal individuals there are serial changes in airway dimension along the long axis of any given bronchus, to measure airway dimensions on a single cross section is not sufficient (125). Brillet et al. have shown that the repeatability of airway dimension measurements on two different CT

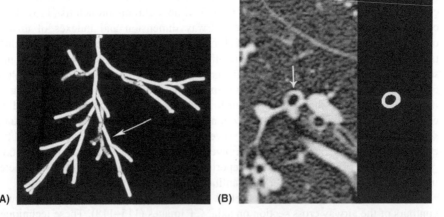

(A)   (B)

Figure 14 Quantification of airway dimensions. High resolution helical multidetector computed tomography scan in the same patient as in Figure 7. (**A**) Sagittal view of the 3D reconstruction of the central axis of the right bronchial tree (right middle and lower lobes). A point (*arrow*) is selected on the bronchial tree, corresponding to a subsegmental bronchus in the anterobasal segment of the right lower lobe (B8-b). (**B**) Cross section of the 8b bronchus strictly perpendicular to its central axis (*left*), and results of automatic segmentation of the inner and outer contours of this bronchial cross section (*right*), permitting measurement of the wall area, lumen area. The percentage of wall area (WA%) was 66%.

acquisitions in a given patient is better if the measurements are obtained from the mean of 10 different cross sections than from a single one (31).

Nakano et al. measured lung attenuation and the dimensions of the right upper lobe apical segmental bronchus in 114 smokers, using the FNHM method. Ninety-four exhibited bronchial obstruction while 20 did not despite having a comparable smoking history (4). They found that the area of lung with low attenuation (LAA%) and changes in airway dimensions (wall thickness and WA%) independently correlated with measures of airflow obstruction, and that LAA% was also related to diffusion capacity. The increase in WA% was related to both an increase in WA and a decrease in lumen area. Some of the smokers with airways obstruction had only an increase in WA%, others had only an increased LAA% and some had both abnormalities (4). These data suggest that individual COPD patients may have either emphysema or airway wall remodeling as their predominant phenotype and that these phenotypes can be separated by CT scanning (126).

The fact that the airway dimensions of a segmental bronchus relate to measures of airflow obstruction is surprising since it has long been recognized that the major site of airway narrowing in COPD is membranous airways with an internal diameter <2 mm. The recent study by Nakano et al. may explain this result: these authors found that the WA% in larger airways, which are clearly identified and accurately measured by CT, was significantly related to the WA in the bronchioles of the same patients measured histologically (127). This result supports the observation of Tiddens et al., who found that cartilaginous airway wall thickening was related to airflow obstruction and to small airway inflammation and suggests that a similar process affects both large and small airways in COPD patients (128). Thickening and narrowing of the larger airways, which are amenable to CT assessment, may serve as a surrogate measure to quantify the small airway inflammatory process. In a series of 52 patients with clinically stable COPD, Hasegawa et al. demonstrated that airway lumen area and WA percents were significantly correlated with FEV_1% predicted (129). More importantly, they also showed that correlation coefficients improved as the airways became smaller in size from the third to sixth generations, demonstrating that, in COPD, airflow limitation is more related to the dimensions of the distal airways than to that of proximal airways (129).

IV. Nuclear Medicine

A. Perfusion +/− Ventilation Scanning

Before surgical treatment of emphysema, ventilation/perfusion scanning usually provides useful information regarding the relative function of each lung and distribution of disease. This may be valuable in selecting the side for single lung transplantation or candidates for LVRS (50). Relative distribution of emphysema is usually demonstrated by matched perfusion and ventilation defects. Perfusion imaging alone may be adequate. The SPECT scan imaging can improve the rendering of perfusion detects but that is not essential (50). Moreover, the role of perfusion scintigraphy in the preoperative evaluation of patients with emphysema remains controversial. According to Wang et al., this technique provides only modest prognostic information in patients who undergo evaluation for LVRS (130). An experience from another group of investigators that was recently reported (131) showed a strong correlation between lung perfusion assessed by HRCT and lung perfusion on scintigraphy, suggesting that perfusion scintigraphy is superfluous in the preoperative evaluation of patients with emphysema with LVRS. Hunsaker et al. found CT and ventilation–perfusion preoperative assessment with either visual scoring or computer-based algorithms are nearly equivalent to predict improvement in FEV_1 measures (132). However, in a series of 45 potential candidates for LVRS, Cederlund et al. demonstrated that emphysema heterogeneity was significantly better classified on the basis of a combination of both CT and lung perfusion scintigraphy than with only one of these techniques (133).

B. Single Photon Emission Computed Tomography

The 3D SPECT radionuclide ventilation scanning is a new approach to obtain quantitative, volumetric maps of regional gas trapping in the lungs (134,135). Equilibrium phase images using Xenon-133 gas are used to render 3D images of the total lung volume whereas washout images are used to create 3D views of gas trapping. These volumetric displays of gas trapping can then be superimposed to the total lung volumes to localize and measure regions of obstructive lung disease. Actually, in patients with diffuse changes of emphysema demonstrated by CT, targeted regions of maximum gas trapping have been shown on the SPECT scans. Theoretically, it should be possible to create fused images obtained from 3D SPECT images and 3D CT-based images of emphysema in order to relate the morphologic changes of emphysema with the functional maps. Suga et al. used dynamic 133Xe SPECT in 34 patients with emphysema and 15 patients with other forms of COPD (136). The 3D voxel-based functional images of the half-clearance time (T1/2, which mainly reflects the initial rapid washout of 133Xe gas from the large airways) and of the mean transit time (MTT, reflecting 133Xe gas washout from the entire lungs, including the small airways and alveoli) were created. T1/2 and MTT values were compared with the regional extent of emphysema assessed by CT. They showed that MTT values were more critically affected in emphysematous lungs than in forms of COPD with less alveolar destruction; in addition, MTT and T1/2 values appeared to be differently correlated with the regional extent of emphysema between these two disorders. They concluded that direct comparison of regional T1/2 and MTT values on functional images might help approaching lung pathology in these disorders (136).

V. MR Imaging

A. Static Measurements

Single breath hold MR imaging using gradient sequence allows 3D reconstructions of the diaphragm and chest walls which can provide accurate measurements of diaphragmatic functional surfaces and volumes displaced by the rib cage and diaphragm (137). This completely noninvasive technique has a potential to improve the study of chest wall mechanics and their structure–function relationships. In addition, MR provides a new reliable method for measurement of lung volumes (82,137). Measurements of changes after lung volume after surgery using MR have been shown to correlate closely to the decrease in lung volumes as determined by phlethysmography (86).

B. Dynamic Measurements

Dynamic MR imaging performed during normal respiratory cycles permits a dynamic evaluation of respiratory mechanics. It is able to reveal asynchronous respiratory motion in patients with emphysema (138,139) and its correction after LVRS (50). Regional interactions between respiratory mechanics and pulmonary emphysema may be assessed by both dynamic MR imaging and 133 Xenon SPECT, used in conjunction (6).

New methods of obtaining high resolution, volumetric displays of regional pulmonary perfusion have also been developed with MR. These include two different approaches. Dynamic gadolinium-enhanced MR imaging permits lung perfusion defects to be detected, and quantitative parameters of regional pulmonary blood flow, including MTTs and blood volume, to be measured and displayed (Fig. 13) (140–143). A spin tagging MR technique, which requires no exogenous contrast agent, may provide 3D images of pulmonary perfusion (144). MR lung perfusion imaging seems to be superior to lung scintigraphy in the evaluation of pulmonary parenchymal perfusion (145).

Pulmonary ventilation MR imaging has proven to be feasible using hyperpolarized 3-helium (He) gas. This technique can provide high signal and high resolution 3D MR images of gas distribution in the lung airspaces (146–151). Defects in gas uptake have been demonstrated in patients with emphysema (148–150,152–154). In addition, with the use of MR methods sensitive to diffusion, the airspace size can also be probed by modifying the pulse sequence such that diffusive motion of the ^{3}He atoms within the airspaces results in a decrease in the signal, from which an apparent diffusion coefficient (ADC) and an average distance associated with the diffusion can be determined (Fig. 15) (148,156). Investigators have demonstrated that the ADC values in the lungs of patients with clinical symptoms of emphysema are increased relative to healthy subjects (Fig. 16) (155,157).

An experimental study in a rat model has also demonstrated significant correlation between ADC values and corresponding morphometric parameters seen in mild emphysema (158). Another experimental study on a canine model of induced emphysema has shown correlations between the diffusivity measurements and resulting

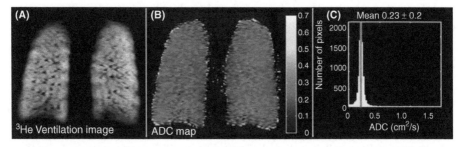

Figure 15 Coronal ventilation (**A**) and apparent diffusion coefficient (ADC) (**B**). ^{3}He magnetic resonance images and the corresponding ADC histogram (**C**) in a representative volunteer. The signal intensities in (**A**) and (**B**) are homogeneous, and (**C**) depicts the low values for the mean ADC (0.21 cm^2/sec) and SD (0.06 cm^2/sec) in this image section. *Abbreviation*: ADC, apparent diffusion coefficient. *Source*: Reproduced from Ref. 155.

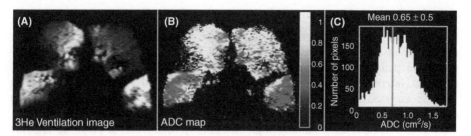

Figure 16 Coronal ventilation (**A**) and apparent diffusion coefficient (ADC) (**B**). ^{3}He magnetic resonance and the corresponding ADC histogram (**C**) in a patient with severe emphysema. Inhomogeneous signal intensities and several ventilation defects are seen in (**A**). Compared with Figure 1B in a volunteer, (**B**) shows a general increase in the ADCs, particularly in the upper portions of the lung, which is reflected by an increase in the mean (0.64 cm^2/sec), and a wider range of ADCs, which is reflected by an increase in the SD (0.27 cm^2) and in the width of the histogram in (**C**). *Abbreviation*: ADC, apparent diffusion coefficient. *Source*: Reproduced from Ref. 155.

acinar airway geometrical characteristics on the one hand, and the local density and air volume calculated from quantitative CT data on the other (159). Fain et al., applying diffusion-weighted ^{3}He MR imaging in asymptomatic smokers found a significant correlation between ADC and pack-years, and negative correlations between ADC and carbon monoxide diffusing capacity (DLCO) and FEV$_1$/forced vital capacity (FVC) (160). Although the use of ^{3}He MR imaging is not permitted in a clinical environment, these experimental results are encouraging in that regional emphysematous changes can be identified at an early stage of the disease when there are no clinical symptoms and before the lung function becomes abnormal. However large-scale clinical studies will be needed to fully determine the utility of this technique for early detection of emphysema.

The same technique of diffusion-weighted MR imaging using hyperpolarized Xenon-129 gas (7) could become an alternative, as this gas is substantially less expansive. The observed sensitivity of this new imaging technique to emphysema progression suggests that diffusion-weighted MR images have the potential to monitor the effects of newly developed drugs designed to slow the destruction process or to restore the damaged alveoli (7).

References

1. de Jong PA, Muller NL, Pare PD, et al. Computed tomographic imaging of the airways: relationship to structure and function. Eur Respir J 2005; 26:140–52.
2. Goldin JG. Quantitative CT of emphysema and the airways. J Thorac Imaging 2004; 19:235–40.
3. Kitaguchi Y, Fujimoto K, Kubo K, et al. Characteristics of COPD phenotypes classified according to the findings of HRCT. Respir Med 2006; 100(10):1742–52.
4. Nakano Y, Muro S, Sakai H, et al. Computed tomographic measurements of airway dimensions and emphysema in smokers. Correlation with lung function. Am J Respir Crit Care Med 2000; 162:1102–8.
5. Madani A, Keyzer C, Gevenois PA. Quantitative computed tomography assessment of lung structure and function in pulmonary emphysema. Eur Respir J 2001; 18:720–30.

6. Suga K, Tsukuda T, Awaya H, et al. Interactions of regional respiratory mechanics and pulmonary ventilatory impairment in pulmonary emphysema: assessment with dynamic MRI and xenon-133 single-photon emission CT. Chest 2000; 117:1646–55.

7. de Lange EE. Science to practice: what is new about detecting emphysema? Radiology 2006; 239:619–20.

8. Laws JW, Heard BE. Emphysema and the chest film: a retrospective radiological and pathological study. Br J Radiol 1962; 35:750–61.

9. Miniati M, Filippi E, Falaschi F, et al. Radiologic evaluation of emphysema in patients with chronic obstructive pulmonary disease. Chest radiography versus high resolution computed tomography. Am J Respir Crit Care Med 1995; 151:1359–67.

10. Thurlbeck WM, Simon G. Radiographic appearance of the chest in emphysema. AJR Am J Roentgenol 1978; 130:429–40.

11. Milne EN, Bass H. The roentgenologic diagnosis of early chronic obstructive pulmonary disease. J Can Assoc Radiol 1969; 20:3–15.

12. Matthay RA, Schwarz MI, Ellis JH, Jr., et al. Pulmonary artery hypertension in chronic obstructive pulmonary disease: determination by chest radiography. Invest Radiol 1981; 16:95–100.

13. Katsura S, Martin CJ. The roenrgenologic diagnosis of anatomic emphysema. Am Rev Respir Dis 1967; 96:700–6.

14. Nicklaus TM, Stowell DW, Christiansen WR, et al. The accuracy of the roentgenologic diagnosis of chronic pulmonary emphysema. Am Rev Respir Dis 1966; 93:889–99.

15. Pratt PC. Role of conventional chest radiography in diagnosis and exclusion of emphysema. Am J Med 1987; 82:998–1006.

16. Sutinen S, Christoforidis AJ, Klugh GA, et al. Roentgenologic criteria for the recognition of nonsymptomatic pulmonary emphysema. Correlation between roentgenologic findings and pulmonary pathology. Am Rev Respir Dis 1965; 91:69–76.

17. Burki NK. Conventional chest films can identify airflow obstruction. Chest 1988; 93:675–6.

18. Pratt PC. Chest radiographs cannot identify airflow obstruction. Chest 1988; 93:1120.

19. Takasugi JE, Godwin JD. Radiology of chronic obstructive pulmonary disease. Radiol Clin North Am 1998; 36:29–55.

20. Reich SB, Weinshelbaum A, Yee J. Correlation of radiographic measurements and pulmonary function tests in chronic obstructive pulmonary disease. AJR Am J Roentgenol 1985; 144:695–9.

21. Thurlbeck WM, Henderson JA, Fraser RG, et al. Chronic obstructive lung disease: comparison between clinical roentgenologic, functional and morphologic criteria in chronic bronchitis, emphysema, asthma and bronchiectasis. Medecine 1970; 49:81–9.

22. Morgan MD, Denison DM, Strickland B. Value of computed tomography for selecting patients with bullous lung disease for surgery. Thorax 1986; 41:855–62.

23. Stern EJ, Webb WR, Weinacker A, et al. Idiopathic giant bullous emphysema (vanishing lung syndrome): imaging findings in nine patients. AJR Am J Roentgenol 1994; 162:279–82.

24. Bates DV, Gordon CA, Paul GI, et al. Chronic bronchitis. Report on the third and fourth stages of the co-ordinated study of chronic bronchitis in the Department of Veterans Affairs, Canada. Med Serv J Can 1966; 22:1–59.

25. Fraser RG, Fraser RS, Renner JW, et al. The roentgenologic diagnosis of chronic bronchitis: a reassessment with emphasis on parahilar bronchi seen end-on. Radiology 1976; 120:1–9.

26. Greene R, Lechner GL. "Saber-sheath" trachea: a clinical and functional study of marked coronal narrowing of the intrathoracic trachea. Radiology 1975; 115:265–8.

27. Greene R. "Saber-sheath" trachea: relation to chronic obstructive pulmonary disease. AJR Am J Roentgenol 1978; 130:441–5.

28. Beigelman-Aubry C, Hill C, Guibal A, et al. Multi-detector row CT and postprocessing techniques in the assessment of diffuse lung disease. Radiographics 2005; 25:1639–52.

29. Grenier PA, Beigelman-Aubry C, Fetita C, et al. New frontiers in CT imaging of airway disease. Eur Radiol 2002; 12:1022–44.

30. Lamers RJ, Thelissen GR, Kessels AG, et al. Chronic obstructive pulmonary disease: evaluation with spirometrically controlled CT lung densitometry. Radiology 1994; 193:109–13.

31. Brillet PY, Fetita C, Beigelman-Aubry C, et al. Quantification of bronchial dimensions at MDCT using dedicated software. Eur Radiol 2007; 17:1483–9.

32. Sashidhar K, Gulati M, Gupta D, et al. Emphysema in heavy smokers with normal chest radiography. Detection and quantification by HCRT. Acta Radiol 2002; 43:60–5.

33. Itoh H, Murata K, Konishi J, et al. Diffuse lung disease: pathologic basis for the high-resolution computed tomography findings. J Thorac Imaging 1993; 8:176–88.
34. Miller RR, Muller NL, Vedal S, et al. Limitations of computed tomography in the assessment of emphysema. Am Rev Respir Dis 1989; 139:980–3.
35. Thurlbeck WM, Muller NL. Emphysema: definition, imaging, and quantification. AJR Am J Roentgenol 1994; 163:1017–25.
36. Webb WR. Radiology of obstructive pulmonary disease. AJR Am J Roentgenol 1997; 169:637–47.
37. Bergin C, Muller N, Nichols DM, et al. The diagnosis of emphysema. A computed tomographic–pathologic correlation. Am Rev Respir Dis 1986; 133:541–6.
38. Foster WL, Jr., Pratt PC, Roggli VL, et al. Centrilobular emphysema: CT–pathologic correlation. Radiology 1986; 159:27–32.
39. Gevenois PA, de Maertelaer V, De Vuyst P, et al. Comparison of computed density and macroscopic morphometry in pulmonary emphysema. Am J Respir Crit Care Med 1995; 152:653–7.
40. Hruban RH, Meziane MA, Zerhouni EA, et al. High resolution computed tomography of inflation-fixed lungs. Pathologic–radiologic correlation of centrilobular emphysema. Am Rev Respir Dis 1987; 136:935–40.
41. Kuwano K, Matsuba K, Ikeda T, et al. The diagnosis of mild emphysema. Correlation of computed tomography and pathology scores. Am Rev Respir Dis 1990; 141:169–78.
42. Muller NL, Staples CA, Miller RR, et al. "Density mask." An objective method to quantitate emphysema using computed tomography. Chest 1988; 94:782–7.
43. Spouge D, Mayo JR, Cardoso W, et al. Panacinar emphysema: CT and pathologic findings. J Comput Assist Tomogr 1993; 17:710–3.
44. Remy-Jardin M, Remy J, Gosselin B, et al. Sliding thin slab, minimum intensity projection technique in the diagnosis of emphysema: histopathologic–CT correlation. Radiology 1996; 200:665–71.
45. Murata K, Itoh H, Todo G, et al. Centrilobular lesions of the lung: demonstration by high-resolution CT and pathologic correlation. Radiology 1986; 161:641–5.
46. Guest PJ, Hansell DM. High resolution computed tomography (HRCT) in emphysema associated with alpha-1-antitrypsin deficiency. Clin Radiol 1992; 45:260–6.
47. Copley SJ, Wells AU, Muller NL, et al. Thin-section CT in obstructive pulmonary disease: discriminatory value. Radiology 2002; 223:812–9.
48. Mura M, Zompatori M, Mussoni A, et al. Bullous emphysema versus diffuse emphysema: a functional and radiologic comparison. Respir Med 2005; 99:171–8.
49. Gierada DS, Glazer HS, Slone RM. Pseudomass due to atelectasis in patients with severe bullous emphysema. AJR Am J Roentgenol 1997; 168:85–92.
50. Slone RM, Gierada DS, Yusen RD. Preoperative and postoperative imaging in the surgical management of pulmonary emphysema. Radiol Clin North Am 1998; 36:57–89.
51. Dirksen A, Dijkman JH, Madsen F, et al. A randomized clinical trial of alpha(1)-antitrypsin augmentation therapy. Am J Respir Crit Care Med 1999; 160:1468–72.
52. Ingenito EP, Berger RL, Henderson AC, et al. Bronchoscopic lung volume reduction using tissue engineering principles. Am J Respir Crit Care Med 2003; 167:771–8.
53. Ingenito EP, Loring SH, Moy ML, et al. Comparison of physiological and radiological screening for lung volume reduction surgery. Am J Respir Crit Care Med 2001; 163:1068–73.
54. Mao JT, Goldin JG, Dermand J, et al. A pilot study of all-trans-retinoic acid for the treatment of human emphysema. Am J Respir Crit Care Med 2002; 165:718–23.
55. Geddes D, Davies M, Koyama H, et al. Effect of lung-volume-reduction surgery in patients with severe emphysema. N Engl J Med 2000; 343:239–45.
56. Flaherty KR, Kazerooni EA, Curtis JL, et al. Short-term and long-term outcomes after bilateral lung volume reduction surgery: prediction by quantitative CT. Chest 2001; 119:1337–46.
57. Slone RM, Pilgram TK, Gierada DS, et al. Lung volume reduction surgery: comparison of preoperative radiologic features and clinical outcome. Radiology 1997; 204:685–93.
58. Mineo TC, Pompeo E, Mineo D, et al. Results of unilateral lung volume reduction surgery in patients with distinct heterogeneity of emphysema between lungs. J Thorac Cardiovasc Surg 2005; 129:73–9.
59. Wisser W, Klepetko W, Kontrus M, et al. Morphologic grading of the emphysematous lung and its relation to improvement after lung volume reduction surgery. Ann Thorac Surg 1998; 65:793–9.
60. Greenberg JA, Singhal S, Kaiser LR. Giant bullous lung disease: evaluation, selection, techniques, and outcomes. Chest Surg Clin N Am 2003; 13:631–49.

61. Cederlund K, Bergstrand L, Hogberg S, et al. Visual grading of emphysema severity in candidates for lung volume reduction surgery. Comparison between HRCT, spiral CT and "density-masked" images. Acta Radiol 2002; 43:48–53.

62. Cederlund K, Bergstrand L, Hogberg S, et al. Visual classification of emphysema heterogeneity compared with objective measurements: HRCT vs. spiral CT in candidates for lung volume reduction surgery. Eur Radiol 2002; 12:1045–51.

63. Aziz ZA, Wells AU, Desai SR, et al. Functional impairment in emphysema: contribution of airway abnormalities and distribution of parenchymal disease. AJR Am J Roentgenol 2005; 185:1509–15.

64. Nakano Y, Sakai H, Muro S, et al. Comparison of low attenuation areas on computed tomographic scans between inner and outer segments of the lung in patients with chronic obstructive pulmonary disease: incidence and contribution to lung function. Thorax 1999; 54:384–9.

65. Haraguchi M, Shimura S, Hida W, et al. Pulmonary function and regional distribution of emphysema as determined by high-resolution computed tomography. Respiration 1998; 65:125–9.

66. Nakano Y, Coxson HO, Bosan S, et al. Core to rind distribution of severe emphysema predicts outcome of lung volume reduction surgery. Am J Respir Crit Care Med 2001; 164:2195–9.

67. Mishima M, Hirai T, Itoh H, et al. Complexity of terminal airspace geometry assessed by lung computed tomography in normal subjects and patients with chronic obstructive pulmonary disease. Proc Natl Acad Sci USA 1999; 96:8829–34.

68. Gierada DS, Slone RM, Bae KT, et al. Pulmonary emphysema: comparison of preoperative quantitative CT and physiologic index values with clinical outcome after lung-volume reduction surgery. Radiology 1997; 205:235–42.

69. Cederlund K, Tylen U, Jorfeldt L, et al. Classification of emphysema in candidates for lung volume reduction surgery: a new objective and surgically oriented model for describing CT severity and heterogeneity. Chest 2002; 122:590–6.

70. Ueda K, Kaneda Y, Sudoh M, et al. Role of quantitative CT in predicting hypoxemia and complications after lung lobectomy for cancer, with special reference to area of emphysema. Chest 2005; 128:3500–6.

71. Gierada DS, Yusen RD, Villanueva IA, et al. Patient selection for lung volume reduction surgery: an objective model based on prior clinical decisions and quantitative CT analysis. Chest 2000; 117:991–8.

72. Dowson LJ, Guest PJ, Hill SL, et al. High-resolution computed tomography scanning in alpha1-antitrypsin deficiency: relationship to lung function and health status. Eur Respir J 2001; 17:1097–104.

73. Sanders C, Nath PH, Bailey WC. Detection of emphysema with computed tomography. Correlation with pulmonary function tests and chest radiography. Invest Radiol 1988; 23:262–6.

74. Bankier AA, De Maertelaer V, Keyzer C, et al. Pulmonary emphysema: subjective visual grading versus objective quantification with macroscopic morphometry and thin-section CT densitometry. Radiology 1999; 211:851–8.

75. Gould GA, MacNee W, McLean A, et al. CT measurements of lung density in life can quantitate distal airspace enlargement—an essential defining feature of human emphysema. Am Rev Respir Dis 1988; 137:380–92.

76. Parr DG, Stoel BC, Stolk J, et al. Validation of computed tomographic lung densitometry for monitoring emphysema in alpha1-antitrypsin deficiency. Thorax 2006; 61:485–90.

77. Mergo PJ, Williams WF, Gonzalez-Rothi R, et al. Three-dimensional volumetric assessment of abnormally low attenuation of the lung from routine helical CT: inspiratory and expiratory quantification. AJR Am J Roentgenol 1998; 170:1355–60.

78. Sakai N, Mishima M, Nishimura K, et al. An automated method to assess the distribution of low attenuation areas on chest CT scans in chronic pulmonary emphysema patients. Chest 1994; 106:1319–25.

79. Madani A, Zanen J, de Maertelaer V, et al. Pulmonary emphysema: objective quantification at multi-detector row CT—comparison with macroscopic and microscopic morphometry. Radiology 2006; 238:1036–43.

80. Kazerooni EA, Whyte RI, Flint A, et al. Imaging of emphysema and lung volume reduction surgery. Radiographics 1997; 17:1023–36.

81. Park KJ, Bergin CJ, Clausen JL. Quantitation of emphysema with three-dimensional CT densitometry: comparison with two-dimensional analysis, visual emphysema scores, and pulmonary function test results. Radiology 1999; 211:541–7.

82. Bae KT, Slone RM, Gierada DS, et al. Patients with emphysema: quantitative CT analysis before and after lung volume reduction surgery. Work in progress. Radiology 1997; 203:705–14.

83. Denison DM, Morgan MD, Millar AB. Estimation of regional gas and tissue volumes of the lung in supine man using computed tomography. Thorax 1986; 41:620–8.

84. Hoffman EA, McLennan G. Assessment of the pulmonary structure–function relationship and clinical outcomes measures: quantitative volumetric CT of the lung. Acad Radiol 1997; 4:758–76.

85. Kinsella M, Muller NL, Abboud RT, et al. Quantitation of emphysema by computed tomography using a "density mask" program and correlation with pulmonary function tests. Chest 1990; 97:315–21.

86. Gierada DS, Hakimian S, Slone RM, et al. MR analysis of lung volume and thoracic dimensions in patients with emphysema before and after lung volume reduction surgery. AJR Am J Roentgenol 1998; 170:707–14.

87. Holbert JM, Brown ML, Sciurba FC, et al. Changes in lung volume and volume of emphysema after unilateral lung reduction surgery: analysis with CT lung densitometry. Radiology 1996; 201:793–7.

88. Kemerink GJ, Lamers RJ, Thelissen GR, et al. Scanner conformity in CT densitometry of the lungs. Radiology 1995; 197:749–52.

89. Bakker ME, Stolk J, Putter H, et al. Variability in densitometric assessment of pulmonary emphysema with computed tomography. Invest Radiol 2005; 40:777–83.

90. Boedeker KL, McNitt-Gray MF, Rogers SR, et al. Emphysema: effect of reconstruction algorithm on CT imaging measures. Radiology 2004; 232:295–301.

91. Parr DG, Stoel BC, Stolk J, et al. Influence of calibration on densitometric studies of emphysema progression using computed tomography. Am J Respir Crit Care Med 2004; 170:883–90.

92. Gierada DS, Yusen RD, Pilgram TK, et al. Repeatability of quantitative CT indexes of emphysema in patients evaluated for lung volume reduction surgery. Radiology 2001; 220:448–54.

93. Moroni C, Mascalchi M, Camiciottoli G, et al. Comparison of spirometric-gated and -ungated HRCT in COPD. J Comput Assist Tomogr 2003; 27:375–9.

94. Shaker SB, Dirksen A, Laursen LC, et al. Volume adjustment of lung density by computed tomography scans in patients with emphysema. Acta Radiol 2004; 45:417–23.

95. Shaker SB, Dirksen A, Laursen LC, et al. Short-term reproducibility of computed tomography-based lung density measurements in alpha-1 antitrypsin deficiency and smokers with emphysema. Acta Radiol 2004; 45:424–30.

96. Zaporozhan J, Ley S, Weinheimer O, et al. Multi-detector CT of the chest: influence of dose onto quantitative evaluation of severe emphysema: a simulation study. J Comput Assist Tomogr 2006; 30:460–8.

97. Stoel BC, Bakker ME, Stolk J, et al. Comparison of the sensitivities of 5 different computed tomography scanners for the assessment of the progression of pulmonary emphysema: a phantom study. Invest Radiol 2004; 39:1–7.

98. Gevenois PA, De Vuyst P, Sy M, et al. Pulmonary emphysema: quantitative CT during expiration. Radiology 1996; 199:825–9.

99. Coxson HO, Rogers RM, Whittall KP, et al. A quantification of the lung surface area in emphysema using computed tomography. Am J Respir Crit Care Med 1999; 159:851–6.

100. Uppaluri R, Mitsa T, Sonka M, et al. Quantification of pulmonary emphysema from lung computed tomography images. Am J Respir Crit Care Med 1997; 156:248–54.

101. Xu Y, Sonka M, McLennan G, et al. MDCT-based 3-D texture classification of emphysema and early smoking related lung pathologies. IEEE Trans Med Imaging 2006; 25:464–75.

102. Remy-Jardin M, Remy J, Boulenguez C, et al. Morphologic effects of cigarette smoking on airways and pulmonary parenchyma in healthy adult volunteers: CT evaluation and correlation with pulmonary function tests. Radiology 1993; 186:107–15.

103. Zompatori M, Sverzellati N, Gentile T, et al. Imaging of the patient with chronic bronchitis: an overview of old and new signs. Radiol Med (Torino) 2006; 111:634–9.

104. King MA, Stone JA, Diaz PT, et al. Alpha 1-antitrypsin deficiency: evaluation of bronchiectasis with CT. Radiology 1996; 199:137–41.

105. Shin MS, Ho KJ. Bronchiectasis in patients with alpha 1-antitrypsin deficiency. A rare occurrence? Chest 1993; 104:1384–6.

106. McMahon MA, O'Mahony MJ, O'Neill SJ, et al. Alpha-1 antitrypsin deficiency and computed tomography findings. J Comput Assist Tomogr 2005; 29:549–53.

107. Baroni RH, Feller-Kopman D, Nishino M, et al. Tracheobronchomalacia: comparison between end-expiratory and dynamic expiratory CT for evaluation of central airway collapse. Radiology 2005; 235:635–41.

108. Boiselle PM, Lee KS, Lin S, et al. Cine CT during coughing for assessment of tracheomalacia: preliminary experience with 64-MDCT. AJR Am J Roentgenol 2006; 187:W175–7.

109. Boiselle PM, Ernst A. Tracheal morphology in patients with tracheomalacia: prevalence of inspiratory lunate and expiratory "frown" shapes. J Thorac Imaging 2006; 21:190–6.

110. Remy-Jardin M, Edme JL, Boulenguez C, et al. Longitudinal follow-up study of smoker's lung with thin-section CT in correlation with pulmonary function tests. Radiology 2002; 222:261–70.

111. Zaporozhan J, Ley S, Eberhardt R, et al. Paired inspiratory/expiratory volumetric thin-slice CT scan for emphysema analysis: comparison of different quantitative evaluations and pulmonary function test. Chest 2005; 128:3212–20.

112. Muller NL, Thurlbeck WM. Thin-section CT emphysema, air trapping, and airway obstruction. Radiology 1996; 199:621–2.

113. Orlandi I, Moroni C, Camiciottoli G, et al. Chronic obstructive pulmonary disease: thin-section CT measurement of airway wall thickness and lung attenuation. Radiology 2005; 234:604–10.

114. Deveci F, Murat A, Turgut T, et al. Airway wall thickness in patients with COPD and healthy current smokers and healthy non-smokers: assessment with high resolution computed tomographic scanning. Respiration 2004; 71:602–10.

115. Webb WR, Gamsu G, Wall SD, et al. CT of a bronchial phantom. Factors affecting appearance and size measurements. Invest Radiol 1984; 19:394–8.

116. Seneterre E, Paganin F, Bruel JM, et al. Measurement of the internal size of bronchi using high resolution computed tomography (HRCT). Eur Respir J 1994; 7:596–600.

117. McNamara AE, Muller NL, Okazawa M, et al. Airway narrowing in excised canine lungs measured by high-resolution computed tomography. J Appl Physiol 1992; 73:307–16.

118. Okazawa M, Muller N, McNamara AE, et al. Human airway narrowing measured using high resolution computed tomography. Am J Respir Crit Care Med 1996; 154:1557–62.

119. Nakano Y, Whittall KP, Kalloger SE, et al. Development and validation of human airway analysis algorithme using multidetector row CT. Proc SPIE 2002; 4683:460–9.

120. Reinhardt JM, D'Souza ND, Hoffman EA. Accurate measurement of intrathoracic airways. IEEE Trans Med Imaging 1997; 16:820–7.

121. King GG, Muller NL, Whittall KP, et al. An analysis algorithm for measuring airway lumen and wall areas from high-resolution computed tomographic data. Am J Respir Crit Care Med 2000; 161:574–80.

122. Berger P, Perot V, Desbarats P, et al. Airway wall thickness in cigarette smokers: quantitative thin-section CT assessment. Radiology 2005; 235:1055–64.

123. Saragaglia A, Fetita C, Preteux F, et al. Accurate 3D quantification of bronchial parameters in MDCT. In: SPIE Conference on Mathematical Methods in Pattern and Image Analysis. Vol. 5916. San Diego, CA, 2005:323–34.

124. Fetita CI, Preteux F, Beigelman-Aubry C, et al. Pulmonary airways: 3-D reconstruction from multislice CT and clinical investigation. IEEE Trans Med Imaging 2004; 23:1353–64.

125. Matsuoka S, Kurihara Y, Yagihashi K, et al. Morphological progression of emphysema on thin-section CT: analysis of longitudinal change in the number and size of low-attenuation clusters. J Comput Assist Tomogr 2006; 30:669–74.

126. Nakano Y, Muller NL, King GG, et al. Quantitative assessment of airway remodeling using high-resolution CT. Chest 2002; 122:271S–5.

127. Nakano Y, Wong JC, de Jong PA, et al. The prediction of small airway dimensions using computed tomography. Am J Respir Crit Care Med 2005; 171:142–6.

128. Tiddens HA, Pare PD, Hogg JC, et al. Cartilaginous airway dimensions and airflow obstruction in human lungs. Am J Respir Crit Care Med 1995; 152:260–6.

129. Hasegawa M, Nasuhara Y, Onodera Y, et al. Airflow limitation and airway dimensions in chronic obstructive pulmonary disease. Am J Respir Crit Care Med 2006; 173:1309–15.

130. Wang SC, Fischer KC, Slone RM, et al. Perfusion scintigraphy in the evaluation for lung volume reduction surgery: correlation with clinical outcome. Radiology 1997; 205:243–8.

131. Cleverley JR, Desai SR, Wells AU, et al. Evaluation of patients undergoing lung volume reduction surgery: ancillary information available from computed tomography. Clin Radiol 2000; 55:45–50.

132. Hunsaker AR, Ingenito EP, Reilly JJ, et al. Lung volume reduction surgery for emphysema: correlation of CT and V/Q imaging with physiologic mechanisms of improvement in lung function. Radiology 2002; 222:491–8.

133. Cederlund K, Hogberg S, Jorfeldt L, et al. Lung perfusion scintigraphy prior to lung volume reduction surgery. Acta Radiol 2003; 44:246–51.

134. Suga K, Kume N, Nishigauchi K, et al. Three-dimensional surface display of dynamic pulmonary xenon-133 SPECT in patients with obstructive lung disease. J Nucl Med 1998; 39:889–93.
135. Suga K, Nishigauchi K, Kume N, et al. Dynamic pulmonary SPECT of xenon-133 gas washout. J Nucl Med 1996; 37:807–14.
136. Suga K, Kawakami Y, Yamashita T, et al. Characterization of 133Xe gas washout in pulmonary emphysema with dynamic 133Xe SPECT functional images. Nucl Med Commun 2006; 27:71–80.
137. Cluzel P, Similowski T, Chartrand-Lefebvre C, et al. Diaphragm and chest wall: assessment of the inspiratory pump with MR imaging-preliminary observations. Radiology 2000; 215:574–83.
138. Iwasawa T, Kagei S, Gotoh T, et al. Magnetic resonance analysis of abnormal diaphragmatic motion in patients with emphysema. Eur Respir J 2002; 19:225–31.
139. Iwasawa T, Yoshiike Y, Saito K, et al. Paradoxical motion of the hemidiaphragm in patients with emphysema. J Thorac Imaging 2000; 15:191–5.
140. Amundsen T, Torheim G, Waage A, et al. Perfusion magnetic resonance imaging of the lung: characterization of pneumonia and chronic obstructive pulmonary disease. A feasibility study. J Magn Reson Imaging 2000; 12:224–31.
141. Berthezene Y, Croisille P, Wiart M, et al. Prospective comparison of MR lung perfusion and lung scintigraphy. J Magn Reson Imaging 1999; 9:61–8.
142. Hatabu H, Gaa J, Kim D, et al. Pulmonary perfusion and angiography: evaluation with breath-hold enhanced three-dimensional fast imaging steady-state precession MR imaging with short TR and TE. AJR Am J Roentgenol 1996; 167:653–5.
143. Hatabu H, Gaa J, Kim D, et al. Pulmonary perfusion: qualitative assessment with dynamic contrast-enhanced MRI using ultra-short TE and inversion recovery turbo FLASH. Magn Reson Med 1996; 36:503–8.
144. Roberts DA, Gefter WB, Hirsch JA, et al. Pulmonary perfusion: respiratory-triggered three-dimensional MR imaging with arterial spin tagging—preliminary results in healthy volunteers. Radiology 1999; 212:890–5.
145. Johkoh T, Muller NL, Kavanagh PV, et al. Scintigraphic and MR perfusion imaging in preoperative evaluation for lung volume reduction surgery: pilot study results. Radiat Med 2000; 18:277–81.
146. Black RD, Middleton HL, Cates GD, et al. In vivo He-3 MR images of guinea pig lungs. Radiology 1996; 199:867–70.
147. Chen XJ, Chawla MS, Hedlund LW, et al. MR microscopy of lung airways with hyperpolarized ³He. Magn Reson Med 1998; 39:79–84.
148. de Lange EE, Mugler JP, III, Brookeman JR, et al. Lung air spaces: MR imaging evaluation with hyperpolarized ³He gas. Radiology 1999; 210:851–7.
149. Kauczor HU, Ebert M, Kreitner KF, et al. Imaging of the lungs using ³He MRI: preliminary clinical experience in 18 patients with and without lung disease. J Magn Reson Imaging 1997; 7:538–43.
150. Kauczor HU, Hofmann D, Kreitner KF, et al. Normal and abnormal pulmonary ventilation: visualization at hyperpolarized He-3 MR imaging. Radiology 1996; 201:564–8.
151. Middleton H, Black RD, Saam B, et al. MR imaging with hyperpolarized ³He gas. Magn Reson Med 1995; 33:271–5.
152. Gierada DS, Saam B, Yablonskiy D, et al. Dynamic echo planar MR imaging of lung ventilation with hyperpolarized (3)He in normal subjects and patients with severe emphysema. NMR Biomed 2000; 13:176–81.
153. Stavngaard T, Sogaard LV, Mortensen J, et al. Hyperpolarized ³He MRI and 81mKr SPECT in chronic obstructive pulmonary disease. Eur J Nucl Med Mol Imaging 2005; 32:448–57.
154. Zaporozhan J, Ley S, Gast KK, et al. Functional analysis in single-lung transplant recipients: a comparative study of high-resolution CT, ³He-MRI, and pulmonary function tests. Chest 2004; 125:173–81.
155. Salerno M, de Lange EE, Altes TA, et al. Emphysema: hyperpolarized helium 3 diffusion MR imaging of the lungs compared with spirometric indexes—initial experience. Radiology 2002; 222:252–60.
156. Saam BT, Yablonskiy DA, Kodibagkar VD, et al. MR imaging of diffusion of (3)He gas in healthy and diseased lungs. Magn Reson Med 2000; 44:174–9.
157. van Beek EJ, Wild JM, Kauczor HU, et al. Functional MRI of the lung using hyperpolarized 3-helium gas. J Magn Reson Imaging 2004; 20:540–54.
158. Peces-Barba G, Ruiz-Cabello J, Cremillieux Y, et al. Helium-3 MRI diffusion coefficient: correlation to morphometry in a model of mild emphysema. Eur Respir J 2003; 22:14–9.

159. Tanoli T, Woods JC, Conradi MS. In vivo lung morphometry with hyperpolarized [3]He diffusion MRI in canines with induced emphysema: disease progression and comparison with computed tomography. J Appl Physiol 2007; 102:477–84.
160. Fain SB, Panth SR, Evans MD, et al. Early emphysematous changes in asymptomatic smokers: detection with [3]He MR imaging. Radiology 2006; 239:875–83.

9

Assessing the Systemic Consequences of COPD

JÁN TKÁČ†
The James Hogg iCAPTURE Center for Cardiovascular and Pulmonary Research,
St. Paul's Hospital, Vancouver, British Columbia, Canada

S. F. PAUL MAN and DON D. SIN
Respiratory Division, University of British Columbia, and The James Hogg iCAPTURE
Center for Cardiovascular and Pulmonary Research, St. Paul's Hospital, Vancouver,
British Columbia, Canada

I. Introduction

Chronic obstructive pulmonary disease (COPD) is an inflammatory disorder associated with important extrapulmonary manifestations. COPD is characterized by progressive expiratory airflow limitation, which is poorly reversible and is associated with chronic airway inflammation and remodeling (1). Inflammation, combined with oxidative stress, apoptosis, and proteolysis, eventually results in the emphysematous destruction of lung parenchyma. In addition, COPD is associated with several systemic complications, including cachexia, weight loss, skeletal muscle dysfunction, osteoporosis, heart failure, atherosclerosis, anxiety, depression, and cancer (1). In mild to moderate COPD (Global Initiative for Chronic Obstructive Lung Disease, GOLD), these extrapulmonary manifestations account for the majority of morbidity and mortality (2). Accordingly, appropriate assessment and clinical management of these systemic complications are essential for the improvement in the health status and prognosis of COPD patients.

II. Extrapulmonary Disorders Associated with COPD

In this section, we summarize several common extrapulmonary manifestations of COPD (i.e., comorbidities), which contribute significantly to the morbidity and mortality of COPD patients.

A. Cardiovascular Disorders

Surprisingly, cardiovascular events are the leading causes of hospitalizations and the second leading causes of mortality in patients with mild to moderate COPD (2).

---

† Currently at Terry Fox Laboratory, British Columbia Cancer Research Centre, Vancouver, British Columbia, Canada.

In GOLD stages 0 to 2, approximately 50% of all hospitalizations are related to cardiovascular events (2), though this percentage decreases in GOLD Stages 3 and 4. Regardless of the severity, cardiovascular events account for 20% to 25% of all deaths in COPD (3).

The Relationship Between FEV_1 and Cardiovascular Disease

COPD patients have reduced forced expiratory volume in one second (FEV_1) and reduced FEV_1 is a significant risk factor for cardiovascular events (4). For instance, the Honolulu Heart Program prospectively followed 5924 generally healthy, middle-aged men (about half were current smokers) for 15 to 18 years and found that compared with those in the highest quintile of FEV_1, individuals in the lowest FEV_1 quintile had an elevated risk of cardiovascular mortality (relative risk, RR, 1.93; 95% confidence interval, CI, 1.46–2.54) (5). In the Tecumseh Cohort study, FEV_1 less than 2.0 L was associated with a fivefold increase in the risk for cardiovascular mortality (RR, 5.03; 95% CI, 3.07–8.22) (6). The Harvard Six Cities Study reported a RR of 2.74 (95% CI, 1.93–3.90) for women and 1.42 (95% CI, 1.07–1.90) for men who were in the lowest FEV_1 quartile compared with those in the highest quartile (7). The Buffalo cohort study reported a RR of 1.96 (95% CI, 0.99–3.88) for women and 2.11 (95% CI, 1.20–3.71) for men, who were in the lowest FEV_1 quintile compared with the highest quintile (8). The Renfrew and Paisley cohort study reported a RR of 1.88 (95% CI, 1.44–2.47) for women and 1.56 (95% CI, 1.26–1.92) for men, who were in the lowest compared with the highest FEV_1 quintile (9). A longitudinal, population-based study of 1861 participants (The First National Health and Nutritional Examination Survey) demonstrated that subjects in the lowest quintile of FEV_1 had the highest risk of cardiovascular mortality (RR, 3.36; 95% CI, 1.54–7.34), independent of smoking status (4). The risk was even higher when only deaths from ischemic heart disease were considered (RR, 5.65; 95% CI, 2.26–14.13). A systematic review of the literature and a meta-analysis that included more than 80,000 subjects showed that reduced FEV_1 nearly doubles the risk for cardiovascular mortality independent of confounding factors such as age, sex, and cigarette smoking (pooled RR, 1.75; 95% CI, 1.54–2.01) (Fig. 1) (4).

Another way to assess the impact of reduced lung function on cardiovascular mortality is to determine attributable risk. Population attributable risk is defined as the percentage of a given illness that could be prevented if the risk factor causing the illness was completely eliminated (10). In one study, the population attributable risk of deaths related to ischemic heart disease (i.e., the percentage of ischemic heart related deaths that could be eliminated if everyone had normal lung function) imposed by reduced FEV_1 was 26% (95% CI, 19–34%) for men and 24% (95% CI, 14–34%) for women, independent of the effects of cigarette smoking (9). In the same study, the comparison of total serum cholesterol (between the lowest quintile and the highest quintiles) produced a population attributable risk of 21% in men and 25% in women for deaths related to ischemic heart disease, suggesting that at the population-level impact of reduced lung function on ischemic heart disease death is as great, if not greater, than the risk imposed by hypercholesterolemia. These and other studies indicate that reduced FEV_1, independent of established risk factors, such as cigarette smoking, total cholesterol and hypertension, is an important risk factor for cardiovascular mortality. Although there are many causes of reduced FEV_1 in the community, approximately

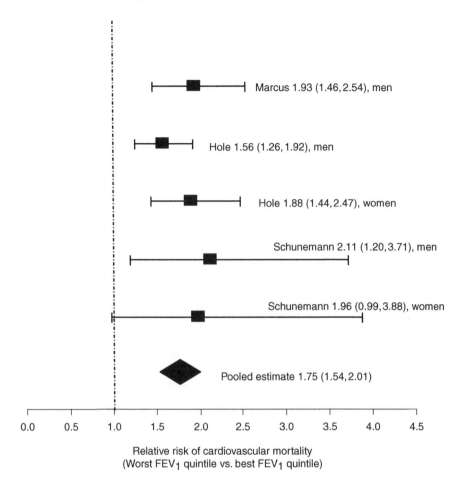

Figure 1 Meta-analysis of studies that reported relative risk of cardiovascular mortality based on FEV_1 quintiles. Reduced FEV_1 nearly doubles the risk for cardiovascular mortality independent of confounding factors such as age, sex, and cigarette smoking. *Abbreviation*: FEV_1, forced expiratory volume in one second. *Source*: From Ref. 4.

80% of adults (45 years and older) with impaired FEV_1 (i.e., <80% predicted) have airways obstruction (11). Thus, reduced FEV_1 among adults is a reasonable surrogate for COPD in population-based studies.

The Relationship Between Rate of FEV₁ Decline and Cardiovascular Disease

Rapid decline in FEV_1 is another phenotypic hallmark of COPD. In the Malmo "Men Born in 1914" Study, the cardiovascular event rate among smokers in the high, middle, and low thirds with regard to the decline in FEV_1 was 56.0, 41.0, and 22.7 events per 1000 person-years, respectively (p for trend = 0.01) (12). In the Baltimore Longitudinal Study of Aging (13), individuals who experienced the most rapid decline in FEV_1 over a 16-year follow-up were three to five times more likely to die from a cardiac cause of death than those who had the slowest decline in FEV_1, after adjustments for age, baseline FEV_1, smoking status, hypertension status, body mass index (BMI), and mean serum cholesterol level. Even among lifetime non-smokers, accelerated decline in FEV_1 was associated with a 5- to 10-fold increase in the risk for cardiac deaths, which suggests that the relationship between changes in FEV_1 and cardiovascular events occurs independently of the effects of smoking. Whether cigarette smoking interacts and modifies the relationship between accelerated decline in FEV_1 and cardiovascular outcomes, however, is unclear.

The Relationship Between FEV₁ to FVC Ratio and Cardiovascular Disease

Although in the general adult population the most common cause of reduced FEV_1 is obstructive airways disease, false positives can occur, since restrictive disorders could also decrease FEV_1. Reduced FEV_1/FVC ratio, on the other hand, is a more specific indicator of airways disease. Sin and Man (14) examined data from 6629 participants of the Third National Health and Nutrition Examination Survey in the United States. They showed that subjects with severe airflow obstruction (defined as $FEV_1 < 50\%$ of predicted and FEV_1/FVC ratio $\leq 70\%$) were 2.1 times more likely to have electrocardiographic evidence of probable or possible myocardial infarction. The odds were also elevated in those with moderate airflow obstruction (defined as FEV_1 50–80% of predicted; odds ratio, 1.4) but not to the same extent as that observed with severe airflow obstruction. Interestingly, participants with severe airflow obstruction were, respectively, 2.18 and 2.74 times more likely to have elevated C-reactive protein ($CRP \geq 2.2$ mg/L) and highly elevated circulating CRP levels (> 10.0 mg/L) than those without airflow obstruction, after adjustments for a variety of factors including age, gender, smoking history, body mass indices, and comorbidities. Participants with moderate airflow obstruction were 1.41 and 1.56 times more likely to have elevated and highly elevated circulating CRP levels. Since CRP is a robust biomarker of systemic inflammation, the results of this study suggest that systemic inflammation may play some role in the relationship between COPD and ischemic heart disease.

In addition to being a risk factor for ischemic heart disease, COPD may act as an effect modifier. In the Malmo "Men Born in 1914" Study (15), Engstrom and coworkers showed that reduced FEV_1/FVC ratio by itself was only a modest independent predictor of coronary events (RR, 1.30). Having arrhythmias on a 24-hour ambulatory ECG recording device in the absence of COPD was not associated with coronary events (RR, 1.01). However, when subjects had both COPD and arrhythmias at baseline, the risk of coronary events increased by over twofold compared with subjects without COPD and without any ectopic rhythm (RR, 2.43; 95% CI, 1.36–4.32). These data suggest that airflow obstruction impacts synergistically on the diseased heart to make it more vulnerable to acute coronary events.

The Relationship Between COPD Symptoms and Cardiovascular Diseases

The most common symptom of COPD is cough with sputum production (1). Jousilahti and colleagues (16) studied 9342 men and 10,102 women, born between 1913 and 1947 in Finland. In this carefully conducted population-based study, a positive response to the question, "do you cough on most days and nights as much as three months each year?" was associated with about a 50% increase in the risk for coronary deaths than those with a negative response to this question, adjusted for age, study year, serum total cholesterol, and amount of smoking (RR, 1.55; 95% CI, 1.26–1.90 in men and

RR 1.41; 95% CI, 0.92–2.16 in women). Even in the absence of spirometric data, having symptoms of COPD increases the risk for cardiovascular events.

The Burden of Cardiovascular Complications in Patients with COPD

The data presented have been largely derived from population-based studies. While these studies are instructive in elucidating the impact of COPD on cardiovascular morbidity and mortality in the general community, these data have limited relevance for patients with COPD. Findings from established COPD cohorts or in those with fixed airflow obstruction would be more salient. A few such studies have been published. In the Tucson Epidemiologic Study of Airways Obstructive Disease (17), only 8% of the decedents who had antemortem spirometric evidence of obstructive airways disease as defined by FEV_1/FVC ratio of less than 65% died directly from their airways disease (as the underlying cause of death). Even among those with severe obstructive airways disease (defined as $FEV_1/FVC < 65\%$ and $FEV_1 < 50\%$ of predicted), less than a quarter died from respiratory failure. Even among those in whom obstructive airways disease was mentioned as a contributing cause of death, cardiovascular causes were listed as the primary cause of death in nearly 50% of the cases, while malignancy was the primary cause in 11% of the cases. Pulmonary causes constituted only 29% of the cases. However, some caution should be exercised in interpreting disease-specific mortality data in COPD. Because the information provided on death certificates was not validated through autopsies, the extent to which diagnostic misclassification confounded the findings is not known. Nevertheless, these data, in the context of previously mentioned studies, suggest that a large proportion of COPD patients die from cardiovascular complications.

The Lung Health Study investigators (2) studied 5887 smokers, aged 35 to 60 years, with mild to moderate airways obstruction. Study participants were randomized to three arms: usual care plus placebo, special intervention for smoking cessation plus ipratropium, and special intervention for smoking cessation plus placebo. During the initial five-year follow-up, 2.5% of the original cohort died and 25% of those died of a cardiovascular event. Approximately, 13% of the cohort experienced at least one hospitalization during the five-year follow-up. Cardiovascular events accounted for 42% of the first hospitalizations and 48% of the second hospitalizations. The rate of hospitalization for lower respiratory tract infection was only a third of that for cardiovascular illnesses. For every 10% decrease in FEV_1, all-cause mortality increased by 14%, cardiovascular mortality increased by 28%, and nonfatal coronary event increased by almost 20%, after adjustments for relevant confounders such as age, sex, smoking status, and treatment assignment.

In more severe cases of COPD, respiratory failure becomes a much more important cause of mortality. However, cardiovascular events still account for a large percentage of deaths even in this group of patients. Towards a Revolution in COPD Health clinical trial followed patients with moderate to severe COPD (FEV_1 60% or less) for three years and treated patients with salmeterol, fluticasone, salmeterol/fluticasone combination, or placebo. There were 784 deaths during this period and each of the deaths was carefully adjudicated by an independent mortality review board, which was blinded to the treatment assignment. It found that 27% of all deaths were directly attributable to cardiovascular events (18). Although the effects of treatment on this outcome are uncertain since the four treatment groups were combined for this analysis, these data, nevertheless, suggest that cardiovascular events account for a large proportion of mortality in COPD patients, even in moderate to severe disease.

In summary, reduced FEV_1 (as well as reduced FEV_1 to FVC ratio) is a risk factor for cardiovascular events. Even relatively small reductions in lung function increases the risk for ventricular arrhythmias, coronary events, and cardiovascular mortality by twofold, independent of the effects of smoking. In patients with mild to moderate COPD, cardiovascular diseases are the leading causes of hospitalization accounting for 40% to 50% of all hospital admissions. They are the second leading causes of mortality, only trailing lung cancer, and account for 25% of all deaths. In general, a 10% decrease in FEV_1 among COPD patients increases the cardiovascular event rate by about 30% (2).

A Model Linking COPD and Cardiovascular Events

The pathways by which COPD contributes to cardiovascular disease have not been fully elucidated. Potential mechanisms include systemic inflammation, oxidative stress, and other pathways. It is postulated that in COPD, persistent pulmonary inflammation promotes the release of pro-inflammatory chemokines and cytokines into the circulation. These mediators then stimulate various end organs including the liver, adipose tissues, and the bone marrow to release excessive amounts of acute-phase proteins, inflammatory cells, and secondary cytokines into the general circulation, resulting in a state of persistent low-grade systemic inflammation. The systemic inflammation in turn adversely impacts the blood vessels, contributing to plaque formation and in certain cases to plaque instability and rupture (19). A simplified model linking COPD with cardiovascular disease is depicted in Figure 2.

Pulmonary and Systemic Inflammation in COPD

In COPD patients, the source of systemic inflammation is most likely the airways. In a landmark study, Hogg and colleagues demonstrated that the small airways of COPD patients are chronically inflamed and that the intensity of the inflammatory process correlates with the severity of COPD (20). Once COPD is established, airway inflammation persists even after many years of smoking cessation (20). The inflammatory process extends beyond the lungs. With disease progression, the inflammatory signal is also present in the systemic circulation. In a meta-analysis of available studies, Gan et al. found that COPD patients had significantly increased levels of circulating CRP compared with those without COPD, independent of confounding factors such as smoking (21). The standardized mean difference in the CRP level between COPD and control subjects was 0.53 U (95% CI, 0.34–0.72) or 1.86 mg/L (95% CI, 0.75–2.97 mg/L). Other biomarkers of systemic inflammation were also elevated in COPD. The standardized mean difference in the plasma fibrinogen was 0.47 U (95% CI, 0.29–0.65) or 0.37 g/L (95% CI, 0.18–0.56 g/L). Circulating leukocytes were also higher in COPD than in control subjects (standardized mean difference, 0.44 U; 95% CI, 0.20–0.67). Likewise serum tumor necrosis factor (TNF)-α levels were higher in COPD than in control subjects (standardized mean difference, 0.59 U; 95% CI, 0.29–0.89).

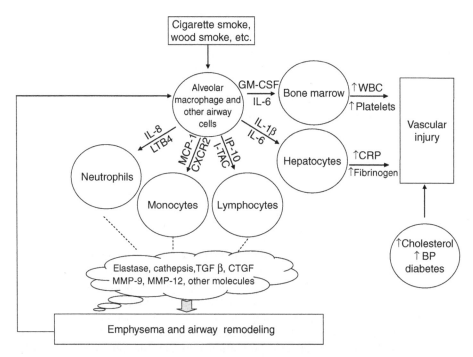

Figure 2 A model of the pathogenesis of chronic obstructive pulmonary disease. Cigarette smoke and other environmental irritants may activate alveolar macrophages and other cells in the airways (e.g., bronchial epithelial cells) of susceptible individuals. These and other cells in the airways produce a variety of signaling molecules, cytokines, and chemokines to activate and recruit pro-inflammatory cells, such as neutrophils, lymphocytes, and monocytes into airway lumen and/or wall. Once activated, these pro-inflammatory cells may release a variety of "toxic" substances, which promote emphysematous changes in the alveoli and inflammatory changes in the airways. Some of these molecules (e.g., IL-6, IL-1β) may "spill" into the systemic circulation, stimulating hepatocytes to produce acute-phase proteins such as C-reactive protein and fibrinogen, and stimulating the bone marrow to synthesize leukocytes and platelets. These pro-inflammatory cells and proteins may then promote vascular injury, in concert with traditional cardiovascular risk factors such as hypercholesterolemia, diabetes, and hypertension. *Abbreviations*: BP, blood pressure; CRP, C-reactive protein; CTGF, connective tissue growth factor; CXCR2, chemokine receptor; GM-CSF, granulocyte macrophage colony-stimulating factor; IL, interleukin; IP-10, interferon-γ-inducible protein-10; I-TAC, interferon-inducible T-cell α-chemoattractant; LTB4, leukotriene B4; MCP, monocyte chemotactic protein; MMP, matrix metalloproteinase; TGF, transforming growth factor; WBC, white blood cells. *Source*: From Ref. 19.

Lung Inflammation Serves as a Substrate for Systemic Inflammation

There are good animal and in vitro models, demonstrating that pulmonary inflammation can lead to systemic inflammation. For instance in a rabbit model, it has been shown that when particles are instilled into the airways of rabbits, alveolar macrophages release inflammatory mediators, which in turn, produce a bone marrow response, inciting a leukocytic and thrombophilic state (22,23). The magnitude of the bone marrow response correlates with the amount of particles phagocytosed by alveolar macrophages in the lung (24). Similarly, when stimulated by cigarette smoke, alveolar macrophages produce factors such as TNF-α, interleukin (IL)-1, IL-6, IL-8, and hematopoietic growth factors such as GM-CSF and G-CSF which are capable of stimulating the proliferation and release of polymorphonuclear leukocytes from the bone marrow (25).

Cigarette smoke also stimulates the release of IL-1, IL-8, G-CSF, and MCP-1 from bronchial epithelial cells via various oxidative pathways, indicating the importance of respiratory epithelium in mediating the inflammatory cascade in COPD (26,27). Additionally, cultures of epithelial cells from the small airways, which are harvested from smokers and patients with COPD, release more transforming growth factor-β_1 than those from non-smokers, which in turn may modulate airway remodeling and fibrosis (28). Collectively, these experimental data indicate that alveolar macrophages and bronchial epithelial cells are critically important in processing inhaled airborne particles and we postulate that they produce mediators that elicit both the local and systemic inflammatory responses.

There are also experimental data demonstrating an important relationship between systemic inflammation and progression of atherosclerosis. Suwa and colleagues showed that when Watanabe Heritable Hyperlipidemic rabbits that develop atherosclerosis naturally were exposed to ambient particles, they demonstrated a brisk systemic inflammatory response. Importantly, the inflammatory response was associated with progression of their atherosclerosis (24). In fact, the extent of the atherosclerotic burden was directly proportional to the concentration of alveolar macrophages that contained the particulate matter (24). Additionally, with airway inflammation, the endothelium became activated, with upregulation of intracellular adhesion molecule-1 and vascular cell adhesion molecule-1 on the endothelium overlying the atherosclerotic plaques (29). These adhesion receptors are critically important for the recruitment of leukocytes such as monocytes and lymphocytes into the atherosclerotic plaques (30).

In summary, there are now convincing experimental data to indicate that airway inflammation from pollution and cigarette smoke can induce a state of systemic inflammation, possibly through activation of alveolar macrophages and bronchial epithelial cells, that influence the progression of pre-existing diseases in distant organ systems such as blood vessels.

Inflammation and Atherosclerosis

The pathogenesis of atherosclerosis is complex and multifactorial. Persistent low-grade systemic inflammation is believed to be one of the centerpiece events leading to plaque formation (31). There are compelling epidemiologic data linking systemic inflammation to atherosclerosis, ischemic heart disease, stroke, and coronary deaths (32,33). Under normal physiologic conditions, the human endothelium does not support leukocyte adhesion, one of the critical steps in the initiation of atherosclerotic plaques (34). However, in an inflammatory state (such as diabetes, COPD, or obesity), the endothelium begins to over-express surface adhesion molecules such as vascular cell adhesion molecule-1 that allow circulating white blood cells to adhere to damaged endothelial surfaces (35). Once the white cells become adherent to the endothelium, they trigger a whole series of inflammatory reactions.

Certain molecules can promote (or amplify) this inflammatory process. The most studied of these molecules is CRP. It is an acute-phase protein that responds to infectious or inflammatory stress. When released into the systemic circulation, CRP can upregulate the production of other inflammatory cytokines, activate the complement system, promote uptake of low-density lipoproteins by macrophages, and foster leukocyte adhesion to vascular endothelium, thereby amplifying the inflammatory cascade. CRP can also upregulate the expression of monocyte chemotactic protein-1 and interact with endothelial cells to stimulate the production of IL-6 and endothelin-1, which in turn amplify the inflammatory signal and incite other structures (e.g., vascular endothelium) to undergo functional changes (36). Other acute-phase proteins released by the liver such as plasma fibrinogen can also be used to predict future cardiovascular events (32).

If systemic inflammation is a key mechanism for atherosclerosis, patients suffering from conditions associated with systemic inflammation should have an excess risk of cardiovascular morbidity and mortality. Indeed, this appears to be the case. There is compelling epidemiologic evidence that patients with rheumatoid arthritis, for example, have an elevated risk of cardiovascular disease. A recently published meta-analysis, evaluating this relationship, indicated that rheumatoid arthritis increases mortality rates by 70%; nearly half of this excess risk is directly attributable to cardiovascular causes (37). Treating rheumatoid arthritis with disease-modifying agents appears to mitigate this risk. In a study by Choi and colleagues, therapy with methotrexate reduced the overall mortality by 60%, primarily by reducing cardiovascular deaths (38). Methotrexate had little impact on other causes of mortality. Similar associations have been observed with systemic lupus erythematosis, another systemic inflammatory disorder (39).

B. Other Pathways Potentially Involved in the Pathogenesis of Cardiovascular Disease in COPD

In addition to persistent, low-grade systemic inflammation, several other pathogenic pathways likely contribute to the increased risk of cardiovascular disease observed in patients with COPD. These include hemostasis, neurohumoral activation, and oxidative stress, which are summarized in this section.

Hemostatic Factors

In addition to inflammation, hemostasis and thrombosis are important cofactors in plaque build up and rupture (40). One of the initial steps in this process is platelet adhesion to collagen. To facilitate adhesion, circulating platelets must first interact with von Willebrand factor (vWF), which slows them down. This allows the platelets to bind to collagen via $\alpha_2\beta_1$ integrin molecule. Increased expression of vWF and/or $\alpha_2\beta_1$ integrin might therefore increase the risk for cardiovascular diseases. Consistent with this notion, an 807 C to T single-nucleotide polymorphism close to the gene coding for the α_2 subunit of the $\alpha_2\beta_1$ integrin molecule, which increases $\alpha_2\beta_1$ integrin density on platelet membranes, has been associated with elevated risk of cardiovascular mortality in female smokers (41). Similarly, raised vWF has been associated with increased cardiovascular disease in a large population-based study (42).

After platelets adhere to cell surface, they become activated and start releasing adenosine diphosphate and thromboxane A2, which in turn recruits additional platelets to the site. The activated platelets also undergo a conformational change in the membranous Glycoprotein IIb–IIIa structure, which becomes a substrate for fibrinogen binding (40). This in turn promotes binding of coagulation factors such as factor Va and VIIIa to the platelet surface. Factor VIIIa becomes the substrate for the synthesis of a VIIIa–IXa–X–Ca^{2+} complex, which catalyzes factor X to Xa. Factor Xa is an important cofactor in the generation of thrombin from pro-thrombin. Thrombin has pleiotropic pro-thrombotic and anti-thrombotic activities. The pro-thrombotic effects of thrombin stimulate the synthesis of a fibrin clot. This process is counter balanced by fibrinolytic molecules such as tissue plasminogen activator (TPA).

Increases in the circulating levels of thrombotic factors may be expected to elevate the risk for cardiovascular disease. Indeed, this appears to be the case. In the Cardiovascular Health Study, for instance, which studied over 5800 men and women, 65 years of age and older, plasma fibrinogen as well as circulating factor VII and VIII levels were associated with increased risk for cardiovascular disease (43). The relationship was particularly notable in men. Elevated circulating levels of plasminogen activator inhibitor (PAI)-1, which neutralizes the effect of TPA, are also associated with cardiovascular disease (44).

COPD patients have increased circulating levels of thrombin, TPA–PAI complex, and β-thromboglobulin, a marker of platelet activation (45). In the FINMONICA study (The Finnish part of the WHO MONICA study), individuals with symptoms of chronic bronchitis had significantly elevated plasma fibrinogen levels (in men 3.70 g/L vs. 3.35 g/L; $p < 0.001$; in women 3.64 g/L vs. 3.44 g/L; $p < 0.001$) compared with individuals without chronic bronchitic symptoms even among non-smokers (46). Overall in men, the mean fibrinogen levels were 11% higher in symptomatic subjects, while in women, they were 6% higher. In another study, Fowkes et al. showed that COPD was a significant risk factor for aortic aneurysm. Most of the excess risk associated with COPD could be nullified when the analytic model accounted for hemostatic markers such as D-dimer (47). During exacerbations, there is a further increase in plasma fibrinogen levels, which may contribute to abnormal hemostasis and thrombosis in such patients (48). Further work is needed to determine the contributions of this pathway to the increased risk of cardiovascular diseases observed in COPD.

Neurohumoral Disturbances

Excess sympathetic nervous activity is significantly related to cardiovascular diseases (49). Excess sympathetic nervous activity increases arterial pressure, induces endothelial dysfunction, and promotes cardiac remodeling. Raised plasma nor-epinephrine levels, a marker and mediator of sympathetic activity, are associated with increased cardiovascular morbidity and mortality in a variety of different conditions (50,51). Patients with heart failure or ischemic heart disease frequently demonstrate excess sympathetic nervous activity, which can be significantly attenuated by the use of β-adrenoceptor blockers. The reduction in the sympathetic nervous activity is associated with improved cardiac function and reduces cardiovascular morbidity and mortality (52).

In advanced COPD, patients demonstrate excess adrenergic activity. Using microneurography of the peroneal nerve, Heindl and colleagues showed that patients with respiratory failure have a marked increase in peripheral sympathetic discharge compared with controls (53). The intensity of the sympathetic nervous activity was inversely related to the patients' oxyhemoglobin saturation ($r=0.54$). Supplemental oxygen attenuated (but did not normalize) the sympathetic nervous activity. Metaiodobenzylguanidine (MIBG), an analog of guanetidine, has similar metabolism to norepinephrine in systemic nervous tissues (54). MIBG has been used to image the heart for assessment of cardiac sympathetic activity. Increased sympathetic nervous activity leads to reduced cardiac to mediastinal activity ratio in the delayed images (54). In a cohort of 28 COPD patients and 7 control subjects, Sakamaki and colleagues showed that COPD patients demonstrated reduced cardiac accumulation of MIBG and a higher washout rate from the heart than control subjects, indicating excess activity of the sympathetic nervous system with increased norepinephrine turnover (55). Interestingly, the MIBG accumulation rate significantly correlated with the intensity of dyspnea of these patients ($p<0.05$). Consistent with the MIBG data, COPD patients had higher plasma norepinephrine levels than did the control subjects (449 pg/mL vs. 69 pg/mL; $p<0.01$).

Oxidative Stress

Oxidative stress induces endothelial dysfunction (56). Oxygen-derived free radicals such as superoxide anion impair endothelial vasomotor function (57). Oxidative stress can impair vasodilatation, endothelial cell growth, and promote plaque build-up and rupture (58). Anti-oxidants, on the other hand, improve endothelial function in patients with coronary artery disease (59). Leukocytes, when activated, can generate a large amount of oxidative stress through the induction of enzymes such as NADPH oxidase, superoxide dismutase, nitric oxide synthase, and myeloperoxidase (60). When the oxidant load exceeds the anti-oxidant capacity of the organ, important proteins, lipids, carbohydrates, and even DNA materials in the local milieu may be modified through oxidation, resulting in tissue injury. Oxidants can also enhance inflammation. Inflammation, in turn, can generate more oxidant species, creating a positive feedback loop (57).

COPD patients experience increased oxidative stress than in the control subjects. The load is further increased in patients who continue to smoke and in patients who experience frequent exacerbations (61). The magnitude of the oxidative stress in these patients appears to be negatively correlated with FEV_1 (as percent predicted) indicating a dose–response relationship (62). Local oxidative stress in the peripheral muscles of COPD patients is associated with reduced muscle strength (63). The etiology of the oxidative burden in COPD is unclear. Hypoxemia, poor nutrition, inflammatory burden, infection, and smoking have all been implicated in the process (64,65). Since COPD patients have perturbed oxidant/anti-oxidant balance in favor of oxidative stress, it is plausible that the excess oxidant load could contribute to the development and progression of atherosclerosis and cardiovascular events. Large clinical studies (specifically in COPD patients) are needed to confirm this hypothesis. A simplified model integrating oxidative stress and inflammation in COPD is shown in Figure 3.

C. Cachexia and Nutritional Abnormalities

Cachexia is defined as excessive weight loss in the setting of ongoing disease, associated with disproportionate muscle wasting (67). Weight loss related to starvation, on the other hand, is associated with a disproportionate reduction in fat mass. Cachexia

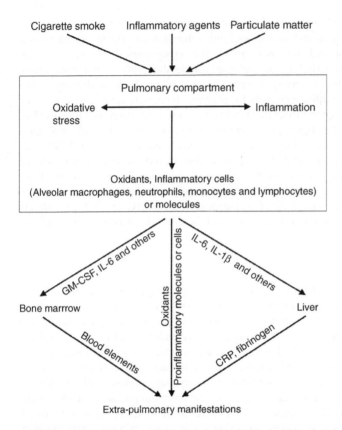

Figure 3 Oxidative stress and inflammation in the lung in chronic obstructive pulmonary disease. Cigarette smoke, infection, and other environmental irritants produce oxidative stress and/or inflammation in the lung. Collectively and individually, inflammatory cells may be activated and/or recruited. Oxidants and products of inflammatory cells or airway cells may affect distant organs by their direct action, or through their action on an intermediate organ, such as the bone marrow or the liver, which in turn release blood elements or CRP and fibrinogen, respectively, into the blood circulation. *Abbreviations*: CRP, C-reactive protein; GM-CSF, granulocyte macrophage colony-stimulating factor; IL, interleukin. *Source*: From Ref. 66.

and weight loss are frequently observed in patients with COPD and are associated with poor functional capacity, reduced health status, and increased mortality (68). Numerous studies from as early as the 1960s (69) have reported that low body weight and weight loss are negatively associated with survival in patients with COPD (68). The prevalence of weight loss in COPD increases with COPD disease progression. In mild to moderate COPD, only 10% to 15% of patients have significant weight loss. In contrast, in severe COPD, nearly 50% of patients have significant weight loss (70). Although cachexia of COPD affects all body compartments, skeletal muscle mass appears to be especially vulnerable. Fat mass, on the hand, is largely spared until the very last stages of the disease. Thus, most patients with moderate to severe COPD have significantly reduced fat-free mass. This perturbation in body composition can also occur in the early stages of the disease and even in the absence of any meaningful reduction in the total body weight (71). Accordingly, while total body weight is a useful surrogate measure to monitor patients for COPD-related cachexia, in certain circumstances, it can be misleading; measurement of fat-free mass may be a more sensitive marker of disease activity and outcomes of COPD patients.

COPD-related cachexia is an important, independent risk factor for morbidity and mortality. In a recent study, Hallin and coworkers found that in a group of patients who were hospitalized due to an exacerbation of COPD, a history of weight loss during a 12-month follow-up period as well as the initial weight of the patients were both independently associated with a higher risk of experiencing a new exacerbation (72). In a study by Schols and colleagues, mortality risk increased significantly once the BMI of patients reached 25 kg/m^2 or below (73). The risk of mortality associated with reduced BMI appears to be modified by the severity of COPD, as measured by FEV_1. In those with mild to moderate COPD ($FEV_1 \geq 50\%$ of predicted), the relationship between BMI and mortality is U-shaped with the extremes of BMI having the worst prognosis, and BMI between 20 and 25 kg/m^2 associated with the best prognosis. In those with severe COPD ($FEV_1 < 50\%$ of predicted), the relationship between BMI and mortality appears to be (inversely) linear. The prognosis progressively worsens with decreasing BMI (74). In the Copenhagen City Heart Study, for instance, COPD mortality was 2.2-fold higher in COPD patients with FEV_1 less than 50% of predicted, who had a BMI less than 20 kg/m^2 compared with those whose BMI was between 20 and 25 kg/m^2 and over sevenfold higher compared with those whose BMI was 30 kg/m^2 or greater (74).

Mechanism of Cachexia

The processes that lead to cachexia in COPD are not well understood. In health, protein degradation and replacement is carefully regulated and controlled. Any significant perturbations of this delicate balance can result over time in cachexia and wasting. Nutritional status and body hormones play significant roles in maintaining this homeostasis. For instance, growth factors such as human growth hormone, insulin-like growth factor-1, and anabolic steroids promote protein synthesis, while glucocorticoids and catecholamines favor catabolism (75). Low testosterone levels have also been associated with COPD cachexia (76) as testosterone promotes myoblastic activity and inhibits the synthesis of pro-inflammatory cytokines such as TNF-α.

More recently, cytokines and chemokines have been implicated in the pathogenesis of cachexia. When patients become clinically ill (from an inflammatory or infectious stimuli), there is a rapid rise in the circulating levels of pro-inflammatory cytokines such as IL-1, IL-2, interferon-γ, and TNF-α. These cytokines especially TNF-α, and IFN-γ can act synergistically to inhibit messenger RNA expression for myosin heavy chain, leading to decreased muscle protein synthesis. These cytokines may also directly or indirectly stimulate proteolysis of myosin heavy chains (77,78). In COPD, the hormonal balance is clearly shifted toward catabolism, especially in the severe to very severe stages of the disease. Patients have reduced testosterone levels, and increased pro-inflammatory cytokine expression both locally in the muscles as well as systemically, and increased catecholamine synthesis (73) presumably related to the underlying inflammatory and oxidative processes in the airways. Moreover, COPD patients frequently take inhaled or systemic glucocorticoids, which further contribute to a catabolic state.

D. Skeletal Muscle Dysfunction and Reduced Exercise Tolerance

With increasing severity of disease, COPD patients complain of reduced exercise capacity and weakness of muscles. Objectively, they display skeletal muscle dysfunction especially in the thighs and upper arms. The skeletal muscle dysfunction of COPD is predominantly driven by a loss in skeletal muscle mass (68). Over time, these patients lose exercise endurance and complain of fatigue and dyspnea with only minimal degree of exertion (79). These symptoms curtail patients' ability to exercise and compromise their cardiac fitness, which further limits their exercise tolerance, creating a vicious downward spiral that can eventually lead to generalized debility and immobility (80). Not surprisingly, skeletal muscle dysfunction contributes to reduced health status of COPD patients and substantially increases the risk of mortality, independent of traditional markers of COPD mortality such as baseline lung function, age, and cigarette smoking (81). Encouragingly, early interventions with exercise programs may restore some of the lost health status related to muscle dysfunction and increase patients' exercise tolerance and stamina (82).

Mechanism of Skeletal Muscle Weakness

Despite the importance of skeletal muscle performance in COPD morbidity and mortality, the pathophysiologic mechanisms responsible for the muscle failure remain largely a mystery. Clearly, with advancing disease, skeletal muscle mass decreases in COPD (83). Biopsy analyses from quadriceps and elsewhere reveal a significant reduction in type I fibers and a relative increase in type II fibers as compared with normal individuals, which probably contributes to increased fatigability and reduced muscle endurance observed in COPD patients (83). Microscopically, these skeletal muscles show accelerated apoptosis, increased oxidative stress, lactic acidosis, and inflammatory changes (84,85), raising the possibility that local inflammatory and oxidative milieu may also play a role in the physiologic changes in COPD skeletal muscles.

However, these changes may also be due to deconditioning and disuse. With COPD progression, patients become more breathless and adopt a more sedentary lifestyle. From disuse, muscles can become progressively weaker, more atrophic and less able to endure oxidative and physical stress (86). These adverse changes in the muscles become exaggerated with hormonal changes (discussed in the previous section), use of corticosteroids, and with poor nutrition (87). On the positive side, even low-intensity pulmonary rehabilitation for a relatively short period of time can recondition the muscles and partially restore their strength (88).

E. Lung Cancer

While strictly speaking, lung cancer cannot be considered an extrapulmonary manifestation of COPD, it is nevertheless an important complication that deserves attention. In fact, lung cancer is the leading cause of mortality in mild to moderate COPD (2). It accounts for over 30% of all deaths. Combined with cancers in other organs, over 50% of patients with mild to moderate COPD die from cancer (2). While cigarette smoking is a major risk factor for both lung cancer and COPD, the effect of COPD on lung cancer risk can occur independently of cigarette smoking (89). Compared with individuals with normal lung function, those with FEV_1 lower than about 70% of predicted are 2.4 times more likely to develop lung cancer, independent of cigarette smoking (89). This excess risk is mostly driven by a predominance of squamous cell carcinoma in COPD patients (90).

Mechanisms of Lung Cancer

The exact mechanisms by which COPD confers an increased risk for lung cancer are unclear. There is some evidence for a familial aggregation of lung cancer and COPD, beyond the shared risk associated with smoking. Linkage analysis has indicated a potential overlap in candidate genes on chromosome 6q and on chromosome 12p for lung cancer and COPD, raising the possibility of shared genetic risk between the two disorders (91–93). Intriguingly, Yang and colleagues found a significant association between lung cancer risk and deficient alleles for the α-1 antitrypsin gene, a known causative risk factor for COPD (94). In this study, haplotypes that included both α-1 antitrypsin gene and genes for neutrophil elastase were even more strongly associated with lung cancer risk suggesting the potential importance of lung proteolysis on the relationship between COPD and lung cancer (94). These results have been replicated by several other groups (95–97). Future work will further elucidate the potential genetic linkage between COPD and lung cancer (97).

Another potential mechanism is by delayed clearance of inhaled carcinogens in COPD patients. With progressive airflow impairment, patients may not be able to fully clear the inhaled carcinogens in a timely manner, which increases the opportunity for carcinogenic materials to effect DNA mutagenesis (98). Additionally, COPD has been associated with increased chronic and persistent oxidative stress (99) and local inflammation, which have also been implicated in the pathogenesis of lung cancer (100).

F. Osteoporosis and Fractures

Reduced bone mass is a common finding in COPD patients. The risk of osteopenia, defined as bone mineral density values less than 1.0 standard deviation, SD (T scores of -1.0) below the mean bone mineral density values of sex-matched Caucasian participants 20 to 29 years of age, increases by 30% in moderate (FEV$_1$ 50–80% of predicted), and 70% in severe COPD (FEV$_1$ less than 50% of predicted) (101). The risk of osteoporosis (T scores of -2.5 or below), increases by 2.1-fold with moderate COPD and 2.4-fold with severe COPD (101). In subjects with severe COPD, the prevalence of osteopenia is 60% and osteoporosis is 10% in men, while in women, the prevalence of osteopenia and osteoporosis is 76% and 33%, respectively (101). Similarly, in a cross-sectional study of 62 patients, Jørgensen and coworkers (102) found that 68% of study participants had osteoporosis or osteopenia.

Not surprisingly, given these data, patients with COPD have increased risk of osteoporotic fractures (RR, 1.61; 95% CI, 1.52–1.71). The risk is amplified in patients who are thin (BMI <20 kg/m^2; RR, 2.54) and in those who experience exacerbations (RR, 2.02). COPD patients are particularly vulnerable to vertebral fractures (103). Their risk is increased four- to eightfold above those without COPD (103). Concomitant use of inhaled corticosteroids may further increase the risk by 10% to 50%, though this relationship is still quite contentious (104,105).

Mechanisms of Osteoporosis

Because pro-inflammatory cytokines can significantly alter bone metabolism, excessive osteoporosis in relation to age could be considered a systemic effect of COPD (71). The etiology of bone loss in COPD is complex but likely includes smoking, vitamin D deficiency, low BMI, hypogonadism, sedentary lifestyle, and use of corticosteroids (106).

G. Psychological Factors in COPD

Mood disorders are common in the general population, particularly in the elderly. In one study, the prevalence for depression in the community was 3% to 4%, while the prevalence for anxiety was 19% in those 65 years of age and older (107). Patients with COPD often report anxiety, depression, and poor health status, especially following hospitalizations and after exacerbations. In a prospective study of 416 COPD patients recruited from five university hospitals in Nordic countries, the investigators found that about half of the studied COPD patients suffered from anxiety and/or depression. Anxiety was more common in women than in men (47% vs. 34%), while current smokers had a higher prevalence of both anxiety (54% vs. 37%) and depression (43% vs. 23%) than non-smokers. Importantly, psychological status (i.e., either depression or anxiety) was independently related to all dimensions of disease-specific health-related quality of life as measured by the St. George's Respiratory Questionnaire (SGRQ). Patients with psychological disorders had worse health status than did those without depression or anxiety (108). Interestingly, COPD severity as measured by the GOLD stages was not related to prevalence of depression and/or anxiety. In all GOLD stages, the prevalence of anxiety and/or depression was similar at about 50%. Patients with anxiety and/or depression suffered from increased risk for hospitalization and rehospitalization (RR, 1.76; 95% CI, 1.16–2.68) (109). Other studies have also shown similar prevalence of psychological disorders in COPD. In a small study of patients with moderate to severe COPD (FEV_1 less than 1.25 L), Light and colleagues reported a prevalence of depression, as assessed by the Beck Depression Scale, of 42% (110) and Withers and colleagues reported a depression rate of 15% and anxiety rate of 29% in patients with FEV_1 of less than 40% of predicted (111). Importantly, in the latter study, those with anxiety and/or depression were more likely to demonstrate functional impairment in walking distances. After pulmonary rehabilitation, however, they demonstrated lower anxiety and depression scores and experienced greater improvements in exercise capacity than patients who did not have significant depression and/or anxiety at baseline (111). Interestingly, in a pilot study, Eiser and colleagues showed that group psychotherapy in severe COPD patients improved functional status of these patients as measured by the distances achieved on a six-minute walk test (112). However, a larger study could not replicate these findings (113). Pulmonary rehabilitation with or without psychotherapy can reduce anxiety and depression in COPD patients (114,115). The precise mechanism by which this occurs is unknown.

III. The Impact of Systemic Consequences of COPD on Mortality

In the past, COPD mortality research has focused on measurements of lung function, especially FEV_1. Although FEV_1 correlates with survival in COPD, the relationship is rather weak probably because FEV_1 does not fully capture the extrapulmonary manifestations of COPD that have been discussed in the previous sections. Prognostic indices that incorporate systemic elements of COPD perform much better than does FEV_1 alone. A recent example is the BMI, airflow obstruction, dyspnea, and exercise capacity (BODE) index. The index is a multi-dimensional instrument that is derived from BMI, FEV_1, modified Medical Research Council dyspnea score, and six-minute walk distance (116). The BODE index is, therefore, an integrated scale that captures respiratory function, cardiovascular fitness, nutritional status, and skeletal muscle performance of COPD patients. A one-point increase in the BODE index is associated with a 34% increase in all-cause mortality (RR, 1.34; 95% CI, 1.26–1.42). Overall, the BODE index is much better than FEV_1 alone in predicting risk of all-cause and respiratory-cause specific mortality.

Health status instruments provide incremental prognostic information beyond FEV_1, in part because they reflect the total burden, including that imposed by systemic components of COPD. In particular, domains such as exercise tolerance and dyspnea provide an assessment of the nutritional and cardiovascular status as well as the fitness level of the COPD patient, which impact on prognosis. In a study by Antonelli-Incalzi and colleagues (117), the presence of systemic disorders was associated with higher scores on SGRQ compared with not having systemic disorders in COPD patients (SGRQ impacts score, β coefficient$=0.137$; $p=0.02$; and SGRQ total score, β coefficient$=0.115$; $p=0.05$). In a three-year follow-up study that included 312 men with COPD, both SGRQ and Short Form-36 physical component (PCS-36) scores were independently associated with mortality after adjustment for age, FEV_1, and BMI (118). In the final adjusted model, poorer SGRQ (standard HR$=1.30$) and PCS-36 (standard HR$=1.32$) scores were associated with approximately 30% increased mortality (118). Furthermore, SGRQ and PCS were independently associated with mortality attributed specifically to respiratory causes.

Peak exercise capacity is another integrated measure of the cardiopulmonary performance of COPD subjects. In one study, the investigators evaluated the relationship between exercise capacity, health status, and mortality in 150 men with COPD, followed-up for five years (119). Univariate analysis showed that SGRQ activity $(p=0.0001)$, impact $(p=0.0023)$, and total $(p=0.0017)$ scores were significantly correlated with mortality. Multivariate analysis showed that SGRQ total score (RR, 1.035; 95% CI, 1.008–1.063; $p=0.012$) and peak oxygen uptake (VO_2; RR, 0.995; 95% CI, 0.993–0.998; $p<0.0001$) were predictive of mortality independently of age and FEV_1. Most importantly, a stepwise Cox analysis found peak VO_2 to be the most significant predictor of mortality (RR, 0.994; 95% CI, 0.992–0.996; $p<0.0001$). Collectively, these data suggest that tools that evaluate both the cardiopulmonary performance of COPD patients (e.g., VO_2 max) provide incremental prognostic information beyond just FEV_1, and in certain settings, perform better than tools that reflect only the ventilatory status of COPD subjects.

IV. Conclusion

COPD can be described as a chronic inflammatory disease of the peripheral airways, the progression of which is often characterized by the development of extrapulmonary diseases. These systemic manifestations such as cardiovascular diseases, cancer, skeletal muscle dysfunction, and osteoporosis, contribute a great deal to reduced quality of life and increased mortality in COPD patients. While the mechanisms for the association of COPD with these systemic disorders have not been fully worked out, local and systemic inflammation, oxidative stress, hemostatic disturbances and perturbations in the neurohumoral states are some of the likely candidate pathways by which these extrapulmonary effects of COPD are effected. Future work will undoubtedly shed more light on the processes and mechanisms for the extrapulmonary manifestations of COPD. In the meantime, when assessing COPD patients, physicians must be mindful of these extra-pulmonary manifestations of COPD including cardiovascular disease, osteoporosis, cachexia, muscle weakness, anxiety, and depression. In addition to a careful history and physical examination, appropriate investigations are needed to ascertain these comorbidities in COPD patients. Once detected, these extra-pulmonary manifestations of COPD should be treated aggressively, as they add to the overall morbidity and mortality of COPD patients. In general, smoking cessation and pulmonary rehabilitation can be recommended to patients to modify some of these processes.

Acknowledgments

The work is supported in part by the Canadian Institutes of Health Research and the GlaxoSmithKline/St. Paul's Hospital Foundation Professorship in COPD.

References

1. Pauwels RA, Buist AS, Calverley PM, Jenkins CR, Hurd SS. GOLD Scientific Committee. Global strategy for the diagnosis, management, and prevention of chronic obstructive pulmonary disease. NHLBI/WHO Global Initiative for Chronic Obstructive Pulmonary Disease (GOLD) workshop summary. Am J Respir Crit Care Med 2001; 163:1256–76.
2. Anthonisen NR, Connett JE, Kiley JP, Altose MD, Bailey WC, Buist AS, Conway WA, Jr., Enright PL, Kanner RE, O'Hara P, et al. Effects of smoking intervention and the use of an inhaled anticholinergic bronchodilator on the rate of decline of FEV1. The Lung Health Study. J Am Med Assoc 1994; 272(19):1497–505.
3. Sin DD, Anthonisen NR, Soriano JB, Agusti AG. Mortality in COPD: role of comorbidities. Eur Respir J 2006; 28:1245–57.
4. Sin DD, Wu L, Man SF. The relationship between reduced lung function and cardiovascular mortality: a population-based study and a systematic review of the literature. Chest 2005; 127(6):1952–9.
5. Beaty TH, Newill CA, Cohen BH, Tockman MS, Bryant SH, Spurgeon HA. Effects of pulmonary function on mortality. J Chronic Dis 1985; 38:703–10.
6. Higgins MW, Keller JB. Predictors of mortality in the adult population of Tecumseh. Arch Environ Health 1970; 21:418–24.
7. Speizer FE, Fay ME, Dockery DW, Ferris BG, Jr. Chronic obstructive pulmonary disease mortality in six U.S. cities. Am Rev Respir Dis 1989; 140:S49–55.
8. Schunemann HJ, Dorn J, Grant BJ, Winkelstein W, Jr., Trevisan M. Pulmonary function is a long-term predictor of mortality in the general population: 29-year follow-up of the Buffalo Health Study. Chest 2000; 118:656–64.
9. Hole DJ, Watt GC, Davey-Smith G, Hart CL, Gillis CR, Hawthorne VM. Impaired lung function and mortality risk in men and women: findings from the Renfrew and Paisley prospective population study. Br Med J 1996; 313:711–5.
10. Greenland S. Attributable fractions: bias from broad definition of exposure. Epidemiology 2001; 12(5):518–20.

11. Mannino DM, Aguayo SM, Petty TL, Redd SC. Low lung function and incident lung cancer in the United States: data from the First National Health and Nutrition Examination Survey follow-up. Arch Intern Med 2003; 163(12):1475–80.
12. Engstrom G, Hedblad B, Janzon L, Valind S. Respiratory decline in smokers and ex-smokers—an independent risk factor for cardiovascular disease and death. J Cardiovasc Risk 2000; 7:267–72.
13. Tockman MS, Pearson JD, Fleg JL, et al. Rapid decline in FEV1. A new risk factor for coronary heart disease mortality. Am J Respir Crit Care Med 1995; 151:390–8.
14. Sin DD, Man SF. Why are patients with chronic obstructive pulmonary disease at increased risk of cardiovascular diseases? The potential role of systemic inflammation in chronic obstructive pulmonary disease. Circulation 2003; 107:1514–9.
15. Engström G, Wollmer P, Hedblad B, Juul-Möller S, Valind S, Janzon L. Occurrence and prognostic significance of ventricular arrhythmia is related to pulmonary function: a study from "men born in 1914", Malmö, Sweden. Circulation 2001; 103:3086–91.
16. Jousilahti P, Vartiainen E, Tuomilehto J, Puska P. Symptoms of chronic bronchitis and the risk of coronary disease. Lancet 1996; 348:567–72.
17. Janssens JP, Herrmann F, MacGee W, Michel JP. Cause of death in older patients with anatomo-pathological evidence of chronic bronchitis or emphysema: a case-control study based on autopsy findings. J Am Geriatr Soc 2001; 49:571–6.
18. McGarvey LP, John M, Anderson JA, Zvarich M, Wise RA. Ascertainment of cause-specific mortality in COPD: operations of the TORCH Clinical Endpoint Committee. Thorax 2007; 62:411–5.
19. Sin DD, Man SF. Chronic obstructive pulmonary disease: a novel risk factor for cardiovascular disease. Can J Physiol Pharmacol 2005; 83:8–13.
20. Hogg JC, Chu F, Utokaparch S, et al. The nature of small-airway obstruction in chronic obstructive pulmonary disease. N Engl J Med 2004; 350(26):2645–53.
21. Gan WQ, Man SF, Senthilselvan A, Sin DD. Association between chronic obstructive pulmonary disease and systemic inflammation: a systematic review and a meta-analysis. Thorax 2004; 59(7):574–80.
22. Terashima T, Wiggs B, English D, Hogg JC, van Eeden SF. Phagocytosis of small carbon particles by alveolar macrophages stimulates the release of PMN from the bone marrow. Am J Respir Crit Care Med 1997; 155:1441–7.
23. Mukae H, Hogg JC, English D, Vincent R, van Eeden SF. Phagocytosis of particulate air pollutants by human alveolar macrophages stimulates the bone marrow. Am J Physiol Lung Cell Mol Physiol 2000; 279(5):L924–31.
24. Suwa T, Hogg JC, Quinlan KB, Ohgami A, Vincent R, van Eeden SF. Particulate air pollution induces progression of atherosclerosis. J Am Coll Cardiol 2002; 39:935–42.
25. Fujii T, Hayashi S, Hogg JC, Vincent R, van Eeden SF. Particulate matter induces cytokine expression in human bronchial epithelial cells. Am J Respir Cell Biol Med 2001; 25:265–71.
26. Mio T, Romberger DJ, Thompson AB, Robbins RA, Heires A, Rennard SI. Cigarette smoke induces interleukin-8 release from human bronchial epithelial cells. Am J Respir Crit Care Med 1997; 155:1770–6.
27. Masubuchi T, Koyama S, Sato E, et al. Smoke extract stimulates lung epithelial cells to release neutrophil and monocyte chemotactic activity. Am J Pathol 1998; 153:1903–12.
28. Takizawa H, Tanaka M, Takami K, et al. Increased expression of transforming growth factor-beta1 in small airway epithelium from tobacco smokers and patients with chronic obstructive pulmonary disease (COPD). Am J Respir Crit Care Med 2001; 163:1476–83.
29. Cybulsky MI, Iiyama K, Li H, et al. A major role for VCAM-1, but not ICAM-1, in early atherosclerosis. J Clin Invest 2001; 107:1255–62.
30. Li H, Cybulsky MI, Gimbrone MA, Jr., Libby P. An atherogenic diet rapidly induces VCAM-1, a cytokine-regulatable mononuclear leukocyte adhesion molecule, in rabbit aortic endothelium. Arterioscler Thromb 1993; 13:197–204.
31. Ross R. Atherosclerosis—an inflammatory disease. N Engl J Med 1999; 340:115–26.
32. Danesh J, Whincup P, Walker M, et al. Low grade inflammation and coronary heart disease: prospective study and updated meta-analyses. Br Med J 2000; 321:199–204.
33. Ridker PM. Clinical application of C-reactive protein for cardiovascular disease detection and prevention. Circulation 2003; 107:363–9.
34. Lusis AJ. Atherosclerosis. Nature 2000; 407:233–41.
35. Verma S, Li SH, Badiwala MV, et al. Endothelin antagonism and interleukin-6 inhibition attenuate the proatherogenic effects of C-reactive protein. Circulation 2002; 105:1890–6.

36. Yeh ET, Anderson HV, Pasceri V, Willerson JT. C-reactive protein: linking inflammation to cardiovascular complications. Circulation 2001; 104:974–5.

37. Van Doornum S, McColl G, Wicks IP. Accelerated atherosclerosis: an extraarticular feature of rheumatoid arthritis? Arthritis Rheum 2002; 46:862–73.

38. Choi HK, Hernan MA, Seeger JD, Robins JM, Wolfe F. Methotrexate and mortality in patients with rheumatoid arthritis: a prospective study. Lancet 2002; 359:1173–7.

39. Roman MJ, Shanker BA, Davis A, et al. Prevalence and correlates of accelerated atherosclerosis in systemic lupus erythematosus. N Engl J Med 2003; 349:2399–406.

40. Wu KK, Thiagarajan P. Role of endothelium in thrombosis and hemostasis. Annu Rev Med 1996; 47:315–31.

41. Roest M, Banga JD, Grobbee DE, et al. Homozygosity for 807 T polymorphism in alpha(2) subunit of platelet alpha(2)beta(1) is associated with increased risk of cardiovascular mortality in high-risk women. Circulation 2000; 102(14):1645–50.

42. Wiman B, Andersson T, Hallqvist J, Reuterwall C, Ahlbom A, deFaire U. Plasma levels of tissue plasminogen activator/plasminogen activator inhibitor-1 complex and von Willebrand factor are significant risk markers for recurrent myocardial infarction in the Stockholm Heart Epidemiology Program (SHEEP) study. Arterioscler Thromb Vasc Biol 2000; 20(8):2019–23.

43. Tracy RP, Arnold AM, Ettinger W, Fried L, Meilahn E, Savage P. The relationship of fibrinogen and factors VII and VIII to incident cardiovascular disease and death in the elderly: results from the cardiovascular health study. Arterioscler Thromb Vasc Biol 1999; 19(7):1776–83.

44. Lyon CJ, Hsueh WA. Effect of plasminogen activator inhibitor-1 in diabetes mellitus and cardiovascular disease. Am J Med 2003; 115:62S–8.

45. Ashitani J, Mukae H, Arimura Y, Matsukura S. Elevated plasma procoagulant and fibrinolytic markers in patients with chronic obstructive pulmonary disease. Intern Med 2002; 41(3):181–5.

46. Jousilahti P, Salomaa V, Rasi V, Vahtera E. Symptoms of chronic bronchitis, haemostatic factors, and coronary heart disease risk. Atherosclerosis 1999; 142(2):403–7.

47. Fowkes FG, Anandan CL, Lee AJ, et al. Reduced lung function in patients with abdominal aortic aneurysm is associated with activation of inflammation and hemostasis, not smoking or cardiovascular disease. J Vasc Surg 2006; 43(3):474–80.

48. Wedzicha JA, Seemungal TA, MacCallum PK, et al. Acute exacerbations of chronic obstructive pulmonary disease are accompanied by elevations of plasma fibrinogen and serum IL-6 levels. Thromb Haemost 2000; 84(2):210–5.

49. Mancia G, Grassi G, Giannattasio C, Seravalle G. Sympathetic activation in the pathogenesis of hypertension and progression of organ damage. Hypertension 1999; 34(4 Pt 2):724–8.

50. Benedict CR, Shelton B, Johnstone DE, et al. Prognostic significance of plasma norepinephrine in patients with asymptomatic left ventricular dysfunction. SOLVD Investigators. Circulation 1996; 94(4):690–7.

51. Zoccali C, Mallamaci F, Parlongo S, et al. Plasma norepinephrine predicts survival and incident cardiovascular events in patients with end-stage renal disease. Circulation 2002; 105(11):1354–9.

52. McMurray JJ, Pfeffer MA. Heart failure. Lancet 2005; 365(9474):1877–89.

53. Heindl S, Lehnert M, Criee CP, Hasenfuss G, Andreas S. Marked sympathetic activation in patients with chronic respiratory failure. Am J Respir Crit Care Med 2001; 164(4):597–601.

54. Wieland DM, Wu J, Brown LE, Mangner TJ, Swanson DP, Beierwaltes WH. Radiolabeled adrenergi neuron-blocking agents: adrenomedullary imaging with [^{131}I]iodobenzylguanidine. J Nucl Med 1980; 21(4):349–53.

55. Sakamaki F, Satoh T, Nagaya N, Kyotani S, Nakanishi N, Ishida Y. Abnormality of left ventricular sympathetic nervous function assessed by (123)I-metaiodobenzylguanidine imaging in patients with COPD. Chest 1999; 116(6):1575–81.

56. Elahi MM, Matata BM. Free radicals in blood: evolving concepts in the mechanism of ischemic heart disease. Arch Biochem Biophys 2006; 450(1):78–88.

57. Cai H, Harrison DG. Endothelial dysfunction in cardiovascular diseases: the role of oxidant stress. Circ Res 2000; 87(10):840–4.

58. Sugiyama S, Kugiyama K, Aikawa M, Nakamura S, Ogawa H, Libby P. Hypochlorous acid, a macrophage product, induces endothelial apoptosis and tissue factor expression: involvement of myeloperoxidase-mediated oxidant in plaque erosion and thrombogenesis. Arterioscler Thromb Vasc Biol 2004; 24(7):1309–14.

59. Azen SP, Qian D, Mack WJ, et al. Effect of supplementary antioxidant vitamin intake on carotid arterial wall intima-media thickness in a controlled clinical trial of cholesterol lowering. Circulation 1996; 94(10):2369–72.
60. Daugherty A, Dunn JL, Rateri DL, Heinecke JW. Myeloperoxidase, a catalyst for lipoprotein oxidation, is expressed in human atherosclerotic lesions. J Clin Invest 1994; 94(1):437–44.
61. Rahman I, Morrison D, Donaldson K, MacNee W. Systemic oxidative stress in asthma, COPD, and smokers. Am J Respir Crit Care Med 1996; 154(4 Pt 1):1055–60.
62. Nadeem A, Raj HG, Chhabra SK. Increased oxidative stress and altered levels of antioxidants in chronic obstructive pulmonary disease. Inflammation 2005; 29(1):23–32.
63. Couillard A, Maltais F, Saey D, et al. Exercise-induced quadriceps oxidative stress and peripheral muscle dysfunction in patients with chronic obstructive pulmonary disease. Am J Respir Crit Care Med 2003; 167(12):1664–9.
64. Koechlin C, Maltais F, Saey D, et al. Hypoxaemia enhances peripheral muscle oxidative stress in chronic obstructive pulmonary disease. Thorax 2005; 60(10):834–41.
65. Owen CA. Proteinases and oxidants as targets in the treatment of chronic obstructive pulmonary disease. Proc Am Thorac Soc 2005; 2(4):373–85.
66. Man SF, Sin DD. Effects of corticosteroids on systemic inflammation in chronic obstructive pulmonary disease. Proc Am Thorac Soc 2005; 2:78–82.
67. Morley JE, Thomas DR, Wilson MM. Cachexia: pathophysiology and clinical relevance. Am J Clin Nutr 2006; 83(4):735–43.
68. Schols AMWJ. Nutrition in chronic obstructive pulmonary disease. Curr Opin Pulm Med 2000; 6:110–5.
69. Vandenbergh E, Van de Woestijne KP, Gyselen A. Weight changes in the terminal stages of chronic obstructive pulmonary disease. Am Rev Respir Dis 1967; 95:556–66.
70. Creutzberg EC, Schols AM, Bothmer-Quaedvlieg FCM, Wouters EFM. Prevalence of an elevated resting energy expenditure in patients with chronic obstructive pulmonary disease in relation to body composition and lung function. Eur J Clin Nutr 1998; 52:396–401.
71. Agusti AGN. Systemic effects of chronic obstructive pulmonary disease. Proc Am Thorac Soc 2005; 2:367–70.
72. Hallin R, Koivisto-Hursti U-K, Lindberg E, Janson C. Nutritional status, dietary energy intake and the risk of exacerbations in patients with chronic obstructive pulmonary disease (COPD). J Respir Med 2006; 100:561–7.
73. Schols AM, Slangen J, Volovics L, Wouters EF. Weight loss is a reversible factor in the prognosis of chronic obstructive pulmonary disease. Am J Respir Crit Care Med 1998; 157(6):1791–7.
74. Landbo C, Prescott E, Lange P, Vestbo J, Almdal TP. Prognostic value of nutritional status in chronic obstructive pulmonary disease. Am J Respir Crit Care Med 1999; 160(6):1856–61.
75. Wing SS, Goldberg AL. Glucocorticoids activate the ATP-ubiquitin-dependent proteolytic system in skeletal muscle during fasting. Am J Physiol 1993; 264:E668–76.
76. Laghi F. Low testosterone in chronic obstructive pulmonary disease: does it really matter? Am J Respir Crit Care Med 2005; 172(9):1069–70.
77. Guttridge DC, Mayo MW, Madrid LV, Wang CY, Baldwin AS, Jr. NF-kappaB-induced loss of MyoD messenger RNA: possible role in muscle decay and cachexia. Science 2000; 289(5488):2363–6.
78. Acharyya S, Ladner KJ, Nelsen LL, et al. Cancer cachexia is regulated by selective targeting of skeletal muscle gene products. J Clin Invest 2004; 114(3):370–8.
79. Sin DD, Jones RL, Mannino DM, Paul Man SF. Forced expiratory volume in 1 second and physical activity in the general population. Am J Med 2004; 117:270–3.
80. Montes de Oca M, Rassulo J, Celli BR. Respiratory muscle and cardiopulmonary function during exercise in very severe COPD. Am J Respir Crit Care Med 1996; 154:1284–9.
81. Marquis K, Debigare R, Lacasse Y, et al. Midthigh muscle cross-sectional area is a better predictor of mortality than body mass index in patients with chronic obstructive pulmonary disease. Am J Respir Crit Care Med 2002; 166:809–13.
82. Sin DD, McAlister FA, Man SF, Anthonisen NR. Contemporary management of chronic obstructive pulmonary disease: scientific review. J Am Med Assoc 2003; 290:2301–12.
83. Mador MJ, Bozkanat E. Skeletal muscle dysfunction in chronic obstructive pulmonary disease. Respir Res 2001; 2:216–24.
84. Agusti AGN, Sauleda J, Miralles C, et al. Skeletal muscle apoptosis and weight loss in chronic obstructive pulmonary disease. Am J Respir Crit Care Med 2002; 166:485–9.

85. Agusti AGN, Morla M, Sauleda J, et al. NF-kappaB activation and iNOS upregulation in skeletal muscle of patients with COPD and low body weight. Thorax 2004; 59:483–7.

86. Serres I, Gautier V, Varray A, Prefaut C. Impaired skeletal muscle endurance related to physical inactivity and altered lung function in COPD patients. Chest 1998; 113(4):900–5.

87. Casaburi R. Skeletal muscle function in COPD. Chest 2000; 117(5 Suppl. 1):267S–71.

88. Clark CJ, Cochrane LM, Mackay E, Paton B. Skeletal muscle strength and endurance in patients with mild COPD and the effects of weight training. Eur Respir J 2000; 15(1):92–7.

89. Wasswa-Kintu S, Gan WQ, Man SF, Pare PD, Sin DD. Relationship between reduced forced expiratory volume in one second and the risk of lung cancer: a systematic review and meta-analysis. Thorax 2005; 60(7):570–5.

90. Malhotra S, Lam S, Man SF, Gan WQ, Sin DD. The relationship between stage 1 and 2 non-small cell lung cancer and lung function in men and women. BMC Pulm Med 2006; 6:2.

91. Merlo A, Gabrielson E, Mabry M, Vollmer R, Baylin SB, Sidransky D. Homozygous deletion on chromosome 9p and loss of heterozygosity on 9q, 6p, and 6q in primary human small cell lung cancer. Cancer Res 1994; 54(9):2322–6.

92. Bailey-Wilson JE, Amos CI, Pinney SM, Petersen GM, de Andrade M, Wiest JS, Fain P, Schwartz AG, You M, Franklin W, et al. A major lung cancer susceptibility locus maps to chromosome 6q23-25. Am J Hum Genet 2004; 75(3):460–74.

93. Takeuchi S, Mori N, Koike M, et al. Frequent loss of heterozygosity in region of the KIP1 locus in non-small cell lung cancer: evidence for a new tumor suppressor gene on the short arm of chromosome 12. Cancer Res 1996; 56(4):738–40.

94. Yang P, Wentzlaff KA, Katzmann JA, et al. Alpha1-antitrypsin deficiency allele carriers among lung cancer patients. Cancer Epidemiol Biomarkers Prev 1999; 8(5):461–5.

95. Park JY, Chen L, Lee J, Sellers T, Tockman MS. Polymorphisms in the promoter region of neutrophil elastase gene and lung cancer risk. Lung Cancer 2005; 48(3):315–21.

96. Taniguchi K, Yang P, Jett J, et al. Polymorphisms in the promoter region of the neutrophil elastase gene are associated with lung cancer development. Clin Cancer Res 2002; 8(4):1115–20.

97. Schwartz AG, Ruckdeschel JC. Familial lung cancer: genetic susceptibility and relationship to chronic obstructive pulmonary disease. Am J Respir Crit Care Med 2006; 173(1):16–22.

98. Yanai M, Hatazawa J, Ojima F, Sasaki H, Itoh M, Ido T. Deposition and clearance of inhaled 18FDG powder in patients with chronic obstructive pulmonary disease. Eur Respir J 1998; 11(6):1342–8.

99. Maestrelli P, Paska C, Saetta M, et al. Decreased haem oxygenase-1 and increased inducible nitric oxide synthase in the lung of severe COPD patients. Eur Respir J 2003; 21(6):971–6.

100. Barthelemy-Brichant N, David JL, Bosquee L, et al. Increased TGFbeta1 plasma level in patients with lung cancer: potential mechanisms. Eur J Clin Invest 2002; 32(3):193–8.

101. Sin DD, Man JP, Man SF. The risk of osteoporosis in Caucasian men and women with obstructive airways disease. Am J Med 2003; 114(1):10–4.

102. Jørgensen NR, Schwarz P, Holme I, Henriksen BM, Petersen LJ, Backer V. The prevalence of osteoporosis in patients with chronic obstructive pulmonary disease: a cross sectional study. Respir Med 2007; 101:177–85.

103. de Vries F, van Staa TP, Bracke MS, Cooper C, Leufkens HG, Lammers JW. Severity of obstructive airway disease and risk of osteoporotic fracture. Eur Respir J 2005; 25(5):879–84.

104. Lee TA, Weiss KB. Fracture risk associated with inhaled corticosteroid use in chronic obstructive pulmonary disease. Am J Respir Crit Care Med 2004; 169(7):855–9.

105. Suissa S, Baltzan M, Kremer R, Ernst P. Inhaled and nasal corticosteroid use and the risk of fracture. Am J Respir Crit Care Med 2004; 169(1):83–8.

106. Biskobing DM. COPD and osteoporosis. Chest 2002; 121:609–20.

107. Eiser N. Anxiety and depression in COPD. In: Similowski T, Whitelaw WA, Derenne J-P, eds. Clinical Management of Chronic Obstructive Pulmonary Disease. New York: Marcel Dekker Inc., 2002:549–82.

108. Gudmundsson G, Gislason T, Janson C, et al. Depression, anxiety and health status after hospitalisation for COPD: a multicentre study in the Nordic countries. Respir Med 2006; 100(1):87–93.

109. Gudmundsson G, Gislason T, Janson C, et al. Risk factors for rehospitalisation in COPD: role of health status, anxiety and depression. Eur Respir J 2005; 26(3):414–9.

110. Light RW, Merrill EJ, Despars JA, Gordon GH, Mutalipassi LR. Prevalence of depression and anxiety in patients with COPD. Relationship to functional capacity. Chest 1985; 87(1):35–8.

111. Withers NJ, Rudkin ST, White RJ. Anxiety and depression in severe chronic obstructive pulmonary disease: the effects of pulmonary rehabilitation. J Cardiopulm Rehabil 1999; 19(6):362–5.

112. Eiser N, West C, Evans S, Jeffers A, Quirk F. Effects of psychotherapy in moderately severe COPD: a pilot study. Eur Respir J 1997; 10(7):1581–4.
113. de Godoy DV, de Godoy RF. A randomized controlled trial of the effect of psychotherapy on anxiety and depression in chronic obstructive pulmonary disease. Arch Phys Med Rehabil 2003; 84(8):1154–7.
114. Guell R, Resqueti V, Sangenis M, et al. Impact of pulmonary rehabilitation on psychosocial morbidity in patients with severe COPD. Chest 2006; 129(4):899–904.
115. Garuti G, Cilione C, Dell'Orso D, et al. Impact of comprehensive pulmonary rehabilitation on anxiety and depression in hospitalized COPD patients. Monaldi Arch Chest Dis 2003; 59(1):56–61.
116. Celli BR, Cote CG, Marin JM, et al. The body-mass index, airflow obstruction, dyspnea, and exercise capacity index in chronic obstructive pulmonary disease. N Engl J Med 2004; 350(10):1005–12.
117. Antonelli-Incalzi R, Imperiale C, Bellia V, et al. Do GOLD stages of COPD severity really correspond to differences in health status? Eur Respir J 2003; 22:444–9.
118. Domingo-Salvany A, Lamarca R, Ferrer M, et al. Health-related quality of life and mortality in male patients with chronic obstructive pulmonary disease. Am J Respir Crit Care Med 2002; 166:680–5.
119. Oga T, Nishimura K, Tsukino M, Sato S, Hajiro T. Analysis of the factors related to mortality in chronic obstructive pulmonary disease: role of exercise capacity and health status. Am J Respir Crit Care Med 2003; 167:544–9.

10

The Pulmonary Vasculature of COPD

JOAN ALBERT BARBERÀ
Servei de Pneumologia, Hospital Clínic, Universitat de Barcelona, Barcelona, Spain

I. Introduction

Pulmonary hypertension is a frequent complication of chronic obstructive pulmonary disease (COPD). Its presence is associated with shorter survival, more frequent exacerbation episodes, and greater need of health resources. At present, there is no specific and effective treatment for this condition in COPD. However, recent advances in the understanding of the pathobiology of pulmonary hypertensive states, along with the development of effective treatments for pulmonary arterial hypertension, have opened a new perspective that might be relevant in COPD.

II. Epidemiology

The actual prevalence of pulmonary hypertension in COPD is not known, because it has not been screened systematically using right heart catheterization in the wide clinical spectrum of COPD. Hemodynamic data currently available are limited to patients with advanced disease. Three recent studies have provided data in large series of patients, most of them in Global Initiative for Chronic Obstructive Lung Disease Stage IV.

Scharf et al. (1) evaluated 120 patients with severe emphysema [forced expiratory volume in one second (FEV_1), 27% pred.], screened for lung volume reduction surgery (LVRS). In this population, the incidence of pulmonary hypertension, defined as a mean pulmonary artery pressure (PAP) > 20 mmHg, was very high (91%), although in the majority of patients (86%) it was mild to moderate (20–35 mmHg). Only in 5% of patients, PAP exceeded 35 mmHg. The correlation between PAP and lung function was very weak [FEV_1 (r^2 0.11) and PaO_2 (r^2 0.03)], although statistically significant. PAP was more closely related to pulmonary artery occlusion pressure (r^2 0.32), which was slightly increased in the majority of patients, likely suggesting the potential effect of gas trapping in raising pulmonary capillary pressure.

Chaouat et al. (2) evaluated retrospectively the results of 998 pulmonary hemodynamic studies performed in COPD patients. They identified 27 patients with severe pulmonary hypertension, defined as a PAP > 40 mmHg. Sixteen of them had another disease capable of causing pulmonary hypertension. In the remaining 11 (1.1% of the whole group), COPD was the only cause. Interestingly, this subset of patients had moderate airway obstruction (FEV$_1$, 50% pred.), severe hypoxemia, hypercapnia, and very low carbon monoxide diffusion capacity (DLCO). Survival was shorter than in the other patients. These findings indicate that there is a subset of COPD patients with "out of proportion" pulmonary hypertension that share some clinical features with idiopathic pulmonary arterial hypertension.

Thabut et al. (3) evaluated 215 patients with severe COPD (FEV$_1$, 24% pred.), candidates to LVRS, or lung transplantation. Pulmonary hypertension, defined as a PAP > 25 mmHg, was present in 50% of the patients, although in the majority of them it was mild (26–35 mmHg). In 9.8% pulmonary hypertension was moderate (36–45 mmHg) and in 3.7% severe (> 45 mmHg). A cluster analysis identified a subset of patients characterized by moderate impairment of airway function and high levels of PAP, along with severe arterial hypoxemia, thus supporting the concept of the existence of a subgroup of COPD patients with out of proportion pulmonary hypertension.

In patients with moderate disease stages, the prevalence of pulmonary hypertension is considered to be low. Yet, in these patients pulmonary hypertension might not be present at rest but develop during exercise. Indeed, patients with exercise-induced pulmonary hypertension are more prone to develop resting pulmonary hypertension at long term (4). The exact prevalence of exercise pulmonary hypertension in patients with moderate COPD is unknown, but it might be elevated. In a study conducted in 131 patients with moderate COPD (FEV$_1$, 45% pred.) who did not have pulmonary hypertension at rest, 58% of the patients developed pulmonary hypertension during exercise (4).

Furthermore, histological evaluation of lung tissue samples from patients with mild-to-moderate COPD have revealed significant vascular changes in the majority of cases (5–7), although the clinical significant of these anatomical abnormalities remains to be established.

Overall, it can be concluded that pulmonary hypertension is common in patients with severe COPD; that in patients with moderate-to-severe disease it might not be apparent at rest but develop during exercise; and that there is a subgroup of patients (1–3% depending on the series) who show severe pulmonary hypertension, out of proportion to the degree of airway impairment.

The presence of pulmonary hypertension in COPD is associated with shorter survival rate. In a longitudinal seven-year study of 50 patients with COPD, Burrows et al. (8) showed that their survival was inversely related to pulmonary vascular resistance (PVR), and that the correlation of survival with PVR was similar to that shown with FEV$_1$. In a 15-year follow-up study conducted in 200 patients, Traver et al. (9) showed that, after correcting for age, the presence or absence of cor pulmonale was one of the best predictors of mortality. In 1981, Weitzenblum et al. (10) showed in 175 patients with COPD that those with PAP > 20 mmHg had shorter survival than those whose PAP was normal. It should be noted that these studies were conducted before long-term oxygen therapy (LTOT) was introduced as a regular treatment for chronic respiratory failure in COPD. In a more recent study by Oswald-Mammoser et al. (11), performed in 84 patients receiving LTOT, these authors showed that PAP was the single best predictor of mortality. The five-year survival rate was 36% in patients with PAP > 25 mmHg, whereas in patients with PAP < 25 mmHg the survival rate was 62% (11). Interestingly, in this study neither the FEV$_1$ nor the degree of hypoxemia or hypercapnia had prognostic value (11).

Furthermore, two recent studies have shown that echocardiographic signs of right ventricular dysfunction (12), and electrocardiographic signs of right ventricular hypertrophy or right atrial overload (13), are predictive of survival in COPD.

In addition to the prognostic significance in relation to survival, the presence of pulmonary hypertension in COPD is also associated with a poorer clinical evolution and more frequent use of health care resources (14). In a group of 64 patients admitted to the hospital because of an exacerbation, Kessler et al. (14) showed that the presence of a PAP > 18 mmHg was one of the best predictors of an increased risk of hospitalization for acute exacerbation in the subsequent months. Interestingly, in this series, parameters commonly used to assess disease severity, namely FEV_1 or PaO_2, were not related to the risk of hospitalization (14). These findings suggest that patients with an abnormal pulmonary vascular bed might have lesser functional reserve to overcome the potential complications that occur during exacerbations, hence requiring hospital admission more frequently.

III. Pathology

In COPD, pulmonary vessels can undergo profound fibrocellular changes that lead to an enlargement of the vessel wall, an active process broadly defined as vascular remodeling. Pulmonary vascular remodeling in COPD affects preferentially small and precapillary arteries and has been identified at different degrees of COPD severity.

In patients with end-stage COPD and pulmonary hypertension or cor pulmonale, *postmortem* studies have shown deposition of longitudinal muscle, fibrosis, and elastosis that produce the enlargement of the intima in pulmonary muscular arteries (15,16). In the arterioles there is development of a medial coat of circular smooth muscle, bounded by a new elastic lamina, with deposition of longitudinal muscle and fibrosis of the intima (15,16).

In lung tissue specimens obtained at LVRS, Santos et al. (17) showed significant enlargement of the intima, when compared with patients with mild COPD and control nonsmokers. Conversely, medial thickness was slightly reduced in patients with severe emphysema, when compared with patients with milder disease (17).

In patients with mild-to-moderate disease, morphometric studies of pulmonary muscular arteries have shown enlargement of the intimal layer with reduction of the lumen size (Fig. 1) (5,6,18). Intimal enlargement occurs in muscular arteries of different sizes, although it is more pronounced in small arteries with an external diameter less than 500 μm (5,18). In addition, the number of small pulmonary muscular arteries, with diameter < 200 μm, is increased (19), indicating muscularization of arterioles. Intimal hyperplasia results from proliferation of poorly differentiated smooth muscle cells and deposition of elastic and collagen fibers (20) (Fig. 1). Changes in the media of muscular arteries are less conspicuous and the majority of morphometric studies have failed to show differences in the thickness of the muscular layer when comparing patients with mild-to-moderate COPD with control subjects (5,6,18).

Structural changes in pulmonary arteries are not restricted to patients with an established diagnosis of COPD. Indeed, intimal thickening, the magnitude of which does not differ from that seen in patients with mild COPD, also occurs in heavy smokers who have normal lung function (6).

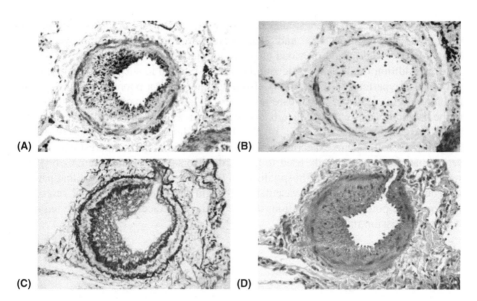

Figure 1 Serial sections of a pulmonary muscular artery from a patient with chronic obstructive pulmonary disease. Artery shows prominent intimal hyperplasia and luminal narrowing. Immunostaining for α-smooth muscle (**A**) denotes intimal proliferation of smooth muscle cells, although not all them showed immunoreactivity to desmin (**B**) a contractile filament expressed in mature smooth muscle cells, indicating a poorly differentiated state. Staining for elastic (**C**) and collagen (**D**) fibers revealed marked elastosis and fibrosis in the intima.

IV. Pathophysiology and Natural History of Pulmonary Hypertension

In COPD pulmonary hypertension is considered to be present when mean PAP exceeds the upper normal limit of 20 mmHg (10,21). In general, the degree of pulmonary hypertension in COPD is of low-to-moderate magnitude, rarely exceeding 35 to 40 mmHg. Both right atrial pressure and pulmonary capillary wedge pressure tend to be normal, as well as the cardiac output (8,21,22). This hemodynamic profile contrasts with other causes of pulmonary hypertension (idiopathic pulmonary arterial hypertension, congenital heart disease, thromboembolic disease) where PAP can reach extremely high values, close to those of the systemic circulation, and the cardiac output is usually reduced.

Pulmonary hypertension in COPD progresses over time and its severity correlates with the degree of airflow obstruction and the impairment of pulmonary gas exchange (1,23). However, the rate of progression of pulmonary hypertension in COPD is slow and usually PAP is only moderately elevated, even in patients who have advanced disease (1). Weitzenblum et al. (23) studied the evolution of PAP in a group of 93 patients with COPD for about five years. They found that PAP increased at an average rate of 0.6 mmHg/yr (23). The rate of increase of PAP was slightly higher in patients who did not have pulmonary hypertension at the beginning of the study when compared with those who already had pulmonary hypertension (23). Nevertheless, the evolution of PAP was more closely linked to the evolution of arterial blood gases than to the initial PAP value (23).

An intriguing question is when pulmonary hypertension commences in the natural history of COPD. Kessler et al. (4) assessed the evolution of pulmonary hemodynamics in patients with moderate COPD without pulmonary hypertension at rest, although 58% of the patients developed it during exercise. In a second study, performed seven years later, PAP had increased by 2.6 mmHg, with an annual rise of 0.4 mmHg/yr. In this second study, 25% of the patients already had pulmonary hypertension at rest. Interestingly, the incidence of resting pulmonary hypertension was greater in the group of patients who at the initial catheterization developed pulmonary hypertension during exercise (32%) than in those without exercise-induced pulmonary hypertension (16%). A logistic regression analysis showed that the PAP value during exercise was an independent predictor for the subsequent development of pulmonary hypertension (4). These results indicate that in COPD changes in pulmonary circulation may start several years before pulmonary hypertension is apparent at rest, and that exercise testing might be useful to show-up abnormalities of pulmonary circulation. These observations are consistent with morphometric studies showing conspicuous changes in the structure of pulmonary muscular arteries in patients with mild COPD (5,6).

A. Hypoxic Pulmonary Vasoconstriction

Pulmonary arteriolar constriction in response to hypoxia reduces perfusion in poorly ventilated or nonventilated lung units and diverts it to better ventilated units, thereby restoring ventilation–perfusion (V_A/Q) equilibrium and increasing PaO_2. Hypoxic vasoconstriction plays an important role in matching pulmonary blood flow to alveolar ventilation in COPD where hypoxemia and hypercapnia are predominantly due to V_A/Q mismatching (24).

Studies using the multiple inert gas elimination technique (25) have shown that in COPD the inhibition of hypoxic pulmonary vasoconstriction with O_2 breathing worsens V_A/Q distributions in patients with different degrees of disease severity (24). In general terms, the contribution of hypoxic vasoconstriction to V_A/Q matching tends to be greater in patients with less severe COPD (5,26). Indeed, hypoxic pulmonary vasoconstriction is less active in patients with severe structural impairment of pulmonary muscular arteries (5). Furthermore, in isolated pulmonary artery rings it has been shown that the magnitude of contraction induced by the hypoxic stimulus is inversely related to the endothelial function and directly related to the arterial PO_2 (27), suggesting that the impairment of endothelial function is associated with an altered response to hypoxic stimulus that further worsens gas exchange. The contribution of hypoxic vasoconstriction to gas exchange in COPD should be taken into account when administering drugs that might potentially inhibit such a response since they may also impair gas exchange (28–31).

B. Right Ventricular Function

In patients with COPD and pulmonary hypertension, the PAP is not markedly elevated and the rate of progression of pulmonary hypertension is slow. Therefore, the right ventricle has time to adapt to such a modest increase in afterload. When PAP is chronically elevated, the right ventricle dilates and both end-diastolic and end-systolic volumes increase. The stroke volume of the right ventricle is usually maintained, whereas the ejection fraction decreases. Subsequent hypertrophy of the right ventricular wall in persistent pulmonary hypertension reduces its tension and hence the afterload.

The reduction in right ventricular ejection fraction (RVEF) is inversely related to PAP (32). Nonetheless, a decrease in RVEF does not mean that there is true ventricular dysfunction (33). Assessments of end-systolic pressure–volume relationships have shown that in clinically stable COPD patients contractility of the right ventricle lies within normal limits, irrespective of the PAP value (34,35). However, during exacerbations, when PAP increases markedly, the contractility of the right ventricle is reduced in patients presenting clinical signs of right heart failure (36,37).

Cardiac output in COPD is usually preserved and might rise during exacerbation episodes (38,39), even when there are apparent signs of right heart failure. Therefore, the usual definition of heart failure as a reduction in cardiac output does not apply in this condition. In fact, the true occurrence of right heart failure in COPD has been questioned and currently there is controversy about the concept of cor pulmonale (36). It has been proposed that this term should be abandoned in favor of a more precise definition based on the objective evidence of right ventricular hypertrophy, enlargement, functional abnormality, or failure (36).

C. Peripheral Edema

Peripheral edema may be a sign of venous congestion secondary to upstream transmission of right ventricular filling pressures. However, in advanced COPD edema is more related to hypercapnia rather than to raised jugular pressures (40,41). Some patients may present peripheral edema without hemodynamic signs of right heart failure or significant changes in PAP (42,43). This has lead to the reconsideration of peripheral edema formation in COPD (36,37,41,44,45).

In COPD, peripheral edema results from a complex interaction between the hemodynamic changes and the balance between edema-promoting and edema-protective mechanisms. In patients with pulmonary hypertension associated with chronic respiratory failure, both hypoxemia and hypercapnia aggravate venous congestion by further activating the sympathetic nervous system, which is already stimulated by right atrial distension. Sympathetic activation decreases renal plasma flow, stimulates the renin–angiotensin–aldosterone system, and promotes tubular absorption of bicarbonate, sodium, and water. Vasopressin also contributes to edema formation. It is released when patients become hyponatremic and its plasma levels rise in patients with hypoxemia and hypercapnia (44).

Atrial natriuretic peptide is released from distended atrial walls and may act as an edema-protective mechanism since it has vasodilator, diuretic, and natriuretic effects. Nevertheless, these effects are usually insufficient to counterbalance the edema-promoting mechanisms.

Peripheral edema may develop or worsen during exacerbation episodes. Analyzing the changes from stable conditions that took place during an exacerbation episode, Weitzenblum et al. (39) identified a subgroup of patients with more marked peripheral edema that was attributed to hemodynamic signs of right heart failure (increase in end-diastolic pressure). Compared with patients with normal end-diastolic pressure, patients with right heart failure had more marked increase in PAP, and more severe hypoxemia and hypercapnia. This suggests that worsening of pulmonary hypertension during exacerbations contributes to edema formation.

D. Exercise

Exercise produces an abnormal increase in PAP, especially in patients who have pulmonary hypertension at rest (8). Patients who appear to be more prone to the development of pulmonary hypertension may show an abnormal increase in PAP during exercise years before pulmonary hypertension is apparent at rest (4). Different studies have identified a number of mechanisms for exercise-induced pulmonary hypertension in COPD, including hypoxic vasoconstriction, reduction of the capillary bed by emphysema, extramural compression by increased alveolar pressure, or impaired release of endothelium-derived relaxing factors (5,30,46,47) that may combine and contribute to the development of pulmonary hypertension during exercise. In COPD, PAP during exercise is greater than predicted by the PVR equation, suggesting active pulmonary vasoconstriction on exertion (30). The latter may be due to the enhancement of hypoxic pulmonary vasoconstriction by decreased mixed venous PO_2, increased tone of the sympathetic nervous system, and/or decreased arterial pH (48). During exercise, patients may develop dynamic hyperinflation due the expiratory flow limitation that results in increased alveolar pressure, which is transmitted to the capillary wedge pressure (49). Furthermore, increased ventilation during exercise, in the presence of airflow obstruction, results in significant swings of intrathoracic pressure that may reduce cardiac output by altering systemic venous return or by increasing left ventricular afterload (50). Impairment of endothelial release of vasorelaxing agents like nitric oxide (NO) may also contribute to an impaired dilator response to increases in flow (51). However, in a group of COPD patients who developed pulmonary hypertension during exercise, the exogenous supply of NO did not block the abnormal increase in PAP, suggesting that the defective release of NO is not a major player in exercise-induced pulmonary hypertension in COPD (52).

Since pulmonary hypertension may develop at moderate levels of exercise, it has been suggested that repeated episodes of pulmonary hypertension during daily activities like stairs climbing, or even walking, could contribute to the development of right ventricular hypertrophy (53).

V. Pathobiology

The field of vascular biology has experienced a tremendous progress over the last decades, since the seminal studies by Furchgott and Zawadzki identifying the key role of endothelium in the regulation of vascular homeostasis (54). Endothelial dysfunction is a common disturbance in hypertensive states of both systemic and pulmonary circulation. Vascular actions of endothelium are mediated through the balanced release of potent vasoactive mediators, such as NO, prostacyclin, endothelin-1 (ET-1), and angiotensin. Some of these mediators also possess antiproliferative and anti-inflammatory properties.

Endothelial dysfunction has been shown in pulmonary arteries of both end-stage (55) and early mild (6) COPD patients. Impairment of endothelial function results from changes in the expression and release of vasoactive mediators. Endothelium-derived NO is a potent endogenous vasodilator with antiproliferative properties in the vessel wall. In pulmonary arteries of COPD patients with pulmonary hypertension, the expression of endothelial nitric oxide synthase (eNOS) is reduced (56). Interestingly, in smokers eNOS expression is also reduced (57), likely explaining endothelial dysfunction shown at early disease states (6). Prostacyclin, which is also synthesized by endothelial cells, exerts similar actions than NO. Nana-Sinkam et al. (58) have recently shown that the expression of prostacyclin synthase is reduced in pulmonary arteries of patients with severe emphysema.

ET-1 is a potent vasoconstrictor that also exerts a mitogenic effect on arterial smooth muscle cells. Its expression is increased in pulmonary arteries of patients with COPD and pulmonary hypertension (59), but not in patients with mild-to-moderate disease (57,60).

These findings indicate that endothelial dysfunction, with changes in the expression and release of endothelium-derived vasoactive mediators that regulate cell growth, is a common feature in COPD. It may appear early in the natural history of the disease and conform the basis for further changes in vascular structure and function induced by additional factors. Different factors might be at the origin of pulmonary endothelial damage in COPD.

Hypoxia is a potential mechanism that may explain endothelial cell damage and vascular remodeling in COPD. Hypoxia may downregulate eNOS expression and induce smooth muscle cell and adventitial fibroblast proliferation (61,62). In addition, hypoxia elicits the contraction of pulmonary arteries. However, the role of hypoxia as the major etiological factor for pulmonary vascular impairment in COPD is being reconsidered. First, COPD patients show wide variation in the individual response of the pulmonary circulation to changes in inspired oxygen concentration (5,63), and the correlation between PaO_2 and PAP is weak (1). Second, LTOT does not reverse pulmonary hypertension completely (64). Third, structural abnormalities and endothelial dysfunction in pulmonary arteries can be observed in patients with mild COPD who do not have hypoxemia and also in smokers with normal lung function (5–7). Therefore, hypoxia does not completely explain changes occurring in pulmonary circulation of COPD.

Inflammation might play a role in the pathogenesis of pulmonary vascular abnormalities associated with COPD, although its precise effect has not been established yet. The inflammatory infiltrate of small airways is associated with intimal hyperplasia of pulmonary muscular arteries (5). Further, there is an increased number of CD8 + T-lymphocytes infiltrating the adventitia of pulmonary arteries in patients with mild-to-moderate COPD (7). Inflammatory cells are a source of cytokines and growth factors that may target the endothelial cells and contribute to the development of structural and functional abnormalities of the vessel wall. Indeed, the number of inflammatory cells infiltrating the pulmonary arteries is inversely related to the endothelial function and directly related to intimal hyperplasia (7). Smokers with normal lung function also exhibit an increased number of CD8 + T-cells with a reduction of the CD4 + /CD8 + ratio in the arterial adventitia, when compared with nonsmokers (7). This suggests that cigarette smoking might induce inflammatory changes in pulmonary arteries at stages when there are no detectable alterations in the lung function examination.

Cigarette smoke products might exert a direct effect on pulmonary vessel structure and function. Smokers with normal lung function show prominent changes in pulmonary arteries, such as smooth muscle cell proliferation (6,20), impairment of endothelial function (6), reduced expression of eNOS (57), increased expression of vascular endothelial growth factor (VEGF) (17), and CD8 + T-cell infiltrate (7). Most of these changes are indistinguishable from those seen in COPD patients, and differ clearly from nonsmokers. Some of these observations have been replicated in a guinea pig model chronically exposed to cigarette smoke (65). In that model, exposure to cigarette smoke induces muscularization of precapillary vessels and increased PAP (66). Interestingly, vascular abnormalities are detectable after two months of cigarette smoke exposure, when there is no evidence of emphysema (66), thereby implicating that cigarette smoke–induced vascular abnormalities may antecede the development of pulmonary emphysema (67). Furthermore, in that model cigarette smoke exposure induces rapid changes in gene expression of VEGF, VEGF receptor-1, ET-1, and inducible NOS (68), mediators that regulate vascular cell growth and vessel contraction, and that are likely involved in the pathogenesis of pulmonary vascular changes of COPD.

Cigarette smoking is a well-known risk factor for the development of vascular disease. Active and passive exposure to tobacco smoke produces endothelial dysfunction in both coronary and systemic arteries (69). Exposure of pulmonary artery endothelial cells to cigarette smoke extract causes the inhibition of both eNOS and prostacyclin synthase at the level of protein content and mRNA expression (58,70). Cigarette smoke contains a number of products that have the potential to produce endothelial injury, among those the aldehyde acrolein seems to play a prominent role since it reduces the expression of prostacyclin synthase in endothelial cells (58).

In summary, there is emerging evidence suggesting that the initial event in the natural history of pulmonary hypertension in COPD could be pulmonary endothelial injury by cigarette smoke products with the subsequent downregulation of eNOS and prostacyclin synthase expression, and impairment of endothelial function. When disease progresses, sustained exposure to hypoxemia and inflammation may induce further pulmonary vascular remodeling, thus amplifying the initial effects of cigarette smoke (Fig. 2).

VI. Evaluation and Diagnosis of Pulmonary Hypertension in COPD

Recognition of pulmonary hypertension in COPD is difficult, especially in its mildest form. Symptoms due to pulmonary hypertension, such as dyspnea or fatigue, are difficult to differentiate from the clinical picture of COPD. Furthermore, the identification of some clinical signs may be obscured by chest hyperinflation or the large swings in intrathoracic pressure. Usually, the main suspicion is based on the presence of peripheral edema, but as discussed earlier, this may not be a sign of right ventricular failure in COPD. Cardiac sounds may be disturbed by the presence of bronchial rales or overinflated lungs. Thus, the typical auscultatory findings of pulmonary hypertension (ejection click or increased pulmonary component of the second heart sound, and pansystolic murmur of tricuspid regurgitation) are uncommon in COPD patients.

A. Conventional Examinations

Chest Radiography

The most characteristic radiographic pattern of pulmonary hypertension is the increase of the vascular hilum size with oligohemia in the peripheral lung fields. Other signs of pulmonary hypertension are cardiomegaly due to an enlarged right ventricle and

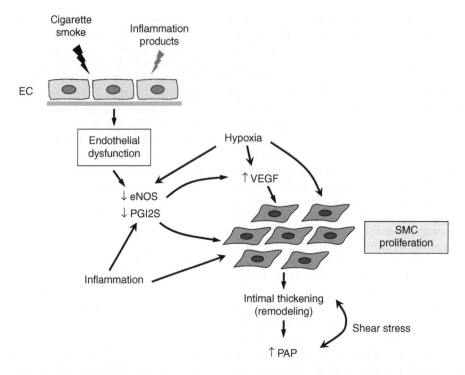

Figure 2   Pathobiology of pulmonary hypertension in chronic obstructive pulmonary disease (COPD). Cigarette smoke products or inflammation may initiate the sequence of changes by producing endothelial dysfunction. *Abbreviations*: EC, endothelial cell; eNOS, endothelial nitric oxide synthase; PAP, pulmonary artery pressure; PGI2S, prostacyclin synthase; SMC, smooth muscle cells; VEGF, vascular endothelial growth factor.

enlarged pulmonary trunk. Widening of the hilium can be estimated by the hiliar thoracic index, which is defined by the ratio of the transhiliar width (distance between the start of divisions of the right and left main pulmonary arteries) to the transverse diameter of the thorax (71). A ratio greater than 0.36 suggests pulmonary hypertension (71,72). Another potential indicator is the widening of the descending right pulmonary artery diameter (usually under 16 mm) to over 18 mm. The enlarged right ventricle accounts for an increased cardiothoracic ratio above 0.5 and, on the lateral view, the encroachment of the retrosternal airspace. However, it must be noted that the sensitivity of chest radiography to detect pulmonary hypertension is low (73), and that in COPD these radiological signs may be difficult to identify.

Electrocardiogram

The sensitivity of the electrocardiogram to detect right ventricular hypertrophy is relatively low and electrocardiographic changes are not closely related to the severity of pulmonary hypertension (72). Electrocardiographic changes associated with pulmonary hypertension include: (*i*) a P-pulmonale pattern suggesting right atrial overload in leads II, III, and aVF; (*ii*) an $S_1S_2S_3$ pattern; (*iii*) an S_1Q_3 pattern; (*iv*) incomplete right bundle branch block; (*v*) right ventricular hypertrophy, as defined by a QRS axis of $+120°$ or more, a predominant R wave in V1, or an R/S amplitude ratio in V5 and V6 < 1 (at least two of these three criteria are sufficient to raise suspicion of right ventricular hypertrophy); and (*vi*) low voltage QRS (13,72). Incalzi et al. (13) assessed the prognostic value of these electrocardiographic changes in 217 patients with COPD, who were followed up to 13 years after an exacerbation episode. Both the $S_1S_2S_3$ pattern and signs of right atrial overload were associated with shorter survival rates (13). Oswald-Mammoser et al. (73) compared the sensitivity and specificity of different noninvasive techniques for predicting the presence of pulmonary hypertension in COPD. Electrocardiographic changes had a specificity of 86% and a sensitivity of 51% in detecting pulmonary hypertension. These values compared favorably with chest radiography (73). Given the simplicity and low cost of ECG, it is recommended to use it for identifying those patients more likely to suffer pulmonary hypertension.

Lung Function Testing

Lung function tests are necessary for the diagnosis of COPD. Unfortunately, there are no specific patterns of pulmonary function impairment associated with the development of pulmonary hypertension. Pulmonary hypertension has little effect per se on lung mechanics or gas exchange. In conditions of preserved lung parenchyma, pulmonary hypertension can reduce carbon monoxide diffusion capacity (DLCO). However, in COPD the decrease of DLCO cannot be attributed to pulmonary hypertension since it can be explained by lung emphysema.

B. Echocardiography

Echocardiography is an important diagnostic step in any patient with suspected pulmonary hypertension. It is noninvasive, easily available; it allows the assessment of right ventricular hypertrophy and/or dilatation; ejection flow dynamics; and may also provide an estimate of PAP (74). However, this method presents technical difficulties in COPD patients because overinflated chests may alter sound wave transmission.

Two-dimensional echocardiography provides information on the morphology and dynamics of cardiac structures and it is also essential for the diagnosis of associated left heart disease. Typical signs of pulmonary hypertension are right ventricular and atrial enlargement with a normal or reduced left ventricular cavity, and eventually reversal of the normal septal curvature. In the presence of tricuspid regurgitation, continuous wave Doppler echocardiography may provide an estimate of systolic PAP. However, tricuspid regurgitation is not always present in COPD, its incidence ranges from 24% to 66% (74–76), thus limiting the possibility to estimate PAP in a number of patients. In a recent study by Arcasoy et al. (77) conducted in 374 lung transplant candidates, estimation of systolic PAP was possible in 166 patients (44%). However, when compared with right heart catheter measurements, 52% of PAP estimations were found to be inaccurate and 48% of patients were misclassified as having pulmonary hypertension by echocardiography. Overall, positive and negative predictive values of systolic PAP estimation for the diagnosis of pulmonary hypertension were 52% and 87%, respectively (77).

Systolic indices of tricuspid valve annular motion measured by tissue Doppler imaging appear to be useful for the prediction of right ventricular failure in patients with COPD (78). Furthermore, exercise echocardiography allows the identification of abnormal ventricular septal motion with distortion of left ventricle in COPD, findings that may help detect occult right ventricular dysfunction (79).

C. Right Heart Catheterization

Right heart catheterization is the gold standard for the diagnosis of pulmonary hypertension. The procedure allows direct measurements of PAP, cardiac output, and PVR. It can be also used to assess the acute effects of therapeutic interventions. Right heart catheterization is a safe procedure in expert hands, but because of its invasive nature, it is not routinely recommended in the assessment of patients with COPD. Nevertheless, in selected cases right heart catheterization might be indicated: patients with severe pulmonary hypertension (i.e., estimated systolic PAP > 50 mmHg) that might be suitable from specific treatment; patients with frequent episodes of right ventricular failure; and in the preoperative evaluation of candidates to lung transplant or LVRS (80).

VII. Treatment

A. Vasodilators

Treatment with vasodilators (i.e., calcium channel blockers) improves symptoms, exercise tolerance, and survival in patients with pulmonary arterial hypertension (81). Accordingly, there is a rationale for the use of vasodilators in COPD in order to decrease PAP and improve both right ventricular function and oxygen delivery, as these effects might increase exercise tolerance and, eventually, survival.

Calcium channel blockers have been extensively evaluated for the treatment of pulmonary hypertension in COPD. The acute administration of nifedipine has been shown to reduce PAP and increase cardiac output in COPD patients studied both at rest and during exercise (30,31,82). However, nifedipine inhibits hypoxic pulmonary vasoconstriction (83), and in COPD this effect worsens V_A/Q relationships and lowers arterial PO_2 (28,30). Similar effects of nifedipine have been shown in exercise-induced pulmonary hypertension. Agustí et al. (30) showed that nifedipine reduced the increase in PVR induced by exercise, but at the same time it worsened V_A/Q distributions and arterial oxygenation. The deleterious effect of vasodilators on V_A/Q distributions in COPD has been also shown with felodipine (84), atrial natriuretic factor (85), and acetylcholine (86).

Clinical results of long-term treatment with calcium channel blockers in COPD have been disappointing. Despite that slight hemodynamic improvement has been observed in some studies (87), in others both pulmonary hemodynamics and clinical status either deteriorated or remained unchanged after several weeks or months of treatment (88,89). In a recent study, Morrell et al. (90) evaluated the effect of the angiotensin II antagonist losartan in a double-blind, placebo-controlled study of 12 months duration. Losartan exerted no significant benefit on systolic PAP, exercise capacity or symptoms in COPD patients with pulmonary hypertension (90).

The effects of selective pulmonary vasodilators have also been investigated in COPD. Inhaled NO acts as a selective vasodilator of the pulmonary circulation, due to its inactivation when combined with hemoglobin, for which it has a very high affinity. The effect of inhaled NO in COPD has been evaluated by several investigators. When inhaled NO is administered in low concentrations it does not seem to exert any effect on gas exchange, whereas it decreases PAP in a dose-dependent manner (86). When administered in high concentrations (i.e., 40 ppm), it usually decreases PAP and exerts variable effects on gas exchange (26,86), although in general terms it usually decreases PaO_2 (26,52,91). Such a deleterious effect on gas exchange results from worsening of V_A/Q distributions, as shown by an increased perfusion in poorly ventilated lung units with low V_A/Q ratio (26). This finding is consistent with inhibition of hypoxic pulmonary vasoconstriction by NO (92) in poorly ventilated alveolar units to which the gas has access too.

The effects of inhaled NO on gas exchange in COPD appear to be different during exercise than at rest. Roger et al. (52) showed that in COPD, inhaled NO decreased PVR both at rest and during exercise. However, whereas PaO_2 decreased during exercise while breathing room air, no change was shown during NO inhalation. Furthermore, at rest NO inhalation worsened V_A/Q distributions, while during exercise it promoted better V_A/Q matching (52). Such a different effect of inhaled NO during exercise was explained by enhanced distribution of the gas to well-ventilated lung units with faster time constants, which are more efficient in terms of gas exchange. In clinical terms, these findings may imply that if inhaled NO could be delivered specifically to well-ventilated alveolar units with fast time constants, the beneficial vasodilator effect of NO would not be offset by its deleterious impact on gas exchange. This notion has lead to the development of the so-called "spiked" or "pulsed" delivery of NO (93). With this system a small bolus of NO is administered at the beginning of inspiration, with the aim that it will be specifically distributed to alveolar units with fast time constants.

Yoshida et al. (94) showed that combined administration of low doses of NO and oxygen resulted in a significant improvement of pulmonary hemodynamics and provided better oxygenation that when breathing oxygen alone. Whereas the hemodynamic effects of combined NO and oxygen appear to be related to the NO dose, the amelioration in gas exchange seems to have a ceiling effect at a concentration of 5 ppm (95). Vonbank et al. (96) evaluated the combined effect of oxygen and pulsed NO inhalation, compared with oxygen alone, in a randomized study of three months duration. Compared with oxygen alone, the combined inhalation of NO and oxygen caused a significant decrease in mean PAP and PVR, without decreasing arterial oxygenation (96).

Overall, it can be concluded that in COPD systemic vasodilators may produce a slight reduction in PAP and increase cardiac output, but their administration is usually accompanied by gas exchange worsening, and there is no evidence that long-term treatment is of clinical benefit. For these reasons they are not recommended for the treatment of pulmonary hypertension associated with COPD (97). Selective vasodilators, like inhaled NO, exert similar hemodynamic and gas exchange effects. For this reason they should be employed using systems of *pulsed* delivery and in combination with oxygen in patients with chronic respiratory failure. Despite some preliminary promising data (96), the long-term effect of selective vasodilators in terms of survival and symptom relieve remains to be established.

B. Long-Term Oxygen Therapy

Chronic hypoxemia plays a key role in the development of pulmonary hypertension in COPD. Therefore, its correction with supplemental oxygen seems to be an appropriate treatment. In patients with advanced COPD, acute administration of oxygen exerts little effect on pulmonary hemodynamics (26,37,98) or RVEF (35), in patients studied at rest under stable clinical conditions. During acute exacerbation episodes, when PAP increases significantly, controlled administration of oxygen also results in minimal or no change of PAP (98,99). By contrast, when oxygen is administered during exercise it often improves pulmonary hemodynamics (8) and RVEF (100).

The administration of LTOT has been shown to improve survival in COPD patients with chronic hypoxemia. In the two classical studies that showed survival benefits in patients treated with LTOT, the Medical Research Council (MRC) (101) and the Nocturnal Oxygen Therapy trial (NOTT) (102), pulmonary hemodynamic measurements were performed before initiating LTOT and after a long period of follow-up. In the MRC study, PAP remained unaltered in patients receiving LTOT (more than 15 hr/day), whereas in the control group PAP rose by a mean of 2.7 mmHg/yr (101). In the NOTT study, 117 patients were reevaluated after six months of treatment. Whereas in patients receiving continuous LTOT (more than 18 hr/day) PAP decreased by an average of 3 mmHg, it did not change in the group receiving nocturnal LTOT (10–12 hr/day) (102). It should be noted that despite the hemodynamic improvement shown in some patients, in the majority of them PAP values recorded in the follow-up study did not return to normal levels. These results indicate that LTOT may slow down the evolution of pulmonary hypertension in COPD and that it might even reverse its progression when oxygen is administered continuously. Nevertheless, both the MRC and the NOTT studies showed that the decrease in mortality in patients receiving LTOT was not related to changes in pulmonary hemodynamics (101,102). Indeed, the NOTT study clearly demonstrated that ameliorating pulmonary hypertension did not result in improved mortality (102).

The beneficial effects of LTOT on the progression of pulmonary hypertension in COPD were confirmed by Weitzenblum et al. (64) in a small group of patients who were followed for long periods of time before and after initiating LTOT. Before the onset of LTOT, PAP rose by an average of 1.5 mmHg/yr. By contrast, patients receiving LTOT showed a progressive decrease of PAP (-2.2 mmHg/yr) (Fig. 3) (64). It should be noted, however, that despite this improvement the normalization of PAP was rarely observed in the study performed 31 months after initiating LTOT (64). Furthermore, necropsic studies have failed to show significant differences in the structural abnormalities of pulmonary vessels in patients receiving LTOT for long periods of time, when compared with patients who did not receive oxygen treatment (15).

Considering that the hemodynamic response to oxygen administration might be widely variable in COPD, Ashutosh et al. (63) evaluated the long-term effects of oxygen therapy according to its acute effects on pulmonary hemodynamics. These authors showed that survival benefit of LTOT was greater in patients who showed a significant decrease in PAP during the acute administration of oxygen (acute responders) (63).

In summary, LTOT appears to be the more appropriate treatment for pulmonary hypertension in hypoxemic COPD patients since its administration slows down, and sometimes reverses, the progression of pulmonary hypertension. Nevertheless, PAP rarely returns to normal values and the structural abnormalities of pulmonary vessels remain unaltered. It is likely that, in agreement with other forms of pulmonary hypertension (81), a subgroup of patients who are acute responders to oxygen administration might obtain greater benefit from LTOT.

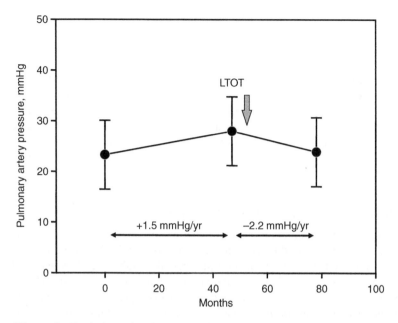

Figure 3 Evolution of pulmonary artery pressure (PAP) in 16 patients with chronic obstructive pulmonary disease (COPD), before and after the onset of long-term oxygen therapy (LTOT). From the initial to the second hemodynamic study PAP increased 4.7 mmHg, at an average rate of 1.5 mmHg/yr. In the third study, performed 31 months after initiating LTOT, PAP decreased from 28 to 23.9 mmHg. These results suggest that LTOT can reverse the progression of pulmonary hypertension in a high percentage of patients with severe COPD, but that normalization of PAP is rarely observed. *Source*: Adapted from Ref. 64.

C. Diuretics

Diuretics are usually administered to COPD patients with peripheral edema in order to reduce sodium and water retention and hence right ventricular workload. Nevertheless, diuretics should be given with caution since they may induce metabolic alkalosis that may aggravate arterial hypercapnia (103). Furthermore, excessive intravascular volume depletion might compromise adequate filling of the afterloaded right ventricle and promote further blood viscosity in polycytemic patients (72). Diuretic treatment is usually instituted with low doses of loop diuretics, such as furosemide (20–40 mg/day). Monitoring of plasma electrolytes is mandatory and potassium or magnesium supplementation may be necessary.

D. Other Treatments

Digitalis has been used for the management of cor pulmonale for many years. However, there is no evidence to support the use of cardiac glycosides in the treatment of right ventricular failure secondary to pulmonary hypertension, unless there is concurrent left ventricular failure (104) or atrial fibrillation (105). Furthermore, cardiac glycosides can induce pulmonary vasoconstriction (44) and the risk of digitalis toxicity is increased in patients with arterial hypoxemia or diuretic-induced hypokalemia.

Bronchodilators may exert some beneficial effects on pulmonary hemodynamics in patients with COPD. Theophylline reduces slightly PVR and improves both right and left ventricular ejection fractions (106). Nevertheless, patients with right ventricular failure have decreased clearance of theophylline, and their plasma levels should be closely controlled. Short-acting β-agonists given by intravenous route exert little effect on PAP. Nevertheless, they increase cardiac output and ventricular performance and, as a result, usually reduce PVR (107,108). However, these effects are frequently accompanied by worsening of arterial oxygenation, due to the inhibitory effect of these drugs on hypoxic pulmonary vasoconstriction (29,108). Such a detrimental effect of β-adrenergic agonists on gas exchange are not seen when they are administered by inhalation (108).

E. New Targeted Therapy for Pulmonary Hypertension

Experience accumulated in pulmonary arterial hypertension, mainly in the idiopathic form and in some associated conditions, indicates that targeted therapy of pulmonary hypertension, addressed to revert or compensate the unbalanced release of endothelium-derived vascular mediators, improves symptoms, exercise performance, pulmonary hemodynamics, and survival (109). Based on this experience and taking into account that the pathogenesis of pulmonary hypertension in COPD shares some common pathways with that of pulmonary arterial hypertension, it is conceivable that drugs that may correct the endothelial vasoconstrictor–dilator imbalance could be of clinical benefit in COPD (48,110).

There are currently three types of drugs that have been successfully used in pulmonary arterial hypertension: prostanoids, endothelin receptor antagonists, and phosphodiesterase-5 inhibitors (111). Prostanoids must be administered by intravenous, subcutaneous, or inhaling route. Stevens et al. (112) reported the use of intravenous epoprostenol in two patients with severe COPD who had severe pulmonary hypertension. In this study, after seven months of treatment one patient had died and the other is still alive (112). There is one case report describing the use of bosentan, a dual endothelin receptor antagonist, in a patient with COPD and associated pulmonary hypertension (113).

Madden et al. (114) reported the use of sildenafil, a phosphodiesterase-5 inhibitor, in seven patients with chronic lung disease, four of them having COPD. After eight weeks, all but one COPD patient experienced improvement in PAP, cardiac output, and exercise tolerance (114). Alp et al. (115) evaluated the acute and long-term effects of sildenafil in six patients with COPD. The acute administration of sildenafil reduced significantly PAP and PVR. Three months of oral therapy resulted in hemodynamic improvement and increased exercise tolerance, as assessed by the six-minute walk test (115).

Overall, these reports suggest a potential role of new targeted therapy in the treatment of pulmonary hypertension associated with COPD. Yet, these preliminary observations should be considered with caution, and the efficacy and security of new targeted therapy for treating pulmonary hypertension in COPD should be assessed in randomized controlled trials before a definitive recommendation could be made. Furthermore, physiological studies must evaluate the role of targeted therapy on pulmonary gas exchange in COPD, since some of these drugs might inhibit hypoxic pulmonary vasoconstriction (116–118), thus entailing the potential risk of worsening gas exchange.

References

1. Scharf SM, Iqbal M, Keller C, Criner G, Lee S, Fessler HE. Hemodynamic characterization of patients with severe emphysema. Am J Respir Crit Care Med 2002; 166:314–22.
2. Chaouat A, Bugnet AS, Kadaoui N, et al. Severe pulmonary hypertension and chronic obstructive pulmonary disease. Am J Respir Crit Care Med 2005; 172:189–94.
3. Thabut G, Dauriat G, Stern JB, et al. Pulmonary hemodynamics in advanced COPD candidates for lung volume reduction surgery or lung transplantation. Chest 2005; 127:1531–6.
4. Kessler R, Faller M, Weitzenblum E, et al. "Natural history" of pulmonary hypertension in a series of 131 patients with chronic obstructive lung disease. Am J Respir Crit Care Med 2001; 164:219–24.
5. Barberà JA, Riverola A, Roca J, et al. Pulmonary vascular abnormalities and ventilation–perfusion relationships in mild chronic obstructive pulmonary disease. Am J Respir Crit Care Med 1994; 149:423–9.
6. Peinado VI, Barberà JA, Ramirez J, et al. Endothelial dysfunction in pulmonary arteries of patients with mild COPD. Am J Physiol 1998; 274:L908–13.
7. Peinado VI, Barberà JA, Abate P, et al. Inflammatory reaction in pulmonary muscular arteries of patients with mild chronic obstructive pulmonary disease. Am J Respir Crit Care Med 1999; 159:1605–11.
8. Burrows B, Kettel LJ, Niden AH, Rabinowitz M, Diener CF. Patterns of cardiovascular dysfunction in chronic obstructive lung disease. N Engl J Med 1972; 286:912–8.
9. Traver GA, Cline MG, Burrows B. Predictors of mortality in chronic obstructive pulmonary disease. A 15-year follow-up study. Am Rev Respir Dis 1979; 119:895–902.
10. Weitzenblum E, Hirth C, Ducolone A, Mirhom R, Rasaholinjanahary J, Ehrhart M. Prognostic value of pulmonary artery pressure in chronic obstructive pulmonary disease. Thorax 1981; 36:752–8.
11. Oswald-Mammosser M, Weitzenblum E, Quoix E, et al. Prognostic factors in COPD patients receiving long-term oxygen therapy. Importance of pulmonary artery pressure. Chest 1995; 107:1193–8.
12. Burgess MI, Mogulkoc N, Bright-Thomas RJ, Bishop P, Egan JJ, Ray SG. Comparison of echocardiographic markers of right ventricular function in determining prognosis in chronic pulmonary disease. J Am Soc Echocardiogr 2002; 15:633–9.
13. Incalzi RA, Fuso L, De Rosa M, et al. Electrocardiographic signs of chronic cor pulmonale: a negative prognostic finding in chronic obstructive pulmonary disease. Circulation 1999; 99:1600–5.
14. Kessler R, Faller M, Fourgaut G, Mennecier B, Weitzenblum E. Predictive factors of hospitalization for acute exacerbation in a series of 64 patients with chronic obstructive pulmonary disease. Am J Respir Crit Care Med 1999; 159:158–64.
15. Wilkinson M, Langhorne CA, Heath D, Barer GR, Howard P. A pathophysiological study of 10 cases of hypoxic cor pulmonale. Q J Med 1988; 249:65–85.
16. Wright JL, Petty T, Thurlbeck WM. Analysis of the structure of the muscular pulmonary arteries in patients with pulmonary hypertension and COPD: National Institutes of Health Nocturnal Oxygen Therapy Trial. Lung 1992; 170:109–24.
17. Santos S, Peinado VI, Ramirez J, et al. Enhanced expression of vascular endothelial growth factor in pulmonary arteries of smokers and patients with moderate chronic obstructive pulmonary disease. Am J Respir Crit Care Med 2003; 167:1250–6.
18. Magee F, Wright JL, Wiggs BR, Paré PD, Hogg JC. Pulmonary vascular structure and function in chronic obstructive pulmonary disease. Thorax 1988; 43:183–9.
19. Hale KA, Ewing SL, Gosnell BA, Niewoehner DE. Lung disease in long-term cigarette smokers with and without chronic airflow obstruction. Am Rev Respir Dis 1984; 130:716–21.
20. Santos S, Peinado VI, Ramirez J, et al. Characterization of pulmonary vascular remodelling in smokers and patients with mild COPD. Eur Respir J 2002; 19:632–8.
21. Naeije R. Should pulmonary hypertension be treated in chronic obstructive pulmonary disease?. In: Weir EK, Archer SL, Reeves JT, eds. The Diagnosis and Treatment of Pulmonary Hypertension. Mount Kisco: Futura Publishing, 1992:209–39.
22. Fishman AP. State of the art: chronic cor pulmonale. Am Rev Respir Dis 1976; 114:775–94.

23. Weitzenblum E, Sautegeau A, Ehrhart M, Mammosser M, Hirth C, Roegel E. Long-term course of pulmonary arterial pressure in chronic obstructive pulmonary disease. Am Rev Respir Dis 1984; 130:993–8.
24. Barberà JA. Chronic obstructive pulmonary disease. In: Roca J, Rodriguez-Roisin R, Wagner PD, eds. Pulmonary and Peripheral Gas Exchange in Health and Disease. New York: Marcel Dekker, Inc., 2000:229–61.
25. Roca J, Wagner PD. Contribution of multiple inert gas elimination technique to pulmonary medicine. 1. Principles and information content of the multiple inert gas elimination technique. Thorax 1994; 49:815–24.
26. Barberà JA, Roger N, Roca J, Rovira I, Higenbottam TW, Rodriguez-Roisin R. Worsening of pulmonary gas exchange with nitric oxide inhalation in chronic obstructive pulmonary disease. Lancet 1996; 347:436–40.
27. Peinado VI, Santos S, Ramirez J, Roca J, Rodriguez-Roisin R, Barberà JA. Response to hypoxia of pulmonary arteries in COPD: an in vitro study. Eur Respir J 2002; 20:332–8.
28. Mélot C, Hallemans R, Naeije R, Mols P, Lejeune P. Deleterious effect of nifedipine on pulmonary gas exchange in chronic obstructive pulmonary disease. Am Rev Respir Dis 1984; 130:612–6.
29. Ringsted CV, Eliasen K, Andersen JB, Heslet L, Qvist J. Ventilation–perfusion distributions and central hemodynamics in chronic obstructive pulmonary disease. Effects of terbutaline administration. Chest 1989; 96:976–83.
30. Agustí AGN, Barberà JA, Roca J, Wagner PD, Guitart R, Rodriguez-Roisin R. Hypoxic pulmonary vasoconstriction and gas exchange during exercise in chronic obstructive pulmonary disease. Chest 1990; 97:268–75.
31. Simonneau G, Escourrou P, Duroux P, Lockhart A. Inhibition of hypoxic pulmonary vasoconstriction by nifedipine. N Engl J Med 1981; 304:1582–5.
32. Brent BN, Berger HJ, Matthay RA, Mahler D, Pytlik L, Zaret BL. Physiologic correlates of right ventricular ejection fraction in chronic obstructive pulmonary disease: a combined radionuclide and hemodynamic study. Am J Cardiol 1982; 50:255–62.
33. Weitzenblum E, Chaouat A. Right ventricular function in COPD: can it be assessed reliably by the measurement of right ventricular ejection fraction? Chest 1998; 113:567–9.
34. Crottogini AJ, Willshaw P. Calculating the end-systolic pressure–volume relation. Circulation 1991; 83:1121–3.
35. Biernacki W, Flenley DC, Muir AL, MacNee W. Pulmonary hypertension and right ventricular function in patients with COPD. Chest 1988; 94:1169–75.
36. MacNee W. Pathophysiology of cor pulmonale in chronic obstructive pulmonary disease. Part one. Am J Respir Crit Care Med 1994; 150:833–52.
37. MacNee W. Pathophysiology of cor pulmonale in chronic obstructive pulmonary disease. Part two. Am J Respir Crit Care Med 1994; 150:1158–68.
38. Barberà JA, Roca J, Ferrer A, et al. Mechanisms of worsening gas exchange during acute exacerbations of chronic obstructive pulmonary disease. Eur Respir J 1997; 10:1285–91.
39. Weitzenblum E, Apprill M, Oswald M, Chaouat A, Imbs JL. Pulmonary hemodynamics in patients with chronic obstructive pulmonary disease before and during an episode of peripheral edema. Chest 1994; 105:1377–82.
40. Campbell EJM, Short DS. The cause of oedema in "cor pulmonale". Lancet 1960; I:1184–6.
41. Baudouin SV. Oedema and cor pulmonale revisited. Thorax 1997; 52:401–2.
42. MacNee W, Wathen CG, Flenley DC, Muir AD. The effects of controlled oxygen therapy on ventricular function in patients with stable and decompensated cor pulmonale. Am Rev Respir Dis 1988; 137:1289–95.
43. MacNee W, Wathen CG, Hannan WJ, Flenley DC, Muir AL. Effects of pirbuterol and sodium nitroprusside on pulmonary haemodynamics in hypoxic cor pulmonale. Br Med J (Clin Res Ed) 1983; 287:1169–72.
44. Lee-Chiong TL, Matthay RA. The heart in the stable COPD patient. In: Similowski T, Whitelaw WA, Derenne JP, eds. Clinical Management of Chronic Obstructive Pulmonary Disease. New York: Marcel Dekker, Inc., 2002:475–532.
45. Palange P. Renal and hormonal abnormalities in chronic obstructive pulmonary disease (COPD). Thorax 1998; 53:989–91.
46. Wright JL, Lawson L, Paré PD, et al. The structure and function of the pulmonary vasculature in mild chronic obstructive pulmonary disease. Am Rev Respir Dis 1983; 128:702–7.

47. Harris P, Segal N, Bishop JM. The relation between pressure and flow in the pulmonary circulation in normal subjects and in chronic bronchitis. Cardiovasc Res 1968; 2:73–83.

48. Naeije R, Barberà JA. Pulmonary hypertension associated with COPD. Crit Care 2001; 5:286–9.

49. Butler J, Schrijen F, Henriquez A, Polu JM, Albert RK. Cause of the raised wedge pressure on exercise in chronic obstructive pulmonary disease. Am Rev Respir Dis 1988; 138:350–4.

50. Montes de Oca M, Rassulo J, Celli BR. Respiratory muscle and cardiopulmonary function during exercise in very severe COPD. Am J Respir Crit Care Med 1996; 154:1284–9.

51. Rubanyi GM, Romero JC, Vanhoutte PM. Flow-induced release of endothelium-derived relaxing factor. Am J Physiol 1986; 250:H1145–9.

52. Roger N, Barberà JA, Roca J, Rovira I, Gomez FP, Rodriguez-Roisin R. Nitric oxide inhalation during exercise in chronic obstructive pulmonary disease. Am J Respir Crit Care Med 1997; 156:800–6.

53. Weitzenblum E. The pulmonary circulation and the heart in chronic lung disease. Monaldi Arch Chest Dis 1994; 49:231–4.

54. Furchgott RF, Zawadzki JV. The obligatory role of endothelial cells in the relaxation of arterial smooth muscle by acetylcholine. Nature 1980; 288:373–6.

55. Dinh-Xuan AT, Higenbottam T, Clelland C, et al. Impairment of endothelium-dependent pulmonary-artery relaxation in chronic obstructive pulmonary disease. N Engl J Med 1991; 324:1539–47.

56. Giaid A, Saleh D. Reduced expression of endothelial nitric oxide synthase in the lungs of patients with pulmonary hypertension. N Engl J Med 1995; 333:214–21.

57. Barberà JA, Peinado VI, Santos S, Ramirez J, Roca J, Rodriguez-Roisin R. Reduced expression of endothelial nitric oxide synthase in pulmonary arteries of smokers. Am J Respir Crit Care Med 2001; 164:709–13.

58. Nana-Sinkam SP, Lee JD, Sotto-Santiago S, et al. Prostacyclin prevents pulmonary endothelial cell apoptosis induced by cigarette smoke. Am J Respir Crit Care Med 2007; 175:676–85.

59. Giaid A, Yanagisawa M, Langblen D, et al. Expression of endothelin-1 in the lungs of patients with pulmonary hypertension. N Engl J Med 1993; 328:1732–9.

60. Melgosa M, Peinado VI, Santos S, et al. Expression of endothelial nitric oxide synthase (eNOS) and endothelin-1 (ET-1) in pulmonary arteries of patients with severe COPD. Eur Respir J 2003; 22:20s.

61. Rabinovitch M, Gamble W, Nadas AS, Miettinen OS, Reid L. Rat pulmonary circulation after chronic hypoxia: hemodynamic and structural features. Am J Physiol 1979; 236:H818–27.

62. Stenmark KR, Fasules J, Hyde DM, et al. Severe pulmonary hypertension and arterial adventitial changes in newborn calves at 4300 m. J Appl Physiol 1987; 62:821–30.

63. Ashutosh K, Mead G, Dunsky M. Early effects of oxygen administration and prognosis in chronic obstructive pulmonary disease and cor pulmonale. Am Rev Respir Dis 1983; 127:399–404.

64. Weitzenblum E, Sautegeau A, Ehrhart M, Mammosser M, Pelletier A. Long-term oxygen therapy can reverse the progression of pulmonary hypertension in patients with chronic obstructive pulmonary disease. Am Rev Respir Dis 1985; 131:493–8.

65. Wright JL, Churg A. A model of tobacco smoke-induced airflow obstruction in the guinea pig. Chest 2002; 121:188S–91.

66. Wright JL, Churg A. Effect of long-term cigarette smoke exposure on pulmonary vascular structure and function in the guinea pig. Exp Lung Res 1991; 17:997–1009.

67. Yamato H, Churg A, Wright JL. Guinea pig pulmonary hypertension caused by cigarette smoke cannot be explained by capillary bed destruction. J Appl Physiol 1997; 82:1644–53.

68. Wright JL, Tai H, Dai J, Churg A. Cigarette smoke induces rapid changes in gene expression in pulmonary arteries. Lab Invest 2002; 82:1391–8.

69. Celermajer DS, Adams MR, Clarkson P, et al. Passive smoking and impaired endothelium-dependent arterial dilatation in healthy young adults. N Engl J Med 1996; 334:150–4.

70. Su Y, Han W, Giraldo C, Li YD, Block ER. Effect of cigarette smoke extract on nitric oxide synthase in pulmonary artery endothelial cells. Am J Respir Cell Mol Biol 1998; 19:819–25.

71. Chetty KG, Brown SE, Light RW. Identification of pulmonary hypertension in chronic obstructive pulmonary disease from routine chest radiographs. Am Rev Respir Dis 1982; 126:338–41.

72. Wiedemann HP, Matthay RA. Heart Disease. A Textbook of Cardiovascular Medicine. Philadelphia, PA: WB Saunders, 1997.

73. Oswald-Mammosser M, Oswald T, Nyankiye E, Dickele MC, Grange D, Weitzenblum E. Non-invasive diagnosis of pulmonary hypertension in chronic obstructive pulmonary disease. Comparison of ECG, radiological measurements, echocardiography and myocardial scintigraphy. Eur J Respir Dis 1987; 71:419–29.

74. Torbicki A, Skwarski K, Hawrylkiewicz I, Pasierski T, Miskiewicz Z, Zielinski J. Attempts at measuring pulmonary arterial pressure by means of Doppler echocardiography in patients with chronic lung disease. Eur Respir J 1989; 2:856–60.

75. Laaban JP, Diebold B, Zelinski R, Lafay M, Raffoul H, Rochemaure J. Noninvasive estimation of systolic pulmonary artery pressure using Doppler echocardiography in patients with chronic obstructive pulmonary disease. Chest 1989; 96:1258–62.

76. Naeije R, Torbicki A. More on the noninvasive diagnosis of pulmonary hypertension: Doppler echocardiography revisited. Eur Respir J 1995; 8:1445–9.

77. Arcasoy SM, Christie JD, Ferrari VA, et al. Echocardiographic assessment of pulmonary hypertension in patients with advanced lung disease. Am J Respir Crit Care Med 2003; 167:735–40.

78. Turhan S, Dincer I, Ozdol C, et al. Value of tissue Doppler myocardial velocities of tricuspid lateral annulus for the diagnosis of right heart failure in patients with COPD. Echocardiography 2007; 24:126–33.

79. Takakura M, Harada T, Fukuno H, et al. Echocardiographic detection of occult cor pulmonale during exercise in patients with chronic obstructive pulmonary disease. Echocardiography 1999; 16:127–34.

80. Yusen RD, Lefrak SS, Trulock EP. Evaluation and preoperative management of lung volume reduction surgery candidates. Clin Chest Med 1997; 18:199–224.

81. Rich S, Kaufmann E, Levy PS. The effect of high doses of calcium-channel blockers on survival in primary pulmonary hypertension. N Engl J Med 1992; 327:76–81.

82. Muramoto A, Caldwell J, Albert RK, Lakshminarayan S, Butler J. Nifedipine dilates the pulmonary vasculature without producing symptomatic systemic hypotension in upright resting and exercising patients with pulmonary hypertension secondary to chronic obstructive pulmonary disease. Am Rev Respir Dis 1985; 132:963–6.

83. Naeije R, Melot C, Mols P, Hallemans R. Effects of vasodilators on hypoxic pulmonary vasoconstriction in normal man. Chest 1982; 82:404–10.

84. Bratel T, Hedenstierna G, Nyquist O, Ripe E. The use of a vasodilator, felodipine, as an adjuvant to long-term oxygen treatment in COLD patients. Eur Respir J 1990; 3:46–54.

85. Andrivet P, Chabrier PE, Defouilloy C, Brun-Buisson C, Adnot S. Intravenously administered atrial natriuretic factor in patients with COPD. Effects on ventilation–perfusion relationships and pulmonary hemodynamics. Chest 1994; 106:118–24.

86. Adnot S, Kouyoumdjian C, Defouilloy C, et al. Hemodynamic and gas exchange responses to infusion of acetylcholine and inhalation of nitric oxide in patients with chronic obstructive lung disease and pulmonary hypertension. Am Rev Respir Dis 1993; 148:310–6.

87. Sturani C, Bassein L, Schiavina M, Gunella G. Oral nifedipine in chronic cor pulmonale secondary to severe chronic obstructive pulmonary disease (COPD). Chest 1983; 84:135–42.

88. Agostoni P, Doria E, Galli C, Tamborini G, Guazzi MD. Nifedipine reduces pulmonary pressure and vascular tone during short- but not long-term treatment of pulmonary hypertension in patients with chronic obstructive pulmonary disease. Am Rev Respir Dis 1989; 139:120–5.

89. Saadjian AY, Philip-Joet FF, Vestri R, Arnaud AG. Long-term treatment of chronic obstructive lung disease by Nifedipine: an 18-month haemodynamic study. Eur Respir J 1988; 1:716–20.

90. Morrell NW, Higham MA, Phillips PG, Shakur BH, Robinson PJ, Beddoes RJ. Pilot study of losartan for pulmonary hypertension in chronic obstructive pulmonary disease. Respir Res 2005; 6:88.

91. Katayama Y, Higenbottam TW, Diaz de Atauri MJ, et al. Inhaled nitric oxide and arterial oxygen tension in patients with chronic obstructive pulmonary disease and severe pulmonary hypertension. Thorax 1997; 52:120–4.

92. Frostell C, Blomqvist H, Hedenstierna G, Lundberg J, Zapol WM. Inhaled nitric oxide selectively reverses human hypoxic pulmonary vasoconstriction without causing systemic vasodilation. Anesthesiology 1993; 78:427–35.

93. Katayama Y, Higenbottam TW, Cremona G, et al. Minimizing the inhaled dose of NO with breath-by-breath delivery of spikes of concentrated gas. Circulation 1998; 98:2429–32.

94. Yoshida M, Taguchi O, Gabazza EC, et al. Combined inhalation of nitric oxide and oxygen in chronic obstructive pulmonary disease. Am J Respir Crit Care Med 1997; 155:526–9.

95. Germann P, Ziesche R, Leitner C, et al. Addition of nitric oxide to oxygen improves cardiopulmonary function in patients with severe COPD. Chest 1998; 114:29–35.

96. Vonbank K, Ziesche R, Higenbottam TW, et al. Controlled prospective randomised trial on the effects on pulmonary haemodynamics of the ambulatory long term use of nitric oxide and oxygen in patients with severe COPD. Thorax 2003; 58:289–93.

97. Pauwels RA, Buist AS, Calverley PMA, Jenkins CR, Hurd SS. Global strategy for the diagnosis, management, and prevention of chronic obstructive pulmonary disease. NHLBI/WHO Global Initiative for Chronic Obstructive Lung Disease (GOLD) Workshop Summary. Am J Respir Crit Care Med 2001; 163:1256–76.
98. DeGaute JP, Domenighetti G, Naeije R, Vincent JL, Treyvaud D, Perret C. Oxygen delivery in acute exacerbation of chronic obstructive pulmonary disease. Effects of controlled oxygen therapy. Am Rev Respir Dis 1981; 124:26–30.
99. Lejeune P, Mols P, Naeije R, Hallemans R, Melot C. Acute hemodynamic effects of controlled oxygen therapy in decompensated chronic obstructive pulmonary disease. Crit Care Med 1984; 12:1032–5.
100. Olvey SK, Reduto LA, Stevens PM, Deaton WJ, Miller RR. First pass radionuclide assessment of right and left ventricular ejection fraction in chronic pulmonary disease. Effect of oxygen upon exercise response. Chest 1980; 78:4–9.
101. Report of the Medical Research Council Working Party. Long term domiciliary oxygen therapy in chronic hypoxic cor pulmonale complicating chronic bronchitis and emphysema. Lancet 1981; i:681–5.
102. Nocturnal Oxygen Therapy Trial Group. Continuous or nocturnal oxygen therapy in hypoxemic chronic obstructive lung disease. A clinical trial. Ann Intern Med 1980; 93:391–8.
103. Brijker F, Heijdra YF, van den Elshout FJ, Folgering HT. Discontinuation of furosemide decreases PaCO2 in patients with COPD. Chest 2002; 121:377–82.
104. Mathur PN, Powles P, Pugsley SO, McEwan MP, Campbell EJ. Effect of digoxin on right ventricular function in severe chronic airflow obstruction. A controlled clinical trial. Ann Intern Med 1981; 95:283–8.
105. Polic S, Rumboldt Z, Dujic Z, Bagatin J, Deletis O, Rozga A. Role of digoxin in right ventricular failure due to chronic cor pulmonale. Int J Clin Pharmacol Res 1990; 10:153–62.
106. Matthay RA, Berger HJ, Loke J, Gottschalk A, Zaret BL. Effects of aminophylline upon right and left ventricular performance in chronic obstructive pulmonary disease: noninvasive assessment by radionuclide angiocardiography. Am J Med 1978; 65:903–10.
107. Mols P, Ham H, Naeije N, et al. How does salbutamol improve the ventricular performance in patients with chronic obstructive pulmonary disease? J Cardiovasc Pharmacol 1988; 12:127–33.
108. Ballester E, Roca J, Ramis L, Wagner PD, Rodriguez-Roisin R. Pulmonary gas exchange in severe chronic asthma. Response to 100% oxygen and salbutamol. Am Rev Respir Dis 1990; 141:558–62.
109. Humbert M, Sitbon O, Simonneau G. Treatment of pulmonary arterial hypertension. N Engl J Med 2004; 351:1425–36.
110. Higenbottam T. Pulmonary hypertension and chronic obstructive pulmonary disease: a case for treatment. Proc Am Thorac Soc 2005; 2:12–9.
111. Galie N, Torbicki A, Barst R, et al. Guidelines on diagnosis and treatment of pulmonary arterial hypertension. The task force on diagnosis and treatment of pulmonary arterial hypertension of the European Society of Cardiology. Eur Heart J 2004; 25:2243–78.
112. Stevens D, Sharma K, Szidon P, Rich S, McLaughlin V, Kesten S. Severe pulmonary hypertension associated with COPD. Ann Transplant 2000; 5:8–12.
113. Maloney JP. Advances in the treatment of secondary pulmonary hypertension. Curr Opin Pulm Med 2003; 9:139–43.
114. Madden BP, Allenby M, Loke TK, Sheth A. A potential role for sildenafil in the management of pulmonary hypertension in patients with parenchymal lung disease. Vascul Pharmacol 2006; 44:372–6.
115. Alp S, Skrygan M, Schmidt WE, Bastian A. Sildenafil improves hemodynamic parameters in COPD— an investigation of six patients. Pulm Pharmacol Ther 2006; 19:386–90.
116. Archer SL, Mike D, Crow J, Long W, Weir EK. A placebo-controlled trial of prostacyclin in acute respiratory failure in COPD. Chest 1996; 109:750–5.
117. Zhao L, Mason NA, Morrell NW, et al. Sildenafil inhibits hypoxia-induced pulmonary hypertension. Circulation 2001; 104:424–8.
118. Modesti PA, Vanni S, Morabito M, et al. Role of endothelin-1 in exposure to high altitude: Acute Mountain Sickness and Endothelin-1 (ACME-1) study. Circulation 2006; 114:1410–6.

11

How the COPD Patient Should Be Assessed for Comorbidities

JOAN B. SORIANO
Program of Epidemiology and Clinical Research, Fundació Caubet-CIMERA Illes Balears, International Centre for Advanced Respiratory Medicine, Mallorca, Illes Balears, Spain

JAUME SAULEDA
Servei de Pneumologia and Unidad de Investigación, Hospital Universitari Son Dureta, Palma de Mallorca, Mallorca, Illes Balears, Spain

I. Introduction

Chronic obstructive pulmonary disease (COPD) represents an important and increasing burden throughout the world. Classically, COPD has been considered a respiratory condition only, mainly caused by tobacco smoking. Indeed COPD affects various domains within the lungs. However, COPD is a syndrome with important manifestations beyond the lungs. The so-called systemic effects of COPD are significant extrapulmonary effects that can be considered not organ specific, including weight loss, nutritional abnormalities, and skeletal muscle dysfunction. All are comprehensively reviewed elsewhere in this book. The focus of this chapter is on organ-specific comorbidities. Comorbidities are defined here as diseases that occur apart from COPD in a given patient, including an increased risk of cardiovascular disease, cancers, neurologic and skeletal defects, and others. Because some comorbidities can be either common and/or severe enough, they should be screened and managed accordingly, to give a holistic medical care to our patients, some in primary care and some at the specialized level. Further, not only comorbidities are important during the life of COPD individuals. COPD-related mortality is probably underestimated because of the difficulties associated with identifying the precise cause of death and little is known about the underlying mechanisms of COPD mortality. The effects of comorbidities at the time of death and on specific causes of death in COPD are also explored. Mechanistically, the links between COPD and comorbid conditions are not fully understood. Independent from tobacco, chronic systemic and pulmonary inflammations are present in all stages of COPD, suggesting a potential link through this pathway. Comorbidities are common in COPD and should be actively identified. Comorbidities often complicate the management of COPD, and vice versa.

COPD is a leading but under-recognized cause of morbidity and mortality worldwide. No other disease that is responsible for comparable burden worldwide is neglected by health care providers as much as COPD. Undisputed, the most important causal factor of COPD is cigarette smoking, and although more people smoke today than at any other time in human history, it is actually aging and the changing demographics worldwide that is driving the COPD tidal wave even faster than the increase in smoking worldwide (1). Overall, the magnitude of the COPD problem in the general population is reaching epidemic proportions, with a prevalence estimated to be ~1% across all ages rising steeply to 8% to 10% or higher amongst those aged ≥40 years. Mortality is escalating, particularly in women. To date, many authors have comprehensively reviewed the historical data on the epidemiology and burden of COPD in detail elsewhere, but interestingly little or no attention has been given to comorbidities in COPD (2–8).

II. GOLD and ATS/ERS Guidelines

Consensus was finally achieved in international COPD guidelines with the agreement on spirometry thresholds to diagnose COPD and grade its severity, both by the Global Initiative for Chronic Obstructive Lung Disease (GOLD) (9,10), and the American Thoracic Society (ATS)/European Respiratory Society (ERS) guidelines on standards for the diagnosis and management of patients with COPD (11). Both guidelines, apart from the listing of diseases that exclude a diagnosis of COPD (bronchiectasis, cystic fibrosis, and fibrosis due to tuberculosis), have also included brief paragraphs on comorbidities.

The current GOLD guidelines have 25 entries on comorbidities. GOLD reports that to achieve the four goals of COPD (namely, assess and monitor the disease, reduce risk factors, manage stable COPD, and manage exacerbations) any treatment strategy is difficult to implement because adverse effects can happen due to common comorbidities. Specifically, GOLD states that comorbidities such as heart disease and rheumatic disease may also contribute to restriction of activity. When treating COPD patients monitoring of comorbidities such as bronchial carcinoma, tuberculosis, sleep apnea, and left heart failure should be considered, and that diagnostic tools [chest X ray, electrocardiogram (EKG), etc.] should be used whenever symptoms suggest any of these conditions. Finally, GOLD states that significant comorbidities are indicators for hospital assessment or admission for exacerbations of COPD (9,10).

On the other hand, the ATS/ERS guidelines contain 18 entries on comorbidities. Briefly, they state that comorbidity is a frequent problem in COPD. Other illnesses, such as bronchiectasis, lung cancer, heart failure, osteoporosis, and malnutrition are frequent in patients with COPD. Comorbidities like those of the heart or peripheral vasculature, neurological, or other related to cigarette smoke exposure should be noted. To optimize treatment, comorbidities that might exacerbate symptoms like heart failure or sleep apnea should be treated. Comorbidities are associated with poor outcomes after bullectomy and lung volume reduction surgery. Although COPD is currently the most common indication for lung transplant (12), some comorbidities are relative contraindications (osteoporosis, psychiatric conditions) or even absolute contra-indications (advanced liver or kidney disease, HIV infection, malignancy within two years except basal or squamous cell carcinoma of the skin) for lung transplant in COPD. Depressive symptoms are also common, especially in patients with severe disease, who are at a 2.5 times greater risk. It is therefore important to search for symptoms of depression and treat them appropriately. It is suggested that when unstable COPD patients show up with a COPD exacerbation in the hospital, criteria for hospitalization may include the coexistence of cardiac arrhythmia, congestive heart failure, uncontrolled diabetes mellitus, liver or kidney failure, as the most common comorbidities. These guidelines conclude that assessment of comorbidities is key for an integrated care at any level of COPD progression, and should be a reason for referral to a more specialized care (11).

III. Comorbidities in General: Definitions

Unfortunately, there is no universally accepted definition of comorbidity. Traditionally, comorbidity has been defined as a disease coexisting with the primary disease of interest, though there are a plethora of examples where this definition has been significantly modified or ignored. The full exploration of mechanisms of comorbidity requires an interdisciplinary approach to investigating the diagnosis, assessment, and underlying models of comorbidity. A more precise specification of comorbidities might help to identify common diagnostic markers relevant in the etiology of specific disorders as well as in comorbid conditions.

In COPD, the definition becomes even more problematic as certain coexisting illnesses may be a consequence of the patients' underlying COPD. Examples of these "comorbid" conditions include cardiovascular diseases, lung cancer, and osteoporosis. For the purposes of this chapter, we define comorbidities as the presence of one or more distinct disorders (or diseases) in addition to COPD, regardless of whether the comorbid conditions are/are not directly related to COPD, and irrespective of whether they are/are not part of the spectrum of the natural history of COPD. Within this case definition, conditions such as ischemic heart disease (IHD), cancer, and osteoporosis but also angina, fractures, or cataracts would be considered comorbid conditions of COPD.

Generally, the assessment of comorbidities can be done in several ways. Qualitatively, simply a chart review can differentiate with a yes/no answer whether a patient only suffers from COPD or from anything else. Quantitatively, the listing of conditions can produce a figure of 0, one or more comorbidities. A number of quantitative/qualitative indices are described next, including Charlson's, Deyo's, and Ghali's scores.

A. Charlson Index

The Charlson index was originally an automated method designed to quantify for analytical purposes, the comorbid conditions that might alter the risk of mortality in hospitalized patients (13). It is based on 17 weighted, diagnostic categories identified from the International Classification of Diseases (ICD)-9 discharge diagnoses, listed in Table 1. An important limitation to consider is that the relationship between the Charlson index and mortality is often assumed to be linear. However, this assumption is unlikely to be valid as the impact of the Charlson index on mortality is probably exponential. Other limitations include the relative complexity of the weighting and scoring system, and perhaps current advances in management of some conditions (liver disease, AIDS, etc.) makes it relatively obsolete.

Table 1 The Charlson Comorbidity Index

Group	Comorbidity list	Score per comorbidity
Group a	MI, CHF, peripheral vascular disease, CVD, dementia, COPD, connective tissue disease, ulcer disease, mild liver disease, and diabetes	1
Group b	Advanced diabetes, hemiplegia, renal disease, and malignancies	2
Group c	Moderate or severe liver disease	3
Group d	AIDS or metastatic malignancies	6
		Add total points to get Charlson score

Abbreviations: CHF, congestive heart failure; COPD, chronic obstructive pulmonary disease; CVD, cardiovascular disease; MI, myocardial infarction.

B. The Deyo Index

The Deyo index is another such scoring system commonly used for research involving hospital administrative databases, ICD-9 diagnoses, and procedural codes (14). Deyo's index is a simplification of the Charlson index. It uses the same listing of conditions as Charlson, but unweighted, and often is shown stratifying comorbidities numerically with 0, 1, 2, or 3+ comorbidities.

C. The Ghali Index

Ghali et al. studied approaches to comorbidity risk adjustment by comparing a new system to ICD-9 Clinical Modification (CM) adaptations of the Charlson comorbidity index (15). This model using a new index to predict mortality had better validity than a model based on the original Charlson index.

IV. Mechanisms on Tobacco and Other Risk Factors

Tobacco is considered the most important causal factor in developing COPD. In 1964, the U.S. Surgeon's general report identified smoking as the most important cause of chronic bronchitis. This statement was expanded in the next report published in 1967, implicating tobacco in the etiology of emphysema as well (16).

Classically, the relative risk (RR) of tobacco in developing COPD was quantified as 7 to 10 and the population attributable risk as 90%. However, not only cigarette smoking produces COPD. There is little doubt that other types of tobacco smoking like pipe, cigarillos, or other produce the same type of lung response.

Perhaps, more controversial is the acceptance of the role of other inhaled particles, like marijuana smoking, biomass, passive smoking, or outdoor pollution. Recently, due to better estimates and the substitution of causes, the population attributable risk of tobacco on COPD has been downgraded to about 50% (1). It seems there is still room for consensus in between clinicians and epidemiologists.

Cigarette smoking is also a causal or predisposing factor for some COPD comorbidities, and some conditions can arise in the presence of tobacco, but others independently. Sophisticated simulations excluding smokers or adjusting for total tobacco smoking have concluded that independently of tobacco, COPD is associated with other conditions. A key related issue that must be considered when measuring the role of comorbidities in COPD is causation and independence of effects from smoking. For example, do comorbidities make patients more susceptible to the consequences of COPD?, does COPD increase their susceptibility to these comorbidities?, or is it a combination of both? Unfortunately, the exact nature of these causal pathways is unknown. However, there is good evidence that COPD is a risk factor for lung cancer (17), and that COPD precedes cardiovascular mortality (18). The possibility of reverse causation is also possible in certain patients for cardiovascular disease, but not for lung cancer. Clearly more work is required to establish the potential mechanisms and causal pathways that link comorbid conditions and COPD mortality.

V. Brief on Systemic Inflammation

COPD is characterized by an abnormal/excessive inflammatory response of the lung parenchyma to inhaled irritants and toxins, mostly tobacco smoking, and by the presence of systemic inflammation. Systematic reviews have identified studies investigating the relationship between stable COPD (of any severity), forced expiratory volume in the first second (FEV_1), or forced expiratory vital capacity (FVC) with levels of systemic inflammatory markers, including C-reactive protein (CRP), fibrinogen, circulating leukocytes, and the proinflammatory cytokine tumor necrosis factor TNF-α (19,20). This increased inflammatory response is inversely related with the degree of airflow obstruction (21). Similar findings are seen during COPD exacerbations (20). The relationship between systemic inflammation and comorbidities in COPD has been poorly studied. Systemic inflammation has been associated with several comorbidities in COPD such as cardiovascular diseases (22), cachexia (23), airway dysplasia (24), muscle weakness, and osteoporosis (25). The clinical relevance of these phenomena is poorly understood but recent evidence suggests a positive association between the presence of systemic inflammation and poor quality of life and decreased exercise capacity (26). Moreover, cardiovascular disease (27), weight loss, and loss of fat-free mass (28) are predictors of mortality in patients with COPD. Thus, comorbidities are relevant parameters for the clinical assessment of COPD patients. Due to this probable link between systemic inflammation and many extrapulmonary complications, several authors recommend the need for studies to determine whether attenuation of the systemic inflammatory process is able to modify risks and outcomes in COPD (29).

Lung-specific measurements such as FEV_1 predict mortality in COPD and in the general population (30). As comprehensively described elsewhere, strong epidemiological evidence appears to point to reduced FEV_1 as a marker for cardiovascular mortality. To our knowledge, there is no report on the quantity and quality of comorbidities associated with different degrees of airflow limitation.

VI. Measurements of Comorbidities in COPD

A. General Population Assessments

There are few general population assessments that systematically review the distribution of COPD comorbidities. Patient data from the U.K. General Practice

Research Database were analyzed to quantify baseline rates of comorbidities in 2699 patients with COPD (46% were current smokers) compared with age-, gender-, practice-, and time-matched controls (21% were current smokers) (31). Angina, cataracts, and osteoporosis all had a frequency of greater than 1% within the first year after COPD diagnosis. Furthermore, compared with controls, COPD patients had a significantly increased risk of comorbidities and other medical events (Fig. 1). It was concluded that COPD is associated with many comorbidities, particularly those related to cardiovascular-, bone-, and other smoking-related conditions, that previously had not been systematically documented. Comorbidities were also assessed in a chart review study of 200 COPD patients compared with 200 matched controls (32). Patients with COPD were randomly selected from a total of 1522 COPD patients enrolled in a health maintenance organization in 1997. Compared with controls, patients with COPD had a longer smoking history (49.5 vs. 34.9 pack-years; $p=0.002$). This chart review revealed that patients with COPD had a higher prevalence of certain comorbid conditions including coronary artery disease, congestive heart disease, other cardiovascular disease, local malignant neoplasm (includes any history of nonmeta-static cancer except basal cell and squamous cell skin carcinoma), neurological disease other than stroke with hemiplegia, ulcers, and gastritis. Patients in the COPD cohort had an average of 3.7 chronic medical conditions (including lung disease) compared with 1.8 chronic medical conditions for the controls ($p<0.001$).

A prospective study of 171 COPD patients hospitalized for an exacerbation of COPD, included comorbidities in its assessment of risk factors for one-year mortality (33). More than two-thirds of patients had at least one comorbid illness and the mean Charlson index score was 1.55 ± 0.90. Although the RR of death was significantly associated with the Charlson index [RR$=1.38$; 95% confidence interval (CI): 1.06,

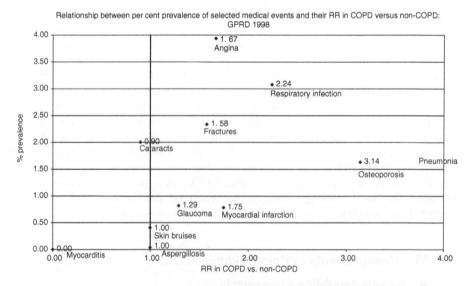

Figure 1 Comparative impact of comorbidities in chronic obstructive pulmonary disease by frequency and relative risk. *Abbreviations*: COPD, chronic obstructive pulmonary disease; GPRD, General Practice Research Database, RR, relative risk. *Source*: Adapted from Ref. 31.

1.80; $p=0.0162$], a multivariate Cox analysis (adjusting for age, number of hospitalization days, FEV_1, $PaCO_2$, and oral corticosteroid use) failed to demonstrate an independent relationship (RR adjusted $= 1.22$; 95% CI: 0.92, 1.62; $p=0.1767$). An important limitation of this analysis was that the relationship between the Charlson index and mortality was assumed to be linear.

Patil et al. (34) used administrative databases to estimate in-hospital mortality and to identify predictors of mortality in 71,130 patients admitted to a hospital with a COPD exacerbation. This cohort included data from the 1996 Nationwide Inpatient Sample for all hospitalizations in a 20% sample of all nonfederal U.S. hospitals. The overall in-hospital mortality was found to be 2.5%. Deyo–Charlson index scores were significantly associated with mortality: individuals with a score of 5 or more (indicating at least four comorbidities) were over five times more likely to die in-hospital compared with COPD patients without comorbidities, adjusted for a wide range of confounders including age and sex [adjusted odds ratio (OR) $= 5.70$; 99% CI: 4.08, 7.89].

Perhaps one of the most important studies that demonstrated the impact and prognostic role of comorbidities in COPD was done by Incalzi et al., (35) in their analysis of data from a cohort of 270 COPD patients discharged from hospital after an acute exacerbation of COPD. The Charlson index was used to quantify comorbidity. The researchers found that the most common comorbid conditions were hypertension (28%), diabetes mellitus (14%), and IHD (10%). The median survival was 3.1 years and 228 of the 270 patients died during the five-year follow-up period. The five-year mortality was predicted by $FEV_1 < 590$ mL [hazard ratio (HR) $= 1.49$; 95% CI, 0.97, 2.27], age (HR $= 1.04$; 95% CI: 1.02, 1.05), EKG signs of right ventricular hypertrophy (HR $= 1.76$; 95% CI: 1.3, 2.38), chronic renal failure (HR $= 1.79$; 95% CI: 1.05, 3.02), and EKG signs of myocardial infarction or ischemia (HR $= 1.42$; 95% CI: 1.02, 1.96) with an overall sensitivity of 63% and a specificity of 77%.

A separate study aimed to identify factors affecting short-term prognosis by retrospectively analyzing the records of 590 patients hospitalized for exacerbated COPD from 1981 to 1990 (36). In this study, increased age (OR $= 1.07$; 95% CI: 1.04, 1.11), alveolar–arterial oxygen partial pressure difference of >41 mmHg (OR $= 2.33$; 95% CI: 1.39, 3.90), the presence of ventricular arrhythmias (OR $= 1.91$; 95% CI: 1.10, 3.31), and atrial fibrillation (OR $= 2.27$, 95% CI: 1.14, 4.51) were independent predictors of one-year mortality in this group of COPD patients. These data suggest that indicators of heart dysfunction are particularly important predictors of increased risk of death in patients with COPD and indicate the importance of cardiovascular disease as a factor contributing to COPD mortality.

A recent evaluation of the U.S. National Hospital Discharge Survey analyzed more than 47 million hospital discharges for COPD (8.5% of all hospitalizations) that occurred in the United States from 1979 to 2001 in adults older than 25 years of age (37). The prevalence and in-hospital mortality of many conditions were greater in hospital discharges with any mention of COPD, versus those that did not mention COPD. Of interest, a hospital diagnosis of COPD was associated with a higher rate of age-adjusted in-hospital mortality for pneumonia, hypertension, heart failure, ventilatory failure, and thoracic malignancies. In contrast, a hospital diagnosis of COPD was not associated with a greater prevalence of hospitalization or in-hospital mortality for acute and chronic renal failure, HIV, gastrointestinal hemorrhage, and cerebrovascular disease (37).

VII.   Comorbidities as Specific Causes of Death in COPD Patients

To determine the specific cause of death in COPD patients is a challenge, even by experienced clinicians and when death occurs in inpatients. It is often agreed that patients die with COPD rather than of COPD. In the 1990s, Zielinski et al. from the World Health Organization reviewed deaths in a multicenter study of patients with COPD and noted that, despite the high global death toll for COPD, little was known about its causes or circumstances (38,39). They collected data from 215 severe COPD patients with chronic respiratory failure ($PaO_2 < 60$ mmHg) who died following treatment with long-term oxygen therapy. Three-quarters of patients died in the hospital. In this very sick group of COPD patients, respiratory failure was the leading cause of death, but overall accounted for only a third of the total number of deaths. Cardiovascular causes, pulmonary infection, pulmonary embolism, lung cancer, and other cancers accounted for the remaining two-thirds of the deaths, reinforcing the likely importance of comorbidities in COPD-related mortality. In a more recent report, the Lung Health Study investigators showed that in this cohort of patients with mild COPD, lung cancer, and cardiovascular complications accounted for nearly two-thirds of all deaths during a 15-year follow-up (40). The specific causes of death reported in different series of COPD patients have been recently reviewed elsewhere (41). To summarize, the main cause of mortality in mild or moderate COPD are lung cancer and cardiovascular diseases, while in more advanced COPD ($<60\%$ FEV_1), respiratory failure becomes the predominant cause (Fig. 2). Addressing the potential link between

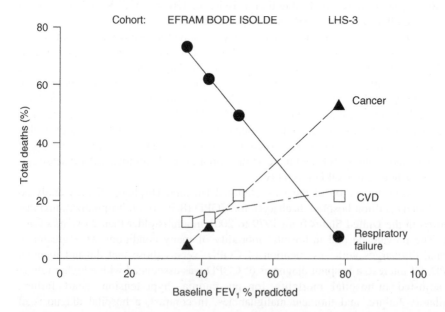

Figure 2   Specific causes of death by severity of chronic obstructive pulmonary disease. *Abbreviations*: CVD, cardiovascular disease; FEV_1, forced expiratory volume in the first second. *Source*: Adapted from Ref. 41.

COPD and causes of death such as cancer and cardiovascular diseases may be of paramount importance in affecting the natural history of COPD beginning from GOLD Stage 0 onwards.

VIII. Comorbidities by Severity of COPD

Current literature is scanty on describing the number and quality of comorbidities with increasing severity of airflow obstruction. On the other hand, most COPD studies have been unable to characterize accurately enough the severity of their COPD population regarding comorbidities. Subsequently, the influence of these comorbidities on the results of clinical trials and on the natural history and severity of the disease are poorly understood (42). However, systemic inflammation which might be intimately related with comorbidity shows a direct relationship with the severity of the disease as previously mentioned, and there are several comorbidities linked with systemic inflammation that clearly show a direct relationship with severity markers of COPD: (*i*) the percentage of COPD patients who loose weight is higher if they present severe airflow obstruction (43); (*ii*) it is well established the association of the lower FEV_1, the higher probability of cardiovascular disease (44). Although cardiovascular (ischemic) disease can be found in all severities of COPD, its frequency correlates with the degree of airflow obstruction; (*iii*) it has been found a direct relationship between osteoporosis and the severity of COPD (45); (*iv*) the intensity of anemia correlates with the severity of COPD (46); (*v*) COPD is a well-known independent risk factor that is associated with primary lung cancer. The likelihood of developing lung cancer within a 10-year period is threefold greater in subjects with mild to moderate COPD versus smokers with normal lung function and nearly 10-fold greater in subjects with severe COPD (47). However, not all studies found this association. For instance in a study by Yeo et al., quality of life, comorbidity, and health service utilization measurements were not significantly different within COPD severity groups (48). Current composite indices to describe the severity of COPD, like the Body mass index (BMI), airflow Obstruction, Dyspnea, and Exercise capacity index (49), have not been explored to determine classification of comorbidities.

IX. Comorbidities in Women with COPD

There has been a dramatic change in the sex ratio of COPD at the population and clinical level. Classical textbooks recommended clinicians to tease out COPD in patients with the triad of elderly, smoking, and male gender. Some large COPD randomized controlled trials (RCT) did not even include women at all. To many, it was therefore surprising to see that in 2000 there were more deaths in the United States from COPD among females than males (4). A demographic change has been observed, with females living longer and smoking harder, therefore being more at risk of developing COPD. It is worth noting worldwide, that in all countries but three (Norway, Sweden and New Zealand), and in these ones only since 2003, females have never smoked as much as males (50). Most recent population surveys identify as many women as men with COPD (51), and recent, large RCTs have no problem in including COPD women.

It is expected that female-specific comorbidities, like gynecological and peri- and postmenopausal disorders will be described within the COPD spectrum.

X. Review of Organ-Specific Comorbidities

Organ-specific comorbidities are summarized here (Fig. 3).

A. Cardiovascular Disease

There is strong epidemiological evidence to conclude that reduced FEV_1, independent of cigarette smoking, cholesterol, and hypertension, is a marker for cardiovascular morbidity and mortality (52). Cardiovascular disease rates have been found increased in patients with COPD. A recent retrospective cohort study in longitudinal health care databases of Saskatchewan, Canada (53), reported increased risks (ORs) of the following conditions when COPD patients ($n = 11,493$) were compared with matched population controls: arrhythmia 1.76, angina 1.61, acute myocardial infarction 1.61, congestive heart failure 3.84, and stroke 1.11. Ischemic disease is characterized by atherosclerosis of coronary arteries. In these vessels there is endothelial dysfunction and an inflammatory process in the atherome plaque with presence of macrophages, T cells and increased proinflammatory cytokines and CRP (54). It is remarkable to observe the similarities of cardiac inflammation with lung inflammation. Cardiac failure has been found in about 20% of COPD patients (55), and it has been related to possible coronary atherosclerosis. Often cardiac failure is difficult to diagnose in chronic respiratory patients due to non-specificity of symptoms. Rutten et al. have suggested a score that combines clinical, EKG, and serum N-terminal fragment of brain-type natriuretic peptide (NTproBNP) to predict the probability to detect left ventricular failure (56).

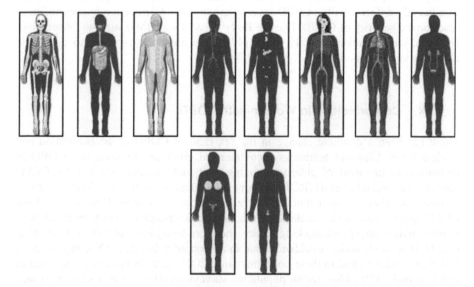

Figure 3 Human body and potential chronic obstructive pulmonary disease comorbidities.

Moreover, the risk of hospitalization and mortality due to cardiovascular causes was increased in COPD patients about 2- and 2.8-fold, respectively (57). In the Lung Health Study, cardiovascular causes accounted for 42% of first and 44% of second hospitalizations in these patients with relatively mild COPD, higher than for respiratory causes (14%) (58).

The underlying mechanisms linking COPD and cardiovascular disease are not fully understood. Cigarette smoking is a common risk factor of both diseases but several studies established that the association between COPD and cardiovascular diseases remains independent of established risk factors (52). Several authors suggest the potential role of systemic inflammation in COPD to explain the increased incidence of cardiovascular morbidity (29). Actually, both systemic inflammation and endothelial dysfunction are key mechanisms for atherosclerosis and patients suffering from conditions associated with systemic inflammation should have an excess risk of cardiovascular morbidity and mortality (59). Due to the fact that systemic inflammation is a common finding in patients with COPD, albeit in mild to moderate degree, it may contribute to increased cardiovascular morbidity and mortality.

Pulmonary embolism has been found increased in patients with COPD, quantified with an OR of five (60). Possible mechanisms and triggers may include sedentary lifestyle, hypercoagulability associated to smoking, and increased procoagulant molecules. In exacerbations of the disease without a clear etiology pulmonary embolism should be ruled out. In the Tillie et al.'s study, pulmonary embolism was found in 25% of COPD exacerbations without known etiology excluding those triggered by respiratory infections (60). However, this elevated frequency was not observed in a recent paper by Rutschmann OT et al. (61), where the prevalence of pulmonary embolism was 6.2% in the 48 COPD patients with exacerbations who had a clinical suspicion of pulmonary embolism and only 1.3% in those patients COPD patients not suspected of pulmonary embolism. With current evidence, screening for pulmonary embolism is not recommended during acute exacerbations of COPD, unless there is clinical suspicion or known risk factors for embolism (62).

B. Lung Cancer

COPD is an independent risk factor for lung cancer, with chronic bronchitis and/or emphysema increasing lung cancer risk by two- to fivefold, compared with incidence rates in smokers without COPD (63) An inverse correlation between the degree of airflow obstruction and lung cancer risk was clearly demonstrated in an analysis of 22-year follow-up data for 5402 participants from the first National Health and Nutrition Examination Survey, including a total of 113 cases of lung cancer (47).

There is also a growing recognition that chronic inflammation may play a salient role in the pathogenesis of lung cancer as a tumor promoter, an idea that was first proposed by Virchow in the 1860s. There are examples elsewhere in the body where chronic inflammation plays a relevant role in triggering cancer. Examples include inflammatory bowel disease and colon cancer, chronic hepatitis and hepatoma, chronic pancreatitis and pancreatic cancer, and Barrett's esophagus and esophageal cancer. Experimental findings suggest that cigarette smoke up-regulates the production of cytokines such as interleukin(IL)-1β, and the Th1 cytokines, which in turn increase cyclooxygenase (COX)-2 enzymatic activity. COX-2 products can promote an inflammatory response by the lymphocytes, leading to the overproduction of cytokines such as IL-6, IL-8, and IL-10. Some of these cytokines can inhibit apoptosis, interfere with cellular repair, and promote angiogenesis. Chronic inflammation may thus be instrumental in amplifying the initial mutagenic damage and promoting tumor growth and metastasis. IL-8, for example, has been demonstrated to up-regulate pro-oncogenes such as B-cell chronic lymphocytic leukemia (BCL)-2 and down-regulate suppressor oncogenes such as p53, thereby inhibiting apoptosis and inducing cell transformation. These cytokines also create a pro-angiogenic environment, which promotes tumor growth. Interestingly, these cytokines have also been implicated in COPD progression. There is a clear link between COPD and lung cancer independently of active smoking (64). Even after patients with COPD stop smoking, the risk of lung cancer remains elevated, though the risk is lower than that of continued smokers (65). Some have suggested that the missing link between reduced FEV_1 and lung cancer is chronic airway inflammation, which is evident in the airways of COPD patients even years after smoking cessation (66,67).

At the molecular level, activation of nuclear factor kappa B (NF-κB) transcription factor may have major relevance for cancer and COPD. Although the precise role of NF-κB in COPD remains speculative, chronic airway inflammation in COPD has been associated with activation of NF-κB in macrophages and epithelial cells. Furthermore, it has been suggested that the synergistic effects of latent infection and cigarette smoking cause chronic airway inflammation through enhanced expression of cytokines and adhesion molecules, possibly through NF-κB-mediated activation. Links between NF-κB and lung cancer have also been reported, including resistance to chemotherapy and regulation of pro-metastatic, pro-angiogenic, and anti-apoptotic genes (68).

C. Diabetes and Glucose Intolerance

It is often stated that diabetes mellitus and hyperglycemia are common in people with COPD. In a general population sample, women with COPD had a 1.8-fold increased risk of developing Type 2 diabetes compared with those without COPD (69). Hyperglycemia is an important event because it is associated with poor outcomes in patients admitted to hospital with exacerbations of the disease (70). There are several potential mechanisms that could explain this association: (*i*) oxidative stress, present in COPD, has been implicated in insulin resistance (71); (*ii*) CRP, IL-6, and TNF-α have been implicated in the pathogenesis of insulin resistance and Type 2 diabetes (72); and, (*iii*) steroid treatment could induce hyperglycemia in both stable state and during exacerbations (73).

D. Other Chronic Respiratory Conditions (Asthma, Rhinitis, Atopy, Bronchiectasis)

Asthma

There are some difficulties to estimate the prevalence of asthma in patients with COPD. This is because a high percentage of these patients with COPD have already demonstrable airway hyperresponsiveness (AHR) (74). It is often considered that in potential COPD patients, post-bronchodilator increases of more than 500 mL in their FEV_1 may indicate an underlying diagnosis of asthma (75). A recent study suggests an asthma prevalence of 3% in patients with COPD that is not any higher than in the general population (76). However, the overlap of asthma with chronic bronchitis and emphysema can be larger in the general population than previously considered in selected clinical series, especially in the elderly (77). The substantial segments of population with, on the one hand COPD and bronchial reversibility, and on the other hand of asthmatics who smoke, have systematically been excluded from clinical trials and many natural history studies. To date, we do not have efficacy or safety evidence of many therapeutic interventions in these large groups of respiratory patients.

Rhinitis and Atopy

There is no evidence that patients with COPD have a higher prevalence of atopy or atopic diseases, such as rhinitis or eczema. Specific and nonspecific immunoglobulin E levels are not elevated in patients with COPD (78).

Bronchiectasis

Most national and international guidelines consider bronchiectasis exclusion criteria to diagnose COPD. However, as bronchiectasis are often not actively searched by thoracic computed tomography (CT) scan, currently the most sensitive method to identify them, it is likely that bronchiectasis are generally underdiagnosed in COPD patients, particularly in smokers where cough and sputum production are assumed to be due to cigarette smoke (42). Therefore, it is expected a high prevalence of radiological bronchiectasis among patients with COPD. CT scanning with a high-resolution algorithm is now the test of choice to confirm a diagnosis of bronchiectasis, found in one-third of these patients then (42). Other studies found higher prevalence but were based on patients referred for investigation of cough and sputum production and most of them were nonsmokers, which may explain the high frequency observed (79).

E. Skeletal Muscle Disorders

Patients with COPD associate respiratory and peripheral muscle weakness.

Respiratory Muscles

Lung hyperinflation secondary to chronic airflow limitation carry a mechanical disadvantage to the respiratory muscles, with decreasing muscle strength and endurance (80). Other factors potentially associated with COPD can impair respiratory muscle function such as undernutrition, dyselectrolytemia, and hypoxemia. Functionally, COPD patients present a switch in Type I diaphragmatic fibers with no changes in fiber size (81). The main negative consequence is respiratory muscle fatigue with dyspnea, exercise intolerance, hypoxemia, and hypercapnia (82). Expiratory muscles have also been found impaired in some patients with COPD (83).

Peripheral Muscles

Peripheral muscle weakness is a common feature in patients with COPD, and it is related with severity of the disease. Several studies have shown muscle fiber atrophy (84), lower proportion of Type I fibers, decreased capillary density, oxidative stress (85), and decreased strength and endurance (86). Several explanatory factors have been suggested, such as inactivity, hypoxemia, dyselectrolytemia, undernutrition, steroids, oxidative stress, and systemic inflammation (87). Muscle weakness has been associated to exercise intolerance (88,89), leg fatigue, increased lactic acidosis, and hypercapnia during exercise (90,91), dyspnea, higher consumption of medical resources (92), poor quality of life (93), and lower survival (94). Muscle dysfunction is located in both upper and lower extremities, and in particular an improvement in the lower limbs has been reported after rehabilitation (95).

F. Osteoporosis and Fractures

Osteoporosis with subsequent fractures is a significant problem in patients with advanced COPD. Compared to non-COPD, patients with COPD seen in primary care were at increased risk for osteoporosis and fractures (RR, 3.1 and 1.6, respectively) (31). Thirty-six to sixty percent of COPD patients have osteoporosis (96), and its proportion increases proportionally with the severity of COPD. The risk factors include smoking, vitamin D deficiency, low BMI, hypogonadism, decreased mobility, systemic inflammation, and glucocorticoid use. It is important to note that patients with oral glucocorticoid therapy have lower bone mineral density. It is not clear this association with inhaled glucocorticoid therapy, but several studies have suggested that high dose of inhaled steroids may be associated with bone loss (97). Others did not find this association (98). However it is important to note that systemic glucocorticoid use alone does not fully explain this comorbidity. The main consequence of osteoporosis are fractures, particularly thoracic vertebral fractures that compromise lung function and hip fractures that decrease mobility and are associated with significant mortality (99).

G. Lower Respiratory Tract Infections and Pneumonia

Respiratory infection is very frequent in patients with COPD. Compared to non-COPD subjects the RR is 2.2 for low tract respiratory infection and 16 for pneumonia (31). Respiratory infections are considered the main cause of COPD exacerbations needing hospital admissions (100), and are associated with a larger decline in lung function, worsening health status, and increasing mortality (101,102). Most of these infections are caused by bacteria mainly *Haemophilus influenzae*, Pneumococcus and *Moraxella catarrhalis* (103,104). These microorganisms may also be cultured in sputum from about 25% of these patients in the absence of respiratory symptoms in stable condition, the so-called colonized COPD patients. This phenomenon might be very relevant because these patients display higher bronchial inflammation, poorer quality of life, more exacerbations, and accelerated lung function decline (105–107). Besides, chronic infection has been related with early atherogenesis mainly in those subjects with active smoking and increased CRP (108).

H. Depression

Depression and anxiety are common in patients with any chronic medical condition (109), but new evidence indicates that they have been grossly neglected and underestimated in COPD patients. Individuals with COPD have a higher prevalence of comorbid depression than either the general population or patients with other chronic illnesses, and the best estimates report a prevalence of approximately 40% in COPD patients, compared with 15% in the general adult population (110). Depression in

COPD patients leads to a lower quality of life, greater objective impairment in function, and decreased adherence to therapeutic interventions. While many depressed COPD patients have been treated empirically with antidepressants, subjecting them to antidepressant side effects, toxicities, and costs, there is a surprising lack of evidence supporting or directing that treatment (111). Most likely, holistic approaches to COPD like pulmonary rehabilitation improve several depression indicators, apart from several COPD outcomes (112).

I. Autoimmune Disorders

There are several lines of evidence suggesting an impaired immune response in patients with COPD (113–115) including increased lymphocyte T-cell accumulation in the lungs, increased bronchus-associated lymphoid tissue, and smoking is associated with an expansion of the population of antigen-presenting cells on the epithelial surface of the lower respiratory tract, increased antinuclear antibodies titers in blood, development of an autoimmune experimental model of emphysema, and identification of anti-endothelial cell antibodies in the serum of patients with end stage emphysema. For all of these previous reasons, it has been hypothesized that COPD could have an autoimmune component (116). To date the prevalence of autoimmune disorders in patients with COPD is unknown. There are two studies suggesting a possible relationship with autoimmune disorders: Birring et al. (117) found in patients with COPD who never smoked had an association with organ autoimmune disease, particularly thyroid disease. Similarly, Wisnieski et al. (118) found an association between hypo-complementemia, and urticarial vasculitis syndrome in patients with COPD. There are several ongoing studies investigating the prevalence of autoantibodies in patients with COPD and more information on this topic will likely be available shortly.

J. Anemia

Preliminary studies suggest that anemia is present in 10% to 15% of patients suffering from severe forms of COPD (119). Anemia has been associated to similar mechanisms present in other chronic diseases, such as the action of cytokines at different levels in hematopoiesis in bone marrow. In patients with COPD, it produces a significant clinical impact such as worsened dyspnea, exercise limitation, increased morbidity, and reduced survival (119).

K. Sleep-Related Disorders

Obstructive Sleep Apnea Syndrome

The association between obstructive sleep apnea syndrome (OSAS) and COPD has been labeled overlap syndrome (120), a term coined more than 20 years ago now virtually abandoned. This syndrome presents with diurnal hypoxemia and hypercapnia, pulmonary hypertension, and *cor pulmonale*. Although some earlier studies suggested that OSAS was more common than expected in patients with COPD (121), recent evidence suggests that the prevalence is not different than in patients without COPD (122,123).

Nocturnal Oxygen Desaturations

In COPD patients there is an increase in episodes of nocturnal oxygen desaturation mainly in those with $FEV_1 < 49\%$ and daytime $PaO_2 > 60$ mmHg, particularly when associated to elevated $PaCO_2$ values and high BMI (121,122). These patients should undergo testing with nocturnal pulse oxymetry in order to identify possible nocturnal oxygen desaturations. In those patients with arterial PO_2 higher than 60 mmHg and sleep desaturation, nocturnal oxygen therapy did not modify the evolution of pulmonary hemodynamics and no effect on survival was observed; however, the small number of deaths in this study precluded any firm conclusion (123).

L.   Other Comorbidities

A number of other comorbidities have been previously associated with COPD, but with a somewhat smaller clinical impact expected. They include cataracts, reportedly increased in patients treated with inhaled steroids (124), glaucoma, peptic ulcer (125), impotence (126), and gastroesophageal reflux (127), among others. Gastroesophageal reflux is increased but this comorbidity is associated with several chronic respiratory disorders associated to changes in thoracic pressures (128). To our knowledge, no COPD research has been focused on deafness and macular degeneration, two of the most common conditions observed in elderly patients seen in primary care without or with COPD (129,130).

XI.   Assessment of Comorbidities in Primary Care

The assessment of comorbidities in primary care might include screening for all the conditions previously described. However, Public Health and Preventive Medicine identify a set of rules before implementing large-scale screening procedures in the general population (131,132). Namely, for a comorbidity to be screened out in COPD patients, the following questions should be answered: (*i*) Is there an effective intervention? (*ii*) Does intervention earlier than usual improve outcome? (*iii*) Is there an effective screening test that recognizes disease earlier than usual? (*iv*) Is the test available and acceptable to the target population? (*v*) Is the disease one that commands priority? and (*vi*) Do the benefits exceed the costs?

Usually, if the answer to these six questions is "yes," then the case for screening is sound. However, for most of these criteria we do not have evidence that this does occur to date. These screening procedures might include (Table 2) (9,133,134):

1. *Anamnesis and physical examination* focused to respiratory disease and eventual comorbidities.
2. *Calculation of BMI*, mainly in those patients who have recently lost weight or in the obese ones.
3. *Pulmonary function tests*, to assess the severity of COPD, and to rule out bronchial hyperresponsiveness, asthma, other obstructive and restrictive disorders.
4. *EKG*, to rule out subclinical cardiopathies. If positive the patient should be referred to a cardiologist.
5. *Blood analysis*, including routine analysis to investigate potential risk factors for cardiovascular diseases (glucose, lipids), hemoglobin (anemia or

Table 2 Suggested List of Diagnostic Tests and Procedures to Assess Comorbidities in COPD

Assessment	Diagnostic test
Primary care	Anamnesis and physical exploration
	Calculation of BMI
	Pulmonary function tests
	EKG
	Blood analysis
	Chest X ray
Specialized care	Echocardiography
	Pulmonary catheterism
	Sleep studies
	Bone densitometry
	CT thoracic scan
	Fiber-optic bronchoscopy
	Sputum culture
	Autoimmune tests
	Muscle function
	Other assessments depending on symptoms and patient characteristics
In the event of a COPD exacerbation	Blood tests
	Chest X ray
	EKG
	Sputum culture
	Hyperglycemia test
	Other tests to rule out lung cancer suspicion, cardiac comorbidities, and infection
	Additional, secondary tests might include echocardiography, CT scan, etc.

Abbreviations: BMI, body mass index; COPD, chronic obstructive pulmonary disease; CT, computed tomography; EKG, electrocardiography.

polycythemia), possibility of infection (white blood cells), and nutritional parameters (proteins and electrolytes).

6. *Chest X ray.* It is very important to rule out lung cancer that is particularly prevalent in patients with mild COPD (133), pulmonary hypertension, and cardiomegaly. Moreover it can detect the occurrence of bronchiectasis, and assessing the bone density it can help to evaluate the possibility of osteopenia/ osteoporosis.

XII. Assessment of Comorbidities in Respiratory Medicine

COPD patients visited by pulmonologists usually have more advanced stage of the disease, and consequently they have more chances to suffer several comorbidities. Besides the previous procedures to be conducted in primary care, the respiratory physician could expand this assessment with the following tests (Table 2):

1. *Echocardiography.* Indicated if there is clinical suspicion of pulmonary hypertension or cardiac comorbidities.

2. *Pulmonary catheterism.* It could be performed in those patients with disproportionate pulmonary hypertension (more than 50 mmHg estimated by EKG) if it is considered for specific treatment.

3. *Sleep studies.* Sleep apnea syndrome and/or nocturnal desaturations should be evaluated in those patients with overweight, hypersomnia, relatively preserved lung function (FEV_1 predicted > 50% predicted) with hypoxemia and/or hypercapnia, and/or *cor pulmonale*.

4. *Bone densitometry.* To be performed only in those patients with suspected osteopenia, particulary elderly women.

5. *Thoracic CT scan.* Mainly it should be performed in those patients with radiological pulmonary abnormalities such as nodule/mass or bronchiectasis.

6. *Fiber-optic bronchoscopy.* It should be performed basically in those patients with a suspected lung neoplasm.

7. *Sputum culture.* Useful to rule out bacterial colonization in those patients with more exacerbations, bronchiectasis, and/or hypersecretors.

8. *Autoimmune tests.* In patients with clinical suspicion of a systemic autoimmune systemic disease and in those with low exposure to tobacco smoking, it should be reasonable to perform basic blood immunology.

9. *Muscle function.* Tests of respiratory muscle function should be performed in patients with symptoms or signs suggesting respiratory muscle dysfunction (normal alveolar–arterial oxygen partial pressure difference or lower FVC without air trapping). In these patients, it should be advisable to assess mouth maximal inspiratory and expiratory pressures. The evaluation of peripheral muscles could be done in patients with low exercise capacity.

10. *Other assessments (ophtalmic, psychiatric, gastrointestinal).* Depending on the symptoms, patients should be referred to the corresponding specialist.

Evaluation of all clinical data and procedures performed during exacerbations of COPD is mandatory, depending on the availability of resources and urgency, to identify the main trigger/s to establish the most appropriate treatment strategy (Table 2). It might include: blood tests, chest X ray, EKG, and sputum culture, to rule out hyperglycemia, anemia/policytemia, or leukocytosis lung cancer suspicion, cardiac comorbidities, and infection. Depending on the results of these studies and the presence of other diseases or conditions, the evaluation could be expanded (EKG, CT scan, etc.).

Overall, the assessment of comorbidities is clinically relevant in patients with COPD for a number of reasons: (*i*) Cardiovascular disease and lung cancer are major causes of death in mild to moderate COPD (41); (*ii*) The number of comorbidites directly correlates with poor quality of life; (*iii*) It correlates with systemic inflammation, and it is associated with systemic effects, prognosis, and quality of life. Thus, evaluating and treating carefully the comorbidities in patients with COPD should improve their quality of life and prognosis, giving them a holistic assessment.

XIII. Treatment Considerations in COPD

Treatment guidelines provide recommendations including the use of multidrug regimens for the treatment of patients with a given disease. However, they are based

Table 3 Potential Interactions and Contraindications in the Management and Treatment of COPD

Interactions of comorbidity treatment with COPD	Interactions of COPD treatments with comorbidities
β-Blockers	β-Agonists
Hypnotics	Anticholinergics
Statins	Methylxanthines
ACE inhibitors and ARA	Steroids
Antibiotics	Rehabilitation

Abbreviations: ACE, angiotensin converting enzyme; ARA, angiotensin receptor antagonists; COPD, chronic obstructive pulmonary disease.

on evidence from clinical trials that excluded COPD patients with several coexisting health conditions (135). All medications have the potential for harm as well as benefit, and due to increased comorbidity in patients with COPD, there are potential interactions that might lead for adverse short- or long-term consequences in these patients with multiple conditions. Then the treatment of comorbidities could influence the natural history of COPD, and the other way round, treatment of COPD could influence other associated health conditions (Table 3).

A. Interactions of Comorbidity Treatment with COPD

β-Blockers

Patients with COPD frequently have associated cardiac comorbidity requiring β-blockers. This treatment is known to worsen FEV_1 and AHR in patients with asthma (136). This is an important issue because both characteristics determine several outcomes of COPD. There are several studies showing deleterious effects of nonselective β-blockers over lung function. This effect does not occur in cardiac selective β-blockers (137). Thus, cardio-selective β-blockers can generally be administered safely to patients with heart failure and COPD.

Hypnotics

Patients with COPD often have sleep complaints reducing their quality of life. Many of the traditional sedatives and hypnotics to be used in any COPD population include benzodiazepines, imidazopyridines, pyrazolopyrimidines and, less commonly, anti-depressants and phenothiazines. Clinical trials support the role of numerous agents in treating insomnia, but do not always provide reassurance that these therapies can be used safely, particularly in the patients with severe COPD with hypercapnia (138). Therefore, when prescription of a sedative is to be made, extra caution is required for those patients at increased risk of adverse respiratory effects, such as those with advanced disease and hypercapnia in whom pharmacological therapy of insomnia is often best avoided.

Statins

Patients with COPD have an increased risk of IHD, and statins reduce mortality and morbidity in IHD. In a hypothesis-generating exercise, statins and other cardiovascular drugs were associated with better outcomes in COPD patients (139). In a retrospective, observational study of 854 COPD patients discharged from hospital, treatment with statins was associated with improved survival after discharge. Inhaled corticosteroids appeared to increase the survival benefit associated with statin use (140). In this case the interaction might be positive.

ACE Inhibitors and ARA

This is another example of potential positive interaction. Treatment of patients with COPD is often complicated by the coexistence of systemic arterial hypertension and left ventricular failure (141). They are frequently treated with angiotensin converting enzyme (ACE) inhibitors or angiotensin receptor antagonists (ARA). These drugs have an additional anti-inflammatory effect (142). Then, inflammation already present in COPD could benefit from these drugs. It has been demonstrated with this approach, that patients with cardiopathy and COPD reduce exacerbations of the disease and improve the cardiovascular components of morbidity and mortality in these patients (143). Importantly, when combining statins and ACE inhibitors or ARA, this combination in a retrospective cohort study found a reduction in COPD hospitalization and total mortality (142). This combination also reduced myocardial infarction in a subset of patients characterized by high cardiovascular risk. These studies suggest a cardioprotective effect of statins, ACE, and ARA in COPD patients. But, apart from potential benefits when treating undiagnosed cardiovascular disease, this approach affect pulmonary disease itself as suggested by a reduction of hospitalizations secondary to COPD. The authors of these studies propose clinical trials to validate their observations.

Antibiotics

Excessive, irrational treatment with antibiotics in COPD patients could change the bacterial flora of these patients, facilitating the existence of multiple-drug–resistant bacteria (MDRB). In 8% of severe exacerbations of COPD that require mechanical ventilation, MDRB bacteria have been found (144). Then in these patients is very important to optimize antibiotic treatment in case of any infection elsewhere.

B. Interactions of COPD Treatment with Comorbidity

Inhaled β-Agonists

Short- and long-term inhaled β-agonists are often used in the management of patients with COPD. COPD patients, again as previously discussed, frequently have cardiovascular disease, and then β-adrenergic agonists exert physiologic effects that are the opposite of those of β-blockers used to treat cardiopathy. The initiation of β-agonist treatment increases heart rate and reduces potassium concentrations compared with placebo (145). β(2)-agonist used in patients with chronic obstructive airway disease might increase the risk for adverse cardiovascular events (146). In the recently reported Toward a Revolution in COPD Health study results, the best cardiovascular morbidity and mortality were observed in the individuals randomized to salmeterol (147). In conclusion, these drugs should be used carefully in patients with

COPD and cardiovascular disease. Anecdotally, it has been reported a few cases of acute glaucoma in the course of treatment with aerosols of salbutamol (148).

Anticholinergics

Antimuscarinics are usually considered with having a good cardiovascular safety in most studies, although a recent case control study showed association with supraventricular tachycardia (149). Similarly to nebulized salbutamol, it has been reported a few cases of acute glaucoma in the course of treatment with aerosols of ipratropium bromide (148) and also one case associated with tiotropium (150). Because patients with COPD can have glaucoma, it is very important to protect their eyes during the nebulization. Also patients with COPD are elderly and most of them are at risk to suffer prostate hypertrophy, which potentially could be impaired by ipratropium bromide (151).

Methylxanthines

This second line of treatment has shown increased cardiovascular side effects and should be used carefully in patients with COPD and cardiovascular disease. These drugs produce frequent nausea and this is an important issue in those patients with chronic conditions such as gastroesophageal reflux and those who require taking oral medications. Therefore, the benefits of theophylline in stable COPD have to be weighed against the risk of their adverse effects. However recent findings showed that low doses of methylxanthines activate hystone deacetylases, and these drugs have regained further therapeutic interest (152).

Steroids

Systemic steroids have been proved useful in exacerbations of COPD (153). However they have several significant side effects, namely hyperglycemia, osteopenia, myopathy, and cataracts (154). All of these side effects concur with the systemic effects of COPD and could worsen them. In frail patients with repeated COPD exacerbations, systemic steroid treatment must be weighed against the risk for serious adverse effects (155). On the other hand, inhaled steroids decrease exacerbations and improve quality of life, and at low doses appear to be safe. However, there is growing evidence that higher doses have a slight increase in the risk of fractures (hip, upper extremities, and vertebral fractures) (156).

Pulmonary Rehabilitation

It has proven useful in patients with COPD because it improves both quality of life and exercise tolerance (157). However, it could be a contraindication in patients with severe osteoporosis with bone fractures, mainly, vertebra and hip.

XIV. Concluding Remarks

Comorbidities are a regular feature of general practice and specialist care in general. However, to date evidence-based diagnostic and treatment strategies generally overlook comorbidities (158). Despite the support that disease-specific guidelines give, these guidelines may introduce more problems than they solve when used in patients with comorbidities (159). Treatment or even diagnosis of a disease might interact negatively with the treatment or natural course of a coexisting disease. Comorbidities may become harder to manage when COPD is present, either because COPD adds to the total level of disability or because COPD therapy adversely affects the comorbid disorder. Until more integrated guidance about disease management for specific comorbid problems becomes available, the focus should be on identification and management of these individual problems in line with local treatment guidance. Comorbidities are common in COPD and should be actively identified. Comorbidities often complicate the management of COPD, and conversely.

References

1. Chapman KR, Mannino DM, Soriano JB, et al. Epidemiology and costs of chronic obstructive pulmonary disease. Eur Respir J 2006; 27:188–207.
2. Viegi G, Scognamiglio A, Baldacci S, Pistelli F, Carrozzi L. Epidemiology of chronic obstructive pulmonary disease. Respiration 2001; 68:4–192.
3. Anto JM, Vermeire P, Vestbo J, Sunyer J. Epidemiology of chronic obstructive pulmonary disease. Eur Respir J 2001; 17:982–94.
4. Mannino DM, Homa DM, Akinbami LJ, Ford ES, Redd SC. Chronic obstructive pulmonary disease surveillance—United States, 1971–2000. MMWR Surveill Summ 2002; 51:1–16.
5. Mannino DM. COPD: epidemiology, prevalence, morbidity and mortality, and disease heterogeneity. Chest 2002; 121(5 Suppl.):121S–6.
6. Mannino DM. Chronic obstructive pulmonary disease: definition and epidemiology. Respir Care 2003; 48:1185–91.
7. Pauwels RA, Rabe KF. Burden and clinical features of chronic obstructive pulmonary disease (COPD). Lancet 2004; 364:613–20.
8. Doherty DE, Briggs DD, Jr. Chronic obstructive pulmonary disease: epidemiology, pathogenesis, disease course, and prognosis. Clin Cornerstone 2004; (Suppl. 2):S5–16.
9. Pauwels RA, Buist AS, Calverley PM, Jenkins CR, Hurd SS, GOLD Scientific Committee. Global strategy for the diagnosis, management, and prevention of chronic obstructive pulmonary disease. NHLBI/WHO Global Initiative for Chronic Obstructive Lung Disease (GOLD) workshop summary. Am J Respir Crit Care Med 2001; 163:1256–76.
10. GOLD Guidelines 2006. (Accessed April 4, 2007 at www.goldcopd.com)
11. Celli BR, MacNee W, ATS/ERS Task Force. Standards for the diagnosis and treatment of patients with COPD: a summary of the ATS/ERS position paper. Eur Respir J 2004; 23:932–46.
12. United Network for Organ Sharing (UNOS) online database. www.unos.org (last accessed August 31, 2007).
13. Charlson ME, Pompei P, Ales KL, MacKenzie CR. A new method of classifying prognostic comorbidity in longitudinal studies: development and validation. J Chronic Dis 1987; 40:373–83.
14. Deyo RA, Cherkin DC, Ciol MA. Adapting a clinical comorbidity index for use with ICD-9-CM administrative databases. J Clin Epidemiol 1992; 45:613–9.
15. Ghali WA, Hall RE, Rosen AK, Ash AS, Moskowitz MA. Searching for an improved clinical comorbidity index for use with ICD-9-CM administrative data. J Clin Epidemiol 1996; 49(3):273–8.
16. Davis RM, Novotny TE. The epidemiology of cigarette smoking and its impact on chronic obstructive pulmonary disease. Am Rev Respir Dis 1989; 140(3 Pt 2):S82–4.
17. Wasswa-Kintu S, Gan WQ, Man SF, Pare PD, Sin DD. Relationship between reduced forced expiratory volume in one second and the risk of lung cancer: a systematic review and meta-analysis. Thorax 2005; 60:570–5.
18. Sin DD, Wu L, Man SF. The relationship between reduced lung function and cardiovascular mortality: a population-based study and a systematic review of the literature. Chest 2005; 127:1952–9.
19. Gan WQ, Man SF, Senthilselvan A, Sin DD. Association between chronic obstructive pulmonary disease and systemic inflammation: a systematic review and a meta-analysis. Thorax 2004; 59:574–80.

20. Franciosi LG, Page CP, Celli BR, et al. Markers of disease severity in chronic obstructive pulmonary disease. Pulm Pharmacol Ther 2006; 19:189–99.
21. Sin DD, Man SF. Skeletal muscle weakness, reduced exercise tolerance, and COPD: is systemic inflammation the missing link? Thorax 2006; 61:1–3.
22. Sin DD, Man SF. Why are patients with chronic obstructive pulmonary disease at increased risk of cardiovascular diseases? The potential role of systemic inflammation in chronic obstructive pulmonary disease Circulation 2003; 107:1514–9.
23. Agusti A. Thomas A. Neff lecture. Chronic obstructive pulmonary disease: a systemic disease. Proc Am Thorac Soc 2006; 3:478–81.
24. Sin DD, Man SF, McWilliams A, Lam S. Progression of airway dysplasia and C-reactive protein in smokers at high risk of lung cancer. Am J Respir Crit Care Med 2006; 173:535–9.
25. Bolton CE, Ionescu AA, Shiels KM, et al. Associated loss of fat-free mass and bone mineral density in chronic obstructive pulmonary disease. Am J Respir Crit Care Med 2004; 170:1286–93.
26. Broekhuizen R, Wouters EF, Creutzberg EC, Schols AM. Raised CRP levels mark metabolic and functional impairment in advanced COPD. Thorax 2006; 61:17–22.
27. Pistelli R, Lange P, Miller DL. Determinants of prognosis of COPD in the elderly: mucus hypersecretion, infections, cardiovascular comorbidity. Eur Respir J Suppl 2003; 40:10s–4.
28. Vestbo J, Prescott E, Almdal T, et al. Body mass, fat-free body mass, and prognosis in patients with chronic obstructive pulmonary disease from a random population sample: findings from the Copenhagen City Heart Study. Am J Respir Crit Care Med 2006; 173:79–83.
29. Sevenoaks MJ, Stockley RA. Chronic obstructive pulmonary disease, inflammation and co-morbidity—a common inflammatory phenotype? Respir Res 2006; 7:70.
30. Sorlie PD, Kannel WB, O'Connor G. Mortality associated with respiratory function and symptoms in advanced age. The Framingham Study. Am Rev Respir Dis 1989; 140:379–84.
31. Soriano JB, Visick GT, Muellerova H, Payvandi N, Hansell AL. Patterns of comorbidities in newly diagnosed COPD and asthma in the primary care. Chest 2005; 128:2099–107.
32. Mapel DW, Hurley JS, Frost FJ, Petersen HV, Picchi MA, Coultas DB. Health care utilization in chronic obstructive pulmonary disease. A case-control study in a health maintenance organization. Arch Intern Med 2000; 160:2653–8.
33. Groenewegen KH, Schols AM, Wouters EF. Mortality and mortality-related factors after hospitalization for acute exacerbation of COPD. Chest 2003; 124:459–67.
34. Patil SP, Krishnan JA, Lechtzin N, Diette GB. In-hospital mortality following acute exacerbations of chronic obstructive pulmonary disease. Arch Intern Med 2003; 163:1180–6.
35. Incalzi RA, Fuso L, De Rosa M, et al. Co-morbidity contributes to predict mortality of patients with chronic obstructive pulmonary disease. Eur Respir J 1997; 10:2794–800.
36. Fuso L, Incalzi RA, Pistelli R, et al. Predicting mortality of patients hospitalized for acutely exacerbated chronic obstructive pulmonary disease. Am J Med 1995; 98:272–7.
37. Holguin F, Folch E, Redd SC, Mannino DM. Comorbidity and mortality in COPD-related hospitalizations in the United States, 1979 to 2001. Chest 2005; 128:2005–11.
38. Zielinski J, MacNee W, Wedzicha J, et al. Causes of death in patients with COPD and chronic respiratory failure. Monaldi Arch Chest Dis 1997; 52:43–7.
39. Zielinski J. Circumstances of death in chronic obstructive pulmonary disease. Monaldi Arch Chest Dis 1998; 53:324–30.
40. Anthonisen NR, Skeans MA, Wise RA, Manfreda J, Kanner RE, Connett JE. The effects of a smoking cessation intervention on 14.5-year mortality: a randomized clinical trial. Ann Intern Med 2005; 142:233–9.
41. Sin DD, Anthonisen NR, Soriano JB, Agusti AGN. Mortality in COPD: role of comorbidities. Eur Respir J 2006; 28:1245–57.
42. Weiss ST, DeMeo DL, Postma DS. COPD: problems in diagnosis and measurement. Eur Respir J Suppl 2003; 41:4s–12.
43. Wouters EF. Nutrition and metabolism in COPD. Chest 2000; 117(5 Suppl. 1):274S–80.
44. Gan WQ, Man SF, Sin DD. The interactions between cigarette smoking and reduced lung function on systemic inflammation. Chest 2005; 127:558–64.
45. de VF, van Staa TP, Bracke MS, Cooper C, Leufkens HG, Lammers JW. Severity of obstructive airway disease and risk of osteoporotic fracture. Eur Respir J 2005; 25:879–84.
46. Krishnan G, Grant BJ, Muti PC, et al. Association between anemia and quality of life in a population sample of individuals with chronic obstructive pulmonary disease. BMC Pulm Med 2006; 6:23.

47. Mannino DM, Aguayo SM, Petty TL, Redd SC. Low lung function and incident lung cancer in the United States: data from the First National Health and Nutrition Examination Survey follow-up. Arch Intern Med 2003; 163:1475–80.

48. Yeo J, Karimova G, Bansal S. Co-morbidity in older patients with COPD—its impact on health service utilisation and quality of life, a community study. Age Ageing 2006; 35(1):33–7.

49. Celli BR, Cote CG, Marin JM, et al. The body-mass index, airflow obstruction, dyspnea, and exercise capacity index in chronic obstructive pulmonary disease. N Engl J Med 2004; 350:1005–12.

50. Mackay J, Eriksen M, eds. The Tobacco Atlas. Geneva: World Health Organization, 2002. (Accessed July 4, 2006 at http://www.who.int/tobacco/statistics/tobacco_atlas/en/print.html)

51. Rennard S, Decramer M, Calverley PM, et al. Impact of COPD in North America and Europe in 2000: subjects' perspective of Confronting COPD International Survey. Eur Respir J 2002; 20:799–805.

52. Sin DD, Man SF. Chronic obstructive pulmonary disease as a risk factor for cardiovascular morbidity and mortality. Proc Am Thorac Soc 2005; 2:8–11.

53. Curkendall SM, DeLuise C, Jones JK, et al. Cardiovascular disease in patients with chronic obstructive pulmonary disease, Saskatchewan Canada cardiovascular disease in COPD patients. Ann Epidemiol 2006; 16:63–70.

54. Buffon A, Biasucci LM, Liuzzo G, D'Onofrio G, Crea F, Maseri A. Widespread coronary inflammation in unstable angina. N Engl J Med 2002; 347:5–12.

55. Rutten FH, Cramer MJ, Lammers JW, Grobbee DE, Hoes AW. Heart failure and chronic obstructive pulmonary disease: an ignored combination? Eur J Heart Fail 2006; 8(7):706–11.

56. Rutten FH, Moons KG, Cramer MJ, et al. Recognising heart failure in elderly patients with stable chronic obstructive pulmonary disease in primary care: cross sectional diagnostic study. Br Med J 2005; 331:1379.

57. Huiart L, Ernst P, Suissa S. Cardiovascular morbidity and mortality in COPD. Chest 2005; 128:2640–6.

58. Anthonisen NR, Connett JE, Kiley JP. Effects of smoking intervention and the use of an inhaled anticholinergic bronchodilator on the rate of decline of FEV_1. The Lung Health Study. J Am Med Assoc 1994; 272:1497–505.

59. Mannino DM, Watt G, Hole D, et al. The natural history of chronic obstructive pulmonary disease. Eur Respir J 2006; 27:627–43.

60. Tillie-Leblond I, Marquette CH, Perez T, et al. Pulmonary embolism in patients with unexplained exacerbation of chronic obstructive pulmonary disease: prevalence and risk factors. Ann Intern Med 2006; 144:390–6.

61. Rutschmann OT, Cornuz J, Poletti PA, et al. Should pulmonary embolism be suspected in exacerbation of chronic obstructive pulmonary disease? Thorax 2007; 62:121–5.

62. Wedzicha JA, Hurst JR. Chronic obstructive pulmonary disease exacerbation and risk of pulmonary embolism. Thorax 2007; 62:103–4.

63. Sherman CB. Health effects of cigarette smoking. Clin Chest Med 1991; 12:643–58.

64. Jacobs DR, Jr., Adachi H, Mulder I, et al. Cigarette smoking and mortality risk: twenty-five-year follow-up of the Seven Countries Study. Arch Intern Med 1999; 159:733–40.

65. Pride NB, Soriano JB. Chronic obstructive pulmonary disease in the United Kingdom: trends in mortality, morbidity, and smoking. Curr Opin Pulm Med 2002; 8:95–101.

66. Lapperre TS, Postma DS, Gosman MM, et al. Relation between duration of smoking cessation and bronchial inflammation in COPD. Thorax 2006; 61:115–21.

67. Hogg JC, Chu F, Utokaparch S, et al. The nature of small-airway obstruction in chronic obstructive pulmonary disease. N Engl J Med 2004; 350:2645–53.

68. Dennis PA, Van Waes C, Gutkind JS, et al. The biology of tobacco and nicotine: bench to bedside. Cancer Epidemiol Biomarkers Prev 2005; 14:764–7.

69. Rana JS, Mittleman MA, Sheikh J, et al. Chronic obstructive pulmonary disease, asthma, and risk of type 2 diabetes in women. Diabetes Care 2004; 27:2478–84.

70. Baker EH, Janaway CH, Philips BJ, et al. Hyperglycaemia is associated with poor outcomes in patients admitted to hospital with acute exacerbations of chronic obstructive pulmonary disease. Thorax 2006; 61:284–9.

71. Rosen P, Nawroth PP, King G, Moller W, Tritschler HJ, Packer L. The role of oxidative stress in the onset and progression of diabetes and its complications: a summary of a Congress Series sponsored by UNESCO-MCBN, the American Diabetes Association and the German Diabetes Society. Diabetes Metab Res Rev 2001; 17:189–212.

72. Pradhan AD, Manson JE, Rifai N, Buring JE, Ridker PM. C-reactive protein, interleukin 6, and risk of developing type 2 diabetes mellitus. J Am Med Assoc 2001; 286:327–34.

73. Sayiner A, Aytemur ZA, Cirit M, Unsal I. Systemic glucocorticoids in severe exacerbations of COPD. Chest 2001; 119:726–30.

74. Hansen EF, Vestbo J. Bronchodilator reversibility in COPD: the roguish but harmless little brother of airway hyperresponsiveness? Eur Respir J 2005; 26:6–7.

75. O'Brien C, Guest PJ, Hill SL, Stockley RA. Physiological and radiological characterisation of patients diagnosed with chronic obstructive pulmonary disease in primary care. Thorax 2000; 55:635–42.

76. Chen Y, Stewart P, Dales R, Johansen H, Bryan S, Taylor G. In a retrospective study of chronic obstructive pulmonary disease inpatients, respiratory comorbidities were significantly associated with prognosis. J Clin Epidemiol 2005; 58:1199–205.

77. Soriano JB, Davis KJ, Coleman B, Visick G, Mannino D, Pride NB. The proportional Venn diagram of obstructive lung disease: two approximations from the United States and the United Kingdom. Chest 2003; 124:474–81.

78. Barnes PJ. Against the Dutch hypothesis: asthma and chronic obstructive pulmonary disease are distinct diseases. Am J Respir Crit Care Med 2006; 174:240–3.

79. Smith IE, Jurriaans E, Diederich S, Ali N, Shneerson JM, Flower CD. Chronic sputum production: correlations between clinical features and findings on high resolution computed tomographic scanning of the chest. Thorax 1996; 51:914–8.

80. Polkey MI, Kyroussis D, Hamengard C-H, Mills GH, Green M, Moxham J. Diaphragm strength in chronic obstructive pulmonary disease. Am J Respir Crit Care Med 1996; 154:1310–7.

81. Levine S, Kaiser L, Leferovich J, Tikunov B. Cellular adaptations in the diaphragm in chronic obstructive pulmonary disease. N Engl J Med 1997; 337:1799–806.

82. Grassino A, Clanton T. Respiratory muscle fatigue. Semin Respir Med 1991; 12:305–21.

83. Ninane V. "Intrinsic" PEEP(PEEPi): role of expiratory muscles. Eur Respir J 1997; 10:516–8.

84. Whittom F, Jobin J, Simard PM, et al. Histochemical and morphological characteristics of the vastus lateralis muscle in patients with chronic obstructive pulmonary disease. Med Sci Sports Exerc 1998; 30:1467–74.

85. Sauleda J, García-Palmer FJ, Wiesner R, et al. Cytochrome oxidase activity and mitochondrial gene expression in skeletal muscle of patients with chronic obstructive pulmonary disease. Am J Respir Crit Care Med 1998; 157:1413–7.

86. Bernard S, Leblanc P, Whittom F, et al. Peripheral muscle weakness in patient with chronic obstructive pulmonary disease. Am J Respir Crit Care Med 1998; 158:629–34.

87. Maltais F, Leblanc P, Jobin J, Casaburi R. Peripheral muscle dysfunction in chronic obstructive pulmonary disease. Clin Chest Med 2000; 21:665–77.

88. Wang XN, Williams TJ, McKennna MJ, et al. Skeletal muscle oxidative capacity, fiber type, and metabolites after lung transplantation. Am J Respir Crit Care Med 1999; 160:57–63.

89. Rabinovich RA, Ardite E, Troosters T, et al. Reduced muscle redox capacity after endurance training in patients with chronic obstructive pulmonary disease. Am J Respir Crit Care Med 2001; 164:1114–8.

90. Maltais F, Simard AA, Simard C, et al. Oxidative capacity of the skeletal muscle and lactic acid kinetics during exercise in normal subjects and in patients with COPD. Am J Respir Crit Care Med 1996; 153:288–93.

91. Casaburi R, Patessio A, Ioli F, Zanaboni S, Donner CF, Wasserman K. Reductions in exercise lactic acidosis and ventilation as a result of exercise training in patients with obstructive lung disease. Am Rev Respir Dis 1991; 143:9–18.

92. Decramer M, Gosselink R, Troosters T, Verschueren M, Evers G. Muscle weakness is related to utilization of health care resources in COPD patients. Eur Respir J 1997; 10:417–23.

93. Simpson K, Killian K, McCartney N, Stubbing DG, Jones NL. Randomised controlled trial of weightlifting exercise in patients with chronic airflow limitation. Thorax 1992; 47:70–5.

94. Schols AM, Slangen J, Volovics L, Wouters EF. Weight loss is a reversible factor in the prognosis of chronic obstructive pulmonary disease. Am J Respir Crit Care Med 1998; 157(6 Pt 1):1791–7.

95. Hernandez N, Orozco-Levi M, Belalcazar V, et al. Dual morphometrical changes of the deltoid muscle in patients with COPD. Respir Physiol Neurobiol 2003; 134:219–29.

96. Biskobing DM. COPD and osteoporosis. Chest 2002; 121:609–20.

97. Scanlon PD, Connett JE, Wise RA, et al. Loss of bone density with inhaled triamcinolone in Lung Health Study II. Am J Respir Crit Care Med 2004; 170:1302–9.

98. Suissa S, Baltzan M, Kremer R, Ernst P. Inhaled and nasal corticosteroid use and the risk of fracture. Am J Respir Crit Care Med 2004; 169:83–8.

99. Myers AH, Robinson EG, Van Natta ML, Michelson JD, Collins K, Baker SP. Hip fractures among the elderly: factors associated with in-hospital mortality. Am J Epidemiol 1991; 134:1128–37.

100. Burge S, Wedzicha JA. COPD exacerbations: definitions and classifications. Eur Respir J Suppl 2003; 41:46s–53.
101. Donaldson GC, Seemungal TA, Bhowmik A, Wedzicha JA. Relationship between exacerbation frequency and lung function decline in chronic obstructive pulmonary disease. Thorax 2002; 57:847–52.
102. Soler-Cataluna JJ, Martinez-Garcia MA, Roman SP, Salcedo E, Navarro M, Ochando R. Severe acute exacerbations and mortality in patients with chronic obstructive pulmonary disease. Thorax 2005; 60:925–31.
103. Monso E, Ruiz J, Rosell A, et al. Bacterial infection in chronic obstructive pulmonary disease. A study of stable and exacerbated outpatients using the protected specimen brush. Am J Respir Crit Care Med 1995; 152(4 Pt 1):1316–20.
104. Miravitlles M, Espinosa C, Fernandez-Laso E, Martos JA, Maldonado JA, Gallego M. Relationship between bacterial flora in sputum and functional impairment in patients with acute exacerbations of COPD. Study Group of Bacterial Infection in COPD. Chest 1999; 116:40–6.
105. Monso E. Bronchial colonization in chronic obstructive pulmonary disease: what's hiding under the rug. Arch Bronconeumol 2004; 40:543–6.
106. Wilkinson TM, Patel IS, Wilks M, Donaldson GC, Wedzicha JA. Airway bacterial load and FEV_1 decline in patients with chronic obstructive pulmonary disease. Am J Respir Crit Care Med 2003; 167:1090–5.
107. Patel IS, Seemungal TAR, Wilks M, Lloyd-Owen SJ, Donaldson GC, Wedzicha JA. Relationship between bacterial colonisation and the frequency, character, and severity of COPD exacerbations. Thorax 2002; 57:759–64.
108. Kiechl S, Werner P, Egger G, et al. Active and passive smoking, chronic infections, and the risk of carotid atherosclerosis: prospective results from the Bruneck Study. Stroke 2002; 33:2170–6.
109. Katon W, Lin EH, Kroenke K. The association of depression and anxiety with medical symptom burden in patients with chronic medical illness. Gen Hosp Psychiatry 2007; 29:147–55.
110. Norwood R, Balkissoon R. Current perspectives on management of co-morbid depression in COPD. COPD 2005; 2:185–93.
111. Horn EK, van Benthem TB, Hakkaart-van Roijen L, et al. Cost-effectiveness of collaborative care for chronically ill patients with comorbid depressive disorder in the general hospital setting, a randomised controlled trial. BMC Health Serv Res 2007; 7:28.
112. Paz-Diaz H, Montes de Oca M, Lopez JM, Celli BR. Pulmonary rehabilitation improves depression, anxiety, dyspnea and health status in patients with COPD. Am J Phys Med Rehabil 2007; 86:30–6.
113. Inoue S, Nakamura H, Otake K, et al. Impaired pulmonary inflammatory responses are a prominent feature of streptococcal pneumonia in mice with experimental emphysema. Am J Respir Crit Care Med 2003; 167:764–70.
114. Voelkel N, Taraseviciene-Stewart L. Emphysema: an autoimmune vascular disease? Proc Am Thorac Soc 2005; 2:23–5.
115. Taraseviciene-Stewart L, Burns N, Kraskauskas D, Nicolls MR, Tuder RM, Voelkel NF. Mechanisms of autoimmune emphysema. Proc Am Thorac Soc 2006; 3:486–7.
116. Agusti A, MacNee W, Donaldson K, Cosio M. Hypothesis: does COPD have an autoimmune component? Thorax 2003; 58:832–4.
117. Birring SS, Brightling CE, Bradding P, et al. Clinical, radiologic, and induced sputum features of chronic obstructive pulmonary disease in nonsmokers: a descriptive study. Am J Respir Crit Care Med 2002; 166:1078–83.
118. Wisnieski JJ, Baer AN, Christensen J, et al. Hypocomplementemic urticarial vasculitis syndrome. Clinical and serologic findings in 18 patients. Medicine (Baltimore) 1995; 74:24–41.
119. Similowski T, Agusti A, MacNee W, Schonhofer B. The potential impact of anaemia of chronic disease in COPD. Eur Respir J 2006; 27:390–6.
120. Flenley DC. Sleep in chronic obstructive lung disease. Clin Chest Med 1985; 6:651–61.
121. Guilleminault C, Cummiskey J, Motta J. Chronic obstructive airflow disease and sleep studies. Am Rev Respir Dis 1980; 122:397–406.
122. Weitzenblum E, Chaouat A. Sleep and chronic obstructive pulmonary disease. Sleep Med Rev 2004; 8:281–94.
123. Bednarek M, Plywaczewski R, Jonczak L, Zielinski J. There is no relationship between chronic obstructive pulmonary disease and obstructive sleep apnea syndrome: a population study. Respiration 2005; 72:142–9.

124. Gartlehner G, Hansen RA, Carson SS, Lohr KN. Efficacy and safety of inhaled corticosteroids in patients with COPD: a systematic review and meta-analysis of health outcomes. Ann Fam Med 2006; 4:253–62.

125. Wakabayashi O, Suzuki J, Miura A, et al. The etiology of peptic ulceration in patients with chronic pulmonary emphysema. Nippon Shokakibyo Gakkai Zasshi 1994; 91:2174–82.

126. Koseoglu N, Koseoglu H, Ceylan E, Cimrin HA, Ozalevli S, Esen A. Erectile dysfunction prevalence and sexual function status in patients with chronic obstructive pulmonary disease. J Urol 2005; 174:249–52.

127. Rascon-Aguilar IE, Pamer M, Wludyka P, et al. Role of gastroesophageal reflux symptoms in exacerbations of COPD. Chest 2006; 130:1096–101.

128. Mokhlesi B, Morris AL, Huang CF, Curcio AJ, Barrett TA, Kamp DW. Increased prevalence of gastroesophageal reflux symptoms in patients with COPD. Chest 2001; 119:1043–8.

129. Eckstein D. Common complaints of the elderly. Hosp Pract 1976; 11:67–74.

130. van den Ouweland FA, Grobbee DE, De Jong PT, Hofman A. Causes and prevention of chronic diseases in the elderly; the Erasmus Rotterdam health and the elderly study. Ned Tijdschr Geneeskd 1991; 135:574–7.

131. Wilson JMG, Jungner G. Principles and practice of screening for disease. Public Health Papers No. 34. Geneva: World Health Organization, 1968.

132. Khoury MJ, McCabe LL, McCabe ER. Population screening in the age of genomic medicine. N Engl J Med 2003; 348:50–8.

133. Celli BR, MacNee W, Agusti AG, et al. Standards for the diagnosis and treatment of patients with COPD: a summary of the ATS/ERS position paper. Eur Respir J 2004; 23:932–46.

134. Barbera JA, Peces-Barba G, Agusti AG, et al. Guía clínica para el diagnóstico y el tratamiento de la enfermedad pulmonar obstructiva crónica. Arch Bronconeumol 2001; 37:297–316.

135. Tinetti ME, Bogardus ST, Jr., Agostini JV. Potential pitfalls of disease-specific guidelines for patients with multiple conditions. N Engl J Med 2004; 351:2870–4.

136. van der Woude HJ, Zaagsma J, Postma DS, Winter TH, van HM, Aalbers R. Detrimental effects of beta-blockers in COPD: a concern for nonselective beta-blockers. Chest 2005; 127(3):818–24.

137. Salpeter SS, Ormiston T, Salpeter E, Poole P, Cates C. Cardioselective beta-blockers for chronic obstructive pulmonary disease. Cochrane Database Syst Rev 2002:CD003566.

138. George CF, Bayliff CD. Management of inomnia in patients with chronic obstructive pulmonary disease. Drugs 2003; 63:379–87.

139. Mancini GB, Etminan M, Zhang B, Levesque LE, FitzGerald JM, Brophy JM. Reduction of morbidity and mortality by statins, angiotensin-converting enzyme inhibitors, and angiotensin receptor blockers in patients with chronic obstructive pulmonary disease. J Am Coll Cardiol 2006; 47:2554–60.

140. Soyseth V, Brekke PH, Smith P, Omland T. Statin use is associated with reduced mortality in COPD. Eur Respir J 2007; 29:279–83.

141. Dart RA, Gollub S, Lazar J, Nair C, Schroeder D, Woolf SH. Treatment of systemic hypertension in patients with pulmonary disease: COPD and asthma. Chest 2003; 123:222–43.

142. Mancini GB, Khalil N. Angiotensin II type 1 receptor blocker inhibits pulmonary injury. Clin Invest Med 2005; 28:118–26.

143. Mancini GJ. The 'double dip' hypothesis: simultaneous prevention of cardiovascular and pulmonary morbidity and mortality using angiotensin II type 1 receptor blockers. Can J Cardiol 2005; 21:519–23.

144. Nseir S, Di PC, Cavestri B, et al. Multiple-drug-resistant bacteria in patients with severe acute exacerbation of chronic obstructive pulmonary disease: prevalence, risk factors, and outcome. Crit Care Med 2006; 34:2959–66.

145. Salpeter SR, Ormiston TM, Salpeter EE. Cardiovascular effects of beta-agonists in patients with asthma and COPD: a meta-analysis. Chest 2004; 125:2309–21.

146. Salpeter SR, Buckley NS. Systematic review of clinical outcomes in chronic obstructive pulmonary disease: beta-agonist use compared with anticholinergics and inhaled corticosteroids. Clin Rev Allergy Immunol 2006; 31:219–30.

147. Calverley PM, Anderson JA, Celli B, et al. Salmeterol and fluticasone propionate and survival in chronic obstructive pulmonary disease. N Engl J Med 2007; 356:775–89.

148. Lellouche N, Guglielminotti J, de Saint-Jean M, Alzieu M, Maury E, Offenstadt G. Acute glaucoma in the course of treatment with aerosols of ipratropium bromide and salbutamol. Presse Med 1999; 28:1017.

149. Huerta C, Lanes SF, Garcia Rodriguez LA. Respiratory medications and the risk of cardiac arrhythmias. Epidemiology 2005; 16:360–6.

150. Oksuz H, Tamer C, Akoglu S, Duru M. Acute angle-closure glaucoma precipitated by local tiotropium absorption. Pulm Pharmacol Ther 2006 (Epub ahead of print).
151. Pras E, Stienlauf S, Pinkhas J, Sidi Y. Urinary retention associated with ipratropium bromide. DICP 1991; 25:939–40.
152. Ito K, Ito M, Elliott WM, et al. Decreased histone deacetylase activity in chronic obstructive pulmonary disease. N Engl J Med 2005; 352:1967–76.
153. Davies L, Angus RM, Calverley PM. Oral corticosteroids in patients admitted to hospital with exacerbations of chronic obstructive pulmonary disease: a prospective randomised controlled trial. Lancet 1999; 354:456–60.
154. McEvoy CE, Niewoehner DE. Adverse effects of corticosteroid therapy for COPD—a critical review. Chest 1997; 111:732–43.
155. McEvoy CE, Niewoehner DE. Corticosteroids in chronic obstructive pulmonary disease. Clinical benefits and risks. Clin Chest Med 2000; 21:739–52.
156. Man SF, Sin DD. Inhaled corticosteroids in chronic obstructive pulmonary disease: is there a clinical benefit? Drugs 2005; 65:579–91.
157. Lacasse Y, Wong E, Guyatt GH, King D, Cook DJ, Goldstein RS. Meta-analysis of respiratory rehabilitation in chronic obstructive pulmonary disease. Lancet 1996; 348:1115–9.
158. Boyd CM, Darer J, Boult C, Fried LP, Boult L, Wu AW. Clinical practice guidelines and quality of care for older patients with multiple comorbid diseases. J Am Med Assoc 2005; 294:716–24.
159. van Weel C, Schellevis FG. Comorbidity and guidelines: conflicting interests. Lancet 2006; 367:550–1.

12

Goals of COPD Treatments and Measurement of Their Efficacy: From Clinical Trials to Real-World Practice

VÉRONIQUE PEPIN, FRANÇOIS MALTAIS, and YVES LACASSE
Centre de Pneumologie, Hôpital Laval, Ste-Foy, Quebec, Canada

I. Introduction

The results of clinical trials should translate in clinical practice. This is one of the paradigms of evidence-based medicine (1). Assuming that the study design is likely to lead to valid results, knowledge transfer from clinical trials to clinical practice requires that (*i*) the study population be well defined, (*ii*) the intervention described with sufficient details to be replicated, and (*iii*) the outcomes be relevant to clinical practice. In this regard, the Global Initiative for Chronic Obstructive Lung Disease Workshop clearly defined treatment objectives that include (*i*) prevention of disease progression, (*ii*) relief of symptoms, (*iii*) improvement in exercise tolerance and health status, (*iv*) prevention and treatment of complications and exacerbations, and, ultimately, (*v*) reduction in mortality attributable to the disease (2).

These objectives offer an important framework for trialists who must select study outcomes that correspond to clinicians' expectations. This chapter critically reviews the measurements properties (especially validity and responsiveness) of instruments commonly used in clinical trials involving patients with chronic obstructive pulmonary disease (COPD).

II. Outcomes in Epidemiological and Clinical Studies

A. Incidence–Prevalence

In interpreting the studies of prevalence and incidence of COPD, one must first question the validity of the diagnosis of COPD. Halbert et al. issued in 2003 a critical evaluation of the published literature addressing the epidemiology of COPD (3). Thirty-two sources of COPD prevalence rates were identified and broadly grouped into one of four categories according to the methods used to classify patients: (*i*) spirometry with or without clinical examination; (*ii*) presence of respiratory symptoms; (*iii*) patient-reported disease; and (*iv*) expert opinions. Overall, COPD prevalence rates ranged from $<1\%$ to $>18\%$ depending on the methods used to estimate prevalence. This emphasizes that, in interpreting the studies of prevalence and incidence of COPD, one must first question the validity of the diagnosis of COPD.

Spirometry

Spirometry is likely to provide the most reliable data regarding the prevalence of COPD. When spirometry was rigorously measured, the prevalence of COPD ranged from 4% to 10% (3). An important report on the prevalence of COPD, based on the spirometric measurement, came from the National Health and Nutrition Examination Survey (NHANES III) (1980–1994) of 20,050 U.S. adults (4). About 6.8% of this population had reduced lung function [a forced expiratory volume in one second $(FEV_1) < 80\%$ predicted and an FEV_1/forced vital capacity $(FVC) < 0.7$]. Of these individuals, 63.3% had not been diagnosed with obstructive lung disease. Of those with an $FEV_1 < 50\%$ predicted, 44.0% did not have such a diagnosis. Undiagnosed airflow obstruction was associated with health impact. The prevalence of respiratory symptoms increased even among those with mild impairment, and the presence of symptoms increased consistently with increasing severity of the FEV_1 impairment (5). NHANES III also emphasized that spirometry was not used widely in clinical practice.

Respiratory Symptoms

In Halbert's review, the symptom-based diagnosis of COPD yielded higher rates than spirometry alone, although the diagnosis was limited to chronic bronchitis defined by Medical Research Council criteria (6). A recent study raised concerns regarding the accuracy of the COPD prevalence derived from self-reported symptoms or diagnosis (7). The primary objective of this study was to determine the degree to which new, self-reported, diagnosis of chronic bronchitis and a physician-confirmed diagnosis of chronic bronchitis satisfied the symptom criteria of cough and sputum production for at least three months per year for at least two consecutive years. Data were drawn from the Tucson Epidemiologic Study of Obstructive Lung Disease, a longitudinal population study that enrolled a stratified sample of 1655 households in Tucson, Arizona in the mid-1970s. Participants were administered standardized questionnaires during 12 different surveys 1 to 1.5 years apart. The study population included 4034 individuals, of which 481 (11.9%) were given the diagnosis of chronic bronchitis, on the basis of either self-reported diagnosis (i.e., a positive answer to the following question: "Since the last questionnaire, have you had chronic bronchitis?") or a physician-confirmed diagnosis. Concordance of the diagnosis with symptom criteria for chronic bronchitis proved to be poor. The authors concluded that responses to respiratory questionnaires did not provide an accurate clinical diagnosis.

Patient-Reported Diseases

The 1994 to 1995 Canadian National Population Health Survey reflected several limitations in data collection, including the computation of prevalence rates from self-reported surveys (8). Estimates of the prevalence of COPD were derived from the individual's response to the following question: "Do you have chronic bronchitis or emphysema diagnosed by a health professional?" The respondents' answers were not validated by further investigation. We emphasized that the information reported should be thought of as the perceived prevalence. If individuals with non-obstructive bronchitis were included, then the survey might have overestimated the true prevalence of COPD in the community. However, as the survey could not capture undiagnosed individuals or those unaware of their diagnosis, the true prevalence might have been underestimated. The direction of the bias, if any, is uncertain. Nonetheless, we concur with Halbert's view that the burden of COPD is most likely underestimated (3).

B. Mortality

Few interventions really reduced mortality in randomized trials in COPD. The interventions that did so targeted major pathophysiological processes that are still often poorly understood. Long-term oxygen therapy in patients with severe hypoxemia is one among them (9,10). Lung-volume-reduction surgery reduces mortality in highly selected patients with severe emphysema (11). Non-invasive positive pressure ventilation improves survival in patients presenting with acute respiratory failure (12). There is still debated evidence that inhaled corticosteroids combined with long-acting β_2 agonists reduce mortality in patients with COPD (13). Smoking cessation also reduced mortality in patients with mild COPD (14). Finally, although pneumococcal and influenza vaccinations have long been thought to reduce mortality in COPD, the evidence comes only from nonrandomized studies (15). In all cases, the outcome consisted of all-cause mortality and COPD encompassed only for a limited proportion of causes of death.

All-cause mortality is often preferred over disease-specific mortality because of the difficulty in classifying causes of death and the notorious lack of validity of death certificates in patients with COPD (16). In clinical trials, causes of mortality are usually adjudicated by an independent committee unaware of the intervention received by the patient during the trial.

Although mortality related to COPD represents an important point of comparison in the burden of the disease around the world, several factors limit the comparison of epidemiological data related to COPD-specific mortality. These include (*i*) the lack of standardization of death certification and coding practices; (*ii*) international differences in diagnostic practices; (*iii*) availability and quality of medical care; (*iv*) differences in the completeness and coverage of deaths data; (*v*) incorrect or systematic biases in diagnosis; and (*vi*) misinterpretation of the International Classification of Diseases' rules for selection of the underlying cause of death (17,18). We accessed in 2004 the WHO mortality database and computed the COPD-specific mortality rates for the population aged ≥ 55 years. The mortality rates are presented for men and women in Figure 1A and B respectively. These figures show much heterogeneity in the death rates across the selected countries. The 30-fold difference between the highest and lowest reported mortality rates is considerably greater than that normally expected, illustrating the limitations of the data and the difficulty, in clinical practice, in confidently attributing death to COPD in a given individual.

C. Hospitalizations

Although there is usually no ambiguity on what constitutes a hospitalization, causes of hospitalizations (like causes of death) are often difficult to ascertain. In addition, criteria for hospitalization may vary from one site to another (19), depending on the

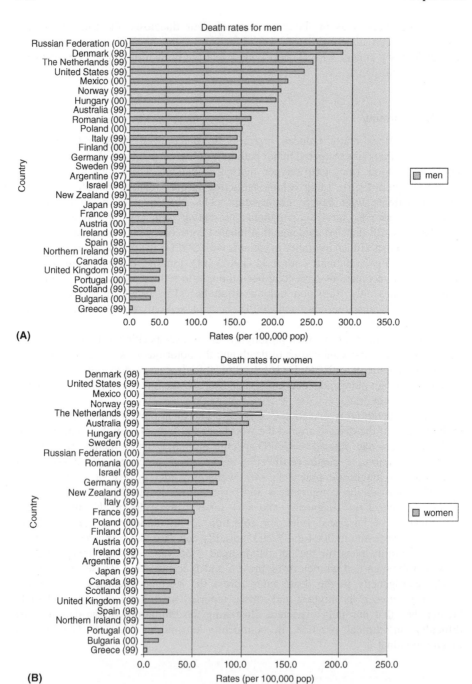

Figure 1   Age-adjusted death rates for chronic obstructive pulmonary disease by country and sex in individuals aged ≥55 years. Year of data is shown in parentheses. Death rates for (**A**) men and (**B**) women.

available resources. Mean lengths of stay may also vary from one site to another because of clinical or administrative reasons.

D. Exacerbations

COPD is characterized by periods of clinical instability called "acute exacerbations" [acute exacerbation of chronic obstructive pulmonary disease (AECOPD)]. AECOPD represent important events in the course of the disease for several reasons. They are associated with deterioration of quality of life (20) and often lead to hospitalizations (21). Repeated AECOPD result in further decline in lung function and contribute to disease progression (22). Mortality is also related to the frequency of severe exacerbations requiring hospitalization (23–25).

No consensus has been reached on a clear definition of "exacerbation" (26,27). An example is from the Canadian Thoracic Society that refers to such episodes as "a sustained worsening dyspnea, cough, or sputum production leading to an increase in the use of maintenance medications and/or supplementation with additional medications" (28). Such definition is "symptom based." Others would require that new symptoms lead to a clinical event (such as the prescription of medication or hospitalization) before counting them as an AECOPD (event-based definition). In clinical trials, the distinction between "symptom-based" and "event-based" exacerbations is important since symptom-based AECOPD are often unreported.

Our understanding of what is an AECOPD is still incomplete. No sputum of plasma biomarkers can identify the presence or severity of an exacerbation (27). Recurrent exacerbations (i.e., AECOPD occurring with an intervening period of "usual health") and "relapsed exacerbations" (where clinical deterioration occurs and additional intervention is necessary within the course of an exacerbation) probably represent different clinical conditions. Both should probably be distinguished. This is certainly an important area for future research.

E. Cost of COPD

COPD represents a significant burden of health care systems wherever it has been assessed (29–37). For instance, the Confronting COPD Survey provided important and detailed information on the economics of COPD (36). In this survey, more than 200,000 households were screened by random-digit dialing in eight countries, including Canada. In the Canadian cohort of the Confronting COPD Survey (3265 individuals; mean age: 63 years; 44% female), the annual direct cost of the disease was estimated at $1997 per patient (37). The economic burden of COPD was particularly high in terms of inpatient care: although only 14% of patients reported being hospitalized in the last 12 months, hospital stays accounted for over half (53%) of the total direct costs per patient. Outpatient treatment for COPD accounted for over 30% of total direct costs, the majority of which was for home oxygen therapy. Overall, home oxygen therapy accounted for 17% of the entire annual direct costs. Home oxygen therapy comes in second place (only after hospitalizations) among the most expensive health care resources for COPD (37).

Difficulties in the interpretation of economic data are numerous however. Costs differ from one jurisdiction to another, and the validity of such data is short lived.

III. Outcomes in Clinical and Physiological Studies

A. Spirometry Revisited

The impact of pharmacotherapy in patients with COPD has been traditionally assessed by spirometry and FEV_1, which is still the most widely used primary outcome in COPD clinical trials (Table 1) (38–50). In general, clinicians are looking at acute changes in FEV_1 induced by therapy that is beyond random variation of the measurement. These so-called reversibility criteria vary according to different medical societies. The American Thoracic Society suggests that a ≥ 200 mL increase in FEV_1 that represent $\geq 12\%$ in baseline FEV_1 value should be considered significant. Its European counterpart prefers to use a reversibility criteria based on relative change in the predicted normal value (change in $FEV_1 > 9\%$ predicted normal value). Other FEV_1-based parameters commonly used in clinical trials include chronic changes in pre- (43,44) and post-dosing FEV_1 (48), longitudinal decline in FEV_1 (47), and area under the curve of FEV_1 over time (40,41).

Is Acute Improvement in FEV₁ Following Bronchodilation Common in COPD?

COPD is often deemed as an irreversible disease. Based on this, the acute response to bronchodilation is often considered a useful parameter differentiating COPD from asthma. In addition, North American and European regulatory agencies often require that only patients showing no irreversible disease (showing no reversibility criteria on spirometry) be enrolled in clinical trials for the purpose of registering a new inhaler therapy (47,51). In light of the various studies looking at the issue of bronchodilator reversibility in COPD, this attitude may not be warranted.

In one study, in which 361 patients with COPD were randomized to receive either salmeterol, ipratropium, or placebo for 12 weeks, the bronchodilator responsiveness was assessed at baseline (40). In that study, patients were selected on the basis of moderate to severe airflow obstruction in the presence of a significant smoking history (≥ 10 packs/yr). Patients with a known history of asthma were excluded, but acute bronchodilator reversibility was not part of the inclusion/exclusion criteria. Using a reasonable operational definition of COPD, these authors reported that 65% of patients showed a significant improvement in FEV_1 (≥ 200 mL increase in FEV_1 and $\geq 12\%$ in baseline value) after 200 µg of albuterol. In the responsive patients, the increase in FEV_1 was 300 to 400 mL or 28% to 30% of baseline FEV_1. In subsequent large clinical trials involving patients with COPD and moderate to severe airflow obstruction, the proportion of patients exhibiting significant bronchodilator reversibility was 40% to 60% (41,42,49). These studies clearly indicate that, in contrast to common belief, a significant portion of patients with COPD show some degree of responsiveness to bronchodilators. Of note, the FEV_1 was markedly reduced in these trials (40–50% predicted value). In comparison, the proportion of patients with significant reversibility was much smaller in the Lung Health Study, in which the average FEV_1 at study entry was 75% to 80% predicted. It would therefore seem that the proportion of patients with significant bronchodilator reversibility is related to baseline disease severity.

Even patients initially showing irreversible airflow obstruction may show significant reversibility on subsequent testing. For example, in a secondary analysis of the ISOLDE trial (52), Calverley and colleagues reported that, in patients with COPD preselected based on irreversible COPD (increase in $FEV_1 < 10\%$ predicted normal value after albuterol), the mean change in FEV_1 on a subsequent visit was 128 mL following inhalation of albuterol and 191 mL when ipratropium was added to albuterol. Day-to-day variation in the bronchomotor tone is a reasonable physiological explanation for the observation that bronchodilator responsiveness may fluctuate over time. This study is also useful in pointing out that the absence of reversibility to one drug does not imply irreversibility to other class of bronchodilator.

Another spirometric variable that can be used to quantify treatment effect is FVC. In general, changes in FVC parallel those of FEV_1, although they are usually of greater magnitude (42,45,46,53). In addition, the improvement in FVC may be more sensitive to detect improvement in expiratory flows than changes in FEV_1 (54). The main limitation of FVC in assessing reversibility is its strong time dependence in the context of a forced expiratory maneuvre whose time is not predetermined and highly variable. Relating the changes in FEV_1 to those of FVC may also be instructive about the mechanism of improvement in airflow. In a portion of patients, a disproportionate increase in FEV_1 over FVC is seen as indicated by a concomitant increase in the FEV_1/FVC ratio. This type of response can be explained by better airway conductance and is termed a flow response (54). In a larger portion of patients, a different pattern is seen: the increase in FEV_1 is relatively smaller than that of FVC and a reduced FEV_1/FVC ratio is seen. In this situation, the increased FEV_1 can be explained by a volume recruitment due to relief of gas trapping, a response refereed to as a volume response (54).

Several important messages arise from this discussion. One has to be cautious in labeling a patient with COPD with an irreversible condition. Significant improvement in FEV_1 following bronchodilation is not uncommon in patients with COPD. In fact, approximately 50% of patients show significant reversibility to bronchodilator according to accepted reversibility criteria. It is also important to avoid making treatment decision based on the acute responsiveness to bronchodilator because of the spontaneous fluctuation in bronchomotor tone.

B. Inspiratory Capacity, Lung Volumes, and Hyperinflation

There are obvious limitations to spirometry. Because of dynamic airway compression during forced expiratory maneuvres, the true available expiratory flow could be underestimated. Spirometric indices of airflow obstruction correlate poorly with patient-centered outcome such as dyspnea, exercise tolerance, and quality of life. Lastly, significant improvement in patients' clinical condition with pharmacotherapy can occur despite the absence of change in FEV_1 (54).

Resting hyperinflation is a major consequence of chronic airflow obstruction. Recent studies have emphasized the strong link between resting hyperinflation and the clinical consequences of COPD, such as dyspnea and exercise intolerance (55,56). Based on this rationale, the impact of bronchodilation on resting lung volume has been scrutinized in several studies (53,57–60).

In a very informative study, O'Donnell and colleagues measured the changes in resting lung volumes in patients with otherwise poorly reversible airflow obstruction (defined as an improvement in FEV_1 following albuterol $< 10\%$ predicted) and resting hyperinflation [functional residual capacity (FRC) $> 120\%$ predicted] (61). One important finding of this study was that an improvement in one or more lung volume(s) occurred in the majority (83%) of patients after a single dose of inhaled salbutamol.

Table 1 Examples of Clinical Trials Using Spirometry as the Primary Outcome

Study	Duration	Reversibility criteria	Medication	Primary outcome	Changes in primary outcome with therapy
Combivent Aerosol Study (38)	12 weeks		Combivent, albuterol, ipratropium	Increase in FEV$_1$ over baseline	31–33% increase in FEV$_1$ (post-dosing) over baseline with Combivent
Boyd et al. (39)	16 weeks		Salmeterol 100 µg b.i.d., salmeterol 50 µg b.i.d., placebo	Changes in FEV$_1$ versus placebo	7% increase in FEV$_1$ (post-dosing) with active treatment compared to placebo
Mahler et al. (40)	12 weeks	No	Salmeterol 50 µg b.i.d., ipratropium, placebo	Changes in FEV$_1$ versus placebo (AUC)	200 mL improvement in FEV$_1$ (post-dosing) in active treatment groups compared to placebo
Dahl et al. (41)	12 weeks	No	Formoterol 12 µg b.i.d., 24 µg b.i.d., placebo	Changes in FEV$_1$ versus placebo (AUC)	200–300 mL improvement in FEV$_1$ (post-dosing) in active treatment groups compared to placebo
Rennard et al. (42)	12 weeks	No	Salmeterol 50 µg b.i.d., ipratropium, placebo	Changes in FEV$_1$ versus placebo (AUC)	Improved FEV$_1$ with active treatment compared to placebo
Casaburi et al. (43)	1 year	No	Tiotropium 18 µg i.d. versus placebo	Changes in FEV$_1$ versus placebo	120–150 mL improvement in FEV$_1$ (pre-dosing) in active treatment compared to placebo
Vincken et al. (44)	1 year	No	Tiotropium 18 µg i.d. versus ipratropium	Changes in FEV$_1$ versus ipratropium	120–150 mL improvement in FEV$_1$ (pre-dosing) in active treatment compared to ipratropium
Donohue et al. (45)	6 months	No	Tiotropium 18 µg versus salmeterol versus placebo	Changes in FEV$_1$ versus placebo	80–140 mL improvement in FEV$_1$ (pre-dosing) in active treatment compared to placebo

Study	Duration		Treatment	Outcome	Result
Van Noord et al. (46)	6 weeks	No	Tiotropium 18 μg versus formoterol 12 μg i.d. versus tiotropium+formoterol 12 μg b.i.d	Changes in average FEV$_1$ over 12 and 24 hours between treatment group	100 mL improvement in average FEV$_1$ over 12 hour tiotropium+formoterol versus tiotropium
Burge et al. (47)	3 years	Yes (increase in FEV$_1$ > 10% predicted normal value)	Fluticasone 500 μg b.i.d. versus placebo	Decline in post-bronchodilator FEV$_1$ (mL/yr)	9 mL/yr difference in the decline in FEV$_1$ between treatment groups (NS)
Calverley et al. (48)	1 year		Salmeterol 50 μg b.i.d., fluticasone 500 μg b.i.d., salmeterol/fluticasone 50/500 b.i.d., placebo	Changes in pre-bronchodilator FEV$_1$ at 1 year	133 mL improvement in pre-dose FEV$_1$ with combination therapy compared to placebo
Hanania et al. (49)	6 months		Salmeterol 50 μg b.i.d., fluticasone 250 μg b.i.d., salmeterol/fluticasone 50/250 b.i.d., placebo	Changes in pre- and post-bronchodilator FEV$_1$ at 6 months	164 mL improvement in pre-dose FEV$_1$ with combination therapy compared to placebo
Szafranski et al. (50)	1 year	No	Formoterol 12 μg b.i.d., budesonide 200 μg b.i.d., formoterol/budesonide 12/200 b.i.d., placebo	Exacerbation rate and changes in FEV$_1$	

Abbreviations: AUC, area under the curve; FEV$_1$, forced expiratory volume in one second; NS, not significant.

In patients with severe airflow obstruction, the fall in residual volume averaged 500 mL or 22% of baseline value. Physiologically, this volume response to bronchodilator is thought to reflect improved small airway function and lung emptying that is not captured by the FEV_1 (54,62). The possibility to induce lung deflation with broncho-dilators in patients initially thought to have an irreversible disease underlines that most patients with COPD may indeed respond favorably to pharmacotherapy.

Although clinical trials using changes in lung volumes as important clinical outcomes are now performed (Table 2), resting lung volume measurements are still not part of the routine assessment of patients with COPD, in part because they are cumbersome to perform. Inspiratory capacity, which mirrors FRC and can be obtained using a simple spirometer, could represent an attractive surrogate of hyperinflation in COPD. It should be appreciated that the ability of inspiratory capacity to accurately mirror the post-bronchodilator changes in FRC may be confounded by the reduction in total lung capacity that may occur with bronchodilation (61). In this situation, the magnitude of lung deflation with bronchodilator will be underestimated by measuring inspiratory capacity. Despite this potential limitation, a reduced inspiratory capacity is a strong determinant of exercise intolerance in patients with COPD (55), while increasing inspiratory capacity with bronchodilation improves exercise tolerance and lessens dyspnea (55,56,64).

In the near future, inspiratory capacity will likely be incorporated in the assessment of the response to pharmacotherapy in COPD. An important step toward this progress will be the definition of what is a significant and clinically meaningful change in inspiratory capacity. Although such a threshold is not currently defined, O'Donnell suggest that an increase of 10% predicted, representing 300 to 400 mL, is likely to be of clinical significance since it usually translates into reduction in dyspnea and improved exercise capacity (55,56).

C. Exercise Tolerance

Exercise testing provides a global, dynamic, and non-invasive evaluation of the integrative response of several major systems (cardiovascular, pulmonary, muscular, etc.) to a standardized external stimulus (65). It is a key approach to monitor response to treatment because it allows clinicians and researchers to objectively assess exercise tolerance and exertional dyspnea, two pivotal outcomes in patients with COPD (65). It offers exclusive information that cannot reliably be predicted from resting measures and is more strongly correlated with quality of life than either spirometry or oxygenation (65). The use of exercise testing for clinical purposes has risen dramatically in the past decades, largely as a result of an increased awareness of its value and of advances in technology which have made exercise systems more "user-friendly" (65).

Exercise testing can be conducted in a laboratory setting using calibrated exercise equipment or in the field as walking or stair-climbing tests. The most popular devices for laboratory-based exercise tests are the treadmill and the cycle ergometer (65). The treadmill has the advantage of subjecting patients to a familiar form of activity, although walking on a treadmill is different from walking on regular ground (66,67). Walking also typically allows patients to achieve a slightly higher peak oxygen consumption than cycling because it involves more muscle groups (65). Cycling predominantly solicits the quadriceps muscle group and therefore increases the

Table 2 Examples of Clinical Trials Using Lung Volumes as an Important Outcome

Study	Duration (weeks)	Reversibility criteria	Medication	Primary outcome	Changes in primary outcome with therapy
Celli et al. (53)	4		Tiotropium versus placebo	Changes in inspiratory capacity	220 mL increase in inspiratory capacity with tiotropium
O'Donnell et al. (58)	6		Tiotropium versus placebo	Change in endurance time	300 mL reduction in pre-dose FRC with tiotropium
Maltais et al. (59)	6		Tiotropium versus placebo	Change in endurance time	170 mL reduction in pre-dose FRC with tiotropium
Van Noord et al. (63)	6 (3 treatment periods in a crossover design)		Tiotropium versus tiotropium + formoterol		Combination therapy improved resting hyperinflation over tiotropium alone

Abbreviation: FRC, functional residual capacity.

likelihood that the test will end prematurely [before peak oxygen uptake (VO_{2peak}) is achieved] because of localized leg fatigue (68). On the other hand, cycle ergometers have the advantage of being less expensive, requiring less space, and making less noise than treadmills (65). In addition, cycling induces less movement from the arms and torso, which makes it easier to obtain high-quality ECG, blood pressure measurements, and inspiratory capacity maneuvres (65).

Field tests have the advantage of requiring minimal equipment and less technical expertise than laboratory-based tests, and are consequently less expensive and easier to administer (69). They are believed to be more reflective of daily living than laboratory-based tests because they employ activities that patients perform on a regular basis (walking on a flat surface, climbing stairs, etc.) (69). However, field tests do not provide specific information with regards to the mechanisms of change after treatment (70), unless upgraded with portable metabolic technology, in which case their cost and labor requirements increase considerably (71–73).

Several different exercise testing protocols are available to evaluate patients with COPD. Most protocols can be categorized as (*i*) maximal, symptom limited, or submaximal, (*ii*) incremental or constant load, and (*iii*) externally paced or self-paced. By definition, an exercise test is considered "maximal" when the patient exercises to the point of volitional fatigue. There is no universally accepted marker for the objective determination of maximal effort in COPD patients (65). However, a number of criteria have been proposed, including the achievement of predicted peak oxygen consumption and/or predicted peak work rate, the presence of a plateau in oxygen consumption despite an increasing workload, evidence of a ventilatory limitation (minute ventilation to maximal ventilatory capacity ratio $\geq 100\%$), a respiratory exchange ratio ≥ 1.15, and a Borg rating of 9 to 10 on a 0 to 10 scale (65). Tests that are terminated because of the appearance of abnormal signs or symptoms are referred to as "symptom limited," while those that are terminated because a predetermined endpoint has been reached (e.g., 85% of age-predicted maximum heart rate), without any signs/symptoms or volitional fatigue, are described as "submaximal."

"Incremental" exercise tests submit patients to an increasing workload (using stepwise or continuous increments), whereas "constant-load" tests impose a fixed work rate, typically determined by using a certain percentage of the patient's peak capacity (e.g., 80% of peak cycling work rate). Finally, exercise tests are described as "externally paced" when the workload is imposed to patients (e.g., shuttle walks) and as "self-paced" when patients get to determine their own work rate (e.g., timed walks). Self-paced tests have the advantage of being easier to perform and more reflective of daily living (69), but are less standardized and more affected by patient motivation and pacing ability than externally paced tests (74). In fact, because self-paced tests let patients determine their own work rate, they have been shown to assess a mixture of maximal and endurance exercise capacity (65,75,76).

There is currently no consensus as to which test should be used to assess exercise tolerance in patients with COPD. According to the latest statement on cardiopulmonary testing from the American Thoracic Society and the American College of Chest Physicians (65), the maximal incremental cycle ergometry test remains the most frequently used in clinical practice. However, constant-load cycling tests as well as field walking tests have gained popularity, largely because they have been shown to be responsive to various treatments in COPD (65). Although several factors need to be taken into account when selecting an exercise test (e.g., reproducibility, practicability, availability, cost, patient acceptance, etc.), foremost consideration should be given to the purpose of the test because the protocol most appropriate for a certain indication (e.g., assessment of functional impairment) is not necessarily optimal for other applications (e.g., exercise evaluation for exercise prescription, identification of exercise-limiting factors, determination of oxygen requirements, etc.). With that in mind, the following section will discuss the value of the most common exercise tests for the purpose of monitoring response to treatment in COPD.

Measurement of Treatment Efficacy: Which Exercise Test Should Be Used?

Incremental exercise tests, constant-load exercise tests, and field walking tests have been used interchangeably to document improvements in exercise tolerance following treatment in COPD (77–79). However, emerging evidence strongly suggests that different exercise tests do not share the same responsiveness to treatment in COPD (67,71,75,76,80–83). The evidence published to date in that regard has focused on bronchodilators (71,75,80,82) and pulmonary rehabilitation (67,76,81,83), two treatments generally known to improve exercise tolerance in COPD patients, but whose effects on exercise tolerance have been found to be variable in magnitude (77,79).

To date, responsiveness to bronchodilation across different exercise tests has been the focus of four randomized, placebo-controlled, double-blind, crossover trials (71,75,80,82). First, Oga and colleagues (75) compared maximal incremental cycle ergometry, constant-load cycling at 80% of peak work rate, and the six-minute walking test (6MWT) with respect to their ability to detect changes in exercise performance after a single dose of oxitropium bromide. Their results indicated that the percent improvement from baseline was much larger for the endurance time to constant-load cycling than for maximal exercise capacity (peak work rate and VO_{2peak} from maximal incremental cycling) and six-minute walking distance (6MWD) (Fig. 2) (75). The same authors followed up with a comparison of two constant-load cycling intensities and reported that a test performed at 80% of peak work rate was more sensitive to the acute effects of salbutamol and ipratropium bromide than a test performed at 60% of peak work rate (80). The difference between the two cycling intensities was largely attributable to the fact that the response to bronchodilation was much less variable for the higher-intensity test than for the lower-intensity test (80).

In a subsequent study conducted in the authors' laboratory (71), the endurance shuttle walk was found to capture larger and more consistent improvements in exercise performance following bronchodilation with ipratropium bromide than constant-load cycling at 80% of peak work rate (Fig. 3) (71). This study was followed up with a head-to-head comparison of the endurance shuttle walk and the 6MWT (82). Results from that trial indicated that the endurance shuttle walk was more responsive to the acute effects of ipratropium bromide than the 6MWT, thereby confirming earlier findings suggesting that the two walking tests did not share the same responsiveness to bronchodilation (Fig. 4) (71,75,82).

One approach proven useful to compare the responsiveness to treatment of measurement tools that use different units (work rate, seconds, meters, etc.) is to calculate their standardized response mean. This parameter, which is obtained by dividing the mean change after treatment by the standard deviation of the change, is a strong indicator of the responsiveness of a measurement tool because it estimates the signal-to-noise ratio (84). It has direct implications in the determination of sample size

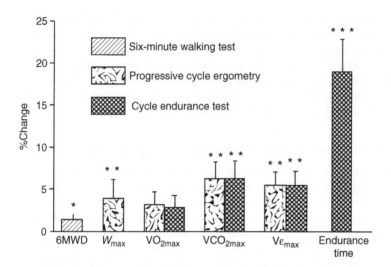

Figure 2 Changes in various measures of exercise performance after oxitropium bromide dose in three exercise tests. Changes are expressed as the %change from placebo. Values are expressed as mean $\pm$ SE. $*p < 0.05$, $**p < 0.01$, $***p < 0.001$ versus placebo. *Abbreviations*: 6MWD, six-minute walking distance; $V\varepsilon_{max}$, maximum ventilation; VCO_{2max}, maximum carbon dioxide uptake; VO_{2max}, maximum oxygen uptake; W_{max}, maximum work rate during progressive cycle ergometry. *Source*: From Ref. 75.

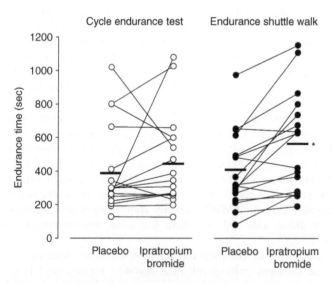

Figure 3 Individual data for changes in endurance time from the placebo to the ipratropium bromide condition for the cycle endurance test (*open circles*) and the endurance shuttle walk (*filled circles*). The group mean for each experimental condition is represented by a horizontal bar. $*p = 0.0015$. *Source*: From Ref. 71.

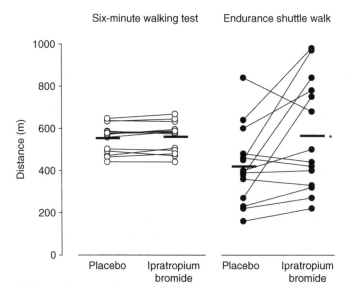

Figure 4 Individual data for changes in distance walked from the placebo to the ipratropium bromide condition for the six-minute walking test (*open circles*) and the endurance shuttle walk (*filled circles*). The group mean for each experimental condition is represented by a horizontal bar. *$p = 0.028$. *Source*: From Ref. 82.

for clinical trials; the larger the standardized response mean, the smaller the sample needed to demonstrate a treatment effect. In the trials reviewed above, the endurance shuttle walk obtained the largest standardized response mean after bronchodilation, with values of 0.93 (71) and 0.66 (82) reported for that measure. The constant-load cycling test performed at 80% of peak work rate initially yielded a standardized response mean of 0.64 (75), but subsequently obtained a much lower value of 0.20 (71). The 6MWT achieved standardized response means of 0.32 (75) and 0.42 (82) respectively. Finally, VO_{2peak} assessed with maximal incremental cycle ergometry achieved a standardized response mean of 0.26 (75).

The above-mentioned findings are consistent with what has been reported in the bronchodilation-related literature. Indeed, in a systematic review of the effects of bronchodilators on exercise capacity in patients with COPD (77), the majority of trials evaluating change in maximal exercise capacity (peak work rate or VO_{2peak}) after bronchodilation found no significant improvement in that measure following treatment (85–92). The same review revealed that investigations of the impact of bronchodilators on 6MWD had yielded inconsistent results (40,74,93–95), with improvements ranging from 0 to 39 m. Perhaps more importantly, none of the studies included in that systematic review reached the minimal clinical important difference for the 6MWT, identified at 54 m by Redelmeier and coworkers (96). This supports the contention that the 6MWT is not highly responsive to bronchodilation in patients with COPD. Fewer studies have assessed the impact of bronchodilators on the endurance time to constant-load cycling, but the 20% improvement reported by Oga et al. (75) and Pepin et al. (71) is consistent in magnitude with values previously reported in two large clinical trials (58,59). Finally, no studies other than the two discussed above (71,82) have used the endurance shuttle walk to measure changes in exercise performance following bronchodilation. Larger clinical trials will have to be conducted to confirm the assertion that this test is highly responsive to bronchodilation.

Different exercise tests have also been found to have various degrees of responsiveness to pulmonary rehabilitation (67,76,83). Several studies have documented large improvements (e.g., 150%) in endurance time to constant-load cycling or treadmill walking after pulmonary rehabilitation, with little or no change in maximal exercise capacity obtained from incremental exercise testing (97–99). Likewise, Revill and colleagues (67) demonstrated that the endurance shuttle walk detected much larger improvements in exercise performance following pulmonary rehabilitation than did the incremental shuttle walk (160% vs. 32% improvement respectively). Subsequently, Ong and coworkers (76) compared progressive cycle ergometry, constant-load cycling at 80% of peak work rate, and the 6MWT with respect to their ability to detect changes in exercise tolerance after pulmonary rehabilitation. Although statistically significant improvements were obtained in all indices of exercise performance, the endurance time to constant-load cycling showed the largest improvement after the six-week program (Fig. 5) (76). The standardized response mean for constant-load cycling in that study was 0.67.

More recently, Eaton and colleagues (81) demonstrated that the endurance shuttle walk was more responsive to pulmonary rehabilitation than the 6MWT (92% vs. 17% improvement respectively). The endurance shuttle walk yielded a standardized response mean of 0.54 in that study, compared to a value of 0.32 for the 6MWT. Finally, another investigation from the authors' laboratory (83) indicated that both endurance time to constant-load cycling and 6MWD improved significantly after pulmonary rehabilitation, but that the magnitude of the change was greater for constant-load cycling than for the 6MWT (187% vs. 113% improvement respectively).

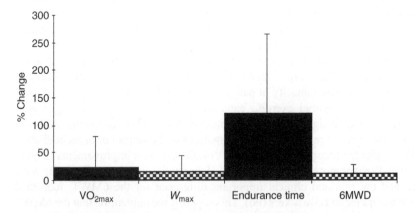

Figure 5 Mean $\pm$ SD changes in various measures of exercise performance after pulmonary rehabilitation, expressed as %change from baseline. *Abbreviations*: 6MWD, six-minute walking distance; VO_{2max}, maximum oxygen uptake; W_{max}, maximum work rate during progressive cycle ergometry. *Source*: From Ref. 76.

The standardized response mean for constant-load cycling in that study was 0.60, while the corresponding value for the 6MWT was 0.77.

Several conclusions can be drawn from this emerging body of evidence. First, there is now convincing data to support the contention that maximal exercise capacity, as measured from incremental exercise testing, is considerably less responsive to COPD treatments than measures of endurance capacity (67,75,76,97–99). It has been suggested that patients with COPD were more affected by reduced ventilatory capacity during incremental exercise than during constant-load exercise (76). However, recent physiological data from the authors' laboratory (82) indicate that the ventilatory response to endurance shuttle walking and six-minute walking reaches, and in some cases exceeds, the response achieved during maximal incremental shuttle walking.

Second, constant-load cycling tests are responsive to both bronchodilation (71,75,80) and pulmonary rehabilitation (76,83). Interestingly, these tests seem to elicit a more heterogeneous response to bronchodilation than walking tests (71). One potential explanation for this phenomenon is that quadriceps muscle fatigue, which is known to be more frequent and more pronounced after cycling than after walking (71,100), has been shown to prevent acute bronchodilation from translating into better exercise tolerance in patients with COPD (101). In other words, in patients predominantly limited by quadriceps muscle fatigue during cycling exercise, the administration of a bronchodilator does not necessarily translate into improvements in exercise tolerance. This may explain the somewhat heterogeneous response to bronchodilation of constant-load cycling tests. On the other hand, given that their ability to detect improvements in exercise tolerance after bronchodilation has been documented in over 400 patients, their responsiveness to bronchodilation can certainly be considered well established.

Third, the 6MWT lacks responsiveness to bronchodilation (75,82), but is somewhat responsive to pulmonary rehabilitation (81,83). Performances on the 6MWT remain remarkably similar between pre- and post-bronchodilation conditions (Fig. 4). Given that the test is self-paced and has a fixed duration, patients must increase walking speed to improve their performance. Yet, in one of the studies conducted in the authors' laboratory, patients were found to replicate the exact same walking pattern under placebo and ipratropium bromide, and consequently did not increase their 6MWD in response to bronchodilation (82). The situation appears to be different in pulmonary rehabilitation, where the six-minute walk has been shown to be somewhat responsive (76,83). One potential explanation is that patients may learn to walk faster during pulmonary rehabilitation, an effect unlikely to be achieved by acute bronchodilation alone. Currently, one of the strongest indications for the 6MWT is to monitor the response to medical treatment (70). One of the main advantages of using the six-minute walk to monitor response to treatment resides in the fact that the minimal clinical important difference is known for that test (96). Nonetheless, the latest evidence certainly questions its use as an evaluative tool to monitor response to bronchodilation.

Finally, the endurance shuttle walk appears to be highly responsive to both bronchodilation and pulmonary rehabilitation in patients with COPD (67,71,81,82). Its response to bronchodilation is more homogeneous than that of constant-load cycling (Fig. 3), likely because quadriceps muscle fatigue does not play a major role as a limiting factor during that test (71). The endurance shuttle walk is also more responsive to both bronchodilation and pulmonary rehabilitation than the six-minute walk, possibly because it is easier for patients to increase endurance time than to increase walking speed in response to treatment. Thus, the evidence accumulated to date regarding the responsiveness to treatment of the endurance shuttle walk is encouraging. However, the minimal clinical important difference as well as normal reference values will have to be provided for that test to improve its clinical interpretability.

In summary, the latest evidence suggests that the exercise tests most commonly used to monitor response to treatment in COPD do not share the same sensitivity to change. Trials conducted thus far suggest that constant-load exercise tests are more responsive to bronchodilation and pulmonary rehabilitation than incremental exercise tests. In addition, externally paced tests (e.g., endurance shuttle walk, constant-load cycling test) tend to be more responsive to treatment than self-paced tests (e.g., 6MWT). The endurance shuttle walk appears to be highly responsive to both bronchodilation and pulmonary rehabilitation, but more investigations will be needed to confirm these findings. Overall, these differences in responsiveness to treatment across different exercise tests likely explain why studies investigating the effects of COPD treatments on exercise tolerance have yielded such heterogeneous results.

D. Quality of Life

End-stage COPD is preceded by years of progressive disability and handicap associated with exercise capacity (102,103) and a variety of symptoms not necessarily confined to the respiratory system. For instance, when specifically asked to describe their symptoms, breathlessness, fatigue, sleep disturbance, irritability, and sense of hopelessness have been among those the most frequently acknowledged (104,105). COPD thus contributes to the impairment of all domains of what is usually referred to as "health-related quality of life," i.e., the patients' perception of performance in at least one of four important domains: (*i*) somatic sensation, (*ii*) physical function, (*iii*) emotional state, and (*iv*) social interaction (106). The term "health-related quality of life" is often used when widely valued aspects of life not directly related to health, such as income and freedom, are not considered (107).

Many investigators have found that measures of lung function and exercise capacity correlate only weakly or moderately with quality of life instruments in chronic lung diseases. Consequently, physiological measures cannot be used as a surrogate outcome for quality of life. Instead, quality of life should be measured directly.

Health-status measurement is a growing field. In early trials (108,109), health-related quality of life was assessed by the means of either more or less structured interviews, questionnaires related to fixed personality traits, or health-status measure instruments borrowed from the psychosocial sciences that had most often been developed to measure psychological status in psychiatric patients. The most important limitation of these early strategies is related to their validity. Recognizing that chronic lung diseases may be important determinants in the deterioration of quality of life, investigators have developed their own questionnaire or adapted existing instruments (110). The availability of disease-specific questionnaires has highlighted the limitations of these strategies. For instance, trials of theophylline in stable COPD in which health-status was measured with nonvalidated diary questionnaires failed to show significant improvement in subjective effects of the drug (110). Subsequently, several trials in which disease-specific questionnaires were used concluded that theophylline was associated with significant changes in quality of life (111–113). Further discussion about quality of life measurement can be found elsewhere in this book.

IV. Conclusion

Patients and clinicians are interested in clinical trials addressing outcomes that are important to them. Physicians and nonphysician health professionals are likely to continue clinical research aimed at improving the comprehensive and integrative care of patients with COPD. Future research includes not only the development on new measures, but also further validation of existing instruments.

References

1. Evidence-Based Medicine Working Group. Evidence-based medicine. A new approach to teaching the practice of medicine. Evidence-Based Medicine Working Group. JAMA 1992; 268:2420–5.
2. Pauwels RA, Buist AS, Calverley PM, et al. Global strategy for the diagnosis, management, and prevention of chronic obstructive pulmonary disease. NHLBI/WHO Global Initiative for Chronic Obstructive Lung Disease (GOLD) Workshop summary. Am J Respir Crit Care Med 2001; 163:1256–76.
3. Halbert RJ, Isonaka S, George D, et al. Interpreting COPD prevalence estimates: what is the true burden of disease? Chest 2003; 123:1684–92.
4. Mannino DM, Gagnon RC, Petty TL, et al. Obstructive lung disease and low lung function in adults in the United States: data from the National Health and Nutrition Examination Survey, 1988–1994. Arch Intern Med 2000; 160:1683–9.
5. Coultas DB, Mapel D, Gagnon R, et al. The health impact of undiagnosed airflow obstruction in a national sample of United States adults. Am J Respir Crit Care Med 2001; 164:372–7.
6. Ciba Guest Symposium Report. Terminology, definitions, and classification of chroic pulmonary emphysema and related contidions. Thorax 1959; 14:286–99.
7. Bobadilla A, Guerra S, Sherrill D, et al. How accurate is the self-reported diagnosis of chronic bronchitis? Chest 2002; 122:1234–9.
8. Lacasse Y, Brooks D, Goldstein RS. Trends in the epidemiology of COPD in Canada, 1980 to 1995. COPD and Rehabilitation Committee of the Canadian Thoracic Society. Chest 1999; 116:306–13.
9. Nocturnal Oxygen Therapy Trial Group (NOTT). Continuous or nocturnal oxygen therapy in hypoxemic chronic obstructive lung disease: a clinical trial. Nocturnal Oxygen Therapy Trial Group. Ann Intern Med 1980; 93:391–8.
10. Medical Research Council Working Party (BMRC). Long term domiciliary oxygen therapy in chronic hypoxic cor pulmonale complicating chronic bronchitis and emphysema. Report of the Medical Research Council Working Party. Lancet 1981; 1:681–6.
11. Fishman A, Martinez F, Naunheim K, et al. A randomized trial comparing lung-volume-reduction surgery with medical therapy for severe emphysema. N Engl J Med 2003; 348:2059–73.
12. Ram FS, Picot J, Lightowler J, et al. Non-invasive positive pressure ventilation for treatment of respiratory failure due to exacerbations of chronic obstructive pulmonary disease. Cochrane Database Syst Rev 2004; (3):CD004104.
13. Calverley PM, Anderson JA, Celli B, et al. Salmeterol and fluticasone propionate and survival in chronic obstructive pulmonary disease. N Engl J Med 2007; 356:775–89.
14. Anthonisen NR, Skeans MA, Wise RA, et al. The effects of a smoking cessation intervention on 14.5-year mortality: a randomized clinical trial. Ann Intern Med 2005; 142:233–9.
15. Nichol KL, Baken L, Nelson A. Relation between influenza vaccination and outpatient visits, hospitalization, and mortality in elderly persons with chronic lung disease. Ann Intern Med 1999; 130:397–403.
16. Ernst P, Bourbeau J, Rainville B, Benayoun S. Underestimation of COPD as a cause of death. Eur Respir J 2000; 16(Suppl. 31):13S (Abstract).
17. Hurd SS. International efforts directed at attacking the problem of COPD. Chest 2000; 117:336S–8.
18. WHO. World Health Organization mortality database, 2004. www.who.int/whosis/mort/download/en/index.html (last accessed August 31, 2007).
19. The COPD Guidelines Group of the Standards of Care Committee of the BTS. BTS guidelines for the management of chronic obstructive pulmonary disease. Thorax 1997; 52(Suppl. 5):S1–28.

20. Seemungal TA, Donaldson GC, Paul EA, et al. Effect of exacerbation on quality of life in patients with chronic obstructive pulmonary disease. Am J Respir Crit Care Med 1998; 157:1418–22.

21. Garcia-Aymerich J, Monso E, Marrades RM, et al. Risk factors for hospitalization for a chronic obstructive pulmonary disease exacerbation. EFRAM study. Am J Respir Crit Care Med 2001; 164:1002–7.

22. Donaldson GC, Seemungal TA, Bhowmik A, et al. Relationship between exacerbation frequency and lung function decline in chronic obstructive pulmonary disease. Thorax 2002; 57:847–52.

23. Patil SP, Krishnan JA, Lechtzin N, et al. In-hospital mortality following acute exacerbations of chronic obstructive pulmonary disease. Arch Intern Med 2003; 163:1180–6.

24. Roberts CM, Barnes S, Lowe D, et al. Evidence for a link between mortality in acute COPD and hospital type and resources. Thorax 2003; 58:947–9.

25. Soler-Cataluna JJ, Martinez-Garcia MA, Roman SP, et al. Severe acute exacerbations and mortality in patients with chronic obstructive pulmonary disease. Thorax 2005; 60:925–31.

26. Pauwels R, Calverley P, Buist AS, et al. COPD exacerbations: the importance of a standard definition. Respir Med 2004; 98:99–107.

27. Donaldson GC, Wedzicha JA. COPD exacerbations 1: epidemiology. Thorax 2006; 61:164–8.

28. O'Donnell DE, Aaron S, Bourbeau J, et al. Canadian Thoracic Society recommendations for management of chronic obstructive pulmonary disease. Can Respir J 2003; 10(Suppl. A):11A–165.

29. Ruchlin HS, Dasbach EJ. An economic overview of chronic obstructive pulmonary disease. Pharmacoeconomics 2001; 19:623–42.

30. Wilson L, Devine EB, So K. Direct medical costs of chronic obstructive pulmonary disease: chronic bronchitis and emphysema. Respir Med 2000; 94:204–13.

31. Sullivan SD, Ramsey SD, Lee TA. The economic burden of COPD. Chest 2000; 117:5S–9.

32. Ward MM, Javitz HS, Smith WM, et al. Direct medical cost of chronic obstructive pulmonary disease in the U.S.A. Respir Med 2000; 94:1123–9.

33. Guest JF. The annual cost of chronic obstructive pulmonary disease to the U.K.'s National Health Service. Dis Manag Health Outcome 1999; 5:93–100.

34. Rutten-van Molken MP, Postma MJ, Joore MA, et al. Current and future medical costs of asthma and chronic obstructive pulmonary disease in The Netherlands. Respir Med 1999; 93:779–87.

35. Jacobson L, Hertzman P, Lofdahl CG, et al. The economic impact of asthma and chronic obstructive pulmonary disease (COPD) in Sweden in 1980 and 1991. Respir Med 2000; 94:247–55.

36. Rennard S, Decramer M, Calverley PM, et al. Impact of COPD in North America and Europe in 2000: subjects' perspective of Confronting COPD International Survey. Eur Respir J 2002; 20:799–805.

37. Chapman KR, Bourbeau J, Rance L. The burden of COPD in Canada: results from the Confronting COPD survey. Respir Med 2003; 97(Suppl. C):S23–31.

38. Combivent Inhalation Aerosol Study Group. In chronic obstructive pulmonary disease, a combination of ipratropium and albuterol is more effective than either agent alone. An 85-day multicenter trial. Chest 1994; 105:1411–9.

39. Boyd G, Morice AH, Pounsford JC, et al. An evaluation of salmeterol in the treatment of chronic obstructive pulmonary disease (COPD). Eur Respir J 1997; 10:815–21.

40. Mahler DA, Donohue JF, Barbee RA, et al. Efficacy of salmeterol xinafoate in the treatment of COPD. Chest 1999; 115:957–65.

41. Dahl R, Greefhorst LA, Nowak D, et al. Inhaled formoterol dry powder versus ipratropium bromide in chronic obstructive pulmonary disease. Am J Respir Crit Care Med 2001; 164:778–84.

42. Rennard SI, Anderson W, ZuWallack R, et al. Use of a long-acting inhaled beta2-adrenergic agonist, salmeterol xinafoate, in patients with chronic obstructive pulmonary disease. Am J Respir Crit Care Med 2001; 163:1087–92.

43. Casaburi R, Mahler DA, Jones PW, et al. A long-term evaluation of once-daily inhaled tiotropium in chronic obstructive pulmonary disease. Eur Respir J 2002; 19:217–24.

44. Vincken W, van Noord JA, Greefhorst AP, et al. Improved health outcomes in patients with COPD during 1 yr's treatment with tiotropium. Eur Respir J 2002; 19:209–16.

45. Donohue JF, van Noord JA, Bateman ED, et al. A 6-month, placebo-controlled study comparing lung function and health status changes in COPD patients treated with tiotropium or salmeterol. Chest 2002; 122:47–55.

46. van Noord JA, Aumann JL, Janssens E, et al. Comparison of tiotropium once daily, formoterol twice daily and both combined once daily in patients with COPD. Eur Respir J 2005; 26:214–22.

47. Burge PS, Calverley PM, Jones PW, et al. Randomised, double blind, placebo controlled study of fluticasone propionate in patients with moderate to severe chronic obstructive pulmonary disease: the ISOLDE trial. Br Med J 2000; 320:1297–303.

48. Calverley P, Pauwels R, Vestbo J, et al. Combined salmeterol and fluticasone in the treatment of chronic obstructive pulmonary disease: a randomised controlled trial. Lancet 2003; 361:449–56.

49. Hanania NA, Darken P, Horstman D, et al. The efficacy and safety of fluticasone propionate (250 μg)/salmeterol (50 μg) combined in the Diskus inhaler for the treatment of COPD. Chest 2003; 124:834–43.

50. Szafranski W, Cukier A, Ramirez A, et al. Efficacy and safety of budesonide/formoterol in the management of chronic obstructive pulmonary disease. Eur Respir J 2003; 21:74–81.

51. Rennard SI, Schachter N, Strek M, et al. Cilomilast for COPD: results of a 6-month, placebo-controlled study of a potent, selective inhibitor of phosphodiesterase 4. Chest 2006; 129:56–66.

52. Calverley PM, Burge PS, Spencer S, et al. Bronchodilator reversibility testing in chronic obstructive pulmonary disease. Thorax 2003; 58:659–64.

53. Celli B, ZuWallack R, Wang S, et al. Improvement in resting inspiratory capacity and hyperinflation with tiotropium in COPD patients with increased static lung volumes. Chest 2003; 124:1743–8.

54. Newton MF, O'Donnell DE, Forkert L. Response of lung volumes to inhaled salbutamol in a large population of patients with severe hyperinflation. Chest 2002; 121:1042–50.

55. O'Donnell DE, Lam M, Webb KA. Measurement of symptoms, lung hyperinflation, and endurance during exercise in chronic obstructive pulmonary disease. Am J Respir Crit Care Med 1998; 158:1557–65.

56. O'Donnell DE, Lam M, Webb KA. Spirometric correlates of improvement in exercise performance after anticholinergic therapy in chronic obstructive pulmonary disease. Am J Respir Crit Care Med 1999; 160:542–9.

57. Pellegrino R, Sterk PJ, Sont JK, et al. Assessing the effect of deep inhalation on airway calibre: a novel approach to lung function in bronchial asthma and COPD. Eur Respir J 1998; 12:1219–27.

58. O'Donnell DE, Fluge T, Gerken F, et al. Effects of tiotropium on lung hyperinflation, dyspnoea and exercise tolerance in COPD. Eur Respir J 2004; 23:832–40.

59. Maltais F, Hamilton A, Marciniuk D, et al. Improvements in symptom-limited exercise performance over 8 h with once-daily tiotropium in patients with COPD. Chest 2005; 128:1168–78.

60. Aliverti A, Rodger K, Dellaca RL, et al. Effect of salbutamol on lung function and chest wall volumes at rest and during exercise in COPD. Thorax 2005; 60:916–24.

61. O'Donnell DE, Forkert L, Webb KA. Evaluation of bronchodilator responses in patients with "irreversible" emphysema. Eur Respir J 2001; 18:914–20.

62. Pellegrino R, Rodarte JR, Brusasco V. Assessing the reversibility of airway obstruction. Chest 1998; 114:1607–12.

63. van Noord JA, Aumann JL, Janssens E, et al. Effects of tiotropium with and without formoterol on airflow obstruction and resting hyperinflation in patients with COPD. Chest 2006; 129:509–17.

64. Di Marco F, Milic-Emili J, Boveri B, et al. Effect of inhaled bronchodilators on inspiratory capacity and dyspnoea at rest in COPD. Eur Respir J 2003; 21:86–94.

65. American Thoracic Society, American College of Chest Physicians. ATS/ACCP Statement on cardiopulmonary exercise testing. Am J Respir Crit Care Med 2003; 167:211–77.

66. Stevens D, Elpern E, Sharma K, et al. Comparison of hallway and treadmill six-minute walk tests. Am J Respir Crit Care Med 1999; 160:1540–3.

67. Revill SM, Morgan MD, Singh SJ, et al. The endurance shuttle walk: a new field test for the assessment of endurance capacity in chronic obstructive pulmonary disease. Thorax 1999; 54:213–22.

68. Gibbons RJ, Balady GJ, Bricker JT, et al. ACC/AHA 2002 guideline update for exercise testing: summary article. A report of the American College of Cardiology/American Heart Association Task Force on Practice Guidelines (Committee to Update the 1997 Exercise Testing Guidelines). J Am Coll Cardiol 2002; 40:1531–40.

69. Solway S, Brooks D, Lacasse Y, et al. A qualitative systematic overview of the measurement properties of functional walk tests used in the cardiorespiratory domain. Chest 2001; 119:256–70.

70. ATS Committee on Proficiency Standards for Clinical Pulmonary Function Laboratories. ATS statement: guidelines for the six-minute walk test. Am J Respir Crit Care Med 2002; 166:111–7.

71. Pepin V, Saey D, Whittom F, et al. Walking versus cycling: sensitivity to bronchodilation in chronic obstructive pulmonary disease. Am J Respir Crit Care Med 2005; 172:1517–22.

72. Palange P, Forte S, Onorati P, et al. Ventilatory and metabolic adaptations to walking and cycling in patients with COPD. J Appl Physiol 2000; 88:1715–20.

73. Troosters T, Vilaro J, Rabinovich R, et al. Physiological responses to the 6-min walk test in patients with chronic obstructive pulmonary disease. Eur Respir J 2002; 20:564–9.

74. Eiser N, Willsher D, Dore CJ. Reliability, repeatability and sensitivity to change of externally and self-paced walking tests in COPD patients. Respir Med 2003; 97:407–14.

75. Oga T, Nishimura K, Tsukino M, et al. The effects of oxitropium bromide on exercise performance in patients with stable chronic obstructive pulmonary disease. A comparison of three different exercise tests. Am J Respir Crit Care Med 2000; 161:1897–901.

76. Ong KC, Chong WF, Soh C, et al. Comparison of different exercise tests in assessing outcomes of pulmonary rehabilitation. Respir Care 2004; 49:1498–503.

77. Liesker JJ, Wijkstra PJ, Ten Hacken NH, et al. A systematic review of the effects of bronchodilators on exercise capacity in patients with COPD. Chest 2002; 121:597–608.

78. Troosters T, Casaburi R, Gosselink R, et al. Pulmonary rehabilitation in chronic obstructive pulmonary disease. Am J Respir Crit Care Med 2005; 172:19–38.

79. Lacasse Y, Wong E, Guyatt GH, et al. Meta-analysis of respiratory rehabilitation in chronic obstructive pulmonary disease. Lancet 1996; 348:1115–9.

80. Oga T, Nishimura K, Tsukino M, et al. Exercise responses during endurance testing at different intensities in patients with COPD. Respir Med 2004; 98:515–21.

81. Eaton T, Young P, Nicol K, et al. The endurance shuttle walking test: a responsive measure in pulmonary rehabilitation for COPD patients. Chronic Respir Dis 2006; 3:3–9.

82. Pepin V, Whittom F, Brodeur J, et al. Six-minute walking versus shuttle walking: responsiveness to bronchodilation in chronic obstructive pulmonary disease. Proc Am Thorac Soc 2006; 3:A225.

83. Laviolette L, Bourbeau J, Lacasse Y, et al. Changes in the 6-minute walking distance and in cycle endurance time after pulmonary rehabilitation and one year folow-up in COPD. Proc Am Thorac Soc 2006; 3:A317.

84. Liang MH. Longitudinal construct validity: establishment of clinical meaning in patient evaluative instruments. Med Care 2001; 38:84–90.

85. Tsukino M, Nishimura K, Ikeda A, et al. Effects of theophylline and ipratropium bromide on exercise performance in patients with stable chronic obstructive pulmonary disease. Thorax 1998; 53:269–73.

86. Tobin MJ, Hughes JA, Hutchison DC. Effects of ipratropium bromide and fenoterol aerosols on exercise tolerance. Eur J Respir Dis 1984; 65:441–6.

87. Brown SE, Prager RS, Shinto RA, et al. Cardiopulmonary responses to exercise in chronic airflow obstruction. Effects of inhaled atropine sulfate. Chest 1986; 89:7–11.

88. Ikeda A, Nishimura K, Koyama H, et al. Dose response study of ipratropium bromide aerosol on maximum exercise performance in stable patients with chronic obstructive pulmonary disease. Thorax 1996; 51:48–53.

89. Dullinger D, Kronenberg R, Niewoehner DE. Efficacy of inhaled metaproterenol and orally-administered theophylline in patients with chronic airflow obstruction. Chest 1986; 89:171–3.

90. Iversen ET, Sorensen T, Heckscher T, et al. Effect of terbutaline on exercise capacity and pulmonary function in patients with chronic obstructive pulmonary disease. Lung 1999; 177:263–71.

91. Eaton ML, MacDonald FM, Church TR, et al. Effects of theophylline on breathlessness and exercise tolerance in patients with chronic airflow obstruction. Chest 1982; 82:538–42.

92. Fink G, Kaye C, Sulkes J, et al. Effect of theophylline on exercise performance in patients with severe chronic obstructive pulmonary disease. Thorax 1994; 49:332–4.

93. Connolly CK, Chan NS. Salbutamol and ipratropium in partially reversible airway obstruction. Br J Dis Chest 1987; 81:55–61.

94. Hay JG, Stone P, Carter J, et al. Bronchodilator reversibility, exercise performance and breathlessness in stable chronic obstructive pulmonary disease. Eur Respir J 1992; 5:659–64.

95. Spence DP, Hay JG, Carter J, et al. Oxygen desaturation and breathlessness during corridor walking in chronic obstructive pulmonary disease: effect of oxitropium bromide. Thorax 1993; 48:1145–50.

96. Redelmeier DA, Bayoumi AM, Goldstein RS, et al. Interpreting small differences in functional status: the six-minute walk test in chronic lung disease patients. Am J Respir Crit Care Med 1997; 155:1278–82.

97. Casaburi R, Patessio A, Ioli F, et al. Reductions in exercise lactic acidosis and ventilation as a result of exercise training in patients with obstructive lung disease. Am Rev Respir Dis 1991; 143:9–18.

98. Ries AL, Kaplan RM, Limberg TM, et al. Effects of pulmonary rehabilitation on physiologic and psychosocial outcomes in patients with chronic obstructive pulmonary disease. Ann Intern Med 1995; 122:823–32.

99. Niederman MS, Clemente PH, Fein AM, et al. Benefits of a multidisciplinary pulmonary rehabilitation program. Improvements are independent of lung function. Chest 1991; 99:798–804.

100. Man WD, Soliman MG, Gearing J, et al. Symptoms and quadriceps fatigability after walking and cycling in chronic obstructive pulmonary disease. Am J Respir Crit Care Med 2003; 168:562–7.

101. Saey D, Debigare R, LeBlanc P, et al. Contractile leg fatigue after cycle exercise: a factor limiting exercise in patients with chronic obstructive pulmonary disease. Am J Respir Crit Care Med 2003; 168:425–30.

102. Killian KJ, LeBlanc P, Martin DH, et al. Exercise capacity and ventilatory, circulatory, and symptom limitation in patients with chronic airflow limitation. Am Rev Respir Dis 1992; 146:935–40.

103. Jones NL, Jones G, Edwards RH. Exercise tolerance in chronic airway obstruction. Am Rev Respir Dis 1971; 103:477–91.

104. Kinsman RA, Yaroush RA, Fernandez E, et al. Symptoms and experiences in chronic bronchitis and emphysema. Chest 1983; 83:755–61.

105. Guyatt GH, Townsend M, Berman LB, et al. Quality of life in patients with chronic airflow limitation. Br J Dis Chest 1987; 81:45–54.

106. Shipper H, Clinch J, Powell V. Definition and conceptual issues. In: Spilker B, ed. Quality of Life Assessment in Clinical Trials. New York: Raven Press Ltd, 1990:11–24.

107. Guyatt GH, Feeny DH, Patrick DL. Measuring health-related quality of life. Ann Intern Med 1993; 118:622–9.

108. McGavin CR, Gupta SP, Lloyd EL, et al. Physical rehabilitation for the chronic bronchitic: results of a controlled trial of exercises in the home. Thorax 1977; 32:307–11.

109. Cockcroft AE, Saunders MJ, Berry G. Randomised controlled trial of rehabilitation in chronic respiratory disability. Thorax 1981; 36:200–3.

110. Alexander MR, Dull WL, Kasik JE. Treatment of chronic obstructive pulmonary disease with orally administered theophylline. A double-blind, controlled study. J Am Med Assoc 1980; 244:2286–90.

111. Jaeschke R, Guyatt GH, Singer J, et al. Mechanism of bronchodilator effect in chronic airflow limitation. CMAJ 1991; 144:35–9.

112. Jaeschke R, Guyatt GH, Willan A, et al. Effect of increasing doses of beta agonists on spirometric parameters, exercise capacity, and quality of life in patients with chronic airflow limitation. Thorax 1994; 49:479–84.

113. McKay SE, Howie CA, Thomson AH, et al. Value of theophylline treatment in patients handicapped by chronic obstructive lung disease. Thorax 1993; 48:227–32.

PART III: PHARMACOLOGICAL TREATMENTS OF COPD

13

Choosing the Right Bronchodilator

DONALD A. MAHLER

Section of Pulmonary and Critical Care Medicine, Dartmouth Medical School, Dartmouth-Hitchcock Medical Center, Lebanon, New Hampshire, U.S.A.

I. Introduction

The most important benefits of bronchodilator medications in patients with chronic obstructive pulmonary disease (COPD) are relaxation of bronchial smooth muscle, which increases lung function and improves lung emptying during tidal breathing. For a long time the major outcome measure to evaluate the efficacy of a bronchodilator has been forced expiratory volume in one second (FEV_1). However, the goals of treating COPD have shifted from improving physiological measures to improving clinical outcomes. There are several reasons for this paradigm shift. First, the individual patient is interested primarily in being able to breathe easier with activities, have a better quality of life, and avoid respiratory tract infections. Second, studies have demonstrated that bronchodilator reversibility (i.e., the acute changes in FEV_1 after inhalation of albuterol or ipratropium) does not predict the clinical benefits of long-acting bronchodilators as experienced directly by the patient (1,2). Moreover, studies have demonstrated that improvements in breathlessness and exercise tolerance are more importantly related to enhanced lung emptying rather than the magnitude of the increase in expiratory airflow. Third, there is no current evidence that bronchodilator therapy slows the progression of the disease as traditionally measured by the changes in FEV_1 over time (3). Although the mean change in post-bronchodilator FEV_1 over three years was significantly lower with salmeterol compared with placebo in the Toward a Revolution in COPD Health (TORCH) trial, living function was a tertiary end point (4). Fourth, bronchodilators do not affect survival in patients with COPD (4,5). Consequently, international guidelines for the management of patients with COPD emphasize patient-centered outcomes, relief of breathlessness, improving health status, preventing exacerbations, and increasing exercise capacity—as the major goals of therapy (6–8).

Although short-acting bronchodilators (β_2-agonists and anticholinergic antagonists) are recommended as initial therapy to be used *as needed for intermittent symptoms*, some physicians have continued to prescribe one or both of these medications as maintenance treatment for patients with COPD. However, there is clear and consistent evidence that inhaled *long-acting* bronchodilators, which have duration of action of 12 to 24 hours, are superior to short-acting medications, which last four to six hours, for improving both lung function and patient-centered outcomes in patients with COPD.

In this chapter, I review the available data from randomized controlled trials (RCTs) and review articles, which have examined the efficacy of long-acting bronchodilators in the treatment of patients with COPD. I also comment on the role of combining the two classes of long-acting bronchodilators in patients with persistent symptoms, and describe the possible role of theophylline as an "add-on" therapy for patients with COPD.

II. Goals of Treatment

The goals of treating patients with COPD are outlined in Part III of this publication. The major guidelines clearly emphasize symptom relief as a "key" objective. For example:

■ the American Thoracic Society/European Respiratory Society Task Force has stated that, "Effective medications for COPD are available and all patients who are symptomatic merit a trial of drug treatment" (6).
■ the global initiative for chronic obstructive lung disease (GOLD) has commented, "Bronchodilator medications are central to the symptomatic management of COPD (Evidence A). They are given on an as-needed basis or on a regular basis to prevent or reduce symptoms" (8).
■ the Canadian Thoracic Society has recommended that, "For patients whose symptoms persist despite reasonable short-acting bronchodilator therapy, a long-acting bronchodilator should be used" (7).

Before describing the effects of long-acting bronchodilators on the goals of effective COPD management, I review briefly the characteristics of long-acting β_2-agonists (LABA) and tiotropium, a long-acting muscarinic antagonist.

III. Long-Acting β_2-Agonists

The β_2-agonists activate β_2-receptors that release the enzyme, adenylate cyclase, in airway smooth muscle, which increases intracellular cyclic adenosine monophosphate (cAMP). cAMP promotes relaxation of bronchial smooth muscle. Both LABAs, formoterol and salmeterol, provide bronchodilation for ≥ 12 hours and have been approved for twice daily use. In addition, Johnson and Rennard (9) have proposed that LABAs exert nonsmooth muscle effects, such as stimulation of mucociliary transport, cytoprotection of the respiratory mucosa, and attenuation of neutrophil recruitment and activation. However, the clinical relevance of these mechanisms remains to be determined.

Although inhaled β_2-agonists are generally well tolerated by patients with COPD, the most common side effects involve the cardiovascular and central nervous systems. Cardiovascular adverse effects may include tachycardia, palpitations, premature ventricular contractions, and atrial fibrillation. Hypokalemia may develop as a result of intracellular shifts of potassium into skeletal muscle. However, evidence from RCTs and from analyses of different studies shows a good cardiovascular safety profile with LABAs in patients with COPD (4,10–13). A study by Cazzola and colleagues (14) showed that single doses of 12 µg of formoterol and 50 µg of salmeterol "allowed a relatively higher safety margin than 24 µg formoterol" based on 24-hour Holter monitoring in 12 patients with COPD, who had preexisting cardiac arrhythmias and hypoxemia. LABAs may stimulate the central nervous system and cause irritability, difficulty sleeping, and tremor. Other adverse effects may include gastrointestinal symptoms.

A. Formoterol Fumarate

Formoterol was developed in an effort to increase the affinity of the agonist for the β_2-adrenergic receptor. Formoterol is able to reach the receptor from the aqueous phase, which accounts for its rapid onset of action within 5 to 10 minutes of inhalation (15). Although the exact mechanism for the prolonged duration of action is unknown, it may involve interaction with the membrane lipid bilayer. Peak effect for bronchodilation occurs at approximately one to two hours (15,16). Formoterol is considered as a *full* β_2-agonist based on its ability to completely activate β_2-adenoreceptors (17). One potential clinical benefit of a full agonist is greater bronchoprotective effect in the presence of a bronchoconstrictive stimulus, such as methacholine (17). However, a full agonist may allow more rapid receptor desensitization and has the potential to cause more severe side effects, such as greater tachycardia and reduction in serum potassium, than a partial agonist (17).

The doses of formoterol are 9 µg (two puffs of 4.5 µg) delivered via the Turbuhaler® and 12 µg metered-dose inhaler or dry powder capsules via the breath-activated Aerolizer®. Arformoterol, the R,R isomer of formoterol, is an inhaled solution delivered via nebulization at a dose of 15 µg (18). Randomized controlled studies have demonstrated the physiological and/or clinical benefits of formoterol compared with placebo, ipratropium bromide, and/or theophylline (15,19–22).

B. Salmeterol Xinofoate

Salmeterol was designed to have prolonged binding to the β_2-adrenergic receptor along with repeated stimulation of the active site. Due to its lipophilic properties, salmeterol partitions into the phospholipid membrane and diffuses laterally to approach the β_2-adrenergic receptor through the cell membrane (23). The side chain of salmeterol binds to a discrete hydrophobic domain called the exosite, which prevents the molecule from dissociating from the receptor. Salmeterol is considered as a *partial* β_2-agonist, because it only partially activates the β_2-adenoreceptors (17). However, the clinical relevance of this is unclear as a higher dose of a partial agonist can be used as long as the therapeutic ratio of desired effect to undesirable side effects is the same. As noted above, partial agonists may have fewer side effects than full agonists (17).

Salmeterol xinafoate is deliverd via a dry powder Diskus® device, which contains a double-foil blister strip of powdered medication. Each blister contains 50 µg which is dispersed upon inhalation by the patient into lower respiratory tract. Although salmeterol does not have a rapid onset of action, significant improvements in FEV_1 have been demonstrated within 30 minutes of inhalation (10,11). Peak effect for bronchodilation is two hours. Randomized controlled studies have demonstrated the physiological and/or clinical benefits of salmeterol compared with placebo and ipratropium bromide (10,11).

IV. Long-Acting Muscarinic Antagonist

Tiotropium bromide is a quaternary anticholinergic agent that has a unique kinetic selectivity for the M_1 and M_3 muscarinic (M) receptor subtypes (located in large and medium-sized airways) compared with the M_2 receptor (located on the postganglionic parasympathetic nerve endings) (24). Stimulation of the M_1 and M_3 receptors release acetylcholine, which causes bronchial smooth muscle contraction; in contrast, the M_2 receptor inhibits acetylcholine release. Tiotropium binds to all three muscarinic receptor subtypes, but dissociates rapidly from M_2 receptors. Compared with ipratropium bromide, tiotropium dissociates 100 times more slowly than from M_1 and M_3 receptors (i.e., blocking acetylcholine release) and provides bronchodilation for ≥ 24 hours (25).

The dose of tiotropium is 18 μg delivered via dry powder capsule placed into a breath-actuated HandiHaler taken once a day. Peak effect for bronchodilation is two hours (25,26). Randomized controlled studies have demonstrated the physiological and/or clinical benefits of tiotropium compared with placebo and ipratropium bromide (25,26). Comparative trials of tiotropium versus salmeterol will be discussed later in this chapter.

Tiotropium has been well tolerated in clinical trials (27). The most common side effect was dryness of the mouth which occurred in approximately 10% to 16% of study patients; this frequency was slightly greater than that observed with ipratropium (25). Serial electrocardiograms in 6- and 12-month placebo-controlled trials and 24-hour electrocardiographic (Holter) monitoring in a six-week placebo-controlled trial showed no significant differences between tiotropium and placebo for heart rate or arrhythmias (28).

V. Effect of Long-Acting Bronchodilators on Goals of Treatment

The effects of long-acting bronchodilators are considered based on the goals of treatment as proposed in the Global Initiative for GOLD and by recommendations from the American Thoracic Society/European Respiratory Society Task Force and from the Canadian Thoracic Society (6–8).

A. Relieve Symptoms

Respiratory Symptoms

Different types of scales or questionnaires have been used to quantify individual or "total" symptoms in RCTs of long-acting bronchodilators (29). One approach has been to ask the patient to rate the severity of symptoms (e.g., ability to perform usual daily activities; breathlessness over the past 24 hours; waking at night due to respiratory symptoms; cough; sputum production) on a 0 to 3 or a 0 to 4 category scale as part of daily diary. Of the six studies performed to evaluate LABAs using this methodology, four trials reported a statistically significant improvement in symptoms with LABAs (Table 1). However, it is uncertain whether the magnitude of these changes on a numerical scale represents a clinically meaningful ben efit for patients with COPD.

Table 1 Effects of Long-Acting β_2-Agonists on Respiratory Symptoms/Dyspnea, Health Status, and/or Number of Exacerbations

Author (year)	Duration	Number	FEV$_1$	Δ Symptoms	Δ Health status	Δ Exacerbations
Formoterol						
Dahl et al. (2001) (15)	12 weeks	194 F12	47	↓[a] Total symptom scores	−5.1[a] SGRQ	NR
		192 F24	47	↓[a] Total symptom scores	−3.3[a] SGRQ	NR
Aalbers et al. (2002) (19)	12 weeks	200 P	46			
		171 F4.5	53	+0.7 TDI	NR	NR
		166 F9	54	+0.5 TDI	NR	NR
		177 F18	55	+1.1[a] TDI	NR	NR
		173 P	54			
Wadbo et al. (2002) (21)	12 weeks	61 F18	34	−0.21[a] 0–4 scale	−1.5 SGRQ	NR
		60 P	33			
Rossi et al. (2002) (22)	1 year	211 F12	47	−08 Total symptom score	−4.4[a] SGRQ	↓[a] Mild exacerbation
		214 F24	47	−0.7 Total symptom score	−3.0[a] SGRQ	↓[a] Mild and moderate exacerbations
Calverley et al. (2003) (30)	12 months	220 P	49	−0.21[a] 0–4 scale	−4.1[a] SGRQ	No difference
		255 F9	36			
		256 P	36			
Szafranski et al. (2003) (32)	12 months	201 F9	36	NR	−3.6 SGRQ	↓ 2% Severe exacerbations
Campbell et al. (2005) (20)	6 months	205 P	36	−0.27[a] CSS	0.8 SGRQ	↑ 2% Severe exacerbations
		1 F9	53			
		73 P	54			

(Continued)

Table 1 Effects of Long-Acting β₂-Agonists on Respiratory Symptoms/Dyspnea, Health Status, and/or Number of Exacerbations (*Continued*)

Author (year)	Duration	Number	FEV$_1$	Δ Symptoms	Δ Health status	Δ Exacerbations
Salmeterol						
Jones (1997) (71)	16 weeks	94 S 95 P	47 45	NR	−5.4^a SGRQ	NR
Mahler et al. (1999) (11)	12 weeks	135 S 143 P	41 42	0.1 TDI	5.0 CRQ	↓ 37%^{a,b}
Rennard et al. (2001) (10)	12 weeks	132 S 135 P	1.22 L 1.30 L	No difference	3.5 CRQ	↓ 5%^{b}
Mahler et al. (2002) (33)	6 months	160 S 181 P	40 41	+0.5 TDI	3.8 CRQ	NR
Brusasco et al. (2003) (34)	6 months	177 S 400 P	38 39	+0.7^a TDI	−1.3 SGRQ	↓ 17%
Hanania et al. (2003) (35)	6 months	177 S 185 P	42 42	+0.7^a TDI	2.0 CRQ	NR
Calverly et al. (2003) (31)	2 months	372 S 361 P	44 44	−0.07 0–4 scale	−0.1 SGRQ	↓ 20%^{a}
Calverley et al. (2007) (4)	3 years	1521 S 1524 P	44 44	NR	−1.0 SGRQ	↓ 15%

^{a} $p < 0.05$.
^{b} Data from Ref. 36.
Abbreviations: Δ, difference between long-acting β₂-agonist and placebo treatments, values for FEV$_1$ are percent predicted unless otherwise listed; CRQ, Chronic Respiratory Questionnaire; CSS, combined symptom score; FEV$_1$, forced expiratory volume in one second as percent predicted; F4.5, formoterol 4.5 µg; F9, formoterol 9 µg; F12, formoterol 12 µg; F18, formoterol 18 µg; F24, formoterol 24 µg; NR, not reported; Number, number of subjects; P, placebo; S, salmeterol; SGRQ, St. George's Respiratory Questionnaire; TDI, transition dyspnea index.

Dyspnea Related to Activities of Daily Living

RCTs have demonstrated inconsistent effects of LABAs on relief of breathlessness as measured by the multidimensional Transition Dyspnea Index (TDI), a comprehensive assessment of the impact of daily activities on changes in dyspnea (Table 1) (37). For example, Aalbers and colleagues (19) reported greater improvement in breathlessness with formoterol at a dose of 18 μg dose (Δ TDI = 1.1 units; $p = 0.002$) compared with placebo; with the 4.5 or 9 μg doses, the changes in breathlessness were lower (Δ TDI = 0.7 and 0.5 units, respectively; $p > 0.05$ for both doses). In identical RCTs used for registration of salmeterol in the United States the changes in the TDI at the end of 12 weeks compared to placebo were small and did not reach statistical significance (10,11). In three 6-month studies salmeterol provided modest improvements in breathlessness compared with placebo (Δ TDI = 0.5, 0.7, and 0.7 units; $p < 0.05$ in each study) (33–35). However, the magnitudes of improvement were less than the one unit change considered to be the minimal clinically important difference (38,39).

In five separate RCTs ranging from 12 weeks to one year in duration tiotropium provided consistent and clinically meaningful changes (range of Δ TDI: $+1.1$ to $+1.7$ units) in breathlessness related to activities of daily living compared to placebo or ipratropium (Table 2) (25,26,34,40,44).

Dyspnea During Exercise

In general, treatment with LABAs have shown no change in breathlessness ratings after patients walked for six minutes (10,11) or completed the shuttle walking test (19,21). However, Grove et al. (45) reported lower Borg scores for perceived exertion after four weeks of treatment with salmeterol compared with placebo in 29 patients with severe COPD ($FEV_1 = 42\%$ predicted).

Constant work cycle ergometry has been recommended as the preferred exercise stimulus to assess the efficacy of bronchodilator therapy than the six minutes walking test (46). In four published trials, patients have reported less breathlessness using the 0 to 10 category-ratio (Borg) scale during constant work exercise with salmeterol and tiotropium compared with placebo treatments (Table 3). However, the decrements in dyspnea at exercise isotime with salmeterol (-0.4 and -0.9 units) did not achieve statistical significance (41,47). In contrast, patients who received tiotropium reported significant reductions in breathlessness ratings at exercise isotime compared with placebo (-0.9 and -1.0 units) (40,48).

The observed improvements in breathlessness with long-acting bronchodilators were correlated, in part, to better lung emptying with bronchodilation as measured by increases in inspiratory capacity during exercise (40,41,47,48).

B. Prevent Disease Progression

In COPD disease progression has been traditionally defined by the accelerated decline in FEV_1. In a meta-analysis of nine placebo-controlled RCTs Stockley and associates (49) found that patients treated with salmeterol 50 μg b.i.d over 12 months had a greater increase in FEV_1 (73 mL difference vs. placebo/usual therapy; $p < 0.001$). In the TORCH trial the adjusted mean change in post-bronchodilator FEV_1 averaged over three years was significantly lower with salmeterol (-0.021 L) compared with placebo (-0.062 L) ($p < 0.001$) (4). Although these results suggest that salmeterol may modify disease progression, a prospective RCT is required to examine this possibility.

Table 2 Effects of Tiotropium Bromide (18 µg/day) on Dyspnea, Health Status, and/or Number of Exacerbations

Author (year)	Duration	Number	FEV_1	Δ TDI	Δ SGRQ	Δ Exacerbation
Vincken et al. (2002) (25)	1 year	356 T	42	$+1.7^a$	-3.3^a	↓ 24%[a]
		179 IB	39			
Casaburi et al. (2002) (26)	1 year	550 T	39	$+1.1^a$	-3.7^a	↓ 20%[a]
		371 P	38			
Brusasco et al. (2003) (34)	6 months	402 T	39	$+1.1^a$	-2.7^a	↓ 28%[a]
		400 P	39			
O'Donnell et al. (2004) (40)	6 weeks	96 T	42	$+1.7^a$	NR	NR
		91 P	42			
Niewoehner et al. (2005) (42)	6 months	914 T	36	NR	NR	↓ 5.7%[a]
		915 P	36			
Verkindre (2005) (44)	12 weeks	46 T	35	$+1.3$	-6.5^a	NR
		54 P	36			
Dusser et al. (2006) (43)	1 year	500 T	48	NR	NR	↓ 35%[a]
		510 P	48			

[a] $p < 0.05$.
Abbreviations: FEV_1, forced expiratory volume in one second at baseline as percent predicted; IB, ipratropium bromide; Number, number of subjects; NR, not reported; P, placebo; Δ SGRQ, difference between tiotropium and placebo treatments on the St. George's Respiratory Questionnaire; T, tiotropium; Δ TDI, difference between tiotropium and placebo treatments on the Transition Dyspnea Index.

The Lung Health Study I showed that ipratropium bromide prescribed three times a day did not alter the decline in FEV_1 over three years in patients with mild COPD (3). However, compliance was less than optimal in the study as patients only took their medication, on average, twice a day (3).

In one year RCTs the baseline FEV_1 was maintained with tiotropium, whereas the expected decline in lung function was observed in the placebo treated group (25,26). A retrospective analysis demonstrated a mean decline of 58 mL/yr in the placebo group and of 12 mL/yr in the tiotropium treated group in trough FEV_1 between days 8 and 344 ($p = 0.005$) (50). Based on these data a prospective investigation Understanding the Potential Long-term Impacts on Function with Tiotropium (UPLIFT) trial is underway to determine whether tiotropium might slow the accelerated decline in FEV_1 over four years compared with placebo (51).

C. Improve Exercise Tolerance

Walking Tests

Four studies have shown that salmeterol did not increase the distance walked in six minutes compared to placebo (10,11,45,52). Investigators of two RCTs reported no increase in the shuttle walking test distance after formoterol (9 and 18 µg twice daily)

Table 3 Comparison of Selected Outcomes with Long-Acting Bronchodilators Versus Placebo During Constant Work Cycle Ergometry

Drug	Duration	Δ Exercise duration	Δ IC	Δ Dyspnea
Formoterol	No studies reported			
Salmeterol				
O'Donnell et al. (2004) (41)	2 weeks crossover design	1.6 minutes[b]	170 mL[b]	0.9
O'Donnell et al. (2006) (47)	6 weeks	1.4 minutes	150 mL[b]	0.4
Tiotropium				
O'Donnell et al. (2004) (40)	6 weeks	1.7 minutes[b]	180 mL[b]	0.9[b]
Maltais et al. (2005) (48)	6 weeks at 2.25 hours[a] at 8 hours[a]	3.9 minutes[b] 2.9 minutes[b]	220 mL[b] 140 mL[b]	1.0[b] 1.0[b]

[a] Testing performed following dosing of tiotropium at 8:00 to 9:00 hours.
[b] $p < 0.05$.
Abbreviations: Δ, difference between long-acting bronchodilator and placebo during constant work exercise; Δ IC and Δ Dyspnea, comparisons are made at a standardized exercise time (isotime).

for 12 weeks compared with placebo (19,21). However, Verkindre and colleagues (44) found that 12 weeks of tiotropium therapy significantly increased the shuttle walking distance compared with placebo ($\Delta = 36 \pm 14$ m; $p < 0.05$). There is concern that the six minutes walking test may not be an appropriate stimulus to evaluate exercise performance with inhaled bronchodilators (46). For example, the six minutes walking test depends entirely on the patient's motivation to walk faster (and thus farther) after treatment, but there is no uniform exercise stimulus. At the present time constant work cycle ergometry has been used as the preferred mode of exercise to investigate the efficacy of bronchodilator medications.

Cycle Ergometry

Recent clinical trials have used constant work exercise at ∼75% of maximal work load as a stimulus to examine the effect of long-acting bronchodilators on exercise performance (Table 3). In a two week cross-over study design patients exercised 1.6 ± 0.6 minutes ($p = 0.018$) longer with salmeterol (two hours post-dose) compared with placebo (41). In a six week parallel-design study O'Donnell and colleagues (47) found an increase of 1.4 minutes in endurance time with post-dose salmeterol compared with placebo ($p > 0.05$).

Tiotropium has shown consistent improvements in cycle endurance time in two separate six week RCTs using similar study designs. O'Donnell et al. (40) reported an increase of 1.7 minutes in exercise time with post-dose (2 hours 15 minutes) tiotropoium compared with placebo treatment ($p < 0.05$). Maltais et al. (48) showed increases of 3.9 and 2.9 minutes at 2 hours 15 minutes and at 8 hours, respectively, following administration of tiotropium compared with placebo ($p < 0.05$).

In conclusion, four RCTs using similar methodology showed improvements in exercise endurance time with both salmeterol and with tiotropium. In these studies the increases in endurance time were correlated with increases in inspiratory capacity at rest and/or at exercise isotime.

D. Improve Health Status

The majority of RCTs evaluating long-acting bronchodilators have used disease-specific instruments, such as the Chronic Respiratory Questionnaire (CRQ) or the St. George's Respiratory Questionnaire (SGRQ), to quantify health status. In 2003 Sin and colleagues (36) published a systematic review of the management of COPD. Based on meta-analysis of placebo-controlled studies with LABAs there was a change of -2.8 units on the SGRQ (95% confidence interval, -4.1 to -1.6) in five studies and $+4.3$ units on the CRQ (95% confidence interval, 1.6–7.0) in two studies. Studies published after the review by Sin and colleagues show similar changes in the SGRQ or the CRQ with either formoterol or salmeterol compared with placebo (Table 1). In the three-year TORCH trial the difference in the SGRQ between salmeterol and placebo was -1.0 units ($p=0.06$) (4).

In three RCTs consistent improvements in health status were observed with tiotropium compared with placebo (Δ SGRQ $= -2.7$, -3.7, and -6.5 units; $p<0.05$ for all three studies) (26,34,44). These results along with one study showing that tiotropium was superior to ipratropium (Δ SGRQ $= -3.3$ units; $p<0.05$) are presented in Table 2.

In summary, both LABAs and tiotropium enhance health status in patients with COPD. However, the reported improvements in the scores on the SGRQ and on the CRQ are generally less than the minimal clinically important differences established for each of these instruments [-4 units for the SGRQ and 10 units (0.5 per question) for the CRQ].

E. Prevent and Treat Complications

There is little if any data on the effects of long-acting bronchodilators related to prevention and/or treatment of complications of COPD such as the development of hypoxemia, pulmonary hypertension, muscle weakness, deconditioning, etc. Nonetheless, the prevention and treatment of complications are important outcomes for future pharmacological studies.

F. Prevent and Treat Exacerbations

A variety of definitions of exacerbations (particularly increases in symptoms and/or health care use) has been used in clinical studies. This fact plus the variable duration of the RCTs makes comparisons between studies and between the long-acting bronchodilators difficult. Nonetheless, meta-analyses and reviews have examined the effect of LABAs and of tiotropium on prevention of exacerbations of COPD. Tables 1 and 2 summarize the clinical trial data.

Based on results of eight studies Sin and colleagues (36) found that LABAs reduced exacerbations by an average of 21% (95% confidence interval, 0.69 to 0.90). However, one-year studies by Calverley et al. (30) and Szafranski et al. (32) showed little or no effect with 9 µg formoterol twice daily compared with placebo on the prevention of exacerbations (Table 1). In a recent meta-analysis of nine studies performed by Stockley and colleagues (49) patients treated with salmeterol were less likely to suffer a moderate/severe exacerbation (34% with salmeterol vs. 39% with placebo/usual therapy; $p < 0.001$). RCTs by Brusasco et al. (34) and Calverley et al. (31) showed similar reductions in the number of COPD exacerbations (17% and 20%, respectively) with 50 µg salmeterol twice daily (Table 1). Calverley and colleagues (4) reported an overall 15% reduction in moderate or severe exacerbations with salmeterol compared with placebo treatments at the end of a three-year RCT ($p < 0.001$).

Pooled data of three studies by Sin and colleagues (36) showed a 26% reduction in exacerbations with tiotropium (Table 2). In two subsequent studies the number of exacerbations was the primary outcome. Niewoehner et al. (42) and Dusser et al. (43) found significant reductions in exaxerbation rates (5.7% and 35%; $p < 0.05$ both studies) with tiotropium. These results were observed irrespective of previous therapy with LABAs and/or inhaled corticosteroids. In a recent meta-analysis of six RCTs Barr and colleagues (53) reported an overall 26% decline in exacerbations with tiotropium. In summary, available studies demonstrate consistent reductions in exacerbations with tiotropium, whereas the effect of LABAs has been variable (Table 1) (54).

G. Reduce Mortality

In a retrospective analysis of the U.K. General Practice Research Database Soriano and colleagues (5) found that salmeterol had no effect on survival in patients with COPD ($p = 0.123$). In the prospective TORCH trial salmeterol exhibited no significant effect on mortality compared with placebo (13.5% vs.15.2% all-cause mortality; $p = 0.18$) (4).

At the present time there is no data available on the impact of tiotropium on mortality. However, such information will be available as part of the four-year UPLIFT trial comparing tiotropium versus placebo (51).

VI. Comparison of Long-Acting β_2-Agonists and Tiotropium

The benefits of tiotropium once daily and salmeterol twice daily have been compared in double-blind, double-dummy, parallel-group study designs (34,55). In the study by Briggs et al. (55) tiotropium demonstrated significantly greater post-dose improvements in FEV_1 and forced vital capacity ratio compared with salmeterol. For example, the mean average FEV_1 over 12 hours was 37 mL higher with tiotropium than salmeterol ($p = 0.03$) (55). However, the morning pre-dose, or trough, FEV_1 was only 18 mL higher with tiotropium ($p = 0.24$).

Brusasco and colleagues (34) reported on the results of two 6-month studies performed in 18 countries in a double-blind, double-dummy, parallel group design. Tiotropium was significantly better than salmeterol metered-dose inhaler for FEV_1, as reflected by peak and trough values as well as the area under the curve from zero to three hours on the last day of the study ($p < 0.05$). In addition, tiotropium was numerically better than salmeterol for reducing the number of COPD exacerbations, improving health status, and relieving breathlessness, although these differences were not statistically significant.

van Noord et al. (56) found that tiotropium produced a significantly greater improvement in average daytime FEV_1 than formoterol 12 µg twice daily (127 mL vs. 86 mL) while the average night-time FEV_1 (43 mL vs. 38 mL) was not different over six weeks of treatment. Overall, these three studies show that tiotropium has greater bronchodilator activity than LABAs.

VII. Combining Long-Acting β₂-Agonists and Tiotropium as Maintenance Therapy

In two separate studies, van Noord and colleagues (56,57) reported that combining tiotropium with formoterol was more effective than single agent therapy. Compared with tiotropium alone add-on formoterol (once or twice a day) improved airflow obstruction, resting hyperinflation as measured by inspiratory capacity, and use of rescue albuterol in an open-label, placebo-controlled trial with two week treatment periods in 95 patients with stable COPD (FEV$_1$ = 38% predicted) (57).

Aaron and colleagues (58) examined the combination of tiotropium with salmeterol versus tiotropium with placebo in a one-year RCT in 449 patients with moderate to severe COPD. The investigators found that tiotropium plus salmeterol did not statistically reduce exacerbations (the primary outcome) or improve lung function or hospitalization rates compared with tiotropium plus placebo (58). However, more than 40% of patients in each of these groups discontinued therapy prematurely. Sensitivity analyses that made alternative assumptions for patients who prematurely withdrew from the trial showed shifts in the point estimates and 95% confidence bounds favoring tiotropium plus salmeterol (58).

VIII. Theophylline

Although theophylline has been used in the treatment of COPD for over 60 years, at the present time it is recommended as third or fourth-line therapy after tiotropium, a LABA, and an inhaled corticosteroid have been prescribed (6,7). The molecular mechanism of bronchodilation is likely explained by phosphodiesterase inhibition (59). Theophylline also appears to have a stimulatory effect on mucociliary clearance (60). Renewed interest has occurred in theophylline in part because it has been shown to possess anti-inflammatory properties (61). In addition, theophylline activates histone deacetylase activity, which suppresses the expression of inflammatory genes (59,62). By this mechanism theophylline may enhance responsiveness to corticosteroids (59,62).

In RCTs theophylline has been shown to improve lung function, decrease hyperinflation, and improve breathlessness in patients with COPD (63,64). ZuWallack and colleagues (65) performed a randomized, double-blind, double-dummy, parallel group trial in 943 patients with COPD comparing salmeterol twice daily, theophyllline twice daily, and the combination of the two medications. As expected, salmeterol plus theophylline provided significantly greater improvements in lung function, greater decreases in dyspnea, and less use of rescue albuterol than either treatment alone ($p < 0.05$). The proportion of patients reporting adverse events was not significantly different among treatment groups (65).

The main limitation of theophylline is the frequency of side effects, which may include headache, nausea and vomiting, abdominal discomfort, gastroesophageal

Table 4 Summary of the Efficacy of Long-Acting Bronchodilators on Various Outcomes

Drug	FEV_1	↓ Hyperinflation	↓ Dyspnea[a]	↑ Health status	↓ Exacerbations[b]
Formoterol	+ +	?	+	+ +	+
Salmeterol	+ +	+ +	+	+ +	+
Tiotropium	+ + +	+ +	+ +	+ +	+ +

The above judgments are based on results reported in Tables 1–3 with greater emphasis placed on studies lasting ≥6 months.

[a] Based on the impact of daily activities on dyspnea ratings using various questionnaires and during cycle ergometry.

[b] Number of exacerbations.

Abbreviations: ?, limited or no published data; +, generally positive effect compared to placebo; + +, consistently positive effect compared to placebo; + + +, superior to long-acting β_2-agonists in head-to-head comparisons.

reflux, and restlessness. If theophylline is prescribed, a low dose is recommended to achieve a plasma concentration of 5 to 10 mg/L (59).

IX. Summary

Numerous studies of long-acting bronchodilators in patients with COPD clearly demonstrate that it is a treatable disease. Based on published data (Tables 1–3) the relative efficacy of formoterol, salmeterol, and tiotropium on the outcomes of FEV_1, hyperinflation, severity of dyspnea, health status, and number of exacerbations are provided in Table 4. The weight of evidence from RCTs demonstrates that maintenance treatment with tiotropium is superior to therapy with LABAs for the outcomes of lung function and the patient-centered outcomes of dyspnea and exacerbations of COPD. In general, tiotropium and LABAs appear to have a similar impact on health status. These data suggest that tiotropium be used as first-line maintenance therapy. This is consistent with the recommendations of various authors who have recently reviewed bronchodilator therapy in patients with COPD (53,54,66–68).

Based on international guidelines for the treatment of COPD a second long-acting bronchodilator should be added if the patient remains symptomatic (6–8). Accordingly, either formoterol or salmeterol should be prescribed if the patient remains symptomatic after a reasonable trial of tiotropium (e.g., four to six weeks). The combined use of different classes of bronchodilators is based on the rationale that these medications act by distinct mechanisms (cholinergic and sympathomimetic pathways) to relax bronchial smooth muscle. Two short-term RCTs (two- and six-week durations) by van Noord et al. (56,57) demonstrate the additive benefits on improving lung function. Although the study by Aaron and colleagues (58) did not show any statistical benefit combining tiotropium and salmeterol, their investigation of concurrent use of two different classes of long-acting bronchodilators was limited by the high percentage of patients who "dropped out": 47% in the tiotropium plus placebo group and 43% in the tiotropium plus salmeterol group. The use of combined therapy with a LABA and an inhaled corticosteroid is addressed in the next chapter.

Long-acting bronchodilators are more efficacious, provide convenience for the patient, and enhance compliance compared with short-acting bronchodilators. Although LABAs and tiotropium are more expensive than the short-acting agents, the reduced number of exacerbations and the subsequent reduced need for hospitalization should provide substantial cost savings (52,69,70).

Finally, theophylline should be considered in a patient who remains symptomatic despite therapy as described above (concurrent use of tiotropium, a LABA, and an inhaled corticosteroid). A low dose should be prescribed initially in order to assess benefits and minimize possible side effects. The dose can be increased based on clinical response and if the patient does not experience any major adverse events. Theophylline should not be prescribed for those patients with clinically significant cardiovascular disease, history of tachyarrhythmias, or a seizure disorder. Care should also be used in prescribing theophylline for those patients who experience gastrointestinal reflux disease.

References

1. Calverley PM, Burge PS, Spencer S, Anderson JA, Jones PW. Bronchodilator reversibility testing in chronic obstructive pulmonary disease. Thorax 2003; 58(8):659–64.
2. Tashkin D, Kesten S. Long-term treatment benefits with tiotropium in COPD patients with and without short-term bronchodilator responses. Chest 2003; 123(5):1441–9.
3. Anthonisen NR, Connett JE, Kiley JP, et al. Effects of smoking intervention and the use of an inhaled anticholinergic bronchodilator on the rate of decline of FEV1. The Lung Health Study. J Am Med Assoc 1994; 272(19):1497–505.
4. Calverley PM, Anderson JA, Celli B, et al. Salmeterol and fluticasone propionate and survival in chronic obstructive pulmonary disease. N Engl J Med 2007; 356(8):775–89.
5. Soriano JB, Vestbo J, Pride NB, Kiri V, Maden C, Maier WC. Survival in COPD patients after regular use of fluticasone propionate and salmeterol in general practice. Eur Respir J 2002; 20(4):819–25.
6. Celli BR, MacNee W, ATS/ERS Task Force. Standards for the diagnosis and treatment of patients with COPD: a summary of the ATS/ERS position paper. Eur Respir J 2004; 23(6):932–46.
7. O'Donnell DE. Executive Summary. Canadian thoracic society recommendations for management of chronic obstructive pulmonary disease—2003. Can Respir J 2003; 10(Suppl. a):5a–58.
8. Rabe KF. GOLD Scientific Committee. Global strategy for the diagnosis, management and prevention of COPD: 2006. Executive summary. www.gold copd.com/guidelines (last accessed August 31, 2007).
9. Johnson M, Rennard S. Alternative mechanisms for long-acting beta(2)-adrenergic agonists in COPD. Chest 2001; 120(1):258–70.
10. Rennard SI, Anderson W, ZuWallack R, et al. Use of a long-acting inhaled beta2-adrenergic agonist, salmeterol xinafoate, in patients with chronic obstructive pulmonary disease. Am J Respir Crit Care Med 2001; 163(5):1087–92.
11. Mahler DA, Donohue JF, Barbee RA, et al. Efficacy of salmeterol xinafoate in the treatment of COPD. Chest 1999; 115(4):957–65.
12. Ferguson GT, Funck-Brentano C, Fischer T, Darken P, Reisner C. Cardiovascular safety of salmeterol in COPD. Chest 2003; 123(6):1817–24.
13. Campbell SC, Criner GJ, Levine BE, et al. Cardiac safety of formoterol 12mug twice daily in patients with chronic obstructive pulmonary disease. Pulm Pharmacol Ther 2007; 20(5):571–9.
14. Cazzola M, Imperatore F, Salzillo A, et al. Cardiac effects of formoterol and salmeterol in patients suffering from COPD with preexisting cardiac arrhythmias and hypoxemia. Chest 1998; 114(2):411–5.
15. Dahl R, Greefhorst LA, Nowak D, et al. Inhaled formoterol dry powder versus ipratropium bromide in chronic obstructive pulmonary disease. Am J Respir Crit Care Med 2001; 164(5):778–84.
16. Cazzola M, Matera MG, Santangelo G, Vinciguerra A, Rossi F, D'Amato G. Salmeterol and formoterol in partially reversible severe chronic obstructive pulmonary disease: a dose–response study. Respir Med 1995; 89(5):357–62.

17. Hanania NA, Sharafkhaneh A, Barber R, Dickey BF. Beta-agonist intrinsic efficacy: measurement and clinical significance. Am J Respir Crit Care Med 2002; 165(10):1353–8.
18. Hanrahan JP, Sahn SA, Fogarty CM, Sciarappa K, Baumgartner RA. Efficacy and safety of arformoterol in COPD: a pospective phase 3 clinical trial. Proc Am Thorac Soc 2006; 3:A847.
19. Aalbers R, Ayres J, Backer V, et al. Formoterol in patients with chronic obstructive pulmonary disease: a randomized, controlled, 3-month trial. Eur Respir J 2002; 19(5):936–43.
20. Campbell M, Eliraz A, Johansson G, et al. Formoterol for maintenance and as-needed treatment of chronic obstructive pulmonary disease. Respir Med 2005; 99(12):1511–20.
21. Wadbo M, Lofdahl CG, Larsson K, et al. Effects of formoterol and ipratropium bromide in COPD: a 3-month placebo-controlled study. Eur Respir J 2002; 20(5):1138–46.
22. Rossi A, Kristufek P, Levine BE, et al. Comparison of the efficacy, tolerability, and safety of formoterol dry powder and oral, slow-release theophylline in the treatment of COPD. Chest 2002; 121(4):1058–69.
23. Rhodes DG, Newton R, Butler R, Herbette L. Equilibrium and kinetic studies of the interactions of salmeterol with membrane bilayers. Mol Pharmacol 1992; 42(4):596–602.
24. Gross NJ. Tiotropium bromide. Chest 2004; 126(6):1946–53.
25. Vincken W, van Noord JA, Greefhorst AP, et al. Improved health outcomes in patients with COPD during 1 year's treatment with tiotropium. Eur Respir J 2002; 19(2):209–16.
26. Casaburi R, Mahler DA, Jones PW, et al. A long-term evaluation of once-daily inhaled tiotropium in chronic obstructive pulmonary disease. Eur Respir J 2002; 19(2):217–24.
27. Kesten S, Jara M, Wentworth C, Lanes S. Pooled clinical trial analysis of tiotropium safety. Chest 2006; 130(6):1695–703.
28. Morganroth J, Golisch W, Kesten S. Eletrocardiographic monitoring in COPD patients receiving tiotropium. COPD 2004; 1(2):181–90.
29. Mahler DA. Measurement of dyspnea: clinical ratings. In: Mahler DA, O'Donnell DE, eds. Dyspnea: Mechanisms, Measurement, and Management. 2nd ed. Boca Raton, FL: Taylor & Francis, 2005:147–65.
30. Calverley PM, Boonsawat W, Cseke Z, Zhong N, Peterson S, Olsson H. Maintenance therapy with budesonide and formoterol in chronic obstructive pulmonary disease. Eur Respir J 2003; 22(6):912–9.
31. Calverley P, Pauwels R, Vestbo J, et al. Combined salmeterol and fluticasone in the treatment of chronic obstructive pulmonary disease: a randomised controlled trial. Lancet 2003; 361(9356):449–56.
32. Szafranski W, Cukier A, Ramirez A, et al. Efficacy and safety of budesonide/formoterol in the management of chronic obstructive pulmonary disease. Eur Respir J 2003; 21(1):74–81.
33. Mahler DA, Wire P, Horstman D, et al. Effectiveness of fluticasone propionate and salmeterol combination delivered via the Diskus device in the treatment of chronic obstructive pulmonary disease. Am J Respir Crit Care Med 2002; 166(8):1084–91.
34. Brusasco V, Hodder R, Miravitlles M, Korducki L, Towse L, Kesten S. Health outcomes following treatment for six months with once daily tiotropium compared with twice daily salmeterol in patients with COPD. Thorax 2003; 58(5):399–404.
35. Hanania NA, Darken P, Horstman D, et al. The efficacy and safety of fluticasone propionate (250 μg)/salmeterol (50 μg) combined in the Diskus inhaler for the treatment of COPD. Chest 2003; 124(3):834–43.
36. Sin DD, McAlister FA, Man SF, Anthonisen NR. Contemporary management of chronic obstructive pulmonary disease: scientific review. J Am Med Assoc 2003; 290(17):2301–12.
37. Mahler DA, Weinberg DH, Wells CK, Feinstein AR. The measurement of dyspnea. Contents, interobserver agreement, and physiologic correlates of two new clinical indexes. Chest 1984; 85(6):751–8.
38. Witek TJ, Jr., Mahler DA. Meaningful effect size and patterns of response of the transition dyspnea index. J Clin Epidemiol 2003; 56(3):248–55.
39. Witek TJ, Jr., Mahler DA. Minimal important difference of the transition dyspnoea index in a multinational clinical trial. Eur Respir J 2003; 21(2):267–72.
40. O'Donnell DE, Fluge T, Gerken F, et al. Effects of tiotropium on lung hyperinflation, dyspnoea and exercise tolerance in COPD. Eur Respir J 2004; 23(6):832–40.
41. O'Donnell DE, Voduc N, Fitzpatrick M, Webb KA. Effect of salmeterol on the ventilatory response to exercise in chronic obstructive pulmonary disease. Eur Respir J 2004; 24(1):86–94.
42. Niewoehner DE, Rice K, Cote C, et al. Prevention of exacerbations of chronic obstructive pulmonary disease with tiotropium, a once-daily inhaled anticholinergic bronchodilator: a randomized trial. Ann Intern Med 2005; 143(5):317–26.
43. Dusser D, Bravo ML, Iacono P. The effect of tiotropium on exacerbations and airflow in patients with COPD. Eur Respir J 2006; 27(3):547–55.

44. Verkindre C, Bart F, Aguilaniu B, et al. The effect of tiotropium on hyperinflation and exercise capacity in chronic obstructive pulmonary disease. Respiration 2006; 73(4):420–7.

45. Grove A, Lipworth BJ, Reid P, et al. Effects of regular salmeterol on lung function and exercise capacity in patients with chronic obstructive airways disease. Thorax 1996; 51(7):689–93.

46. Oga T, Nishimura K, Tsukino M, Hajiro T, Ikeda A, Izumi T. The effects of oxitropium bromide on exercise performance in patients with stable chronic obstructive pulmonary disease. A comparison of three different exercise tests. Am J Respir Crit Care Med 2000; 161(6):1897–901.

47. O'Donnell DE, Sciurba F, Celli B, et al. Effect of fluticasone propionate/salmeterol on lung hyperinflation and exercise endurance in COPD. Chest 2006; 130(3):647–56.

48. Maltais F, Hamilton A, Marciniuk D, et al. Improvements in symptom-limited exercise performance over 8 h with once-daily tiotropium in patients with COPD. Chest 2005; 128(3):1168–78.

49. Stockley RA, Whitehead PJ, Williams MK. Improved outcomes in patients with chronic obstructive pulmonary disease treated with salmeterol compared with placebo/usual therapy: results of a meta-analysis. Respir Res 2006; 7:147.

50. Anzueto A, Tashkin D, Menjoge S, Kesten S. One-year analysis of longitudinal changes in spirometry in patients with COPD receiving tiotropium. Pulm Pharmacol Ther 2005; 18(2):75–81.

51. Decramer M, Celli B, Tashkin DP, et al. Clinical trial design considerations in assessing long-term functional impacts of tiotropium in COPD: the UPLIFT trial. COPD 2004; 1(2):303–12.

52. Boyd G, Morice AH, Pounsford JC, Siebert M, Peslis N, Crawford C. An evaluation of salmeterol in the treatment of chronic obstructive pulmonary disease (COPD). Eur Respir J 1997; 10(4):815–21.

53. Barr RG, Bourbeau J, Camargo CA, Ram FS. Tiotropium for stable chronic obstructive pulmonary disease: a meta-analysis. Thorax 2006; 61(10):854–62.

54. Decramer M. Tiotropium as essential maintenance therapy in COPD. Eur Respir Rev 2006; 15(99):51–7.

55. Briggs DD, Jr., Covelli H, Lapidus R, Bhattycharya S, Kesten S, Cassino C. Improved daytime spirometric efficacy of tiotropium compared with salmeterol in patients with COPD. Pulm Pharmacol Ther 2005; 18(6):397–404.

56. van Noord JA, Aumann JL, Janssens E, et al. Comparison of tiotropium once daily, formoterol twice daily and both combined once daily in patients with COPD. Eur Respir J 2005; 26(2):214–22.

57. van Noord JA, Aumann JL, Janssens E, et al. Effects of tiotropium with and without formoterol on airflow obstruction and resting hyperinflation in patients with COPD. Chest 2006; 129(3):509–17.

58. Aaron SD, Vandemheen KL, Fergusson D, et al. Tiotropium in combination with placebo, salmeterol, or fluticasone-salmeterol for treatment of chronic obstructive pulmonary disease: a randomized trial. Ann Intern Med 2007; 146(8):545–55.

59. Barnes PJ. Theophylline: new perspectives for an old drug. Am J Respir Crit Care Med 2003; 167(6):813–8.

60. Wanner A. Effects of methylxanthines on airway mucociliary function. Am J Med 1985; 79(6A):16–21.

61. Culpitt SV, de Matos C, Russell RE, Donnelly LE, Rogers DF, Barnes PJ. Effect of theophylline on induced sputum inflammatory indices and neutrophil chemotaxis in chronic obstructive pulmonary disease. Am J Respir Crit Care Med 2002; 165(10):1371–6.

62. Barnes PJ. Reduced histone deacetylase in COPD: clinical implications. Chest 2006; 129(1):151–5.

63. Chrystyn H, Mulley BA, Peake MD. Dose response relation to oral theophylline in severe chronic obstructive airways disease. Br Med J 1988; 297(6662):1506–10.

64. Mahler DA, Matthay RA, Snyder PE, Wells CK, Loke J. Sustained-release theophylline reduces dyspnea in nonreversible obstructive airway disease. Am Rev Respir Dis 1985; 131(1):22–5.

65. ZuWallack RL, Mahler DA, Reilly D, et al. Salmeterol plus theophylline combination therapy in the treatment of COPD. Chest 2001; 119(6):1661–70.

66. Cooper CB, Tashkin DP. Recent developments in inhaled therapy in stable chronic obstructive pulmonary disease. Br Med J 2005; 330(7492):640–4.

67. Rodrigo GJ, Nannini LJ. Tiotropium for the treatment of stable chronic obstructive pulmonary disease: a systematic review with meta-analysis. Pulm Pharmacol Ther 2007; 20(5):495–502.

68. Husereau D, Shukla V, Boucher M, Mensinkai S, Dales R. Long acting beta2 agonists for stable chronic obstructive pulmonary disease with poor reversibility: a systematic review of randomised controlled trials. BMC Pulm Med 2004; 4:7.

69. Friedman M, Menjoge SS, Anton SF, Kesten S. Healthcare costs with tiotropium plus usual care versus usual care alone following 1 year of treatment in patients with chronic obstructive pulmonary disorder (COPD). Pharmacoeconomics 2004; 22(11):741–9.

70. Oostenbrink JB, Rutten-van Molken MP, Al MJ, van Noord JA, Vincken W. One-year cost-effectiveness of tiotropium versus ipratropium to treat chronic obstructive pulmonary disease. Eur Respir J 2004; 23(2):241–9.
71. Jones PW, Bosh TK. Quality of life changes in COPD patients treated with salmeterol. Am J Resp Crit Care Med 1997; 155(4):1283–9.

14

When Should We Use Glucocorticoids in COPD?

PETER M. A. CALVERLEY
Division of Infection and Immunity, Department of Respiratory Medicine,
Clinical Sciences Center, University Hospital Aintree, Liverpool, U.K.

I. Introduction

Chronic obstructive pulmonary disease (COPD) is a serious condition characterized by symptoms, particularly breathlessness, that range from the troublesome to the disabling in symptomatic patients with more than mild disease. Episodic exacerbations of these symptoms are commonly reported and contribute to a worsening health status (1) as well as predicting the risk of premature death (2). Lung function decline is accelerated when compared with that seen in older normal individuals free from COPD and has become an accepted marker of disease progression (3). Given these problems, it is not surprising that doctors are prepared to consider all available treatments that might offer the chance of reducing the morbidity associated with this disease, especially when the treatment in question has been highly effective in a related condition like bronchial asthma. Although the data available until quite recently were relatively limited, the use of corticosteroids in the management of COPD has been widespread and has normally occurred despite the lack of specific regulatory approval for these drugs in this condition. Glucocorticosteroids have been used in quite varying ways ranging from high-dose oral treatment given to stable people as a diagnostic test, through oral or systemic treatment of exacerbations to low-dose oral or inhaled corticosteroids (ICSs) in the management of stable disease. More recently, ICSs have been available in combination with long-acting β-agonists (LABAs) and these are now commonly given in single inhalers.

This chapter will review the evidence in support of each of these different uses for corticosteroids, but the intention here is to be synoptic and offer a relatively brief review of the background literature. Other publications are available for the reader who wishes to look at summary details from each of the contributory studies, particularly in relationship to the management of stable disease with supplementary corticosteroids (4,5). This chapter will focus on the most recent and relevant information as a result of which it has become possible to offer some evidence-based guidance about how these agents should be integrated into clinical care. However, before considering this evidence it is worthwhile to briefly review some of the pharmacology and possible mechanisms of action of these drugs.

II. Pharmacology and Mechanisms Action

The glucocorticoids we use therapeutically are synthetic compounds based on the naturally occurring cortisone molecule. The most commonly used preparations are listed in Table 1, which also indicate those that are available in combination inhalers with LABA, to date the only fixed dose combination inhaled treatments that have been tested in COPD. All preparations have good bioavailability and a long half-life. Once-daily dosing is sufficient to achieve stable blood levels. Inhaled preparations are currently advised twice daily, although some preliminary data suggest that it is possible to use mometasone fumarate in a once-daily regime. New truly long-acting once-daily ICSs are being developed but have not entered clinical trials on COPD patients yet. Beclomethasone dipropionate remains the most widely used generic corticosteroid and has recently been reformulated using a novel excipient to increase its duration and action. The majority of clinical studies in COPD have been conducted with either fluticasone propionate (FP) or budesonide which are the two ICSs currently available in combination products. Although widely used in the U.S.A., the disappointing results from the second Lung Health Study has led to a relative decline in the use of triamcinolone in the COPD field (6).

There is remarkably little basic clinical pharmacology available relevant to the use of oral or ICSs in COPD. There are no good dose-ranging studies, although clinically there is a strong suspicion that the dose–response relationship is relatively flat. As a result doses of FP more than 1000 μg per day or budesonide equivalent are not recommended in the management of stable disease. This has been the most commonly studied dose, although whether there are fewer side effects and equivalent efficacy at the 500 μg per day dose is not clear. Observational studies, either in acute exacerbations or with systemic corticosteroids or in the early post-randomization period of clinical trials with ICSs, suggest that changes in forced expiratory volume in one second (FEV_1) are detectable within the first 24 to 48 hours (7). Benefits seem to be cumulative in the stable state but are slower to be attained, at least in population studies, than is the case with long-acting inhaled bronchodilators (8). The data about systemic availability remain difficult to interpret. There is a formidable range of side effects associated with oral corticosteroid therapy and these are listed in Table 2. Local adverse events, specifically a hoarse voice and oral candidiasis, are infrequent and rarely troublesome problems with most ICSs, although the occasional patient has to discontinue treatment because of this. Spontaneous skin bruising has been reported, particularly in patients with mild disease (9) and this must indicate some systemic availability of the inhaled dose. However, this was not seen when specifically sought in patients with more severe

Table 1 Inhaled Corticosteroid Preparations

Drug	Available preparations	Daily dose (μg)	Regimen (hourly)
Beclomethasone dipropionate	MDI, DPI	400–2000	12
Budesonide	MDI, DPI, Neb	400–1600 2000–4000 in exacerbation	12
Fluticasone propionate	MDI, DPI, Neb	200–2000	12
Triamcinolone acetonide	MDI, DPI	400–1200	12
Mometasone furoate	DPI	200–800	12–24
Ciclesonide	MDI	80–160	24

Abbreviations: DPI, dry powder inhaler; MDI, metered dose inhaler; Neb, nebulizer.

Table 2 Side Effects of Corticosteroids

Central obesity, moon face, "buffalo hump"
Striae, thinning of skin
Spontaneous bruising
Glucose intolerance, diabetes mellitus
Osteoporosis
Avascular necrosis
Fluid retention
Peptic ulceration, gastrointestinal bleeding
Cataracts
Peripheral muscle myopathy
Adrenal suppression
Pharyngeal candidiasis[a]
Dysphonia[a]

[a] Only with inhaled form.

COPD (10). Interpreting the skin bruising in the context of patients who receive large doses of corticosteroids intermittently to treat exacerbations is particularly difficult and the same problem applies to tests that examine the integrity of adrenal function. In general these markers of safety have been relatively reassuring which contrasts with the problems reported in patients with much better preserved lung function. Particle deposition within the COPD airways is more central than in individuals with better preserved lung function, although whether this impacts on the efficacy of the drugs is less clear. Nonetheless, with drugs like FP or budesonide absorption into the bronchial circulation increases the chance of metabolism in the liver, which is very efficient for most currently available corticosteroids.

There are real concerns about the hazards of systemic corticosteroids, specifically to the bones and the muscles. Osteoporosis and osteopenia are surprisingly common in COPD patients irrespective of their prior exposure to corticosteroids or their gender. This may reflect part of the systemic impact of the disease and its effects on patient mobility. The steady reduction of prescribing of low-dose oral corticosteroids has been paralleled by a decrease in the number of significantly cushingoid patients with osteoporotic fractures. Concerns remain that there may be an association between ICSs and these events and database studies have suggested that this may be present (11). However, as with all database information it is difficult to avoid confounding by severity and much of these data are relevant in asthma rather than COPD. There are now good data to suggest that oral corticosteroids, even low dose, are bad for skeletal muscle and increase the chance of hospitalization above and beyond that might be anticipated from lung function measures (12). These data have led major international guidelines to advice against the use of oral corticosteroids in long-term maintenance therapy in COPD (13–15).

The mechanism of action of corticosteroids is complex and has been reviewed in detail previously (16). These agents have additional effects on the bronchial circulation (17) and indeed on the circulation in general, which have formed the basis of potency testing based on the vasoconstrictor action (18). However, their action as anti-inflammatory drugs is related to the translocation of the glucocortico-steroid receptor complex into the nucleus of the cell where it is subsequently involved in gene transcription that increases the production of a number of anti-inflammatory proteins.

Additionally, glucocorticoids increase the number of β_2-receptors on the cell surface and this may be particularly relevant when they are used synergistically with LABA drugs. There is an increasing body of evidence that in COPD the cells are effectively corticosteroid resistant (19). Some degree of corticosteroid resistance is seen in all smokers and clinically is thought to be responsible for the reduced efficacy of ICSs in asthmatic patients (20). The key steps seem to involve a failure of a specific enzyme histone deacetylase 2 in COPD patients which restricts access of the corticosteroid receptor complex to the nucleus. The mechanisms here are clearly complex but seem to involve oxidative damage to the enzyme (21). One line of future research aims to try and restore the functioning of this enzyme using other molecules with theophylline in low dose as a possible candidate. Even if this were to be partially successful, it would be an important step forward with a high probability of better more specific compounds to follow. Although there is growing evidence for this, there is no clinical data as yet to suggest a change in our current practice or approaches to patient management.

III. Corticosteroids as an Aid to Diagnosis

The belief that corticosteroid responsiveness was only seen in asthma lead to the use of the so-called "trial of oral corticosteroids" as a diagnostic test for patients with stable COPD who might benefit from regular corticosteroid treatment. More widely used in Europe than North America, this concept extended to bronchodilator reversibility as well and influenced the patients included in the subsequent large clinical trials of corticosteroid treatment. The usual outcome is to report the change in FEV_1 either immediately after the bronchodilator drug or at some time, commonly two weeks, after taking a large dose of corticosteroids, usually the equivalent of 30 to 40 mg or oral prednisone (22). Establishing criteria for what constitutes a significant pulmonary function change has proved difficult, particularly when changes are expressed as a percentage of the baseline value which itself declines as COPD worsens. Hence, a small absolute change, which can fall within the between-day reproducibility of the FEV_1, can appear significant and define a "positive response" (23). The day-to-day reproducibility of this type of testing is relatively poor (24) and neither the short-term bronchodilator or oral corticosteroid response was found to relate to clinically important changes in lung function, exacerbation, frequency, or health status, irrespective of subsequent treatment (25). This depressing conclusion has lead to the U.K. evidence-based COPD guidelines abandoning routine testing with oral cortico-steroids in the evaluation of COPD (15). However, there may be times in specialist practice when a large response to bronchodilators can predict a significant improve-ment in lung function with corticosteroid treatment (26). Moreover, the post-bronchodilator FEV_1 is a useful guide to future prognosis, so testing lung function in this way should not be abandoned entirely, even if small differences in spirometry acutely are of very little value in making therapeutic decisions. A better appreciation of the natural day-to-day variation in airway caliber allows the experienced clinician to set these changes into context, but also explains why we now place much more emphasis on changes in symptoms rather than small and potentially misleading changes in FEV_1 when evaluating the clinical impact of therapy.

IV. Corticosteroids in Exacerbations of COPD

Although short courses of oral corticosteroids have been used for the treatment of exacerbations of COPD for many years, clear evidence to support this practice has only been obtained recently. Albert et al. noted a significant increase in pre-bronchodilator FEV_1 measured over the first six hours of admission in patients treated with corticosteroids compared with placebo, although the post-bronchodilator FEV_1 effect was much smaller (27). In a carefully conducted but small ($n = 17$) study of outpatients with COPD, those whose exacerbations were treated with a tapering dose of oral prednisone (total dose 360 mg) had a significantly higher FEV_1 and PaO_2 at days 3 and 10 compared with the placebo-treated patients. Although symptomatic improvement appeared to be more rapid in the active treatment group, this was not statistically significant for the whole admission (28). Two larger studies of patients admitted to hospital with exacerbations have supported these findings. Niewoehner and colleagues studied 271 patients using a treatment failure endpoint (a combination of death, ventilation, readmission, or treatment intensification) and found that those who received oral corticosteroids were less likely to relapse than those given placebo. However, there was no difference between two weeks and two months of this intensive treatment (29). Post-bronchodilator FEV_1 increased more rapidly and hospital stay was shorter in the 56 patients studied by Davies et al. (30) (Fig. 1). Although the change in FEV_1 was relatively modest, further analysis of the North American data showed that patients with the greatest FEV_1 improvement in the early stages of an exacerbation were less likely to relapse subsequently and confirmed the United Kingdom finding that this was more likely to be the case in the corticosteroid-treated individuals (31). The total dose of oral corticosteroids (30 mg prednisolone daily for two weeks) in the U.K. study was significantly less than the cumulative doses used in the North American trial, but there no clear difference in the magnitude of benefit was seen. Whether it is the dose or duration of treatment that produces these effects remains unclear. Further support for the role of oral corticosteroids in the treatment of exacerbations comes from a study of 147 Canadian patients discharged from the emergency room where treatment with prednisone for 10 days prolonged the time to relapse ($p = 0.04$) and reduced the overall relapse rate from 43% to 27% in the 30 days after discharge (32). As with the earlier studies, the rate of recovery of FEV_1 was more rapid in those receiving corticosteroids, as was the speed with which breathlessness improved when assessed by the transitional dyspnea index.

A further Canadian study found that lung function could be improved to a similar degree with oral and nebulized corticosteroids, although whether this latter expensive therapy can be justified remains doubtful (33). The logistical problems of examining different doses of oral corticosteroids remained formidable in this setting, the only small (and underpowered) study to address this finding that a slightly longer duration of treatment appeared to be beneficial (34). However, in an environment of rapid patient throughout particular care is needed to ensure that oral corticosteroids are stopped after an appropriately brief exposure, in case subsequent excessive side effects develop. This may prove difficult when the patient perceives a significant symptomatic benefit while taking this high-dose therapy, but failure to stop therapy can be very deleterious (see above).

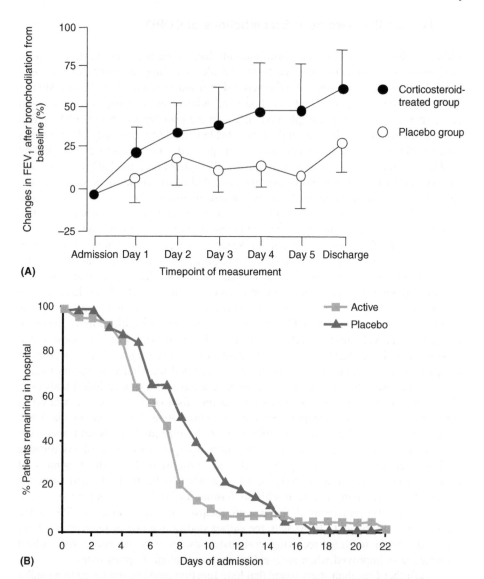

(A)

(B)

Figure 1 In this study post-bronchodilator (**A**) FEV$_1$ improved significantly faster in patients receiving 30 mg oral prednisolone for 10 days than those getting placebo. (**B**) The time to discharge from hospital was significantly shorter in the patients receiving oral corticosteroids for their nonacidotic chronic obstructive pulmonary disease (COPD) exacerbations. *Abbreviation*: FEV$_1$, forced expiratory volume in one second. *Source*: Redrawn from Ref. 30.

V. Corticosteroids in Stable Disease

As noted above, even low-dose oral corticosteroids are no longer recommended for the management of stable COPD, although some older physicians still believe that used in this way these drugs maintain patient well-being and provide a cheap alternative to inhaled therapy which may have greater availability within the lungs. This was certainly the view in the original studies reported in Holland in the 1980s which led many Dutch physicians to be strong advocates of the use of corticosteroids in what they then called "chronic nonspecific lung disease," a combination term that included both chronic asthma and COPD. This confusion in terminology meant that differences in entry criteria to clinical trials led to very different outcomes. A series of studies was reported during the 1990s of varying size and duration which suggested that there may be benefits from using ICSs in COPD (35–38). The most interesting of these was a study from Nijmegen, where patients had been followed for two years before beginning ICSs and were then followed for two years thereafter. There was a suggestion that the pre-bronchodilator FEV_1 improved after institution of corticosteroids in this observational study (39). However, the post-bronchodilator values were less impressive and these are a truer reflection of disease progression.

None of these studies were ideally designed to test the hypothesis that ICSs were beneficial in COPD, nor at the time had the appropriate clinical outcomes been well enough defined to know whether they would have an effect on patients with symptoms. This began to change when a series of relatively large (for the time) randomized control trials were conducted which between them covered almost the whole range of COPD severity from individuals identified within the community by community health surveys (40) to patients with little or no symptoms but more definite airflow obstruction who were recruited to smoking cessation studies (6,9) and in the U.K. study, patients who were already under hospital supervision because of persistent limitations due to their COPD (41). These studies have formed the core of our current data about COPD management, although they have been supplemented by information obtained from the comparisons made in studies primarily directed to the effectiveness of combination treatment (8,10,42). All four of the trials primarily comparing ICSs and placebo mentioned above lasted for three years and were primarily conducted to test the hypothesis that ICSs reduced the decline in lung function. Until recently, trials with combination treatment lasted one year and were looking at impacts on lung function and symptomatic endpoints, although some were even briefer than this. In the subsequent sections, the main clinical outcomes of these trials will be considered.

A. The Effects of Corticosteroids on Lung Function

In some of the large three-year studies, patients randomized to ICSs showed a small but significant increase in post-bronchodilator FEV_1 which occurred early in the study and was maintained throughout the treatment period (9,41). This effect subsequently complicated the analysis of rate of decline of lung function which was undertaken using relatively complicated mixed effects modeling. These models are inherently conservative and are influenced by differential dropout. This was only a problem in the Inhaled Steroids in Chronic Obstructive Lung Disease (ISOLDE) study where significantly more patients who were randomized to placebo withdrew compared with the active therapy. However, the impact of nonrandom dropouts, which probably reflect treatment benefit that is lost in the placebo limb (43), has had major impacts on the outcomes of other trials (see below).

Figure 2 tabulates the changes seen in decline of lung function in the different studies. In all the studies, there was a trend toward lower lung function in the ICS-treated patients, but none of them showed a significant difference. This has led to two meta-

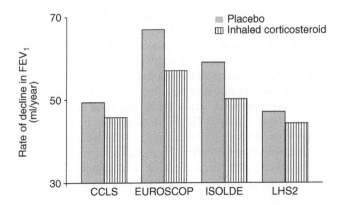

Figure 2 Annual rate of decline in post-bronchodilator forced expiratory volume in one second (FEV₁) in four 3-year trials comparing inhaled corticosteroids with placebo across a range of baseline FEV₁ values.

analyses and third pooled data analysis which is presently in press, which has also included information from three 1-year studies where corticosteroids were compared with placebo. One of the meta-analyses (44) and the pooled data analysis suggested that there was no effect on rate of decline of lung function, although the latter report could be criticized because of the differential treatment exposure. The second meta-analysis was more hopeful and suggested being a little selective with the studies it included that there might be a 10-mL per year difference in the rate of decline of lung function, something which none of the studies individually were powered to detect (45). Data from the very much larger Toward a Revolution in COPD Health (TORCH) trial are now becoming available and although that study was not primarily designed to look at rate of decline of lung function, it contains within it sufficient data for this problem to be properly addressed. Hopefully, when that is reported this controversy can finally be settled. What is clear is that the change in progression of lung function is likely to be small on average in a population of this size.

B. The Effect of Corticosteroids on Exacerbations

The ISOLDE study was the first to try to determine whether ICSs reduce the number of exacerbations in the COPD population (41). Previous studies using nonstandard exacerbation definitions had suggested that this might be possible. The definition adopted by the ISOLDE investigators came to be accepted independently as a sensible way of evaluating exacerbations in a clinical trial population (46) and has now been widely promoted and modified to become one of the acceptable ways of identifying exacerbations as recommended by the recent Global Initiative on Obstructive Lung Disease document. The ISOLDE study focused on episodes that required treatment with oral corticosteroids and/or antibiotics and suggested that there was an approximate 25% reduction in exacerbation numbers. However, the methodology used to express exacerbation data was relatively crude and has subsequently been criticized (47). Reporting mean exacerbation rates in a population where the data are very non-normally distributed is clearly wrong and even the median rate is not very helpful. Several proposals have been made about better ways of addressing these non-normal data with subsequent reports using the Poisson distribution with or without a correction for overdispersion. One of the most recent studies used a further refinement called the "negative binomial method" (48). There are also issues about identifying the length of these exacerbations, which is possible using symptom diary cards but is much harder relying on the patient's case record (49). Whether exacerbation data should be reported in terms of time to first event, number of events in the population at risk or model exacerbation rates per person per year is also contentious and at resent there is no consensus on which way is the best. Each of the above approaches has it advocates, although the last has probably been the most widely used to date. Subsequent studies using FP have reported a reduction in the exacerbation rates relative to placebo (10), but this was not seen in two clinical trials where budesonide was used in patients with more severe disease (42). Exploration of the ISOLDE data suggested that much of the improvement in the rate of decline of health status was attributable to the lower exacerbation numbers and it should be possible to confirm this finding in other studies (1).

C. The Effect of Corticosteroids on Health Status

The most widely reported measure of health state or health-related quality of life has been the St. George's Respiratory Questionnaire, which has the advantage of providing a single total score and having a generally agreed minimum clinically important difference. Traditionally, for a two-point comparison or a cross-sectional comparison within groups, this has been considered to be four units (50), although there has been a suggestion that in longitudinal data this difference may need to be reduced to two units. Data from the large ICS trials could be considered to be equivocal. The original ISOLDE data showed a three-unit difference between placebo and corticosteroid-treated patients, although a more realistic way of viewing this is to say that the treatment delayed deterioration by that amount by approximately 15 months (41). This is likely to be more helpful given that the tendency in COPD patients is to get worse and it is also a conservative estimate, since the patients with the worse health status tend to withdraw soonest as was also seen in the ISOLDE trial (43). Patients treated with budesonide in one of the budesonide combination studies where health status has been initially standardized before study (as was done in the ISOLDE study as well) also showed a benefit with the ICS compared with placebo, such that over the first year the health status was maintained rather than deteriorating by approximately four units (42). This is in keeping with the earlier trial which had been performed in the same way (41) but somewhat at odds in the studies in which there was no standardization of health status and patients were simply withdrawn from their prior medication for two weeks and then randomized to one of the trial therapies (8,10). This shows how small, seemingly insignificant, differences in trial design can lead to quite different outcomes. This is a particular problem when data are simply pooled in a meta-analysis and can lead to the effects of therapy being significantly over or under estimated.

D. The Effect of Withdrawing Corticosteroids

One way of identifying whether corticosteroids are useful in COPD is to stop the treatment and see whether the patient deteriorates. An observational report in the run-in phase of the ISOLDE study suggested that patients who had previously used ICSs were significantly more likely to have an exacerbation if these were stopped (51), a finding supported by a prospective randomized study (52). Differences in treatment, particularly in terms of lung function, were seen in a Dutch study where patients were left on a combination LABA/ICS inhaler or continued on the LABA alone (53). Perhaps the most compelling indirect evidence of this is seen in the large randomized trials where patients who are randomized to placebo withdraw much more readily due to exacerbations and lack of efficacy than those taking active treatment.

VI. Combination Therapy

To date, seven large clinical trials have compared the combination of an ICS and a LABA with the individual components and placebo and have reported most of the same clinical endpoints—exacerbation rate, health status, lung function, and a range of softer endpoints including rescue therapy use and diary card symptoms. Despite differences in design [the most obvious being the intensification of treatment during the run-in phase of one of the Calverley's studies (42)], the outcomes have been fairly consistent. Thus, two U.S. trials over six months reported better lung function compared with placebo and the components of the combination therapy (54,55). In one of these using the higher dose of ICSs, there was improvement in the transitional dyspnea index, but this was not seen in patients in the lower dose ICS study due to an unexpected spontaneous improvement in those randomized to placebo.

The three 1-year studies involving some 3500 patients showed similar significant improvements in FEV_1 to the shorter trials, a significant reduction in exacerbations in the combination therapy compared with placebo and for those trials with the lower baseline FEV_1 significant benefits of the combination compared with the components in this outcome (8,10,42). Likewise, the data about health status tended to be more obviously positive than the patients whose mean FEV_1 was 35% predicted. A variety of other endpoints, including the number of courses of oral corticosteroids and daily diary card symptoms also improved in these studies.

All of this has been put in the shade by the report of the TORCH study which involved over 6000 patients in 42 different countries who were followed for three years (48). The study design was similar to the six-month trials with the principal comparisons being salmeterol 50 μg plus FP 500 μg (SFC) twice daily, each drug in this dose individually twice daily and an identical placebo. The primary endpoint was the difference, if any, in all-cause mortality between placebo and SFC but the other endpoints noted above were also reported. A clinical endpoint committee assigned the cause of death in each case (56) and follow-up at the efficacy population was astonishingly complete with all-bar-one subject having complete survival data at the end of the study. As in the other trials, withdrawal from the study was significantly different between placebo and SFC (Fig. 3) and those previously taking placebo were much more likely to be using one of the active therapies by the end of the study. Altogether 894 patients died with a 15.2% mortality on placebo compared with 12.6% on SFC, a difference that approached but did not quite reach the prespecified p value (0.052) (Fig. 4). This is most likely to be due to the study's lower-than-anticipated mortality in the placebo limb, itself a potential consequence of the large number of people who were able to take active therapy in this intention-to-treat analysis.

TORCH patients receiving SFC had fewer exacerbations than in any other group and maintained their health status on average above baseline values by the end of the

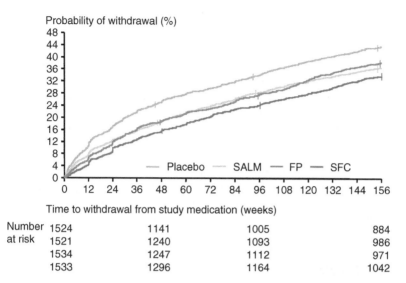

Figure 3 Withdrawal from randomized treatment during the Toward a Revolution in COPD Health (TORCH) study. Significantly more patients withdrew from therapy in the placebo group. Statistical comparisons: SFC, SALM and FP versus placebo $p < 0.001$; SFC versus SALM $p = 0.048$; SFC versus FP $p = 0.01$. Vertical bars are standard errors. *Abbreviations*: CCLS, Copenhagen City Lung Study; FEV_1, forced expiratory volume in one second; ISOLDE, Inhaled Steroids in Chronic Obstructive Lung Disease study; LHS2, Lung Health Study 2; SALM, salmeterol; SFC, salmeterol/fluticasone combination; FP, fluticasone propionate.

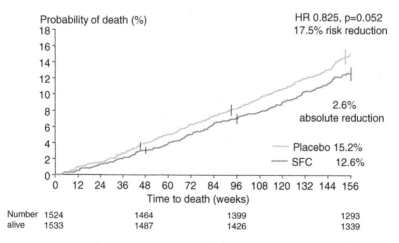

Figure 4 Mortality during the Toward a Revolution in COPD Health trial for patients randomized to placebo and the salmeterol/fluticasone propionate combination. There was an absolute difference in mortality of 2.6% at three years representing a relative risk reduction of death during the three years of 17.5%. After adjustment for interim analysis, the difference approach but did not achieve the prespecified significance level ($p = 0.052$). Vertical bars are standard errors. *Abbreviations*: FP, fluticasone propionate; SALM, salmeterol; SFC, salmeterol/fluticasone combination.

study, something which was not true for other treatments and certainly not for placebo for health status clearly declined over the three years.

One rather smaller but nonetheless important study has also recently been published which has compared the SFC combination as an additional therapy to either long-acting bronchodilatation with the anticholinergic drug tiotropium on its own or in combination with salmeterol (57). This study, which was independently funded by the Canadian Institute for Health Research, was unfortunately underpowered to establish conclusively either equivalence or superiority of one of these treatment limbs. Arguments about how to express the exacerbation rate in a population like this further complicate matters. However, it was clear that patients were least likely to withdraw from treatment if randomized blindly to triple therapy and lung function and health status in these groups of people was also significantly better than the other treatments. Moreover, there was a reduction in hospitalization in this group, lending some support to the current clinical pattern of combining anticholinergic and combination therapy in the most severe patients.

VII. Side Effects

As already noted, oral corticosteroid therapies are associated with significant side effects that occur even when low-dose maintenance oral corticosteroids are given. Whether the same is true when treatment is given by the inhaled route and if so, to what degree and in whom, has been an extremely controversial area. COPD patients are older and have substantial comorbidities, including those such as osteoporosis, cataracts, and glaucoma which have also been associated with corticosteroid therapy (58). Thus, they are potentially a population at risk of harm but where deciding if harm is present is extremely difficult given background fluctuations in the occurrence of these problems anyway. At present, three general statements appear to be true.

1. ICSs are associated with infrequent but sometimes local side effects that have already been described. When metered dose inhalers are used to deliver therapy, a volume spacer device probably decreases the degree of oropharyngeal deposition. In practice, these symptoms are often very troublesome to either patient or doctor.
2. The risks of systemic toxicity with ICSs appear to be low. Earlier reports in patients with better lung function of spontaneous bruising (59) have not been confirmed in studies in more severe disease (10). Many COPD patients do report spontaneous subcutaneous bruising but this seems to track their exposure to oral corticosteroids rather better than that to ICSs. An effect of ICSs cannot be completely excluded because these drugs are often prescribed in patients who already receive courses of oral therapy. This confounding effect also extends to other areas and complicates the analysis of database information where conflicting data about the fracture hazard associated with corticosteroids use has been reported (11,60). In general the outcome of very large studies and particularly the extensive TORCH safety database are reassuring. There was no consistent increase in the number of fracture or reported eye problems and in the subset of U.S. patients where bone minimal density and eye examinations were conducted, there was no clear trend for deterioration in the steroid-treated limbs of the study, although the number of

　　　patients completing the study and the high background of abnormalities at study entry cannot completely exclude some effect that might occur over a longer period of time. Nonetheless, these data together with earlier studies of adrenal function (10) do not point to a large clinical side effect burden.

3. One unanticipated problem, which was identified in the TORCH database for the first time, was that patients receiving ICSs were much more likely to have physician-diagnosed pneumonia during their subsequent follow-up with a relative risk ratio of 1.6 (48). These events were substantially less frequent than exacerbations of the disease, but however the data are considered there is no doubt that either ICSs on their own or in combination with a LABA was associated with more of these events. Unfortunately, there was no requirement to obtain microbiology or a chest X ray when pneumonia was diagnosed nor even to document the physician's basis for making this diagnosis. This substantially limits our understanding of what is going on, although some preliminary data suggest that episodes where the patient reports themselves as being feverish are rather more likely to be diagnosed as being due to pneumonia. Whether this is just an issue of diagnostic labeling or represents a specific pathological problem in a subgroup of COPD patients is an important issue that should be properly addressed in future prospective studies. At present, it would seem sensible to be aware of the risk of pneumonia in patients receiving ICSs and to ensure that they have prophylaxis against this in the form of pneumococcal vaccination and that if an episode does occur, it is investigated appropriately. On the positive side, there did not seem to any increase in hospitalization for mortality related to pneumonia in the SFC-treated patients.

VIII. Conclusion

After 10 years of intensive clinical research, we can at last begin to place corticosteroids therapy in some kind of context in COPD. Now we have reasonable evidence that moderately high doses of oral corticosteroids given for a short period, in my practice no longer than one week, are associated with a more rapid resolution of exacerbations, at least in those patients severe enough to attend hospital. The very small amount of data in ambulatory outpatients would also support using oral corticosteroids here, but it is just as important to stop this treatment as to start it in a timely fashion. Substantial harm can be done to patients by inadvertently leaving them on treatment with oral corticosteroids and after several weeks it can be much harder to withdraw this therapy.

　　　When corticosteroids are used in long-term management, the inhaled route is the best one. At present we have most data about higher doses of inhaled FP or budesonide in this setting. Although there is clear evidence of impact on some endpoints, particularly lung function and probably health status, the role of these drugs in more severe disease is dubious and the results of the TORCH trial suggest that they do not have any important effect on COPD mortality. This contrasts with the situation with combination treatment which is clearly more effective in terms of improving lung function, reducing the number of exacerbations and improving health status. Moreover, there is a possibility of some beneficial effect in terms of life expectancy. This signal was not confined solely to patients with COPD-related deaths nor was the benefit on exacerbations uniquely seen in patients with a prior history of exacerbation at the start of the study. Thus, a case can be made for the more widespread use of this combination treatment in patients with a lung function less than 60% predicted. The most recent data suggest that there may be additional advantage, at least in terms of patient acceptability and well-being, from combining the β-agonist and ICS with a long-acting anticholinergic drug like tiotropium and this will probably become the standard therapy in patients with more severe COPD.

To date, the side effects profile in patients with moderate-to-very severe COPD appears to be quite acceptable with reassuring data about bone mineral density, eye problems, and cardiovascular risk, at least with regard to the LABA. The issue of pneumonia is important and required increased clinical vigilance until such time as we can define more clearly those where this problem might be more troublesome and worth varying the treatment regime.

Thus, the short answer to the question "When should be use glucocorticoids in COPD?" is in moderately large systemic doses by mouth during exacerbations for a defined period and as part of combination treatment with an inhaled LABA in patients with more severe COPD, especially those where exacerbations appear to be troublesome. The availability of patient acceptable devices to deliver these therapies and the prospect of combining them effectively with other treatment means that the place of ICS in COPD management is likely to be secure, although no longer as a treatment used on its own with short-acting bronchodilators. Our next challenge is to follow our colleagues in cardiology and see what else can be added to these existing treatments to further improve the well-being of our COPD patients.

References

1. Spencer S, Calverley PM, Burge PS, Jones PW. Impact of preventing exacerbations on deterioration of health status in COPD. Eur Respir J 2004; 23(5):698–702.
2. Soler-Cataluna JJ, Martinez-Garcia MA, Roman SP, Salcedo E, Navarro M, Ochando R. Severe acute exacerbations and mortality in patients with chronic obstructive pulmonary disease. Thorax 2005; 60(11):925–31.
3. Anthonisen NR, Connett JE, Kiley JP, et al. Effects of smoking intervention and the use of an inhaled anticholinergic bronchodilator on the rate of decline of FEV1. The Lung Health Study. J Am Med Assoc 1994; 272(19):1497–505 (see comments).
4. Calverley PM. The role of corticosteroids in chronic obstructive pulmonary disease. Semin Respir Crit Care Med 2005; 26(2):235–45.
5. Calverley PM. Effect of corticosteroids on exacerbations of asthma and chronic obstructive pulmonary disease. Proc Am Thorac Soc 2004; 1(3):161–6.
6. The Lung Health Study Research Group. Effect of inhaled triamcinolone on the decline in pulmonary function in chronic obstructive pulmonary disease. N Engl J Med 2000; 343:1902–9.
7. Vestbo J, Pauwels R, Anderson JA, Jones P, Calverley P. Early onset of effect of salmeterol and fluticasone propionate in chronic obstructive pulmonary disease. Thorax 2005; 60(4):301–4.
8. Szafranski W, Cukier A, Ramirez A, et al. Efficacy and safety of budesonide/formoterol in the management of chronic obstructive pulmonary disease. Eur Respir J 2003; 21(1):74–81.
9. Pauwels RA, Lofdahl C-G, Laitinen LA, et al. Long-term treatment with inhaled budesonide in persons with mild chronic obstructive pulmonary disease who continue smoking. N Engl J Med 1999; 340(25):1948–53.
10. Calverley P, Pauwels R, Vestbo J, et al. Combined salmeterol and fluticasone in the treatment of chronic obstructive pulmonary disease: a randomised controlled trial. Lancet 2003; 361(9356):449–56.
11. Walsh LJ, Lewis SA, Wong CA, et al. The impact of oral corticosteroid use on bone mineral density and vertebral fracture. Am J Respir Crit Care Med 2002; 166(5):691–5.
12. Schols AM, Wesseling G, Kester AD, et al. Dose dependent increased mortality risk in COPD patients treated with oral glucocorticoids. Eur Respir J 2001; 17(3):337–42.

13. Pauwels RA, Buist AS, Calverley PMA, Jenkins CR, Hurd SS. Global strategy for the diagnosis, management and prevention of chronic obstructive pulmonary disease. Am J Respir Crit Care Med 2001; 163:1256–76.
14. Celli BR, MacNee W. Standards for the diagnosis and treatment of patients with COPD: a summary of the ATS/ERS position paper. Eur Respir J 2004; 23(6):932–46.
15. National Collaborating Centre for Chronic Conditions. Chronic obstructive pulmonary disease. National clinical guideline on management of chronic obstructive pulmonary disease in adults in primary and secondary care. Thorax 2004; 59(Suppl. 1):1–232.
16. Barnes PJ. Scientific rationale for inhaled combination therapy with long-acting beta2-agonists and corticosteroids. Eur Respir J 2002; 19(1):182–91.
17. Horvath G, Wanner A. Inhaled corticosteroids: effects on the airway vasculature in bronchial asthma. Eur Respir J 2006; 27(1):172–87.
18. Brown PH, Teelucksingh S, Matusiewicz SP, Greening AP, Crompton GK, Edwards CRW. Cutaneous vasoconstrictor response to glucocorticoids in asthma. Lancet 1991; 337(8741):576–80.
19. Barnes PJ, Ito K, Adcock IM. Corticosteroid resistance in chronic obstructive pulmonary disease: inactivation of histone deacetylase. Lancet 2004; 363(9410):731–3.
20. Tomlinson JE, McMahon AD, Chaudhuri R, Thompson JM, Wood SF, Thomson NC. Efficacy of low and high dose inhaled corticosteroid in smokers versus non-smokers with mild asthma. Thorax 2005; 60(4):282–7.
21. Ito K, Ito M, Elliott WM, et al. Decreased histone deacetylase activity in chronic obstructive pulmonary disease. N Engl J Med 2005; 352(19):1967–76.
22. Davies L, Nisar M, Pearson MG, Costello RW, Earis JE, Calverley PMA. Oral corticosteroid trials in the management of stable chronic obstructive pulmonary disease. Q J Med 1999; 92(7):395–400.
23. Brand PL, Quanjer PH, Postma DS, et al. Interpretation of bronchodilator response in patients with obstructive airways disease. The Dutch Chronic Non-Specific Lung Disease (CNSLD) Study Group. Thorax 1992; 47(6):429–36.
24. Calverley PM, Burge PS, Spencer S, Anderson JA, Jones PW. Bronchodilator reversibility testing in chronic obstructive pulmonary disease. Thorax 2003; 58(8):659–64.
25. Burge PS, Calverley PM, Jones PW, Spencer S, Anderson JA. Prednisolone response in patients with chronic obstructive pulmonary disease: results from the ISOLDE study. Thorax 2003; 58(8):654–8.
26. Nisar M, Earis JE, Pearson MG, Calverley PM. Acute bronchodilator trials in chronic obstructive pulmonary disease. Am Rev Respir Dis 1992; 146(3):555–9.
27. Albert RK, Martin TR, Lewis SW. Controlled clinical trial of methylprednisolone in patients with chronic bronchitis and acute respiratory insufficiency. Ann Intern Med 1980; 92(6):753–8.
28. Thompson WH, Nielson CP, Carvalho P, Charan NB, Crowley JJ. Controlled trial of oral prednisone in outpatients with acute COPD exacerbation. Am J Respir Crit Care Med 1996; 154(2 Pt 1):407–12.
29. Niewoehner DE, Erbland ML, Deupree RH, et al. Effect of systemic glucocorticoids on exacerbations of chronic obstructive pulmonary disease. N Engl J Med 1999; 340(25):1941–7.
30. Davies L, Angus RM, Calverley PMA. Oral corticosteroids in patients admitted to hospital with exacerbations of chronic obstructive pulmonary disease: a prospective randomised controlled trial. Lancet 1999; 354(9177):456–60.
31. Niewoehner DE, Collins D, Erbland ML. Relation of FEV(1) to clinical outcomes during exacerbations of chronic obstructive pulmonary disease. Department of Veterans Affairs Cooperative Study Group. Am J Respir Crit Care Med 2000; 161(4 Pt 1):1201–5.
32. Aaron SD, Vandemheen KL, Hebert P, et al. Outpatient oral prednisone after emergency treatment of chronic obstructive pulmonary disease. N Engl J Med 2003; 348(26):2618–25.
33. Maltais F, Ostinelli J, Bourbeau J, et al. Comparison of nebulized budesonide and oral prednisolone with placebo in the treatment of acute exacerbations of chronic obstructive pulmonary disease: a randomized controlled trial. Am J Respir Crit Care Med 2002; 165(5):698–703 (JID—9421642).
34. Sayiner A, Aytemur ZA, Cirit M, Unsal I. Systemic glucocorticoids in severe exacerbations of COPD. Chest 2001; 119(3):726–30 (see comments).
35. Renkema TE, Schouten JP, Koeter GH, Postma DS. Effects of long-term treatment with corticosteroids in COPD. Chest 1996; 109(5):1156–62.
36. Paggiaro PL, Dahle R, Bakran I, Frith L, Hollingworth K, Efthimiou J. Multicentre randomised placebo-controlled trial of inhaled fluticasone propionate in patients with chronic obstructive pulmonary disease. International COPD Study Group. Lancet 1998; 351(9105):773–80 (see comments; published erratum appears in Lancet 1998 Jun 27; 351(9120):1968).

37. Bourbeau J, Rouleau MY, Boucher S. Randomised controlled trial of inhaled corticosteroids in patients with chronic obstructive pulmonary disease. Thorax 1998; 53(6):477–82.

38. Wempe JB, Postma DS, Breederveld N, Kort E, van der Mark TW, Koeter GH. Effects of corticosteroids on bronchodilator action in chronic obstructive lung disease. Thorax 1992; 47(8):616–21.

39. Dompeling E, Van Schayck CP, Van Grunsven PM, et al. Slowing the deterioration of asthma and chronic obstructive pulmonary disease observed during bronchodilator therapy by adding inhaled corticosteroids. A 4-year prospective study. Ann Intern Med 1993; 118(10):770–8 (see comments).

40. Vestbo J, Sorensen T, Lange P, Brix A, Torre P, Viskum K. Long-term effect of inhaled budesonide in mild and moderate chronic obstructive pulmonary disease: a randomised controlled trial. Lancet 1999; 353(9167):1819–23.

41. Burge PS, Calverley PM, Jones PW, Spencer S, Anderson JA, Maslen TK. Randomised, double blind, placebo controlled study of fluticasone propionate in patients with moderate to severe chronic obstructive pulmonary disease: the ISOLDE trial. Br Med J 2000; 320(7245):1297–303.

42. Calverley PM, Boonsawat W, Cseke Z, Zhong N, Peterson S, Olsson H. Maintenance therapy with budesonide and formoterol in chronic obstructive pulmonary disease. Eur Respir J 2003; 22(6):912–9.

43. Calverley PM, Spencer S, Willits L, Burge PS, Jones PW. Withdrawal from treatment as an outcome in the ISOLDE study of COPD. Chest 2003; 124(4):1350–6.

44. Alsaeedi A, Sin DD, McAlister FA. The effects of inhaled corticosteroids in chronic obstructive pulmonary disease: a systematic review of randomized placebo-controlled trials. Am J Med 2002; 113(1):59–65.

45. Sutherland ER, Allmers H, Ayas NT, Venn AJ, Martin RJ. Inhaled corticosteroids reduce the progression of airflow limitation in chronic obstructive pulmonary disease: a meta-analysis. Thorax 2003; 58(11):937–41.

46. Rodriguez-Roisin R. Toward a consensus definition for COPD exacerbations.Chest 2000; 117(5 Suppl. 2): 398S–401.

47. Suissa S. Statistical treatment of exacerbations in therapeutic trials of chronic obstructive pulmonary disease. Am J Respir Crit Care Med 2006; 173(8):842–6.

48. Calverley PM, Anderson JA, Celli B, et al. Salmeterol and fluticasone propionate and survival in chronic obstructive pulmonary disease. N Engl J Med 2007; 356(8):775–89.

49. Seemungal TA, Donaldson GC, Bhowmik A, Jeffries DJ, Wedzicha JA. Time course and recovery of exacerbations in patients with chronic obstructive pulmonary disease. Am J Respir Crit Care Med 2000; 161(5):1608–13.

50. Jones PW. Health status measurement in chronic obstructive pulmonary disease. Thorax 2001; 56(11):880–7.

51. Jarad NA, Wedzicha JA, Burge PS, Calverley PMA. An observational study of inhaled corticosteroid withdrawal in stable chronic obstructive pulmonary disease. Respir Med 1999; 93(3):161–8.

52. van der V, Monninkhof E, van der PJ, Zielhuis G, van Herwaarden C. Effect of discontinuation of inhaled corticosteroids in patients with chronic obstructive pulmonary disease: the COPE study. Am J Respir Crit Care Med 2002; 166(10):1358–63.

53. Wouters EF, Postma DS, Fokkens B, et al. Withdrawal of fluticasone propionate from combined salmeterol/fluticasone treatment in patients with COPD causes immediate and sustained disease deterioration: a randomised controlled trial. Thorax 2005; 60(6):480–7.

54. Mahler DA, Wire P, Horstman D, et al. Effectiveness of fluticasone propionate and salmeterol combination delivered via the Diskus device in the treatment of chronic obstructive pulmonary disease. Am J Respir Crit Care Med 2002; 166(8):1084–91.

55. Hanania NA, Darken P, Horstman D, et al. The efficacy and safety of fluticasone propionate (250 microg)/salmeterol (50 microg) combined in the Diskus inhaler for the treatment of COPD. Chest 2003; 124(3):834–43.

56. McGarvey LP, John M, Anderson JA, Zvarich MT, Wise RA, et al. Ascertainment of cause-specific mortality in COPD—operations of the TORCH Clinical Endpoint Committee. Thorax 2007; 62(5):411–5.

57. Aaron SD, Vandemheen KL, Fergusson D, et al. Tiotropium in combination with placebo, salmeterol, or fluticasone–salmeterol for treatment of chronic obstructive pulmonary disease: a randomized trial. Ann Intern Med 2007; 146(8):545–55.

58. Walsh LJ, Wong CA, Oborne J, et al. Adverse effects of oral corticosteroids in relation to dose in patients with lung disease. Thorax 2001; 56(4):279–84.

59. Tashkin DP, Murray HE, Skeans M, Murray RP. Skin manifestations of inhaled corticosteroids in COPD patients: results from Lung Health Study II. Chest 2004; 126(4):1123–33.

60. Johannes CB, Schneider GA, Dube TJ, Alfredson TD, Davis KJ, Walker AM. The risk of nonvertebral fracture related to inhaled corticosteroid exposure among adults with chronic respiratory disease. Chest 2005; 127(1):89–97.

15

Treating and Preventing Infections

SANJAY SETHI
Division of Pulmonary and Critical Care Medicine, Department of Medicine, State University of New York at Buffalo, and Department of Veterans Affairs, Western New York Healthcare System, Buffalo, New York, U.S.A.

I. Introduction

A healthy lung, in spite of repeated exposure to microbial pathogens by inhalation and microaspiration, has a remarkable ability to maintain sterility (1,2). In COPD, this ability is compromised, and infections, both acute and chronic, become a prominent feature of the disease. Acute lower respiratory tract infection in COPD can present as either a tracheobronchial process, usually referred to as exacerbation, or involve the lung parenchyma, with an infiltrate seen on chest X ray, whence it is called pneumonia. Chronic infection in COPD is much more subtle in its clinical manifestations. In fact, whether chronic infection has any clinical significance has been an area of controversy, and is often referred to as "colonization," implying it is innocuous.

Historically, before the realization of the central role of tobacco smoke and other noxious exposures in the development of COPD, infection, along with mucus hypersecretion were thought to play a prominent role in the development of COPD, as embodied in the "British hypothesis." Experimental and epidemiological data generated in the 1970s and 1980s did not clearly support the role of infection and mucus hypersecretion in the pathogenesis of exacerbations and in the chronic phase of the disease (3). This led to infection, especially bacterial, being considered as a mere epiphenomenon of little consequence in both the acute and stable phases of COPD (4). Since then, substantial progress in our understanding of microbial pathogenesis and in research tools to diagnose and evaluate infections has been made. In the last two decades, application of these new tools and understanding to the issues of infection in COPD has revolutionized our understanding of infection in COPD, especially bacterial infection (5,6).

Appreciation of the role of infection in exacerbation and now in stable COPD has led to reexamination of our approach to treatment and prevention of these infections. Though much needs to be done to define our optimal approach to these processes, clinical and translational research has improved our current use of antimicrobials in this disease. The emphasis in this book is on clinical management of COPD, and therefore, treatment and prevention of infection will be discussed in detail in this chapter. A synopsis of our current understanding of pathogenesis of infection in COPD will be presented, and the reader can find additional details in other recent review articles (7,8). For clarity, exacerbations will be discussed initially, followed by chronic infection and then pneumonia, though there is overlap, both clinical and biological, among these entities.

II. Definition and Severity of Exacerbations

There is still considerable debate regarding an exact definition of an exacerbation of COPD (9). This debate exists because of lack of an objective marker to define an exacerbation, which therefore remains a patient-reported, symptom-based, and subjective diagnosis. In our clinical studies, we suspect an exacerbation when a patient with COPD reports a minor increase (or new onset) of two or a major increase (or new onset) of one of the following respiratory symptoms: dyspnea, cough, sputum production, sputum tenacity, and sputum purulence (10). The increase in symptoms should be of at least 24 hours duration and should be of greater intensity than their normal day-to-day variability. Other definitions have required symptoms to be of at least 48 hours and even 72 hours in duration. Furthermore, clinical evaluation should exclude other clinical entities that could present in a similar manner, such as pneumonia, congestive heart failure, upper respiratory infection, noncompliance with medications, etc.

The severity of an exacerbation is a complicated concept because it is constituted by at least two factors: the severity of the underlying COPD and the acute change induced by the exacerbation itself. Therefore, a patient who has got very severe underlying COPD may have significant clinical consequences from a relatively small change from one's own baseline state, while a patient with mild COPD may be able to tolerate a much larger change in symptoms and lung function.

Different notions of severity have been used. Lung function changes are difficult to measure during exacerbations, and often the change with an exacerbation is of the same magnitude as day-to-day variability in these measurements. Severity has also been measured by site of care, with hospitalized exacerbations regarded as severe, outpatient exacerbations as moderate, and self-medicated exacerbations as mild (11). This classification is prone to error as the site of care is dependent on differences among countries and health-care systems as to the threshold for admission as well as patient and physician preferences. Another measure of severity suggested is the intensity of treatment with bronchodilators indicating only mild exacerbations, and treatment with antibiotics and steroids regarded as indicating moderate or severe exacerbations. Again, this approach is beset with problems of preferences and practical approach.

One widely used determination of severity is known as the Anthonisen classification (12). This classification relies on the number of cardinal symptoms and the presence of some supporting symptoms as shown in Table 1. Interestingly, this classification was not designed to be a classification of severity of exacerbations, but has become so over time. This determination of severity is relatively simple and does correlate with benefit with antibiotics, with such benefit seen only in Type 1 and 2 exacerbations. However, there are limitations to the Anthonisen severity classification. It has not been validated against objective measures of severity. The association with benefit with antibiotics has not been reproduced in other studies. Another limitation is the lack of gradation of severity within each symptom, such that an exacerbation with mild dyspnea and mild increase in sputum would be regarded as the same severity in this classification as one with a marked increase in both symptoms.

Table 1 Anthonisen Classification of Chronic Obstructive Pulmonary Disease Exacerbations Based on Cardinal Symptoms

Severity of exacerbation	Type of exacerbation	Characteristics
Severe	Type 1	Increased dyspnea, sputum volume, and sputum purulence
Moderate	Type 2	Any 2 of the above 3 cardinal symptoms
Mild	Type 3	Any 1 of the above 3 cardinal symptoms and 1 or more of the following minor symptoms or signs: (*i*) Cough (*ii*) Wheezing (*iii*) Fever without an obvious source (*iv*) Upper respiratory tract infection in the past 5 days (*v*) Respiratory rate increase > 20% over baseline (*vi*) Heart rate increase > 20% over baseline

Source: From Ref. 12.

It is evident that we need a better definition and objective measures of severity of exacerbations. Ongoing efforts in the development of patient-reported outcomes and biomarkers should provide us with such tools in the future.

III. Pathogenesis of Exacerbations

Increases in plasma fibrinogen, interleukin-6 (IL-6), and C-reactive protein, consistent with a heightened state of systemic inflammation, have been described during exacerbations (13,14). This likely results in the systemic manifestations of exacerbations, including fatigue and, in some instances, fever.

A variety of noninfectious and infectious stimuli can induce an acute increase in airway inflammation in COPD, thereby causing the manifestations of exacerbation (Fig. 1). Epidemiological studies have demonstrated increased respiratory symptoms and respiratory mortality among patients with COPD during periods of increased air pollution (15–17). Indeed, environmental pollutants, such as particulate matter < 10 μm in diameter, and non-particulate gases, such as ozone, nitrogen dioxide, sulfur dioxide, are capable of inducing inflammation in vitro and in vivo (18–20). Infectious agents, including bacteria, viruses, and atypical pathogens, are implicated as causes of up to 80% of acute exacerbations, and are discussed in greater detail below (21).

IV. Microbial Pathogens in COPD

The list of potential pathogens in COPD has expanded considerably in recent years. To the usual suspects, typical respiratory bacterial pathogens and respiratory viruses, atypical bacteria, and fungi have been added (Table 2). Among the typical bacteria, nontypeable *Haemophilus influenzae* (NTHI) is the most common and its role in COPD is the best understood (22). Among the viruses, rhinovirus and respiratory syncytial virus (RSV) have received considerable attention in recent years (23,24). *Pneumocystis*

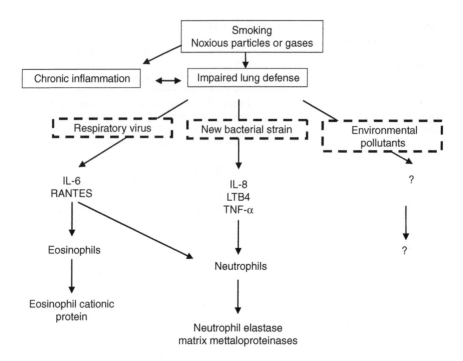

Figure 1 Inflammatory mediators and cells associated with specific causes of exacerbation. Cells and mediators that increase with exacerbation but specific etiologic association has not been made are also listed. *Abbreviations*: ?, unknown; GM-CSF, granulocyte macrophage colony stimulating factor; IL, interleukin; LTB4, leukotriene B-4; TNF-α, tumor necrosis factor-α.

jiroveci has been a recent and somewhat surprising addition to potential pathogens in this disease (25).

Certain shared characteristics of these pathogens provide clues to their predilection for causing infections in COPD. NTHI, *Streptococcus pneumoniae*, and *Moraxella catarrhalis* are the predominant bacterial cause of two other common respiratory mucosal infections: acute otitis media in children and acute sinusitis in children and adults. These mucosal infections have been related to anatomical abnormalities with impaired drainage of secretions, antecedent viral infections, and defects in adaptive immunity. All these predisposing factors likely exist in COPD. These three pathogens are all exclusively human pathogens that are transmitted among individuals. In healthy hosts, their presence is confined to the upper airway and does not cause any clinical manifestations. It is likely that acquisition of these pathogens in a patient with COPD, because of compromised lung defense, allows establishment of infection in the lower respiratory tract, with or without overt clinical manifestations.

Table 2 Microbial Pathogens Associated with Acute and Chronic Infection in COPD

Pathogen class	Proportion of exacerbations (%)	Specific species	Proportion of class of pathogens	Chronic infection
Bacteria	40–50	Nontypeable *Haemophilus influenzae*	30–50%	Major cause
		Streptococcus pneumoniae	15–20%	Uncommon
		Moraxella catarrhalis	15–20%	Uncommon
		Pseudomonas spp. and *Enterobacteriacea*	Isolated in very severe COPD, concomitant bronchiectasis, recurrent exacerbations	In very severe COPD
		Haemophilus parainfluenzae	Isolated frequently, pathogenic significance undefined	Common
		Haemophilus hemolyticus	Isolated frequently, pathogenic significance undefined	Common
		Staphylococcus aureus	Isolated infrequently, pathogenic significance undefined	Uncommon
Viruses	30–40	Rhinovirus	40–50%	Possible
		Parainfluenza	10–20%	Not demonstrated
		Influenza	10–20%	Not demonstrated
		RSV	10–20%	Possible
		Coronavirus	10–20%	Not demonstrated
		Adenovirus	5–10%	Not demonstrated
Atypical bacteria	5–10	*Chlamydia pneumoniae*	90–95%	Likely
		Mycoplasma pneumoniae	5–10%	Not demonstrated
Fungi	?	*Pneumocystis jiroveci*	?	Increased incidence with lower FEV_1

Abbreviations: ?, unknown; COPD, chronic obstructive pulmonary disease; FEV_1, forced expiratory volume at one second; RSV, respiratory syncytial virus.

Respiratory viruses implicated in COPD are able to cause acute tracheobronchial infections in healthy hosts, which are clinically referred to as acute bronchitis. In the setting of COPD, with diminished respiratory reserve, this acute bronchitis has more profound manifestations and serious clinical consequences.

V. Pathogenesis of Infectious Exacerbations

Our understanding of acute exacerbation pathogenesis, especially in relation to bacterial infection, has seen significant progress over the last few years. Both host and pathogen factors are involved in the development of acute bacterial exacerbations (Fig. 2). Acquisition of strains of bacterial pathogens that are new to the host from the environment appears to be the primary event that puts the patient with COPD at risk for an exacerbation (10). Variations among strains of a species in the surface antigenic structure, as is seen with NTHI, *S. pneumoniae*, and *M. catarrhalis*, allow these newly acquired strains to escape the preexisting host immune response that had developed following prior exposure to other strains of the same species of bacteria. These strains can therefore proliferate in the lower airways and induce acute inflammation in the airways. The virulence of the strain and as yet undetermined host factors may determine whether the acute inflammatory response to the pathogen reaches the threshold to cause

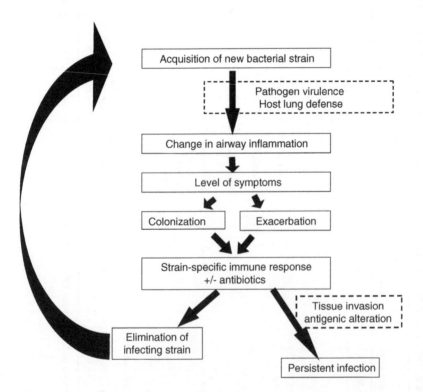

Figure 2 Proposed model of recurrent bacterial exacerbations in chronic obstructive pulmonary disease.

symptoms that present as an exacerbation (26). In many instances, the adaptive immune response results in the development of mucosal and systemic antibodies to the pathogen (27,28). This immune response, in combination with appropriate antibiotics, is able to eliminate or control the infecting bacteria. However, because of antigenic variability among strains of these bacterial species, the antibodies that develop to the infecting strain are quite strain specific and do not provide protection to the host from other strains of the same species that are antigenically distinct. This allows the process of recurrent exacerbations in these patients.

The pathogenesis of acute viral exacerbations is less well understood. However, it appears to be similar to bacterial infections. A common cause of exacerbations, the rhinovirus, demonstrates considerable antigenic variation among its more than 100 serotypes, allowing for recurrent infections. The influenza virus demonstrates drift in the antigenic makeup of its major surface proteins, thereby leading to recurrent infections. In vitro, viruses can damage airway epithelium, stimulate muscarinic receptors, and induce eosinophilic influx. These pro-inflammatory actions could potentially induce the pathophysiological manifestations that characterize acute exacerbation when a viral agent infects the lower airway of a patient with COPD. The pathogenesis of exacerbations with atypical bacterial or *Pneumocystis* infection is poorly understood.

VI. Treatment of Exacerbations

A. Goals of Treatment

Traditionally, the aims of treatment of an exacerbation are the recovery to baseline clinical status and the prevention of complications. Though these goals are undoubtedly important, several new observations raise the question whether these goals are adequate. These include our new understanding of the importance of exacerbations in the course of COPD, the role of infection in exacerbations, the high rates of relapse with an adequate initial clinical response, and the role played by chronic infection in the pathogenesis of COPD. To draw an analogy, confining our goals to short-term resolution of symptoms would be the equivalent of treating acute myocardial infarction with the only aim of resolution of chest pain. Several other important goals of treatment, both clinical and biological, should be considered (Table 3). For instance, clinical success in the treatment of exacerbations has been defined as resolution of symptoms to baseline or improvement of symptoms to a degree that no further treatment is required in the opinion of the treating physician. If symptoms do indeed correlate with exaggerated airway and systemic inflammation, then acceptance of clinical improvement rather than clinical resolution has important implications. Clinical improvement may reflect inadequate treatment, permitting the inflammatory process that underlies the exacerbation to persist for prolonged periods of time (29). Therefore, clinical resolution of symptoms to baseline may actually represent the optimal outcome.

Other important clinical goals of treatment include delaying the next exacerbation, prevention of early relapse, and more rapid resolution of symptoms (30–32). Lengthening the inter-exacerbation interval and prevention of early relapse are being increasingly recognized as important clinical goals of treatment because they ultimately translate to decreasing the frequency of exacerbations, which is now a major

Table 3 Proposed Goals of Treatment of Chronic Obstructive Pulmonary Disease Exacerbation

Goals	Comments
Clinical	
Clinical resolution to baseline	Needs baseline assessment prior to exacerbation onset for comparison
Prevention of relapse	Relapse within 30 days is quite frequent
Increasing exacerbation-free interval	Needs long-term follow-up after treatment
Faster resolution of symptoms	Needs validated symptom assessment tools
Preservation of health-related quality of life	Sustained decrements seen after exacerbations
Biological	
Bacterial eradication	Often presumed in usual antibiotic comparison studies
Resolution of airway inflammation	Shown to be incomplete if bacteria persist
Resolution of systemic inflammation	Persistence of systemic inflammation predicts early relapse
Restoration of lung function to baseline	Incomplete recovery is seen in significant proportion
Preservation of lung function	Needs long-term studies

focus of COPD treatment. Though most patients and physicians would accept faster recovery to baseline as a desirable goal of treatment, acceptance of this goal has been hampered by lack of well-validated instruments to reliably measure the rate of resolution of exacerbations.

Nonclinical goals of treatment are either still in their infancy or, in the case of bacteriological eradication, used only in clinical studies to satisfy regulatory requirements for approval of new antibiotics. If exacerbations are inflammatory events, it would be logical to have resolution of inflammation to baseline as an important goal of treatment. Similarly, exacerbations are in many instances induced by infection; therefore, eradication of the offending infectious pathogen should be a goal of treatment. Practical application of these biological goals of treatment of exacerbations awaits the development of simple, rapid, and reliable measurements of inflammation and infection.

Most exacerbations require a multi-pronged approach that utilizes several therapeutic modalities simultaneously, either to relieve symptoms, to treat the underlying cause, or provide support till recovery occurs (33,34). These therapies include bronchodilators, corticosteroids, and antimicrobials, and in the more severe cases oxygen supplementation and mechanical ventilation for acute respiratory failure. This chapter focuses on the role of antimicrobials in the treatment of exacerbation.

VII. Antibiotics in the Treatment of Exacerbations

The role and choice of antibiotics in the treatment of exacerbations has been a matter of controversy. Recommendations for antibiotic use among published guidelines are often inconsistent, and at times vague (33,35–37). The paucity of well-designed, large randomized controlled trials in this field upon which to base solid recommendations has undoubtedly contributed to the state of affairs (38). Recently, a few well-designed placebo-controlled and antibiotic comparison trials have been reported. In addition, epidemiological studies have consistently identified certain "risk factors," the presence of which in a patient with an acute exacerbation is predictive for failure of treatment or early relapse. There is increasing realization that with the heterogeneity of COPD and of exacerbations, using the same antibiotic in all exacerbations may not provide optimal outcome. It is likely that a proportion of treatment failures in exacerbations are related to ineffective antibiotic treatment. Therefore, patients "at risk" for poor outcome are the logical candidates for aggressive initial antibiotic treatment, with the expectation that such an approach would improve overall outcomes of exacerbation. This "risk-stratification" approach has also been advocated for other community-acquired infections such as pneumonia and acute sinusitis (39,40). Though improved outcomes with risk stratification has not yet been demonstrated in prospective controlled trials, such an approach takes into account concerns of disease heterogeneity, antibiotic resistance, and judicious antibiotic use in exacerbations.

A. Placebo-Controlled Antibiotic Trials

In contrast to the magnitude of the problem of exacerbations of COPD, resulting in significant antibiotic consumption, there are only a handful of placebo-controlled trials in this disease. Two meta-analyses of placebo-controlled trials in exacerbations have been published. In the first such analysis published in 1995, only nine trials met quality criteria and a small but significant beneficial effect of antibiotics over placebo in exacerbation was demonstrated (41). In the second analysis, 11 trials were included, and a much larger beneficial effect on mortality and prevention of clinical failure was demonstrated, especially in moderate to severe exacerbations (42). The numbers needed to treat in severe exacerbations in hospitalized patients to prevent one death was only three patients and that needed to treat for the prevention of one clinical failure was six patients. Diarrhea was the most frequently related adverse effect, with one episode per seven patients treated. Antibiotic treatment was beneficial in resolving sputum purulence; however, a benefit on lung function, including gas exchange, was not observed.

The different results between the two meta-analyses, especially for mortality, can be explained by the addition in the later analysis of a study performed in Tunisia that was published in 2003 (43). In this study, 93 patients with exacerbations of severe underlying COPD requiring ventilator support in an intensive care unit were randomly assigned to receive ofloxacin or placebo in a double-blind manner (43). No systemic corticosteroids were administered. Potential respiratory bacterial pathogens were isolated in tracheobronchial aspirates in 61% of patients. Ofloxacin resulted in a dramatic benefit when compared to placebo, reducing mortality and the need for additional antibiotics by 17.5- and 28.4-fold respectively (Table 4).

Another interesting study, though not included in either meta-analyses, was published in Italian by Allegra et al. in 1991 with an additional analysis later published in English. In this trial, amoxicillin/clavulanate was compared with placebo in 414 exacerbations in 369 patients with a varying severity of underlying COPD (44). A unique feature of this study was the measurement of primary outcome at five days, instead of the traditional two to three weeks. Clinical success (including resolution and improvement) was significantly better with the antibiotic, seen in 86.4% of patients,

Table 4 Results of a Recent Placebo-Controlled Trial in Exacerbations of Chronic Obstructive Pulmonary Disease Requiring Intensive Care Unit Admission

Outcome	Ofloxacin ($n=47$)	Placebo ($n=46$)	Risk reduction	p-value
Hospital mortality	2 (4%)	10 (22%)	17.5 (4.3–30.7)	0.01
Additional antibiotics	3 (6%)	16 (35%)	28.4 (12.9–43.9)	0.0006
Combined primary outcomes	5 (11%)	26 (57%)	45.9 (29.1–62.7)	<0.0001

Source: From Ref. 43.

compared with 50.6% in the placebo arm. Greater benefit with antibiotics as compared to placebo was seen with increasing severity of underlying COPD.

Results of the meta-analyses and these studies, when combined with those of the previous classic large placebo-controlled trial conducted by Anthonisen et al., show that antibiotics are beneficial in the treatment of moderate to severe exacerbations (12,43–45). Furthermore, the benefit with antibiotics is more marked early in the course of the exacerbation, suggesting that antibiotics hasten resolution of symptoms (43,44). There are still important unresolved questions regarding the role of antibiotics in exacerbations. The benefit of antibiotics in mild exacerbations is unproven and warrants a placebo-controlled trial. Whether antibiotics are of benefit in the treatment of exacerbations when a short course of systemic corticosteroids are co-administered has still not been studied in a large well-designed trial. One would suspect that there would be additive benefits when both treatments are used over either treatment alone (42,46).

B. Antibiotic Comparison Trials

Though one can be quite confident that antibiotics are useful in moderate to severe exacerbations of COPD, there is considerable discussion as to antibiotic choice, especially for initial empiric therapy (33,35–37). As most exacerbations nowadays are treated without obtaining sputum bacteriology, this initial empiric choice often becomes the only choice made for antibiotic use in exacerbations. Results of antibiotic comparison trials should guide the recommendations for appropriate empiric antibiotics in exacerbations. However, though a large number of such trials have been conducted, in the vast majority, antibiotic choice does not appear to affect the clinical outcome. Differences in bacteriological eradication rates are seen, with an apparent dissociation between clinical and bacteriological outcomes (47). This is contrary to the expectations that antibiotics with better in vitro and in vivo antimicrobial efficacy and better pharmacodynamic and pharmacokinetic characteristics should show superiority in clinical outcomes. This paradox is likely related to several shortcomings in design of these trials, especially the large proportion of patients with either chronic bronchitis without airflow obstruction or with mild COPD included in these studies (Table 5) (38). Many of these deficiencies are explained by the fact that these trials are performed for regulatory approval of the drugs, and therefore are designed for demonstrating non-inferiority rather than differences between the two antibiotics.

Table 5 Limitations of Published Placebo-Controlled and Comparative Antibiotic Trials in Exacerbations of Chronic Obstructive Pulmonary Disease (COPD)

Limitation of study design	Potential consequences
Small number of subjects	Type 2 error
Subjects with mild or no underlying COPD included	Diminished overall perceived efficacy of antibiotics
Nonbacterial exacerbations included	Type 2 error
Endpoints compared at 3 weeks after onset	(*i*) Spontaneous resolution mitigates differences between arms (*ii*) Clinically irrelevant as most decisions about antibiotic efficacy are made earlier
Speed of resolution not measured	Clinically relevant endpoint not assessed
Lack of long-term follow-up	Time to next exacerbation not assessed
Antibiotic resistance to agents with limited in vitro antimicrobial efficacy	Diminished overall perceived efficacy of antibiotics
Poor penetration of antibiotics used in respiratory tissues	Diminished overall perceived efficacy of antibiotics
Concurrent therapy not controlled	Undetected bias in use of concurrent therapy

Source: From Ref. 38.

Two recent antibiotic comparison trials were designed to show differences among antibiotics and measured some unconventional but clinically relevant endpoints. The gemifloxacin and long-term outcome of bronchitis exacerbations (GLOBE) trial was a prospective, double-blind, randomized trial that compared a fluoroquinolone, gemifloxacin, with a macrolide, clarithromycin (48). End of therapy and long-term outcome assessments were made at the conventional 10- to 14- and 28-day time intervals. In these assessments, in line with most antibiotic comparison trials, there was no statistically significant difference in the two arms in the clinical outcome, with clinical success rates of 85.4% and 84.6% for gemifloxacin and clarithromycin respectively. Bacteriological success, measured as eradication and presumed eradication, was significantly higher with gemifloxacin (86.7%) compared to clarithromycin (73.1%).

Patients who had a successful clinical outcome at 28 days were then offered enrollment in a follow-up period for a total of 26 weeks of observation. In this time period, the primary outcomes were the rate of repeat exacerbations, hospitalizations for respiratory disease, and health-related quality of life measures. Gemifloxacin was associated with a significantly lower rate of repeat exacerbations, with 71% of the gemifloxacin-treated patients remaining exacerbation free at 26 weeks in comparison to 58.5% in the clarithromycin arm. The relative risk reduction for recurrence of exacerbation was 30%. The rate of hospitalization for respiratory tract illness in the 26 weeks was also lower in the gemifloxacin-treated patients than in the clarithromycin-treated patients (2.3% vs. 6.3%, $p=0.059$) (48). Patients who had a recurrent exacerbation in the 26-week period had a lesser improvement in their health-related quality of life when compared to those who remained free of recurrence (49). This trial clearly shows the limitation of the conventional medium-term clinical outcomes to demonstrate differences among antibiotic therapies in exacerbations. If the 26-week follow-up period had not been instituted, significant differences in clinically relevant outcomes of recurrence of exacerbations and respiratory-related hospitalization would have been missed.

Another recent landmark antibiotic comparison trial is the MOSAIC trial. This trial is a large study in which patients were randomized to a fluoroquinolone, moxifloxacin, or to standard therapy (which could be one of the following: amoxicillin, cefuroxime, or clarithromycin) (50). This trial had several unique design features which relate to observations made in this study. A relatively large number of patients were enrolled. In addition, patients were enrolled when stable to establish a baseline as a comparison to reliably distinguish between clinical improvement and resolution following treatment. A substantial proportion of the patients enrolled had one or more risk factors that would predispose to a poor outcome as discussed below. Patients were followed up to nine months after randomization to provide an estimate of recurrence of exacerbation.

Interestingly, in line with usual antibiotic comparison trials, moxifloxacin and standard therapy were equivalent (88% vs. 83%) when clinical success (resolution and improvement) were compared at 7 to 10 days after the end of therapy. However, moxifloxacin therapy was associated with a superior clinical cure rate (defined as resolution of symptoms to baseline, rather than simply improvement) than standard therapy (71% vs. 63%), as well as with superior bacteriological response (91.5% vs. 81%). In addition, when other a priori unconventional endpoints were examined, moxifloxacin was associated with fewer requirements for additional antibiotic therapy (8% vs. 14%) and an extended time to the next exacerbation (131 vs. 104 days) (50). A composite endpoint of clinical failure, requirement of additional antibiotics, and recurrence of exacerbation demonstrated a clear difference between the two arms in the study, with moxifloxacin being superior to standard therapy for up to five months of follow-up (Fig. 3). Again, if the conventional outcome of clinical success would have been measured solely in this study, all the other significant differences in the two arms would have not been discovered.

Results of the GLOBE and MOSAIC trials demonstrate that in vitro microbiological superiority of the fluoroquinolones does translate to greater in vivo effectiveness in treating patients with acute exacerbation. Differences among antibiotics are often not perceptible with the standard regulatory endpoint of clinical success at 7 to 14 days after the end of therapy. However, differences among antibiotics are perceptible when clinically relevant endpoints such as speed of resolution, clinical cure, need for additional antimicrobials, and time to next exacerbation are considered (48,50).

VIII.   Risk Stratification of Patients

Based on the MOSAIC and GLOBE studies results, it would be tempting to prescribe fluoroquinolones for all moderate to severe exacerbations. However, it is clear that such a strategy, though likely to be successful in the short term, would foster antimicrobial resistance to these valuable antibiotics in the long term. Therefore, it would be judicious to make an effort to identify those patients who are most likely to benefit from these antibiotics.

Several studies have now demonstrated that certain patient characteristics when stable and therefore antedate the onset of the exacerbation impact the outcome of the

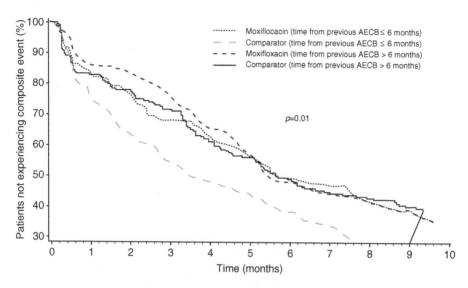

Figure 3 Life-table analysis of time to the first composite event (treatment failure, and/or new exacerbation and/or any further antibiotic treatment) stratified according to the time of the last exacerbation prior to randomization. *Abbreviation*: AECB, acute exacerbation of chronic bronchitis. *Source*: From Ref. 50.

exacerbation (32,51–55). Interestingly, several of these characteristics are relevant to exacerbation outcome in more than one study. These risk factors for poor outcome should be considered in our choice of antibiotics when treating exacerbations. Theoretically, patients at greater risk for poor outcome would have the greatest benefit from early aggressive antibiotic therapy, such as with the fluoroquinolones. These are the patients in whom the consequences of treatment with an antibiotic that turns out to be ineffective against the pathogen causing the exacerbation are likely to be significant, with clinical failures, hospitalizations, and early recurrences likely.

Among the risk factors for poor outcome identified in various studies are age, severity of underlying airway obstruction, presence of co-morbid illnesses (especially cardiac disease), a history of recurrent exacerbations, use of home oxygen, use of chronic steroids, hypercapnia, and acute bronchodilator use (32,51–54). Some of these risk factors are likely to be highly correlated to each other, such as home oxygen use, hypercapnia, and chronic steroid use that reflect increasing severity of underlying COPD. Acute bronchodilator use could be related to the severity of underlying COPD or reflect the wheezy phenotype of exacerbation that may be less responsive to antibiotic treatment. Many of the risk factors discussed above are continuous in severity; however, certain thresholds have been defined in studies that are clinically useful and predictive of poor outcome. These include an age of more than 65 years, forced expiratory volume in one second (FEV_1) less than 50%, and more than three exacerbations in the previous 12 months.

In addition to the risk factors described above, experience in other respiratory infections tells us that recent antibiotic use, within the past three months, places the patient in a high-risk group for harboring antibiotic resistant pathogens and, therefore, having a poor outcome. This has been best described for *S. pneumoniae* among patients with community-acquired pneumococcal pneumonia and, recently, also described for this pathogen among patients with COPD (56,57). Whether such selection for antibiotic resistant strains occurs among NTHI and *M. catarrhalis* after antibiotic exposure is not known.

IX. Risk-Stratification Approach to Antibiotic Therapy in Exacerbation

A risk-stratification approach that has been advocated by several authors for the initial empiric antibiotic treatment of acute exacerbation was based on the risk factors discussed above and the in vitro and in vivo efficacy of antibiotics. Our current treatment algorithm, which is very similar to what others have advocated, is shown in Figure 4 (36). The initial step in the algorithm is the determination of the severity of the exacerbation. Based on the discussion above, we use the Anthonisen criteria of single cardinal symptom exacerbations defined as mild, while the presence of two or all three of the cardinal symptoms defines moderate and severe exacerbations.

Mild exacerbations are managed with symptomatic treatment and antibiotics are not prescribed unless the symptoms progress. In moderate to severe exacerbations, the important step is the differentiation of "uncomplicated" patients from the "complicated" patients. Uncomplicated patients do not have any of the risk factors for poor outcome. Complicated patients have one or more of the following risk factors for poor outcome: age >65 years, $FEV_1 < 50\%$, co-morbid cardiac disease, and three or more exacerbations in the previous 12 months (36). Antibiotic choices for patients with uncomplicated COPD include an advanced macrolide (azithromycin, clarithromycin), a ketolide (telithromycin), a cephalosporin (cefuroxime, cefpodoxime, or cefdinir), doxycycline or trimethoprim/sulfamethoxazole. Amoxicillin is not an appropriate choice with the considerable incidence of β-lactamase production among NTHI and *M. catarrhalis*, two of the major pathogens of exacerbation. In complicated patients, antibiotic choices include a respiratory fluoroquinolone (moxifloxacin, gemifloxacin, or levofloxacin) or amoxicillin-clavulanate.

In choosing an antibiotic, other considerations are also important. In all such patients, exposure to antibiotics within the past three months should be elucidated. Exposure to antibiotic is not confined to those prescribed for respiratory infections, but includes antibiotics prescribed for any indication. The antibiotic chosen should be from a different class of agents from the one prescribed within the past three months. For example, exposure to a macrolide in the past three months should lead to use of a ketolide in an uncomplicated patient. Similarly, recent use of a fluoroquinolone in a complicated patient should lead one to use amoxicillin/clavulanate.

There is a subgroup of the complicated patients who are at risk for infection by *Pseudomonas aeruginosa* and *Enterobacteriaceae* or have a documented infection by these pathogens (58). These patients have usually very severe underlying COPD ($FEV_1 < 30\%$), have developed bronchiectasis, are hospitalized (often requiring intensive care), or have been recently hospitalized or have received multiple courses of antibiotics. In such patients, empiric treatment with ciprofloxacin is appropriate. However, emerged resistance among *P. aeruginosa* to the fluoroquinolones may compromise their efficacy. Therefore, in this subgroup of patients, a sputum (or

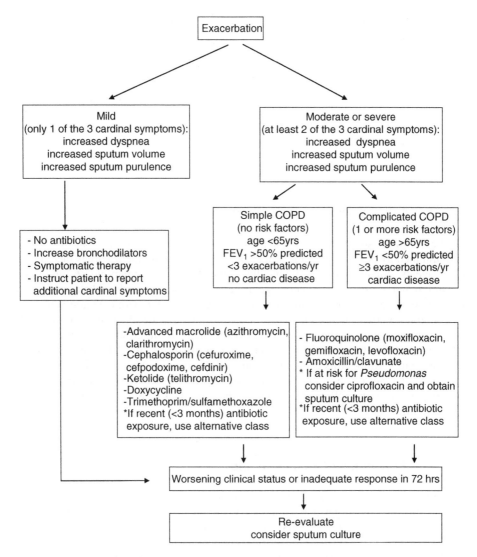

Figure 4 Algorithm outlining a risk-stratification approach to antibacterial therapy of acute exacerbations of COPD. *Abbreviations*: COPD, chronic obstructive pulmonary disease; FEV_1, forced expiratory volume at one second.

tracheobronchial aspirate if intubated) culture should be obtained to allow adjustment of antibiotics based on the in vitro susceptibility of pathogens isolated. However, combination or parenteral antibiotic therapy for *P. aeruginosa* in this setting has never been systematically examined and is of unproven benefit.

In patients who fail initial empiric antimicrobial therapy, it would be appropriate to reexamine the patient to confirm the diagnosis, exclude other conditions that can mimic and/or aggravate exacerbations, namely pneumonia, acute cardiovascular co-morbidities, or pulmonary embolism, consider sputum studies to ascertain for resistant or difficult to treat pathogens, and treat with an alternative agent with better in vitro microbiological efficacy.

Other important considerations in antibiotic prescribing are safety and tolerability of the agent, drug interactions, and finally cost of treatment. Cost of the antibiotic however should not be interpreted in isolation. As shown elegantly by Miravitlles et al., exacerbations with treatment failure of the initial empiric treatment are 10-fold as costly as clinical successes (59). In fact, the overall cost of care could be reduced by half with only a 33% reduction in clinical failure rates. Clinical failure rates are likely to be reduced when antibiotic choice is appropriate and logical, as discussed above.

X. Antiviral Therapy for Exacerbations

Of the various respiratory viruses that cause exacerbations, the only one for which antiviral therapy is available is the influenza virus. The anti-influenza drugs include the older agents, amantadine and rimantadine, and the newer neuraminidase inhibitors, zanamivir and ostelmavir. The latter agents have been shown to reduce the duration and intensity of symptoms of influenza in healthy adults, if started within 48 hours of onset of symptoms. Patients with COPD and influenza infections are likely to derive as much or greater benefit from these agents. However, there is little data available for the efficacy of these drugs in the treatment of exacerbations of COPD related to the influenza virus. Rhinovirus is the most common viral cause of exacerbations and RSV infections can cause substantial morbidity and mortality, comparable to influenza, in elderly patients with COPD (24). However, there is a lack of effective antiviral agents for these infections (60).

XI. Prevention of Exacerbations

Prevention of infectious exacerbations in COPD could be accomplished by medications that do not directly target the pathogens involved in exacerbations. These include agents such as bronchodilators and inhaled corticosteroids that have been shown to decrease the incidence and severity of exacerbations. The utility of these drugs in COPD is discussed elsewhere in this book (see Chapters 13 and 14). Whether the exacerbations prevented are indeed infectious in nature and the mechanisms underlying this preventative effect are unclear.

A. Vaccines

Specific medications that prevent infectious exacerbations include vaccines and antimicrobials. Vaccines available and recommended in patients with COPD are the inactivated trivalent influenza vaccine and the 23-valent pneumococcal polysaccharide vaccine. It should be noted that *H. influenzae* Type B vaccine is not indicated and is likely to be ineffective in COPD. This vaccine is only effective against encapsulated *H. influenzae* serogroup B, while most exacerbations are caused by nonencapsulated *H. influenzae*. Though the conjugated pneumococcal vaccine has been effective in reducing otitis media and invasive pneumococcal disease in children, its role in COPD is not clear and has not been adequately studied.

Trivalent influenza vaccine has been shown to be effective in reducing exacerbations among patients with COPD (61). The data regarding the benefit of pneumococcal vaccine in the prevention of exacerbations of COPD is unclear. No prospective, randomized, placebo-controlled trials have been done with this vaccine in COPD with exacerbations as the primary endpoint. Studies done in elderly patients with pneumonia as the primary endpoint have demonstrated contradictory results, with randomized trials showing little benefit while studies with case–control design showing significant benefits (62). In view of the safety of the vaccine and its benefit in prevention of invasive pneumococcal disease, it is generally recommended that patients with COPD should receive this vaccine. We do need better vaccines for the pneumococcus in the elderly, including subjects with COPD.

B. Prophylactic Antibiotics

As discussed above, about 50% of exacerbations are bacterial in origin and antibiotics are effective in the treatment of exacerbations. This brings up the interesting question about prevention of exacerbations with the use of antibiotics given on a prophylactic basis, especially in those patients who experience recurrent exacerbations. In fact, till 1970, several studies were conducted with prophylactic antibiotics in COPD to prevent exacerbations (5,63). However, these studies would be regarded as poorly designed by today's standards. Limitations of these studies included inclusion of patients with relatively mild disease, at times even without documented COPD. Furthermore, many of these trials used antibiotics that have marginal efficacy against the predominant pathogens in exacerbations of COPD and in doses that would be inadequate to provide adequate suppression or eradication of bacteria from the airways. A Cochrane systematic analysis of these studies demonstrated that antibiotics were of limited benefit in the prevention of exacerbations with a less than 10% reduction in the frequency of exacerbations and a reduction in days lost from work (63). Only some of these studies monitored for the emergence of resistant strains and, interestingly, found emergence of such resistance to be infrequent. With these borderline results of these studies, and because of concerns of fostering bacterial resistance, antibiotic prophylaxis fell in disfavor and has received scant attention since 1970.

Recently, there has been a reemergence of interest in antibiotic prophylaxis to prevent exacerbations of COPD. This has been fueled by the realization both exacerbations and chronic bacterial infection may substantially contribute to the progression of COPD. New antibiotics, such as the macrolides, that have significant anti-inflammatory actions in addition to their antibacterial activity have become available. The success of chronic therapy with the macrolide antibiotics in the prevention of exacerbations and improvement of quality of life in cystic fibrosis has led to a trial, being conducted by the COPD clinical research network in the United States, of a macrolide antibiotic to prevent exacerbations of COPD. This study is ongoing and the results are expected by 2008.

The respiratory fluoroquinolones are very potent broad-spectrum antibiotics that have excellent tissue penetration and are capable of eradicating offending pathogens from the airway rapidly in exacerbations. These properties of these antibiotics are being utilized in an ongoing randomized placebo-controlled trial with intermittent pulses of a fluoroquinolone in an attempt to prevent exacerbations that will be completed in 2007. Results of both these studies will provide a sound basis to either consider or discount antibiotic prophylaxis in COPD.

C. Antiviral Prophylaxis

The situation with antiviral prophylaxis for exacerbations of COPD is very similar to that with treatment of exacerbations. The only antiviral agents available are the anti-influenza drugs that have been shown to be effective in preventing or ameliorating infections with influenza in exposed individuals. There is little data available for the efficacy of these drugs in the prevention of COPD exacerbation in exposed individuals. However, it would be prudent to use one of these agents in these circumstances. Antiviral agents that can prevent rhinovirus and RSV infections are not available.

XII. Chronic Infection in COPD

The presence of microbial pathogens in the lower airway in stable COPD has been referred to as colonization. Though the usage of this term may be an attempt to differentiate from exacerbation, its implication is that the presence of bacteria in the lower airway in stable COPD is innocuous. The definition of "colonization" includes absence of a host response to the pathogen as well as absence of damaging effects to the host. However, the absence of increased symptoms of exacerbation does not satisfy the above criteria. Furthermore, the absence of exacerbation does not imply that this abnormal pathogen presence in the lower airway is innocuous and is not associated with increased airway inflammation with its attendant consequences.

Various microbial pathogens have been implicated in chronic infection in COPD (Table 1). These include typical bacteria such as NTHI and *P. aeruginosa*, atypicals such as *Chlamydia pneumoniae*, viruses such as Adenovirus and RSV, and recently a fungus, *P. jiroveci* (22,23,25,64–67). The contribution of chronic microbial infection to the pathogenesis of COPD has been conceptualized as the "vicious circle hypothesis" (Fig. 5). Chronic microbial infection can contribute to inflammation in COPD directly or indirectly. The microbial pathogen can serve as a primary inflammatory stimulus. Discovery of cell surface receptors such as toll receptors, which interact with specific components of microbial pathogens and engender an inflammatory response, provides a biological basis of chronic inflammation induced by chronic infection. Such a mechanism could be active in the case of typical bacteria such as NTHI and *Pseudomonas*. Another potential mechanism is that the microbial pathogens can alter the host response to tobacco smoke and potentiate the inflammatory and damaging aspects. Such potentiation has been described for the adenovirus.

Demonstration of an inflammatory response or a systemic host response to "colonization" would add credence to the potential pathogenic role of the specific microbial pathogen. Recent studies have demonstrated such phenomena, specifically with typical bacterial pathogens such as NTHI. Bresser and colleagues measured sputum levels of myeloperoxidase, tumor necrosis factor (TNF-α), and interleukin-8 (IL-8) in chronic bronchitis patients who were chronically infected with NTHI. Sputum levels of these inflammatory mediators as well as the degree of plasma protein leakage, measured as sputum to serum ratio of plasma proteins, were significantly higher in the NTHI-infected group compared with noninfected patients (68). In a recent study,

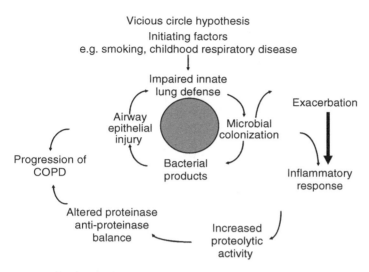

Figure 5 A modified vicious circle hypothesis to explain how microbial infections could contribute to the pathogenesis and progression of chronic obstructive pulmonary disease (COPD).

Banerjee and colleagues studied patients with moderate to severe clinically stable COPD. They showed that patients who were "colonized" with potentially pathogenic bacteria, including NTHI, had a worse health status and an increased inflammatory response, as reflected in higher levels of IL-8, leukotriene B-4, TNF-α, neutrophil elastase, and increased neutrophil chemotaxis compared to those who were not colonized with such bacteria (69).

Sputum mainly reflects the inflammatory process in the larger airways, the trachea, and major bronchi. Bronchoscopic samples sample the peripheral tracheo-bronchial tree, which is the major site of airway obstruction in COPD. Two studies have utilized such sampling to examine the relationship of airway bacterial colonization with inflammation in COPD. Soler and colleagues examined inflammation and colonization in bronchoalveolar lavage samples in patients with stable COPD, smokers without COPD, and in nonsmokers (70). Bacterial colonization was seen in 32% of COPD subjects. Surprisingly, it was also seen in 42% of "healthy smokers" but was absent in nonsmokers. Colonized subjects, with or without COPD, had more bronchial neutrophilia compared to those whose bronchial samples did not yield potentially pathogenic microorganisms. However, smoking-induced inflammation shares the same characteristics as bacterial colonization-associated inflammation. Studies are therefore required in ex-smokers to more reliably demonstrate the association between bacterial colonization and airway inflammation. Such a study was recently completed in which 36% of ex-smokers with stable COPD were found to be "colonized" with bacterial pathogens, predominantly *Haemophilus* spp. None of the ex-smokers without COPD were colonized with bacterial pathogens. Furthermore, colonization was associated with greater numbers of neutrophils as well as higher levels of IL-8 and matrix metalloproteinase-9 in the lavage fluid (Fig. 6) (2). These studies provide evidence that

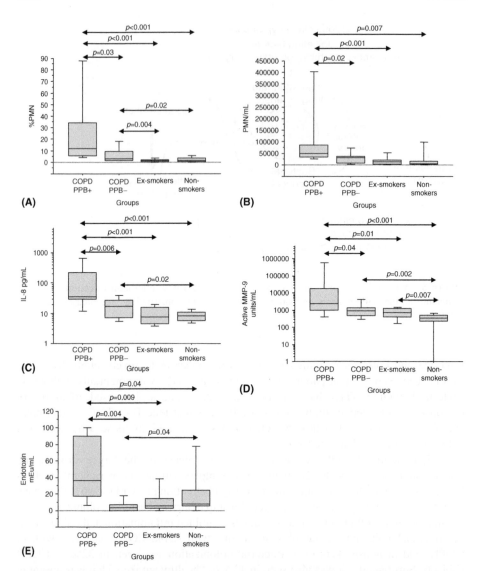

Figure 6 Comparison of bronchoalveolar lavage fluid measurements among patients with COPD colonized (COPD, PPB+) and not colonized with a potential pathogenic bacteria (COPD, PPB−), ex- and nonsmokers. The horizontal lines represent median values, the boxes represent 25th to 75th quartiles and the vertical lines represent 10th to 90th percentile values. Significant differences between groups are represented by double-sided arrows with associated p-values by Mann–Whitney U rank test. (**A**) Relative neutrophil count (PMN%). (**B**) Absolute neutrophil count (PMN). (**C**) IL-8 level (pg/mL). (**D**) Active MMP-9 level (U/mL). (**E**) Endotoxin level (mEU/mL). *Abbreviations*: COPD, chronic obstructive pulmonary disease; IL-8, interleukin-8; MMP-9, matrix metalloproteinase 9; PMN, polymorphonuclear cells; PPB, potential pathogenic bacteria. *Source*: From Ref. 2.

bacterial colonization of the peripheral airways is common in COPD and associated with inflammation. Furthermore, this process of bacterial colonization develops early in the disease and persists in ex-smokers with the disease. Therefore, colonization-induced inflammation has the potential of contributing to the development of COPD at all stages of this disease.

A. Treatment of Chronic Infection

With the relatively recent recognition that colonization of the lower respiratory tract in COPD could have potentially damaging effects, there have not been any recent studies that examine whether treating these infections is possible and of therapeutic value. Prophylactic antibiotics are being utilized in the studies described earlier to determine if the exacerbation frequency is reduced. Those studies should provide us data whether suppression of bacterial colonization is possible and if it translates to any therapeutic benefits or reduction of airway inflammation. Alternative non-antimicrobial approaches should also be considered in this setting. For example, augmentation of innate immunity, either by improving mucociliary clearance or augmenting airway defense mechanisms, such as airway antimicrobial peptides, could be useful to treat chronic infections. This is a fertile area of research and hopefully will translate to future new therapeutic options.

XIII. Community-Acquired Pneumonia in Patients with COPD

COPD is associated with an increased incidence of community-acquired pneumonia (CAP), especially in elderly individuals (71). There is controversy as to whether the prognosis of pneumonia is altered by preexisting COPD, as studies have demonstrated increased mortality with COPD, while others have shown a protective effect (72). An intriguing explanation for the protective effect of COPD is systemic corticosteroid use in these patients, in light of recent studies suggesting that these medications are of potential benefit in this setting (72). Another potential explanation is the abundant exposure these individuals have over a lifetime to these pathogens from colonization and recurrent exacerbations, leading to enough nonspecific immunity from cross-reactive antibodies that systemic disease is less severe in these patients.

COPD does appear to alter the pathogens associated with CAP. The pneumococcus still remains predominant; however, an increased incidence of NTHI and occasionally *M. catarrhalis* is seen (73). The presence of very severe COPD with concomitant bronchiectasis and repeated courses of antibiotics predisposes these patients to pneumonia caused by *P. aeruginosa* (73). However, etiologic diagnosis of pneumonia becomes more difficult in COPD because chronic colonization confounds the interpretation of sputum culture results. COPD and smoking also increase serum titers to *C. pneumoniae*, rendering serologic diagnosis for this infection, especially when single titers are used for diagnosis, difficult to interpret.

COPD does alter significantly the empiric treatment antibiotic regimen recommended for CAP. For less severely ill patients, who are to be treated as outpatients, COPD is a recognized "modifying or risk factor," such that a macrolide or doxycycline is not recommended alone for empiric treatment. Either a respiratory fluoroquinolone or a combination of a macrolide and a β-lactam antibiotic is the recommended regimen (74). Among patients with severe CAP admitted to the intensive care unit, for those who have very severe COPD with possible concomitant bronchiectasis and/or repeated exposures to broad-spectrum antibiotics, it is recommended that empiric treatment includes antibiotics that are likely to be efficacious for *Pseudomonas* pneumonia. This usually entails a regimen of a β-lactam active against this pathogen, in combination with an aminoglycoside or a fluoroquinolone with gram negative activity.

XIV. Conclusions

Substantial progress has been made in understanding the pathogenesis of exacerbations of COPD. The complexity of the host–pathogen interaction that determines the onset and course of exacerbations has become apparent and needs to be explored further. The interaction of the various stimuli capable of inducing exacerbations, such as viruses, bacteria, atypical bacteria, and the environment, needs to be better understood to determine if treatment and prevention strategies can be developed based on these interactions. Though antibiotic treatment for exacerbations is now more evidence based and rational, the impact of the risk-stratification approach on the outcome of exacerbations needs to be evaluated. The interaction of treatment with systemic corticosteroids and antibiotics on the outcome of exacerbations is still not well understood and should be explored in a well-designed trial. Similarly, antibiotic use in mild exacerbations warrants further investigation.

Much excitement now revolves around the potential role of chronic infection in COPD. However, to develop innovative preventive and therapeutic measures for these infections, we need to better understand the host–pathogen interaction. The virulence factors of bacterial pathogens such as NTHI, *S. pneumoniae*, and *M. catarrhalis* are poorly understood in the context of COPD. Understanding what components of these bacterial pathogens are pro-inflammatory, are responsible for tissue invasion, and targets of the host immune response are all important areas of knowledge. Such understanding could allow us to modify the effects of acute and chronic infection, develop effective vaccines and other preventive strategies. Vaccine strategies can be targeted toward prevention of primary infection, abrogation of chronic infection, or immunomodulation of the host response to infection. Our understanding of chronic viral, atypical, and fungal infections in COPD is still in its infancy. Future research should elucidate the significance of such infection and whether specific treatment is effective and beneficial.

References

1. Laurenzi GA, Potter RT, Kass EH. Bacteriologic flora of the lower respiratory tract. N Engl J Med 1961; 265:1273–8.
2. Sethi S, Maloney J, Grove L, Wrona C, Berenson CS. Airway inflammation and bronchial bacterial colonization in chronic obstructive pulmonary disease. Am J Respir Crit Care Med 2006; 173(9):991–8.
3. Fletcher F, Peto R. The natural history of chronic airflow obstruction. Br Med J 1977; 1:1645–8.
4. Tager I, Speizer FE. Role of infection in chronic bronchitis. N Engl J Med 1975; 292(11):563–71.

5. Murphy TF, Sethi S. Bacterial infection in chronic obstructive pulmonary disease. Am Rev Respir Dis 1992; 146:1067–83.
6. Sethi S, Murphy TF. Bacterial infection in chronic obstructive pulmonary disease in 2000: a state-of-the-art review. Clin Microbiol Rev 2001; 14(2):336–63.
7. Veeramachaneni SB, Sethi S. Pathogenesis of bacterial exacerbations of COPD. J Chronic Obstruct Pulm Dis 2006; 3:109–15.
8. White AJ, Gompertz S, Stockley RA. Chronic obstructive pulmonary disease. 6: the aetiology of exacerbations of chronic obstructive pulmonary disease. Thorax 2003; 58(1):73–80.
9. Rodriguez-Roisin R. Toward a consensus definition for COPD exacerbations. Chest 2000; 117(5 Suppl. 2):398S–401.
10. Sethi S, Evans N, Grant BJB, Murphy TF. Acquisition of a new bacterial strain and occurrence of exacerbations of chronic obstructive pulmonary disease. N Engl J Med 2002; 347(7):465–71.
11. Global Initiative for Chronic Obstructive Pulmonary Disease. Global strategy for the diagnosis, management and prevention of chronic obstructive pulmonary disease, 2006. www.goldcopd.com (last accessed August 31, 2007).
12. Anthonisen NR, Manfreda J, Warren CPW, Hershfield ES, Harding GKM, Nelson NA. Antibiotic therapy in exacerbations of chronic obstructive pulmonary disease. Ann Intern Med 1987; 106:196–204.
13. Wedzicha JA, Seemungal TA, MacCallum PK, et al. Acute exacerbations of chronic obstructive pulmonary disease are accompanied by elevations of plasma fibrinogen and serum IL-6 levels. Thromb Haemost 2000; 84(2):210–5.
14. Dev D, Wallace E, Sankaran R, et al. Value of C-reactive protein measurements in exacerbations of chronic obstructive pulmonary disease. Respir Med 1998; 92(4):664–7.
15. Garcia-Aymerich J, Tobias A, Anto JM, Sunyer J. Air pollution and mortality in a cohort of patients with chronic obstructive pulmonary disease: a time series analysis. J Epidemiol Community Health 2000; 54(1):73–4.
16. Sunyer J, Saez M, Murillo C, Castellsague J, Martinez F, Anto JM. Air pollution and emergency room admissions for chronic obstructive pulmonary disease: a 5-year study. Am J Epidemiol 1993; 137(7):701–5.
17. Sunyer J, Schwartz J, Tobias A, Macfarlane D, Garcia J, Anto JM. Patients with chronic obstructive pulmonary disease are at increased risk of death associated with urban particle air pollution: a case-crossover analysis. Am J Epidemiol 2000; 151(1):50–6.
18. Ohtoshi T, Takizawa H, Okazaki H, et al. Diesel exhaust particles stimulate human airway epithelial cells to produce cytokines relevant to airway inflammation in vitro. J Allergy Clin Immunol 1998; 101(6 Pt 1):778–85.
19. Devalia JL, Rusznak C, Herdman MJ, Trigg CJ, Tarraf H, Davies RJ. Effect of nitrogen dioxide and sulphur dioxide on airway response of mild asthmatic patients to allergen inhalation. Lancet 1994; 344(8938):1668–71.
20. Rudell B, Blomberg A, Helleday R, et al. Bronchoalveolar inflammation after exposure to diesel exhaust: comparison between unfiltered and particle trap filtered exhaust. Occup Environ Med 1999; 56:527–34.
21. Sethi S. Infectious etiology of acute exacerbations of chronic bronchitis. Chest 2000; 117:380S–5.
22. Eldika N, Sethi S. Role of nontypeable *Haemophilus influenzae* in exacerbations and progression of chronic obstructive pulmonary disease. Curr Opin Pulm Med 2006; 12(2):118–24.
23. Seemungal T, Harper-Owen R, Bhowmik A, et al. Respiratory viruses, symptoms, and inflammatory markers in acute exacerbations and stable chronic obstructive pulmonary disease. Am J Respir Crit Care Med 2001; 164(9):1618–23.
24. Falsey AR, Hennessey PA, Formica MA, Cox C, Walsh EE. Respiratory syncytial virus infection in elderly and high-risk adults. N Engl J Med 2005; 352(17):1749–59.
25. Morris A, Sciurba FC, Lebedeva IP, et al. Association of chronic obstructive pulmonary disease severity and Pneumocystis colonization. Am J Respir Crit Care Med 2004; 170(4):408–13.
26. Chin CL, Manzel LJ, Lehman EE, et al. *Haemophilus influenzae* from patients with chronic obstructive pulmonary disease exacerbation induce more inflammation than colonizers. Am J Respir Crit Care Med 2005; 172(1):85–91.
27. Murphy TF, Brauer AL, Grant BJ, Sethi S. *Moraxella catarrhalis* in chronic obstructive pulmonary disease: burden of disease and immune response. Am J Respir Crit Care Med 2005; 172(2):195–9.
28. Sethi S, Wrona C, Grant BJB, Murphy TF. Strain specific immune response to *Haemophilus influenzae* in chronic obstructive pulmonary disease. Am J Respir Crit Care Med 2004; 169:448–53.

29. White AJ, Gompertz S, Bayley DL, et al. Resolution of bronchial inflammation is related to bacterial eradication following treatment of exacerbations of chronic bronchitis. Thorax 2003; 58(8):680–5.

30. Anzueto A, Rizzo JA, Grossman RF. The infection-free interval: its use in evaluating antimicrobial treatment of acute exacerbation of chronic bronchitis. Clin Infect Dis 1999; 28(6):1344–5.

31. Aaron SD, Vandemheen KL, Hebert P, et al. Outpatient oral prednisone after emergency treatment of chronic obstructive pulmonary disease. N Engl J Med 2003; 348(26):2618–25.

32. Miravitlles M, Murio C, Guerrero T. Factors associated with relapse after ambulatory treatment of acute exacerbations of chronic bronchitis. DAFNE Study Group. Eur Respir J 2001; 17(5):928–33.

33. Fabbri LM, Hurd SS. Global strategy for the diagnosis, management and prevention of COPD: 2003 update. Eur Respir J 2003; 22(1):1–2.

34. Sethi S. Acute exacerbations of COPD: a "multipronged" approach. J Respir Dis 2002; 23(4):217–55.

35. Bach PB, Brown C, Gelfand SE, McCrory DC. Management of acute exacerbations of chronic obstructive pulmonary disease: a summary and appraisal of published evidence. Ann Intern Med 2001; 134(7):600–20.

36. Balter MS, La Forge J, Low DE, Mandell L, Grossman RF. Canadian guidelines for the management of acute exacerbations of chronic bronchitis. Can Respir J 2003; 10(Suppl. B):3B–32.

37. Murphy TF, Sethi S. Chronic obstructive pulmonary disease: role of bacteria and guide to antibacterial selection in the older patient. Drugs Aging 2002; 19(10):761–75.

38. Sethi S. Bacteria in exacerbations of chronic obstructive pulmonary disease. Phenomenon or epiphenomenon? Proc Am Thorac Soc 2004; 1:109–14.

39. Mandell LA, Bartlett JG, Dowell SF, File TM, Jr., Musher DM, Whitney C. Update of practice guidelines for the management of community-acquired pneumonia in immunocompetent adults. Clin Infect Dis 2003; 37(11):1405–33.

40. Sinus and Allergy Health Partnership. Antimicrobial treatment guidelines for acute bacterial rhinosinusitis 2004. Otolaryngol Head Neck Surg 2004; 130(1):1–45.

41. Saint S, Bent S, Vittinghoff E, Grady D. Antibiotics in chronic obstructive pulmonary disease exacerbations. A meta-analysis. J Am Med Assec 1995; 273(12):957–96.

42. Ram FS, Rodriguez-Roisin R, Granados-Navarrete A, Garcia-Aymerich J, Barnes NC. Antibiotics for exacerbations of chronic obstructive pulmonary disease. Cochrane Database Syst Rev (Online) 2006; (2):CD004403.

43. Nouira S, Marghli S, Belghith M, Besbes L, Elatrous S, Abroug F. Once daily oral ofloxacin in chronic obstructive pulmonary disease exacerbation requiring mechanical ventilation: a randomised placebo-controlled trial. Lancet 2001; 358(9298):2020–5.

44. Allegra L, Blasi F, de Bernardi B, Cosentini R, Tarsia P. Antibiotic treatment and baseline severity of disease in acute exacerbations of chronic bronchitis: a re-evaluation of previously published data of a placebo-controlled randomized study. Pulm Pharmacol Ther 2001; 14(2):149–55.

45. Sachs APE, Koeter GH, Groenier KH, van der Waaij D, Schiphuis J, Jong BMd. Changes in symptoms, peak expiratory flow, and sputum flora during treatment with antibiotics of exacerbations in patients with chronic obstructive pulmonary disease in general practice. Thorax 1995; 50:758–63.

46. Wood-Baker RR, Gibson PG, Hannay M, Walters EH, Walters JA. Systemic corticosteroids for acute exacerbations of chronic obstructive pulmonary disease. Cochrane Database Syst Rev (Online) 2005; (1):CD001288.

47. Obaji A, Sethi S. Acute exacerbations of chronic bronchitis. What role for the new fluoroquinolones? Drugs Aging 2001; 18(1):1–11.

48. Wilson R, Schentag JJ, Ball P, Mandell L. A comparison of gemifloxacin and clarithromycin in acute exacerbations of chronic bronchitis and long-term clinical outcomes. Clin Ther 2002; 24(4):639–52.

49. Spencer S, Jones PW. Time course of recovery of health status following an infective exacerbation of chronic bronchitis. Thorax 2003; 58(7):589–93.

50. Wilson R, Allegra L, Huchon G, et al. Short-term and long-term outcomes of moxifloxacin compared to standard antibiotic treatment in acute exacerbations of chronic bronchitis. Chest 2004; 125(3):953–64.

51. Ball P, Harris JM, Lowson D, Tillotson G, Wilson R. Acute infective exacerbations of chronic bronchitis. QJM 1995; 88:61–8.

52. Dewan NA, Rafique S, Kanwar B, et al. Acute exacerbation of COPD: factors associated with poor treatment outcome. Chest 2000; 117(3):662–71.

53. Groenewegen KH, Schols AM, Wouters EF. Mortality and mortality-related factors after hospitalization for acute exacerbation of COPD. Chest 2003; 124(2):459–67.

54. Adams SG, Melo J, Luther M, Anzueto A. Antibiotics are associated with lower relapse rates in outpatients with acute exacerbations of COPD. Chest 2000; 117:1345–52.

55. Wilson R, Jones P, Schaberg T, Arvis P, Duprat-Lomon I, Sagnier PP. Antibiotic treatment and factors influencing short and long term outcomes of acute exacerbations of chronic bronchitis. Thorax 2006; 61(4):337–42.

56. Vanderkooi OG, Low DE, Green K, Powis JE, McGeer A. Predicting antimicrobial resistance in invasive pneumococcal infections. Clin Infect Dis 2005; 40(9):1288–97.

57. Sethi S, Murphy TF, Cai X, Richter SS, Doern GV. Antibiotic exposure in COPD and the development of penicillin and erythromycin resistance in *Streptococcus pneumoniae*. In: Poster presentation at ICAAC, San Francisco CA, September 2006:C2-0438.

58. Soler N, Torres A, Ewig S, et al. Bronchial microbial patterns in severe exacerbations of chronic obstructive pulmonary disease (COPD) requiring mechanical ventilation. Am J Respir Crit Care Med 1998; 157:1498–505.

59. Miravitlles M, Murio C, Guerrero T, Gisbert R. Pharmacoeconomic evaluation of acute exacerbations of chronic bronchitis and COPD. Chest 2002; 121(5):1449–55.

60. Sethi S, Murphy TF. RSV infection—not for kids only. N Engl J Med 2005; 352(17):1810–2.

61. Poole PJ, Chacko E, Wood-Baker RW, Cates CJ. Influenza vaccine for patients with chronic obstructive pulmonary disease. Cochrane Database Syst Rev (Online) 2006; (1):CD002733.

62. Dear K, Holden J, Andrews R, Tatham D. Vaccines for preventing pneumococcal infection in adults. Cochrane Database Syst Rev (Online) 2003; (4):CD000422.

63. Black P, Staykova T, Chacko E, Ram FS, Poole P. Prophylactic antibiotic therapy for chronic bronchitis. Cochrane Database Systematic Rev (Online) 2003; (1):CD004105.

64. Murphy TF, Brauer AL, Sethi S, Kilian M, Cai X, Lesse AJ. Haemophilus haemolyticus: a human respiratory tract commensal to be distinguished from *Haemophilus influenzae*. J Infect Dis 2007; 195(1):81–9.

65. von Hertzen L, Alakarppa H, Koskinen R, et al. *Chlamydia pneumoniae* infection in patients with chronic obstructive pulmonary disease. Epidemiol Infect 1997; 118:155–64.

66. Matsuse T, Hayashi S, Kuwano K, Keunecke H, Jefferies WA, Hogg JC. Latent adenoviral infection in the pathogenesis of chronic airways obstruction. Am Rev Respir Dis 1992; 146:177–84.

67. Moller LVM, Timens W, van der Bij W, et al. *Haemophilus influenzae* in lung explants of patients with end-stage pulmonary disease. Am J Respir Crit Care Med 1998; 157:950–6.

68. Bresser P, Out TA, van Alphen L, Jansen HM, Lutter R. Airway inflammation in nonobstructive and obstructive chronic bronchitis with chronic *Haemophilus influenzae* airway infection. Comparison with noninfected patients with chronic obstructive pulmonary disease. Am J Respir Crit Care Med 2000; 162(3 Pt 1):947–52.

69. Banerjee D, Khair OA, Honeybourne D. Impact of sputum bacteria on airway inflammation and health status in clinical stable COPD. Eur Respir J 2004; 23(5):685–91.

70. Soler N, Ewig S, Torres A, Filella X, Gonzalez J, Zaubet A. Airway inflammation and bronchial microbial patterns in patients with stable chronic obstructive pulmonary disease. Eur Respir J 1999; 14:1015–22.

71. O'Meara ES, White M, Siscovick DS, Lyles MF, Kuller LH. Hospitalization for pneumonia in the Cardiovascular Health Study: incidence, mortality, and influence on longer-term survival. J Am Geriatr Soc 2005; 53(7):1108–16.

72. Torres A, Menendez R. Mortality in COPD patients with community-acquired pneumonia: who is the third partner? Eur Respir J 2006; 28(2):262–3.

73. Ko FW, Lam RK, Li TS, et al. Sputum bacteriology in patients hospitalized with acute exacerbations of chronic obstructive pulmonary disease and concomitant pneumonia in Hong Kong. Intern Med J 2005; 35(11):661–7.

74. Mandell LA, Wunderink RG, Anzueto A, et al. Infectious diseases society of america/american thoracic society consensus guidelines on the management of community-acquired pneumonia in adults. Clin Infect Dis 2007; 44(Suppl. 2):S27–72.

16

Phosphodiesterase 4 Inhibitors, Mucolytics, and Emerging Pharmacotherapies for COPD

MARK A. GIEMBYCZ
Department of Pharmacology and Therapeutics, Faculty of Medicine, Institute of Infection, Immunity, and Inflammation, University of Calgary, Calgary, Alberta, Canada

I. Introduction

Chronic obstructive pulmonary disease (COPD) is the most common of all respiratory disorders and the prevalence of diagnosed disease is growing at an alarming rate (1) (see Chapter 1, "The Burden of Chronic Obstructive Pulmonary Disease," for more information). Acute exacerbations of COPD are a major concern due to an adverse effect on health status and increased mortality; indeed, it has been estimated that 10% to 30% of the most severely afflicted will die following hospitalization (2). Long-term survival rates after an exacerbation are also poor (3). The World Health Organization predicts that because of the increased prevalence and poor treatment, COPD will become the third most common cause of death worldwide by 2020 and exact an *enormous economic burden* (4). Despite this impending epidemic no drugs, including glucocorticoids, have a major impact on the progression of any aspect of COPD (*cf.* asthma) (5,6). Thus, while smoking cessation intervention reduces the decline in lung function and, along with bronchodilators, provides symptomatic relief, there are unmet needs for patients with COPD, including anti-inflammatory therapy allied with drugs that improve lung function, reduce excessive mucus secretion, arrest remodeling, and normalize airways reactivity. Many new drugs, some with a novel or an unproven mechanism of action, are in development (Table 1). The primary purpose of this chapter to review the clinical data thus far obtained with new chemical entities (NCEs) in late Phase development for COPD that have a realistic chance of reaching the market, specifically, phosphodiesterase (PDE) 4 inhibitors and new mucolytics. In addition, brief mention will be made of novel pharmacotherapeutic approaches that, in the author's opinion, also offer potential promise for the effective treatment of COPD but where development is not so (clinically) advanced.

II. PDE4 Inhibitors

The most advanced NCEs with predicted anti-inflammatory activity that are in development for COPD are inhibitors of PDE4 (Table 1). Since the early 1980s, there has been considerable interest in the therapeutic utility of PDE4 inhibitors for a number of inflammatory diseases and, during the 1990s, this was extended to include COPD.

Table 1 New Drugs in Clinical Development for COPD

Company	Drug	Mode of action	Development stage
Almirall	Arofylline	PDE4I	Phase II/III
Glenmark	Oglemilast (GRC 3886)	PDE4I	Phase III
Pfizer	Tofimilast (CP-325366)	PDE4I	Phase II
ONO	ONO 6126	PDE4I	Phase II
Otsuka	Tetomilast (OPC 6535)	PDE4I	Phase III
Nycomed	Roflumilast	PDE4I	Phase III
GlaxoSmithKline	Cilomilast (SB 207499)	PDE4I	Phase III
GlaxoSmithKline/Elbion	AWD-12-281 (GSK 842470)	PDE4I	Phase II
GlaxoSmithKline	GSK 256066	PDE4I	Phase I
GlaxoSmithKline	GSK 159979 (TD3327)	ULABA	Phase II
GlaxoSmithKline	GSK 579901	ULABA	Phase II
GlaxoSmithKline	GSK 678007	ULABA	Phase II
Sepracor	Arformoterol	ULABA	Phase III
Tanabe Seiyaku	CHF 4226 (TA 2005)	ULABA	Phase II
GlaxoSmithKline	GSK 159802	ULABA	Phase I
GlaxoSmithKline	GSK 642444	ULABA	Phase I
Novartis	Indacaterol (QAB 149)	ULABA	Phase II
GlaxoSmithKline	Allermist (GSK 685698)	GR agonist	Phase II
GlaxoSmithKline	GSK 799943[a]	GR agonist	Phase I
Almirall	LAS 34273	M_3 receptor antagonist	Phase III
GlaxoSmithKline	GSK 202405	M_3 receptor antagonist	Phase II
Arakis/Vectura	AD 237	M_3 receptor antagonist	Phase IIa
GlaxoSmithKline	GSK 656933	$CXCR_2$ antagonist	Phase I
AstraZeneca	AZD 8309	$CXCR_2$ antagonist	Phase I
GlaxoSmithKline	GSK 274150	iNOS inhibitor	Phase II
NicOx	NCX-1020	NO-donating budesonide	Phase I
Sankyo	CS 003	$NK_1/NK_2/NK_3$ receptor antagonist	Phase II
AstraZeneca	AZD 9056	$P2X_7$ ion channel blocker	Phase II
GlaxoSmithKline	GSK 681323	p38 MAPK inhibitor	Phase I
ONO	Pranlukast	$Cys-LT_1/cys-LT_2$ receptor antagonist	Phase II
CoTherix	CTX-100	Hyaluronic acid	Phase I
Inspire	INS365	$P2Y_2$ agonist	Phase I
Edmond pharma/adams respiratory thertherapeurtics	Erdosteine	Mucolytic/free radical scavenger	Marketed (Phase IIb U.S.A.)
GlaxoSmithKiline	Rosiglitazone	PPARγ agonist	Marketed for Type II diabetes

[a] In combination with a (U)LABA.

Abbreviations: Cys-LT, cysteinyl leukotriene; GR, glucocorticoid receptor; iNOS, inducible nitric oxide synthase; MAPK, mitogen-activated protein kinase; NK, neurokinin; NO, nitric oxide; PDE4I, phosphodiesterase 4 inhibitor; PPAR, peroxisome proliferator-activated receptor; ULABA, ultra long-acting β_2-agonist.

Source: From Ref. 7.

The rationale for developing compounds that attenuate PDE4 activity is based on three critical findings: (*i*) PDE4 is the major regulator of cAMP metabolism in almost every proinflammatory and immune cell, and agents that elevate cAMP have a pharmacology consistent with anti-inflammatory activity; (*ii*) PDE4 inhibitors, of varied structural classes, suppress a myriad of in vitro responses such as cytokine generation, NADPH oxidase activity, degranulation, proliferation, mediator generation and chemotaxis; and (*iii*) PDE4 inhibitors are efficacious in animal models of inflammation (8). If these observations hold in humans then, conceptually, PDE4 inhibitors should show a pleiotropic inhibitory profile of activity on proinflammatory and immune cell function. Despite the potential for adverse-events due to the ubiquitous distribution of PDE4 in "non-target" cells (see below), almost all of the main pharmaceutical companies in the world have synthesized and evaluated in the clinic PDE4 inhibitors of varied structural classes, several of which are now in late Phase III development (Table 1). Detailed clinical data relevant for COPD are available for two compounds: cilomilast (Ariflo[®]; Altana Pharma, Konstanz, Germany) and roflumilast (Daxas[®]; GlaxoSmithKline, Stevenage, U.K.), and these are discussed here.

A. Cilomilast Clinical Development Program

Cilomilast has been under development by GlaxoSmithKline (GSK) for over 20 years but only recently was COPD also considered a viable indication for this class of compound (probably because of the poor efficacy of cilomilast in trials of asthma). Cilomilast is an example of a second generation PDE4 inhibitor that was designed to have an improved therapeutic ratio over first generation compounds such as rolipram (9,10), which was initially developed for the treatment of depression (11,12).

To date, 77 Phase I, II, and III studies are known to have been conducted by GSK for the cilomilast clinical development program (13). In COPD, 12 core studies were performed of which two were Phase II dose-ranging studies (#032 and #038) and the remainder Phase III studies assessing efficacy, safety, and mechanism of action (Table 2) (14). In total, 4093 subjects were enrolled in the Phase II and Phase III clinical trials; 2586 were given cilomilast and the remainder (1507) received placebo (14). Data were analyzed on an intention-to-treat basis. The safety of cilomilast in the COPD trials has been evaluated in 1069 subjects over a period of three years (14).

Promising Results from Phase II Studies Prompted Comprehensive Phase III Evaluation

Two Phase II clinical trials have been conducted in outpatients with moderate COPD evaluating the safety, tolerability, and efficacy of cilomilast administered orally (15). In one of those studies (#32), subjects were randomized to receive cilomilast (5, 10 or 15 mg b.i.d) or placebo for six weeks (15,16). At the highest dose, cilomilast produced a progressive and statistically significant increase in trough (pre-dose) forced expiratory volume in one second (FEV_1) from week 1 to the end of the study period (Fig. 1A). At the end of week 6, cilomilast had increased trough FEV_1 by 160 mL, which represented an 11% improvement in lung function when compared to subjects that received placebo (15,16). Similar improvements at week 6, relative to placebo, were observed for the 15 mg b.i.d. dose in forced vital capacity (FVC), peak expiratory

Table 2 Phase III Studies in the Cilomilast Clinical Development Program

Study number	Duration of study	Treatment groups	Dose	Geographical location	Subjects randomized	
					Placebo	Cilomilast
Pivotal efficacy studies						
039	24 weeks	Cilomilast Placebo	15 mg b.i.d	North America	216	431
156	24 weeks	Cilomilast Placebo	15 mg b.i.d	North America	407	418
042	24 weeks	Cilomilast Placebo	15 mg b.i.d	Europe	226	474
091	24 weeks	Cilomilast Placebo	15 mg b.i.d	Europe	242	469
Cardiovascular safety						
168	12 weeks	Cilomilast Placebo	15 mg b.i.d	United States	94	188
Mechanism of action studies						
076	12 weeks	Cilomilast Placebo	15 mg b.i.d	Europe	30	29
110	12 weeks	Cilomilast Placebo	15 mg b.i.d	North America	34	31
111	12 weeks	Cilomilast Placebo	15 mg b.i.d	North America	77	79
Long-term open-label extension studies						
040	Long-term	Cilomilast	15 mg b.i.d	Europe	N/A	714
041	Long-term	Cilomilast	15 mg b.i.d	North America	N/A	355

Abbreviation: N/A, not applicable.
Source: From Ref. 14.

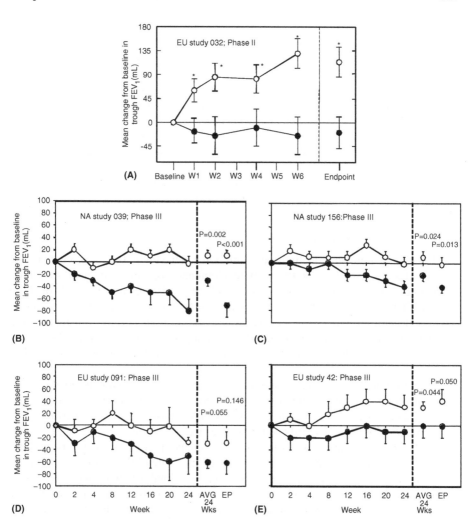

Figure 1 Results of one Phase II (#032) and four Phase III efficacy trials (#039, #156, #091, #042) in Europe and North America of the effect of oral cilomilast on clinic FEV_1 in patients with COPD. In panel (**A**) subjects entered a two-week placebo run-in before being randomized (double-blind) to receive cilomilast (5 mg, $n = 109$; 10 mg, $n = 102$; 15 mg, $n = 107$; b.i.d) or placebo ($n = 106$) for six weeks. At defined times after treatment trough (predose) FEV_1 was measured. Results with 15 mg cilomilast (b.i.d.) are shown. In panels (**B**) to (**E**) subjects entered a four-week placebo run-in before being randomized (double-blind) to receive cilomilast (15 mg. b.i.d; open circle) or placebo (filled) for 24 weeks. At the indicated times after treatment trough (pre-dose) FEV_1 was measured. At the end of the trial the average FEV_1 was calculated and an endpoint measurement made. The *y* axis shows the mean *change from baseline* in clinic FEV_1, which was modest (0 to ~60 mL). *Statistically significant improvement in lung function relative to placebo. *Abbreviation*: FEV_1, forced expiratory volume in one second. *Source*: From Refs. 16, 17 (see text for further details).

flow rate (PEFR), exertional dyspnea, rescue bronchodilator use and resting and post-exercise arterial oxygen saturation (SaO_2) (15,16). Lower doses of cilomilast produced negligible improvements in lung function, which was confirmed in a similar multicenter four week study (#038) (15).

Quality of life assessments using the Medical Outcomes Study 36-item short form health survey (SF-36) and St. George's Respiratory Questionnaire (SGRQ) were also recorded before and after therapy with cilomilast (15 mg b.i.d.) or placebo (16). Consistent improvements approaching those defined as clinically relevant in the total and composite scores of the SGRQ were recorded for those subject that received 15 mg cilomilast when compared to the placebo treatment group, although this did not reach statistical significance (16). Similar improvements with cilomilast were recorded for the physical composite score of the SF-36 (16,18).

Pivotal Phase III Efficacy Studies

The improvement in lung function and health status in the Phase II trials prompted GSK to commit to a comprehensive Phase III development program of six months duration evaluating efficacy, cardiovascular safety, and mechanism of action. In all of these studies, cilomilast was given at the maximum tolerated dose (15 mg b.i.d.), which was the only dose in all Phase II studies that was found to produce improvements in lung function, symptoms, and quality of life that were superior to placebo (15,16,19). In the following sections, the results of the efficacy and mechanism of action studies are reviewed.

Four pivotal, multicenter, randomized, double-blind, placebo-controlled parallel group studies of similar design were conducted evaluating the effect of cilomilast (15 mg b.i.d.) for 24 weeks in subjects with COPD. Two studies were performed in North America (#039 and #156) and two studies were performed in Europe (#042 and #156) (Table 2 for details). The primary efficacy endpoints were change from baseline in trough FEV_1 and change from baseline in the total score of the SGRQ. The primary comparison was the averaged difference between the cilomilast- and placebo-treatment groups over the 24 weeks double-blind period. Secondary measures included COPD exacerbations, FVC, exercise tolerance, exertional dyspnea (modified Borg breathlessness scale), six-minute walking test, and symptoms recorded by each subject on a diary card. Fifteen tertiary efficacy variables were also measured including PEFR, forced expiratory flow (FEF) at 25% and 75% of vital capacity (FEF_{25-75}), FEF at 75% of vital capacity (FEF_{75}), FEV in six seconds (FEV_6), SaO_2, arterial blood gases (PaO_2, $PaCO_2$), and subscales of the SF-36 quality of life health survey. Each study had a four week single-blind placebo run-in followed by 24 weeks of double-blind treatment. Cilomilast (15 mg) was taken orally as a tablet twice a day after breakfast and after the evening meal. A one week safety follow-up was conducted in those subjects who withdrew from the study or who elected not to participate in an open-label extension study. Across the four trials 71% and 76% of cilomilast- and placebo-treated subjects respectively completed the double-blind phase. Key inclusion and exclusion criteria are given in Table 3. Despite the results of the pivotal Phase III studies being in the public domain since 2003, only one trial (#039) has been described and published following peer review (20). Most of the other data presented herein are taken from abstracts and from the Food and Drug Administration Web site (21).

Table 3 Key Inclusion and Exclusion Criteria for the Phase III Studies in the Cilomilast Clinical Development Program

Inclusion	Exclusion
Male or female (40–80 years of age)	Patients with asthma
Diagnosed with COPD as defined by ATS or ERS guidelines	Patients with poorly controlled COPD
Cigarette smoking history (≥ 10 pack years)	Patients with lung cancer or clinically overt bronchiectasis
Pre-bronchodilator FEV_1/FVC ratio ≤ 0.7 at screening	Patients with cardiovascular, neurological, renal, endocrine or hematological abnormalities poorly that were poorly controlled on permitted therapy
Fixed airway obstruction ($\leq 15\%$ or ≤ 200 mL increase in FEV_1 at screening)[a]	Patients with clinically significant gastrointestinal or hepatic abnormalities
Post-bronchodilator FEV_1 between $\geq 30\%$ and $\leq 70\%$ of predicted	Patients with positive fecal occult blood test results between screening and baseline visits
	Patients with clinically significant orthostatic changes in blood pressure or heart rate at screening or baseline visits
	Patients who required treatment with chromones, xanthines, leukotriene modifiers, corticosteroids (oral/inhaled), inhaled long-acting β_2-agonists, oral β_2-agonists and nebulized β_2-agonists/anticholinergics
	Patients receiving treatment with long-term oxygen therapy, patients who required supplemental oxygen on a frequent basis or patients who required nocturnal positive pressure for sleep
	Patients who had participated in a Pulmonary Rehabilitation Program within four weeks prior to screening or who planned to enter such a program during the trial

[a] The study design did not apparently take into account the impact on FEV_1 of regression towards the mean (see text for details).
Abbreviations: ATS, American Thoracic Society; COPD, chronic obstructive pulmonary disease; ERS, European Respiratory Society; FEV_1, forced expiratory volume in one second; FVC, forced vital capacity.
Source: From Ref. 21.

Trial #039

The study was conducted at 102 centers in the United States, Canada and Mexico and subjects were randomized to receive either cilomilast (15 mg b.i.d.) or placebo in 90 of the 102 centers (15). Male (67.6%) Caucasian (96.8%) subjects that were greater than 50 years of age (94.4%) at enrolment dominated the study population (15). At the end of the 24-week treatment period the trough FEV_1 averaged across the study was increased and decreased from baseline by 10 and 30 mL in the cilomilast- and placebo-treatment groups respectively, and the difference between the two treatment groups (40 mL) was statistically significant (Fig. 1B) (15,17,22). Relative to placebo, cilomilast also improved FVC, trough FEF_{25-75}, and trough FEV_6 in the same study population by 110 mL, 40 mL/sec and 90 mL, respectively suggesting that a clinically important impact of cilomilast might have occurred in the small airways (22,23).

It is noteworthy that cilomilast did not improve lung function per se (Fig. 1B) but prevented the decline in FEV_1 seen in subjects taking placebo. Indeed, the statistical significance achieved in this study was driven solely by the rapid deterioration in trough FEV_1 in subjects given placebo when compared to the cilomilast-treatment group where lung function was maintained over the 24-week study period (Fig. 1B) (15,17,22).

Relative to placebo, cilomilast also significantly reduced the risk of a self-managed (Level 1 or mild) exacerbation and of an exacerbation requiring treatment by a physician (Level 2 or moderate) or hospitalization (Level 3 or severe) (22,24). Reanalysis of these data by Kaplan–Meier product limit, Gill–Anderson multiple event regression, and Poisson regression, which assess exacerbation-free survival, the relative risk of an exacerbation and exacerbation rate per patient year respectively has confirmed these findings (25). Significantly, the number of subjects that were exacerbation-free at the end of the treatment period was 69.7% and 81.7% for the placebo and cilomilast-treatment groups, respectively. Furthermore, the relative risk of subjects experiencing at least one Level 2 or Level 3 COPD exacerbation, which are the most clinically relevant, was reduced by 40% in the cilomilast-treatment group when compared to those subjects that were given placebo (17).

Changes in global health status using the SGRQ and SF-36 were made at baseline and six months after therapy with cilomilast (15 mg b.i.d) and placebo (22). In agreement with the lung function data, consistent improvements defined as clinically relevant and statistically significant in the total (-4.1 points) and composite scores (symptoms, activity, and impacts) of the SGRQ were recorded for those subjects that received 15 mg cilomilast when compared to patients that were given placebo. At the end of the study period, significant improvements were also recorded for the physical function and general health perception scores of the SF-36 in the cilomilast-treatment group (22).

Trial #156

The study was conducted at 132 centers in the United States and Canada and subjects were randomized to receive either cilomilast (15 mg b.i.d.) or placebo in 126 of the 132 centers (15). Male (61.7%) Caucasian (92.6%) subjects that were greater than 50 years of age (93.8%) at enrolment dominated the study population (15). The same endpoint measures were made as those described for trial #039.

In general, the results of trial #156 were similar to those obtained from the other North American study (#039). Thus, in the cilomilast and placebo treatment groups trough FEV_1, when averaged over the 24 weeks of study, was increased and decreased by 10 and 20 mL, respectively when compared to baseline, and the difference between the two groups was statistically significant (Fig. 1C) (15,17). Consistent with trial #039, the statistical significance achieved in this study was driven by the deterioration in trough FEV_1 in subjects given placebo, rather that to an improvement in lung function per se in those subjects that received cilomilast (Fig. 1C) (15,17,22).

In contrast to the results of trial #039, no statistically significant difference was found in the relative risk of subjects experiencing either Level 2 or Level 3 exacerbations. Similarly, although a statistically significant improvement in quality of life, as assessed by the SGRQ, was achieved in subjects that received cilomilast relative to placebo, this did not reach the clinically meaningful threshold of -4.0 points (17).

Trial #091

The study was conducted at 110 centers in Belgium, Finland, France, and Italy, The Netherlands, Norway, Portugal, Spain, and the United Kingdom and subjects were randomized to receive either cilomilast (15 mg b.i.d.) or placebo (15). Male (85.5%) Caucasian (97.9%) subjects that were greater than 50 years of age (90.5%) at enrolment dominated the study population (15). The same endpoint measures were made as those described for trial #039.

At the end of the 24-week treatment period, the trough FEV_1 averaged across the study was unchanged relative to baseline in the cilomilast-treatment group while a decline of 30 mL was found in those subjects that were given placebo (Fig. 1D) (15,17). Contrary to both of the North American studies, the mean difference between treatments in change in FEV_1 from baseline did not reach statistical significance (Fig. 1D). Similarly, there was no statistically significant or clinically meaningful improvement in quality of life although treatment with either cilomilast or placebo was associated with a reduction (improvement) of ~two points in the total score of the SGRQ (15,17). The only major secondary measure to show an improvement after treatment with cilomilast was in exacerbation-free rates.

Trial #042

The study was conducted at 98 centers in Australia, New Zealand, Germany, Spain, South Africa, and the United Kingdom and subjects were randomized to receive either cilomilast (15 mg b.i.d.) or placebo (15). Male (79.6%) Caucasian (99.1%) subjects that were greater than 50 years of age (96%) at enrolment dominated the study population (15). The same endpoint measures were made as those described for trial #039.

As shown in Figure 1E, relative to baseline there was no mean change in trough FEV_1 averaged over the 24 weeks of treatment in subjects that were given placebo, while the cilomilast treatment group showed a mean increase of 30 mL (15,17). Although the difference from placebo of 30 mL had a *p* value of 0.044, this was not statistically significant after adjusting for multiple comparisons using the modified Bonferroni procedure of Hochberg. The results of the SGRQ were also not significant between treatment groups (15,17). In fact, the placebo-treated group of subjects showed an average decrease from baseline in the total score of the SGRQ of 4.9 points, which was superior to that produced by cilomilast (4.2 points). Finally, there was no difference between treatment groups in the relative risk of experiencing a Level 2 or Level 3 exacerbation (17).

Disappointing Results of the Phase III Pivotal Efficacy Studies

On balance the data arising from the Phase III pivotal efficacy studies are unremarkable and disappointing. The initial three trials (#039, #042, #091) were designed to demonstrate a difference in FEV_1 between cilomilast- and placebo-treatment groups of 120 mL. This level of lung function improvement was based on the very promising efficacy results obtained in trial #032 of the Phase II dose-ranging study where cilomilast improved trough FEV_1 at week 6 by 130 and 160 mL relative to baseline and placebo, respectively (Fig. 1A). However, using the results of study #39 as an example, the difference from baseline in FEV_1 between the placebo and cilomilast treatment groups was 40 mL, which amounts to only 3% of the mean baseline value and less than

50% of the reversibility effected by inhaled salbutamol (6.5–6.7%). This level of improvement is not clinically important.

The results of the SGRQ should also be considered in context of the scoring system devised by Jones and colleagues (26). Thus, total scores of ≥ -4, ≥ -8 and ≥ -12 indicate that an intervention has produced an effect(s) that is slightly efficacious, moderately efficacious, and very efficacious, respectively. In only one (#039) of the four pivotal efficacy studies was there a clinically meaningful improvement in quality of life, and the total score (-4.1) for that study relative to placebo at endpoint indicated that cilomilast was only slightly efficacious (15).

The poor performance of cilomilast in these efficacy studies is difficult to rationalize given the respectable improvement in FEV_1 obtained in trial #032 (Fig. 1A). However, it is likely that the highest tolerated dose of cilomilast (i.e., 15 mg b.i.d.) falls on the leading edge of the dose–response curve and that it is the low therapeutic ratio of this compound that prevents efficacy from being realized. This possibility could be a major contributing factor to the lack of consistency across Phase II and Phase III efficacy studies and the absence of a dose–response relationship in trial #032, where cilomilast was compared to placebo at 5, 10, and 15 mg (b.i.d.) (18). Other factors that could account for these disappointing results include the large degree of variability in the cilomilast plasma trough concentrations, where the coefficient of variation exceeded 60%, and the fact that the data are highly unbalanced (27).

More difficult to explain is the apparent deterioration (within two to four weeks in study #039) in trough FEV_1 in three of the four Phase III studies in those subjects that received placebo (Fig. 1A,B and C). This is especially confounding given that those results are contrary to the Phase II efficacy data obtained in trial #032, where FEV_1 was unchanged relative to baseline (Fig. 1), and in other long-term clinical trials of COPD where the impact of corticosteroids, theophylline, and short-acting β_2-adrenoceptor agonists on FEV_1 have been examined (see Refs. 28–30). However, it has been implied that this may be only an apparent effect (27) on the basis that trough FEV_1 at baseline is the mean of the number of subjects that were enrolled in the study (216 in the placebo limb of trial #039), whereas all subsequent FEV_1 measurements reflect the mean of a reduced sample size due to subject withdrawal (only 164 subjects completed the double-blind phase). While it is possible that the data are distorted by subject withdrawal ($\sim 25\%$ in trial #039), it is hard to believe that this, alone, accounts for the reported rapid decrement in lung function in the placebo-treatment group in three of the four pivotal efficacy studies. Indeed, the number of withdrawals in the placebo limb of the six-week Phase II dose-ranging trial (#032; Fig. 1) was not too dissimilar (16%) from trial #039, yet lung function in that study was maintained in those subjects that were given placebo (15). One, albeit contentious, explanation that may deserve consideration is that the reduction in FEV_1 in the placebo-treatment group is due to the withdrawal from the study of a sub-group of subjects that were taking corticosteroids prior to enrolment.

Mechanism of Action Studies

Two randomized, placebo-controlled, double-blind, parallel group, exploratory mechanism of action studies of 12-weeks duration have been conducted to assess the effect of cilomilast on inflammatory cell counts in induced sputum (#110) and endobronchial biopsies (#076) (Table 2). The primary endpoint measure was a reduction in sputum neutrophils and in neither study was statistical significance achieved (31,32). However, compared to placebo, statistically significant reductions from baseline in sub-epithelial $CD8^+$ and $CD68^+$ cells were found in bronchial biopsies taken from subjects that received cilomilast indicating an inhibitory effect on T-lymphocytes and cells of the monocyte/macrophage lineage, respectively. Post hoc Poisson regression analysis confirmed these findings and also showed a reduction in the number of sub-epithelial neutrophils and $CD4^+$ cells (32). In contrast, there was no significant treatment-related effect on the number of epithelial neutrophils or on IL-8 and $TNF\alpha$ $mRNA^+$ cells (32). The reason for the discrepancy between the sputum and biopsy data is currently unclear but could reflect an inhibitory effect of cilomilast on proinflammatory cell trafficking and/or, as suggested above, the dose of cilomilast, which may be too low for subtle changes in sputum cell numbers to be detected especially with a small sample size ($n = 29$).

A third 12-week randomized, double-blind, placebo-controlled, parallel group, multicenter mechanism of action study (#111) in subjects with COPD was also conducted. This trial was initiated because there is evidence that FEV_1 alone may have limitations as a clinical outcome measure of efficacy (33,34). As an alternative, it has been advocated that static or dynamic lung volume measurements may provide more instructive information pertaining to the impairment of lung function, especially in subjects who are poorly reversible (35).

Trapping of air in the lungs and subsequent pulmonary hyperinflation is common in subjects with COPD. This condition results from a loss of elastic recoil of the lungs, reduced expiratory muscle strength and airways obstruction, which is partly due to inflammation of the small bronchioles (36,37). Airways obstruction can lead to premature inspiration (i.e., the initiation of inspiration prior to complete expiration of the previous breath) resulting in a state of hyperinflation as more air enters the lungs with each breath than is ejected. Lung hyperinflation is reflected by increases in several lung function parameters including total lung capacity (TLC), functional residual capacity (FRC), and residual volume (RV), the latter two variables reflecting the most detrimental pathophysiological effects. In the context of evaluating new drugs for COPD, it has been shown that inhaled bronchodilators attenuate hyperinflation, producing the greatest benefit in the more severely obstructed and hyperinflated, yet elicit, in the same individuals, only a *very modest* improvement in FEV_1 (35). Accordingly, trial #111 was designed to evaluate the effect of cilomilast on air trapping and measures of hyperinflation in subjects with COPD. The primary efficacy measure was the change in volume of trapped gas at endpoint between the cilomilast and placebo-treatment groups, and was defined as the difference in TLC measured by whole body plethysmography and single breath helium dilution. Changes from baseline in RV and thoracic gas volume (TGV) at FRC were used as indices of hyperinflation. Although the difference in mean volume of trapped air between the two study groups favored cilomilast (by 140 mL) this did not reach statistical significance (34,38). In contrast, there were statistically significant improvements relative to baseline in favor of cilomilast in RV and TGV at FRC indicating a positive impact on lung hyperinflation in the absence of any significant effect on FEV_1 (34,38).

B. Roflumilast Clinical Development Program

There is considerably less information in the public domain on the roflumilast clinical development program despite the fact that many Phase III trials have been conducted.

Indeed, according to the ClinicalTrials.gov Web site several trials are still ongoing examining roflumilast as a monotherapy and in combination with the long-acting muscarinic M_3-receptor antagonist, tiotropium bromide (see Ref. 39). By July 2007, the results of two multicenter, double blind, and placebo-controlled Phase III studies were published following peer review. In one of those, which was conducted in 159 centers across Australia, Austria, Belgium, Canada, France, Germany, Hungary, Ireland, South Africa, Spain. and the United Kingdom, 1411 subjects were randomized to receive roflumilast orally (250 or 500 µg o.d.) or placebo for 24 weeks (40). The primary efficacy endpoint measures were change in post-bronchodilator FEV_1 and health-related quality of life using the SGRQ. Secondary measures included change from baseline in pre-bronchodilator FEV_1, FVC, FEV_6, FEF_{25-75}, and COPD exacerbations. Inclusion and exclusion criteria were comparable to those given in Table 3 for the cilomilast pivotal efficacy studies. Compared to placebo, roflumilast statistically improved lung function at both doses and at all time points over the 24 weeks of treatment at which measurements were made. At the end of the treatment period post-bronchodilator FEV_1 relative to placebo was increased by 74 and 97 mL for the 250 and 500 µg doses, respectively (40), and subjects had experienced fewer exacerbations in the active treatment groups (the mean exacerbation number per patient$= 1.13$, 1.03, and 0.75 for placebo, roflumilast 250 µg and roflumilast 500 µg, respectively). In contrast, there was no significant difference in health-related quality of life as assessed by the SGRQ for any domain whether the effect of roflumilast was compared against baseline or placebo. With regard to secondary outcome measures, significant improvements in pre-bronchodilator FEV_1, post-bronchodilator FVC, FEV_6, and FEF_{25-75} were also reported (40).

Despite the apparently positive outcome of this roflumilast trial in COPD, certain claims made by Rabe and colleagues (40) in that publication have attracted criticisms, some of which merit highlighting here (see Refs. 41–45). Notably, Bergmann (41) attests that if the *raw* data are analyzed (see Ref. 46) there is, in fact, no significant difference at the end of the trial between the placebo and the roflumilast treatment groups. Thus, after 24 weeks of treatment, FEV_1 relative to baseline was increased and decreased by 51 and 45 mL in those subjects that were given roflumilast (500 µg o.d.) and placebo, respectively (40). If those data are corrected for the difference in mean baseline FEV_1 between the placebo and roflumilast treatment groups at the beginning of the trial (these were 1.57 and 1.50 L, respectively), then the absolute difference in FEV_1 at week 24 favors roflumilast by a mere 26 mL [i.e., $(1.5l + 0.051) - (1.57l - 0.45) = 0.026l$]. This is neither statistically nor clinically meaningful. Bergmann (41) also challenges the statistical evaluation of exacerbation rate between the three treatment groups stating that a classical χ^2 test returns a nonsignificant p value of 0.48. Another valid criticism, leveled by Morice (42), is the assertion by Rabe and colleagues that the modest improvement in lung function was due to an anti-inflammatory effect of roflumilast. As indices of inflammation were not measured in this trial, it is remarkable that a statement to this effect is incorporated into the title of the paper. By their own admission (47), the authors of the study extrapolate result from experiments conducted with laboratory animals (which at best can be misleading), and from previously published data where cilomilast was found not to be a directly acting bronchodilator (48).

The results of the other Phase III trial were published in July 2007 (49). In this 159 multicenter, randomized, placebo-controlled, double-blind parallel group study the effect of roflumilast (500 µg o.d.) was compared against placebo in 1513 subjects with severe COPD [Global Initiative for Chronic Obstructive Lung Disease (GOLD) Stages III and IV]. The efficacy endpoint measures were change in post-bronchodilator FEV_1, and exacerbation rate per patient per year. The main secondary variable was health-related quality of life using the SGRQ. Pre-bronchodilator FEV_1, post-bronchodilator FEV_6, FVC, and FEF_{25-75} were also determined. Inclusion and exclusion criteria were broadly comparable to those given in Table 3 for the cilomilast pivotal efficacy studies except that previously prescribed inhaled corticosteroids (ICSs) use was permitted. Compared to placebo, roflumilast improved lung function at all time points over the 52 weeks of treatment at which measurements were made. At the end of the treatment period post-bronchodilator FEV_1 relative to placebo was increased by 39 mL; similar modest improvements in the other indices of lung function relative to placebo were also recorded, demonstrating that these effects can be maintained over a period of one year. However, there was no associated difference in the exacerbation rate between the two treatment groups (0.92 and 0.86 exacerbations/subject/year for placebo and roflumilast respectively) or in health status. Calverley and colleagues (49) also performed a retrospective analysis of exacerbation frequency in those subjects characterized with GOLD Stage IV disease. In that subpopulation, the exacerbation rate was 36% lower in subjects treated with roflumilast when compared to those given placebo (1.01 and 1.59 exacerbations/patient/year respectively).

C. Assessment of the Roflumilast Clinical Development Program

The improvement in lung function effected by roflumilast in both Phase III clinical trials reported herein is modest and of similar magnitude to that evoked by cilomilast and ICSs. While these data are probably of limited clinical significance, the improvement in lung function reported by Calverley and colleagues (49) was evoked in subjects in whom the use ICSs was permitted. Thus, perhaps roflumilast (and other PDE4 inhibitors) can improve lung function beyond that achievable by ICSs alone despite the limited responsiveness of these subjects to bronchodilators (49).

Roflumilast does have an advantage over cilomilast in having a longer half live (~ 16 hours) as its primary metabolite, the N-oxide, is also biologically active (50,51). This superior pharmacokinetic profile allows for once a day dosing, which should translate into improved patient compliance. It is worth noting that a meta-analysis of 13 clinical studies involving 244 subjects found that oral theophylline improves FEV_1 in subjects with stable COPD by approximately 100 mL (30), which is superior to that produced by cilomilast and roflumilast in the Phase III efficacy trials described here. These data may suggest that PDE4 inhibitors could further improve lung function if given at higher doses. Regrettably, most of the second generation PDE4 inhibitors evaluated in the clinical thus far have been given at the highest tolerated dose so this possibility cannot be tested empirically. Whether the therapeutic ratio of this class of compound can be improved is currently unclear. However, clinical trials are ongoing with a variety of new PDE4 inhibitors including oglemilast and tetomilast (Table 1), and the result of those studies could be instructive.

D. Safety and Tolerability of PDE4 Inhibitors

Despite some encouraging data from the pivotal Phase III efficacy studies in COPD, cilomilast, and roflumilast are hampered by a low therapeutic ratio. This limitation became clear early on in the development of these compounds with nausea, diarrhea, abdominal pain, vomiting, and dyspepsia being most common adverse events reported (reviewed in Refs. 10 and 52). Indeed, the number of subjects failing to complete all controlled cilomilast trials conducted by GSK due to an adverse event was positively dose-related across the 2.5, 5, 10, and 15 mg treatment groups (6.9, 12.8, 20.4, and 25.9% withdrawal respectively) with gastrointestinal disturbances being the most prevalent (15). Similarly, the most common adverse events related to roflumilast treatment are diarrhea, nausea (and headache) (40,49). Unfortunately, the unwanted gastrointestinal actions, which are mediated both locally (i.e., in the gastrointestinal tract) and centrally, can be accounted for by the ubiquitous distribution of PDE4 isoforms across many tissues, and represent an extension of the pharmacology of PDE4 inhibitors that is typical of first generation compounds such as rolipram.

Documentation of serious toxicities resulting from the administration of PDE4 inhibitors is relatively sparse. However, the most worrying potential toxicity that may be generic to PDE4 inhibitors is arteritis. This condition is characterized by inflammation, hemorrhage, and necrosis of blood vessels, and is believed to be irreversible in animals. Mechanistically, arteritis is thought to result from hemodynamic changes produced by excessive and prolonged vasodilatation of specific vascular beds, although the means by which PDE4 inhibitors cause certain vessels to become targets of inflammation is unknown. Until recently, it was believed that PDE4 inhibitor-induced arteriopathies were non-primate-specific. However, a recent comprehensive toxico-logical study found that a PDE4 inhibitor, SCH 351591 (Schering Plough), produced, in Cynomolgus monkeys, acute to chronic inflammation of small to medium sized arteries in many tissues and organs (53). Thus, these findings of arteriopathy in primates, which were previously thought to be resistant to this toxicity, have serious implications for human risk, and it is noteworthy that Merck in 2003 abandoned development of their lead PDE4 inhibitor (licensed from Celltech Group) due to an incidence of colitis, raising the possibility that it was secondary to arteritis (54). This finding is a serious issue as COPD is a chronic disease requiring long-term therapy. Accordingly, a wide margin of safety will be needed because toxicity cannot be adequately monitored. Indeed, a major problem for the physician is that presentation of mesenteric ischemia is vague in humans and diagnostic tools are poor. Attempts by GSK to develop biomarkers of arteritis to assist the development of cilomilast have, to date, been unsuccessful. However, perhaps some comfort can be derived from the knowledge that no clinically relevant effects related to arteritis have been produced in patients treated for many years with bronchodilator doses of theophylline [which produces medial necrosis of mesenteric vessels in rats (55,56)] as well as more selective PDE4 inhibitors including rolipram and denbufylline (57).

E. Theophylline and PDE4 Inhibitors: A Comparison of their Safety, Tolerability, Drug Metabolism, and Pharmacokinetics

Despite the adverse-effect profile displayed by roflumilast and cilomilast in trials of COPD, the discovery of PDE4 inhibitors with an improved therapeutic ratio is likely to have distinct advantages over the nonselective PDE inhibitor theophylline. Table 4 shows a comparison of the drug metabolism and pharmacokinetics (DMPK) and clinical safety of theophylline and PDE4 inhibitors for which information is available. Perhaps the most striking difference is in the pharmacokinetics, which has implications for patient compliance and the extent to which the plasma concentration of these drugs requires

Table 4 A Comparison of the Mechanism of Action, DMPK, Safety, and Tolerability of Theophylline and PDE4 Inhibitors

	Theophylline	PDE4 Inhibitors[a]
Mechanism of action	Unclear (inhibition of PI-3Kδ; histone acetylation status) PDE inhibition only at high (>20 mg/L) doses	Selective inhibition of PDE4
DMPK		
Pharmacokinetics	Nonlinear Significant intersubject variability affected by age, smoking status and concomitant medication necessitating plasma monitoring	Linear providing dose proportional systemic exposure Low intersubject variability—no plasma monitoring required
Absorption	Variable, depends on formulation	Oral formulations (o.d. or b.i.d) $t_{max} \sim 1–2$ hours
Bioavailability	Variable, depends on formulation	>80%, unaffected by food or antacids
Half life	7–9 hours	7 hours (cilomilast); 16 hours (roflumilast)
Volume of distribution	500 mL/kg Plasma protein binding ~56%	Low High
Clearance	~400 mL/hr/kg Affected by genetic factors, cigarette smoking, coexisting pathology and drugs that affect hepatic metabolism	Low
Metabolism	~90% metabolized by liver (CYP1A2)	Negligible first pass hepatic metabolism
Drug interactions	High potential for drug interactions including propafenone, mexiletine, enoxacin, ciprofloxacin, cimetidine, propranolol, oral contraceptives, erythromycin, rifampicin, phenytoin, carbamazepine, phenobarbitone, isoprenaline, tobacco smoke	Low potential for drug interactions Can be taken with other drugs prescribed for asthma and COPD
Excretion	10% excreted unchanged via the kidneys	Depends on inhibitor
Dosing adjustment	May be required in cigarette smokers, the elderly, individuals with liver disease and subjects taking concomitant medication Contraindicated in individuals with heart disease, seizure disorders and gastroesophageal reflux	None accept in individuals with moderate hepatic and severe renal impairment Contraindicated in subjects with severe hepatic impairment
Clinical efficacy	Effective in a subset of patients with COPD Non-bronchodilator doses effective in asthma; steroid sparing	Phase III clinical trials ongoing
Safety and tolerability	Serious cardiovascular and CNS side-effects GI irritation, nausea, vomiting, insomnia in 10–15% of patients	No cardiovascular or CNS side-effects Headache, nausea, vomiting, arteriopathy(?)

[a] Details refer to cilomilast and roflumilast, which are in late Phase III clinical trials.

Abbreviations: CNS, central nervous system; COPD, chronic obstructive pulmonary disease; DMPK, drug metabolism and pharmacokinetics; GI, gastrointestinal; PDE, phosphodiesterase.

monitoring. At bronchodilator doses, intra- and intersubject variability to theophylline, together with a low therapeutic ratio, poses a significant clinical problem requiring careful titration with routine plasma monitoring to avoid serious cardiac and central nervous system side effects (58). This is a particular problem with smokers as polycyclic aromatic hydrocarbons present in the vapor phase of cigarette smoke are known to induce drug metabolizing enzymes including CYP1A1 and CYP1A2 (59–61). As theophylline is principally metabolized by CYP1A2 (62,63), dose adjustments are often necessary to compensate for the increased clearance in cigarette smokers (64–66). Age is another factor that has a marked effect on the pharmacokinetics of theophylline. Indeed, the clearance of theophylline decreases 15% to 28% in the elderly when compared to young adults, which probably reflects a decrease in the elimination of theophylline by CYP1A2 (67–69). In contrast, the pharmacokinetics of cilomilast and roflumilast are linear providing dose-proportional systemic exposure that is essentially unaffected by age and cigarette smoking status indicating that no dose adjustments will be necessary in elderly smoking subjects with COPD (10,50,52,58,70–74).

In addition to pharmacokinetic concerns, theophylline is prone to cause adverse events. These are particularly pronounced at plasma concentrations of 20 mg/L or greater although these unwanted actions can be offset by gradually titrating the dose of theophylline until the desired therapeutic level is achieved (75). In contrast, a major benefit of the PDE4 inhibitors in clinical trials is their superior safety and tolerability relative to theophylline. Although nausea and vomiting are not uncommon with second generation PDE4 inhibitors (new compounds need to be developed devoid of these "off-target" actions), they are usually of moderate severity and are reported to be self limiting (16). Moreover, PDE4 inhibitors are generally well tolerated in both short- and long-term dosing trials with a low incidence of serious adverse events; generally, they have no action at adenosine receptors and, with the exception of headache, there is no evidence from human trials of serious adverse cardiovascular activity (10,52) (but see section safety and tolerability of PDE4 inhibitors).

Another significant clinical problem is that theophylline has a high potential for drug interactions (10,52). Thus, in addition to CYP1A2, theophylline is also metabolized, albeit to a lesser extent, by CYP2E1 and CYP3A4. Accordingly, many drug interactions may occur including all of those indicated in Table 4. In contrast, PDE4 inhibitors have, in general, a far reduced propensity for drug interactions. With respect to cilomilast, none of the metabolic pathways involve, to any great extent, cytochrome P450 enzymes (CYP1A2, CYP2D6, CYP3A4) most susceptible to competitive inhibition by other drugs (72). Indeed, the only P450 enzyme implicated (CYP2C8), has few other substrates or inhibitors. Moreover, cilomilast does not inhibit any important hepatic cytochrome P450 enzymes in vitro (72). These data are supported by the finding that, at steady state, cilomilast has no clinically meaningful effect on the pharmacokinetics of digoxin, warfarin, theophylline, or prednisolone (72,76,77). Conversely, neither theophylline nor Maalox Plus, an antacid commonly used in the elderly that contains salts of calcium, magnesium, and/or aluminium that can alter the absorption or bioavailability of some drugs, had significantly influence the pharmacokinetics of cilomilast (78). Similar results have been reported for roflumilast (51,79). Thus, taken together these data demonstrate that the two most clinically advanced PDE4 inhibitors are not contraindicated with commonly prescribed medications for COPD and can be safely coadministered with these drugs. On balance, therefore, provided arteriopathies are not elicited at doses that are required to elicit unambiguous anti-inflammatory activity, then PDE4 inhibitors have significant advantages over theophylline from a pharmacokinetic, adverse-events, and drug interaction perspective.

F. Optimizing the Efficacy of PDE4 Inhibitors

A number of options are available that could result in PDE4 inhibitors with enhanced efficacy and an improved therapeutic ratio. Perhaps the most appealing is to synthesize compounds that are delivered topically (i.e., by inhalation) directly to the site of action. These compounds would not be bioavailable and, thus, systemic consequences including emetic liability and propensity to cause cardiovascular lesions should be minimized. This approach has been used in the past with the development of piclamilast (Rhone-Poulence Rorer—now Sanofi Aventis), AWD 12-241 (Elbion/GlaxoSmithKline), GSK 256066 (GlaxoSmithKline) and tofimilast (Pfizer) but, as yet, no PDE4 inhibitors of this type have reached the market.

Other possibilities of harnessing the therapeutic potential of PDE4 inhibitors are through the development of combination therapies. Indeed, clinical trials are underway with PDE4 inhibitor/muscarinic M_3-receptor antagonist combinations (see Ref. 39) and Union Chimique Belge Pharma have recently published on UCB 101333-3, a 4,6-diaminopyridine derivative, which is a potent dual M_3-receptor antagonist *and* PDE4 inhibitor (80). Such an approach could be more effective than either therapy alone as these drugs should improve lung function by interacting with complementary but mechanistically-distinct processes. Combining an inhaled PDE4 inhibitor with an ICS could also afford greater clinical benefit than either drug given as a monotherapy in the same way that long-acting β_2-agonist (LABA) LABA/ICS combinations deliver superior efficacy. The prospect of triple combination therapies incorporating a ultra long-acting β_2-agonist (ULABA), ICS and inhaled PDE4 inhibitor is also an appealing pharmacotherapeutic strategy. Finally, given that theophylline has been shown to improve FEV_1 in subjects with COPD by at least 100 mL (30), it is tempting to speculate that nonselective PDE inhibitors not based on the xanthine nucleus, which evokes many of the serious side effects reported with theophylline use, may prove to be the best therapeutic strategy for enhancing efficacy. Indeed, concurrent inhibition of multiple PDEs would be expected to exert clinically relevant effects, not achieved by selective PDE4 inhibition, on processes that contribute to the pathogenesis of chronic airflow limitation, including airway remodeling (PDE1-regulated), endothelial cell permeability (PDE2-regulated), airway smooth muscle tone (PDE3-regulated), and remodeling of the pulmonary vasculature (PDE5-regulated) (81).

III. Mucolytics

Mucus hypersecretion is a physiologically protective process that occurs in response to airways inflammation, infection, or after inhalation of irritants. However, the protracted and excessive secretion and retention of mucus within the airways is a pathology that can contribute to chronic airflow limitation seen in COPD. Accordingly, drugs that are able to normalize mucus secretion may play an important role in the management of the bronchitic component of COPD where mucus hypersecretion is a cardinal feature. Theoretically, mucus hypersecretion could be normalized with drugs that resolve airways inflammation or block the processes that govern secretion. Drugs that break down the molecular structure of mucus, thereby reducing its viscosity and aiding expectoration of sputum—so-called mucolytics—offer an alternative and widely adopted approach (82,83).

Many mucolytics have been marketed and continue to be clinically evaluated but therapeutic benefit in COPD has not been established (84); indeed, they neither improve FEV_1 nor arrest the decline in lung function. Consequently, the 2006 GOLD guidelines for the clinical management of COPD do not recommend mucolytics (see Ref. 85). However, in 2004, the National Institute for Clinical Excellence recommended that mucolytic therapy should be "...considered in patients with a chronic cough productive of sputum" and "...continued if there is symptomatic improvement (e.g., reduction in frequency of cough and sputum production)" (86). These recommendations are founded on the results of several meta-analyses (87–91), which were confirmed again in 2006 (92). Thus, relative to placebo, mucolytic therapy was associated with a highly significant reduction in the number of exacerbations, number of days of illness due to COPD, and number of days on prescribed antibiotics. The use of *N*-acetylcysteine, a commonly prescribed mucolytic, has also been significantly associated with a lower risk of hospitalization (93). Collectively, the implication of these finding is that mucolytic therapy is cost-effective, compared to placebo, reducing hospitalization and resource use, as well as the number of working days lost due to illness and associated indirect costs.

These beneficial effects of mucolytics relative to placebo explain the continued interest this class of drug for COPD. One of the more interesting compounds in clinical development is the thiol derivative erdosteine, which entered Phase II trials in the United States in 2006, although it is already marketed in over 30 countries worldwide. Erdosteine has been developed for the treatment of chronic obstructive bronchitis, including acute infective exacerbation of chronic bronchitis. It has been designed to reduce the production and viscosity of mucus, which should translate into improved mucociliary transport and expectoration of sputum (94). Erdosteine is also an antioxidant and is claimed to scavenge free radicals found in cigarette smoke (95).

In a double-blind, placebo-controlled, multicenter (10) study (the EQUALIFE trial), 155 outpatients with moderate COPD ($FEV_1 < 70\%$ predicted; smoking history > 20 pack years) were randomized to receive erdosteine (orally 300 b.i.d) or placebo for eight months (96). The study was performed during the winter season to assess the effect of treatments on exacerbation rate, hospitalization, lung function, six-minute walking test and quality of life; the results were also analyzed from a pharmacoeconomical perspective. One hundred and twenty four subjects completed the study (placebo: $n = 61$; erdosteine: $n = 63$). Subjects in the erdosteine treatment group had significantly fewer exacerbations and were hospitalized less frequently than individuals in the placebo treatment group. Moreover, patients receiving erdosteine showed no reduction in lung function over the duration of the trial and reported a significant improvement in health-related quality of life as assessed by the SGRQ and SF-36 short form survey (96). In addition, at the end of the study the mean total COPD-related costs per patient were lower in the erdosteine treatment group when compared to those individuals who received placebo. It is unclear whether the beneficial effect of erdosteine in this trial is due to its antioxidant and/or mucolytic activity since the findings are consistent with the latest Cochrane review meta-analysis on mucolytic reagents in COPD (92). Regardless, based on the results of the EQUALIFE trial,

Moretti and colleagues (96) suggest that erdosteine is likely to make an important contribution to the therapy of patients with symptomatic COPD.

IV. Other New Chemical Entities for COPD

Other than ULABAs and long-acting muscarinic M_3-receptor antagonists (aka anticholinergics), which are discussed in Chapter 15, there are few novel therapies for COPD that have, thus far, progressed into clinical trials (Table 1). Nevertheless, two novel targets that could be exploited to therapeutic advantage merit discussion here. These are CXC chemokine receptor 2 ($CXCR_2$) and peroxisome proliferator-activated receptor (PPAR)$_\gamma$; drugs that interact with both of these receptors are, or have been, evaluated in the clinic.

A. $CXCR_2$ as a Novel Target

Chemokine receptor antagonists that prevent the recruitment of neutrophils in to the lung are one class of compound that have entered Phase I evaluation and deserve mention here (97). Several, so-called, CXC chemokines have been identified including IL-8 and growth-related oncogene (GRO) α that are potent chemoattractants for neutrophils and exert their activity by interacting with the $CXCR_2$ receptor. Significantly, the level of these chemokines is elevated in subjects with COPD and is correlated with disease severity (98,99). Thus, compounds that antagonize the effect of IL-8, GROα and related chemokines at $CXCR_2$ such as GSK 656933 (GlaxoSmith-Kline) and AZD 8309 (AstraZeneca) may be beneficial in alleviating neutrophilic inflammation in COPD (100). These drugs may have an added advantage as the recruitment of monocytes to the lungs, and ultimate pulmonary macrophage burden, may also be reduced due to coincident expression of $CXCR_2$ on these cells (101).

B. PPARγ as a Novel Target

Another group of compound that merits brief discussion are the thiazolidinediones. Rosiglitazone is one such example that was developed and is now marketed for the treatment of Type II diabetes (102). Compounds within this class bind to a nuclear hormone receptor called PPARγ and promote transcription of a variety of genes and many of these have clear anti-inflammatory potential. The possibility that rosiglitazone or related ligands could afford benefit in disorders other than diabetes is suggested by a wealth of preclinical data (103,104) and studies in asthma and COPD are awaited with interest. The substantive advantage of demonstrating efficacy of rosiglitazone in other inflammatory indications is the speed to which the drug could come to market, since only relative few additional clinical trials would need to be conducted.

V. Concluding Remarks

The decision by the pharmaceutical industry to develop second generation PDE4 inhibitors for the treatment of COPD is based on a conceptually robust hypothesis that is supported by a wealth of preclinical data. Therefore, it is highly likely that if approved and shown to be potentially disease-modifying in clinical trials, PDE4 inhibitors will offer physicians a novel class of drug to treat patients in whom lung function is compromised by emphysema and/or bronchitis. That said, it is the view of this author that neither cilomilast nor roflumilast, given as a monotherapy, will be licensed for use in the European Union or North America for the management of chronic airflow limitation in COPD. Further major refinements in the design and/or use of PDE4 inhibitors are still necessary to improve their therapeutic ratio if major clinical benefit is to be achieved. Several options are available (Discussed in section Optimizing the Efficacy of PDE4 Inhibitors.) and some of these are currently being evaluated in clinical trials. Thus, it is likely that several more years will elapse before we can assess whether the initial optimism in PDE4 inhibitors will be realized.

The ability of mucolytics to reduce exacerbation frequency, hospitalizations, health care resource utilization, and improve health-related quality of life provides a strong rationale for retaining this class of drug in the limited armory of therapies that can be used to treat smoking-related chronic airflow limitation. Thus, despite the fact that current GOLD guidelines do not recommend mucolytics for the clinical management of COPD, current data accrued from a large number of trials suggest that these drugs may, indeed, have therapeutic benefit, especially in the subpopulation of individuals who present with chronic cough productive of sputum, which is indicative of chronic obstructive bronchitis.

Of the other novel therapies being developed for COPD (Table 1), $CXCR_2$ antagonists and $PPAR\gamma$ agonists show particular promise as novel anti-inflammatory therapies. However, it is too soon to gauge whether they will emerge as effective treatment options and, with respect to $CXCR_2$ antagonists, the results of Phase III pivotal efficacy trials are many years away. Thus, in the short term, the pharmacotherapy of COPD is limited to corticosteroids, LABA/corticosteroid combination therapies and drugs that provide symptomatic relief. This is a most unsatisfactory and worrying situation for a disease that afflicts globally 9% to 10% of the population over the age of 40 years (105).

Acknowledgments

The author is an Alberta Heritage Foundation of Medical Research Senior Scholar and is funded by the Canadian Institutes of Health Research.

References

1. Briggs DD. Chronic obstructive pulmonary disease overview: prevalence, pathogenesis, and treatment. J Manag Care Pharm 2004; 10:S3–10.
2. Anto JM, Vermeire P, Vestbo J, et al. Epidemiology of chronic obstructive pulmonary disease. Eur Respir J 2001; 17:982–94.
3. Almagro P, Calbo E, Ochoa dE, et al. Mortality after hospitalization for COPD. Chest 2002; 121:1441–8.
4. Hurd S. The impact of COPD on lung health worldwide: epidemiology and incidence. Chest 2000; 117:1S–4.
5. Alsaeedi A, Sin DD, McAlister FA. The effects of inhaled corticosteroids in chronic obstructive pulmonary disease: a systematic review of randomized placebo-controlled trials. Am J Med 2002; 113:59–65.
6. Barnes PJ. Inhaled corticosteroids are not beneficial in chronic obstructive pulmonary disease. Am J Respir Crit Care Med 2000; 161:342–4.
7. Mealy NE, Bayes M. Treatment of respiratory disorders. Drugs Future 2005; 30:59–112.

8. Torphy TJ. Phosphodiesterase isozymes: molecular targets for novel anti-asthma agents. Am J Respir Crit Care Med 1998; 157:351–70.

9. Torphy TJ, Barnette MS, Underwood DC, et al. Ariflo (SB 207499) a second generation phosphodiesterase 4 inhibitor for the treatment of asthma and COPD: from concept to clinic. Pulm Pharmacol Ther 1999; 12:131–5.

10. Giembycz MA. Cilomilast: a second generation phosphodiesterase 4 inhibitor for asthma and chronic obstructive pulmonary disease. Expert Opin Investig Drugs 2001; 10:1361–79.

11. Zeller E, Stief HJ, Pflug B, et al. Results of a phase II study of the antidepressant effect of rolipram. Pharmacopsychiatry 1984; 17:188–90.

12. Bertolino A, Crippa D, di Dio S, et al. Rolipram versus imipramine in inpatients with major, "minor" or atypical depressive disorder: a double-blind double-dummy study aimed at testing a novel therapeutic approach. Int Clin Psychopharmacol 1988; 3:245–53.

13. GlaxoSmithKline. SB 207499 (Ariflo, Cilomilast)—New Drugs Application (21-573). Pulmonary and Allergy Drug Products Advisory Committee. Summary of Clinical Pharmacology and Biopharmaceutics Findings, 2003. http://www.fda.gov/ohrms/dockets/ac/03/briefing/3976B1_02_E-FDA-Tab%204.pdf (last accessed September 4, 2007).

14. GlaxoSmithKline. SB 207499 (Ariflo, Cilomilast)—New Drugs Application (21-573). Pulmonary and Allergy Drug Products Advisory Committee. Overview of Clinical Development Program, 2003. http://www.fda.gov/ohrms/dockets/ac/03/briefing/3976B1_01_E-Glaxo-Overview%20Clinical%20Dev.pdf (last accessed September 4, 2007).

15. GlaxoSmithKline. SB 207499 (Ariflo, Cilomilast)—New Drugs Application (21-573). Pulmonary and Allergy Drug Products Advisory Committee Briefing Document, 2003. http://www.fda.gov/ohrms/dockets/ac/03/briefing/3976B1_02_D-FDA-%20Tab%203.pdf (last accessed September 4, 2007).

16. Compton CH, Gubb J, Nieman R, et al. Cilomilast, a selective phosphodiesterase-4 inhibitor for treatment of patients with chronic obstructive pulmonary disease: a randomised, dose-ranging study. Lancet 2001; 358:265–70.

17. GlaxoSmithKline. SB 207499 (Ariflo, Cilomilast)—New Drugs Application (21-573). Pulmonary and Allergy Drug Products Advisory Committee. Pivotal Studies, 2003. http://www.fda.gov/ohrms/dockets/ac/03/briefing/3976B1_01_G-Glaxo-Pivotal%20Studies.pdf (last accessed September 4, 2007).

18. Compton C, Gubb J, Cedar E, et al. Ariflo (SB 207499) a second generation, oral PDE4 inhibitor, improves quality of life in patients with COPD. Am J Respir Crit Care Med 1999; 159:A522.

19. GlaxoSmithKline. SB 207499 (Ariflo, Cilomilast)—New Drugs Application (21-573). Pulmonary and Allergy Drug Products Advisory Committee. Clinical Pharmacology, 2003. http://www.fda.gov/ohrms/dockets/ac/03/briefing/3976B1_01_D-Glaxo-Clinical%20Pharmacology.pdf (last accessed September 4, 2007).

20. Rennard SI, Schachter N, Strek M, et al. Cilomilast for COPD: results of a 6-month, placebo-controlled study of a potent, selective inhibitor of phosphodiesterase 4. Chest 2006; 129:56–66.

21. GlaxoSmithKline. SB 207499 (Ariflo, Cilomilast)—New Drugs Application (21-573). Pulmonary and Allergy Drug Products Advisory Committee. Study Design—Pivotal Studies, 2003. http://www.fda.gov/ohrms/dockets/ac/03/briefing/3976B1_01_F-Glaxo-Study%20Design-Pivotal%20Studies.pdf (last accessed September 4, 2007).

22. Edelson JD, Compton C, Nieman R, et al. Cilomilast (Ariflo), a potent, selective inhibitor of phosphodiesterase 4, improves lung function in patients with COPD: results of a 6-month trial. Am J Respir Crit Care Med 2001; 163:A277.

23. Ramsdell J, Edelson J, Compton C, et al. Cilomilast, a potent, selective inhibitor of phosphodiesterase 4, improves small airway function in patients with chronic obstructive pulmonary disease. Eur Respir J 2001; 16:94s.

24. Rodriguez-Roisin R. Toward a consensus definition for COPD exacerbations. Chest 2000; 117:398S–401.

25. Kelsen S, Rennard SI, Chodosh S, et al. COPD exacerbation in a 6-month trial of cilomilast (Ariflo), a potent, selective phosphodiesterase 4 inhibitor. Am J Respir Crit Care Med 2002; 165:A271.

26. Jones PW, Quirk FH, Baveystock CM, et al. A self-complete measure of health status for chronic airflow limitation. The St. George's Respiratory Questionnaire. Am Rev Respir Dis 1992; 145:1321–7.

27. GlaxoSmithKline. SB 207499 (Ariflo, Cilomilast)—New Drugs Application (21-573). Pulmonary and Allergy Drug Products Advisory Committee. Transcript of Hearing held on 5 September 2003 at the Holiday Inn Gaithersburg, Gaithersburg, Maryland, U.S.A., 2003. http://www.fda.gov/ohrms/dockets/ac/03/transcripts/3976T1.doc (last accessed September 4, 2007).

28. van Grunsven PM, van Schayck CP, Derenne JP, et al. Long term effects of inhaled corticosteroids in chronic obstructive pulmonary disease: a meta-analysis. Thorax 1999; 54:7–14.
29. Ram FS, Sestini P. Regular inhaled short acting β_2 agonists for the management of stable chronic obstructive pulmonary disease: Cochrane systematic review and meta-analysis. Thorax 2003; 58:580–4.
30. Ram FS, Jardin JR, Atallah A, et al. Efficacy of theophylline in people with stable chronic obstructive pulmonary disease: a systematic review and meta-analysis. Respir Med 2005; 99:135–44.
31. GlaxoSmithKline. SB 207499 (Ariflo, Cilomilast)—New Drugs Application (21-573). Pulmonary and Allergy Drug Products Advisory Committee. Introduction and Background, 2003. http://www.fda.gov/ohrms/dockets/ac/03/briefing/3976B1_01_B-Glaxo-Intro-Background.pdf (last accessed September 4, 2007).
32. Gamble E, Grootendorst DC, Brightling CE, et al. Anti-inflammatory effects of the phosphodiesterase-4 inhibitor cilomilast (Ariflo) in chronic obstructive pulmonary disease. Am J Respir Crit Care Med 2003; 168:976–82.
33. Belman MJ, Botnick WC, Shin JW. Inhaled bronchodilators reduce dynamic hyperinflation during exercise in patients with chronic obstructive pulmonary disease. Am J Respir Crit Care Med 1996; 153:967–75.
34. GlaxoSmithKline. SB 207499 (Ariflo, Cilomilast)—New Drugs Application (21-573). Pulmonary and Allergy Drug Products Advisory Committee. Supporting Studies, 2003. http://www.fda.gov/ohrms/dockets/ac/03/briefing/3976B1_01_H-Glaxo-Supporting%20Studies.pdf (last accessed September 4, 2007).
35. O'Donnell DE, Revill SM, Webb KA. Dynamic hyperinflation and exercise intolerance in chronic obstructive pulmonary disease. Am J Respir Crit Care Med 2001; 164:770–7.
36. Gibson GJ. Pulmonary hyperinflation: a clinical overview. Eur Respir J 1996; 9:2640–9.
37. Pellegrino R, Brusasco V. On the causes of lung hyperinflation during bronchoconstriction. Eur Respir J 1997; 10:468–75.
38. Zamel N, McClean P, Zhu J, et al. Effect of cilomilast (*Ariflo*) on trapped gas volume and indices of hyperinflation in patients with chronic obstructive lung disease. Am J Respir Crit Care Med 2002; 165:A226.
39. http://www.clinicaltrials.gov/ct/search;jsessionid= 628D4D1FDE10D07C7D6651C13193C47E?term=roflumilast (last accessed September 4, 2007).
40. Rabe KF, Bateman ED, O'Donnell D, et al. Roflumilast: an oral anti-inflammatory treatment for chronic obstructive pulmonary disease: a randomised controlled trial. Lancet 2005; 366:563–71.
41. Bergmann JF. Roflumilast for chronic obstructive pulmonary disease. Lancet 2005; 366:1845–7.
42. Morice AH. Roflumilast for chronic obstructive pulmonary disease. Lancet 2005; 366:1845–7.
43. Eller P, Pechlaner C. Roflumilast for chronic obstructive pulmonary disease. Lancet 2005; 366:1845–6.
44. Boyd AE, Bhowmik A, Rajakulasingam K. Roflumilast for chronic obstructive pulmonary disease. Lancet 2005; 366:1846–7.
45. Vassiliou V. Roflumilast for chronic obstructive pulmonary disease. Lancet 2005; 366:1846–7.
46. Hughes EG. Randomized clinical trials: the meeting place of medical practice and clinical research. Semin Reprod Med 2003; 21:55–64.
47. Rabe KF. Roflumilast for chronic obstructive pulmonary disease. Lancet 2005; 366:1846–7 (author's reply).
48. Grootendorst DC, Gauw SA, Baan R, et al. Does a single dose of the phosphodiesterase 4 inhibitor, cilomilast (15 mg), induce bronchodilation in patients with chronic obstructive pulmonary disease? Pulm Pharmacol Ther 2003; 16:115–20.
49. Calverley PMA, Sanchez-Toril F, McIvor A, et al. Effect of one year treatment with roflumilast in severe chronic obstructive lung disease. Am J Respir Crit Care Med 2007; 176:154–61.
50. Bethke TD, Bohmer GM, Hermann R, et al. Dose-proportional intra-individual single- and repeated-dose pharmacokinetics of roflumilast, an oral, once-daily phosphodiesterase 4 inhibitor. J Clin Pharmacol 2007; 47:26–36.
51. Bethke TD, Giessmann T, Westphal K, et al. Roflumilast, a once-daily oral phosphodiesterase 4 inhibitor, lacks relevant pharmacokinetic interactions with inhaled salbutamol when co-administered in healthy subjects. Int J Clin Pharmacol Ther 2006; 44:572–9.
52. Giembycz MA. Development status of second generation PDE4 inhibitors for asthma and COPD: the story so far. Monaldi Arch Chest Dis 2002; 57:48–64.
53. Losco PE, Evans EW, Barat SA, et al. The toxicity of SCH 351591, a novel phosphodiesterase-4 inhibitor, in Cynomolgus monkeys. Toxicol Pathol 2004; 32:295–308.

54. Data Monitor. Press Release: Merck discontinues development of PDE4 inhibitor compound, 2003. http://www.datamonitor.com/ ~ 90c3cffcaf0546f7ad089c97929631c8 ~ /companies/company/?pid= E915DFB3-6FBF-4C67-AE8F-29EB1160FC4C&nid=816AB3F2-982C-44B3-887C-3451-D89A6362&type=NewsWire&article=1 (last accessed September 4, 2007).

55. Nyska A, Herbert RA, Chan PC, et al. Theophylline-induced mesenteric periarteritis in F344/N rats. Arch Toxicol 1998; 72:731–7.

56. Collins JJ, Elwell MR, Lamb JC, et al. Subchronic toxicity of orally administered (gavage and dosed-feed) theophylline in Fischer 344 rats and B6C3F1 mice. Fundam Appl Toxicol 1988; 11:472–84.

57. GlaxoSmithKline. SB 207499 (Ariflo, Cilomilast)—New Drugs Application (21-573). Pulmonary and Allergy Drug Products Advisory Committee. Non-clinical Findings, 2003. http://www.fda.gov/ohrms/dockets/ac/03/briefing/3976B1_01_C-Glaxo-Nonclinical%20Findings.pdf (last accessed September 4, 2007).

58. Vignola AM. PDE4 inhibitors in COPD—a more selective approach to treatment. Respir Med 2004; 98:495–503.

59. Shimada T, Iwasaki M, Martin MV, et al. Human liver microsomal cytochrome P-450 enzymes involved in the bioactivation of procarcinogens detected by *umu* gene response in *Salmonella typhimurium* TA 1535/pSK1002. Cancer Res 1989; 49:3218–28.

60. Campbell ME, Spielberg SP, Kalow W. A urinary metabolite ratio that reflects systemic caffeine clearance. Clin Pharmacol Ther 1987; 42:157–65.

61. Vistisen K, Poulsen HE, Loft S. Foreign compound metabolism capacity in man measured from metabolites of dietary caffeine. Carcinogenesis 1992; 13:1561–8.

62. Fuhr U, Doehmer J, Battula N, et al. Biotransformation of caffeine and theophylline in mammalian cell lines genetically engineered for expression of single cytochrome P450 isoforms. Biochem Pharmacol 1992; 43:225–35.

63. Sarkar MA, Hunt C, Guzelian PS, et al. Characterization of human liver cytochromes P-450 involved in theophylline metabolism. Drug Metab Dispos 1992; 20:31–7.

64. Jusko WJ. Influence of cigarette smoking on drug metabolism in man. Drug Metab Rev 1979; 9:221–36.

65. Jusko WJ, Schentag JJ, Clark JH, et al. Enhanced biotransformation of theophylline in marihuana and tobacco smokers. Clin Pharmacol Ther 1978; 24:405–10.

66. Hunt SN, Jusko WJ, Yurchak AM. Effect of smoking on theophylline disposition. Clin Pharmacol Ther 1976; 19:546–51.

67. Antal EJ, Kramer PA, Mercik SA, et al. Theophylline pharmacokinetics in advanced age. Br J Clin Pharmacol 1981; 12:637–45.

68. Ohnishi A, Kato M, Kojima J, et al. Differential pharmacokinetics of theophylline in elderly patients. Drugs Aging 2003; 20:71–84.

69. Shin SG, Juan D, Rammohan M. Theophylline pharmacokinetics in normal elderly subjects. Clin Pharmacol Ther 1988; 44:522–30.

70. Zussman BD, Benincosa LJ, Webber DM, et al. An overview of the pharmacokinetics of cilomilast (Ariflo), a new, orally active phosphodiesterase 4 inhibitor, in healthy young and elderly volunteers. J Clin Pharmacol 2001; 41:950–8.

71. Murdoch RD, Zussman B, Schofield JP, et al. Lack of pharmacokinetic interactions between cilomilast and theophylline or smoking in healthy volunteers. J Clin Pharmacol 2004; 44:1046–53.

72. Down G, Siederer S, Lim S, et al. Clinical pharmacology of cilomilast. Clin Pharmacokinet 2006; 45:217–33.

73. Bethke TD, Hunnemeyer A, Hauns B, et al. Smoking has no effect on the pharmacokinetics of roflumilast, a new, orally active selective PDE4 inhibitor. Eur Respir J 2001; 15:156s.

74. Hauns B, Hermann R, Hunnemeyer A, et al. Investigation of a potential food effect on the pharmacokinetics of roflumilast, an oral, once-daily phosphodiesterase 4 inhibitor, in healthy subjects. J Clin Pharmacol 2006; 46:1146–53.

75. Barnes PJ. Theophylline: new perspectives for an old drug. Am J Respir Crit Care Med 2003; 167:813–8.

76. Zussman BD, Kelly J, Murdoch RD, et al. Cilomilast: pharmacokinetic and pharmacodynamic interactions with digoxin. Clin Ther 2001; 23:921–31.

77. Kelly J, Murdoch RD, Clark DJ, et al. Warfarin pharmacodynamics unaffected by cilomilast. Ann Pharmacother 2001; 35:1535–9.

78. Zussman BD, Davie CC, Kelly J, et al. Bioavailability of the oral selective phosphodiesterase 4 inhibitor cilomilast. Pharmacotherapy 2001; 21:653–60.

79. Nassr N, Lahu G, von Richter O, et al. Lack of a pharmacokinetic interaction between steady-state roflumilast and single-dose midazolam in healthy subjects. Br J Clin Pharmacol 2007; 63:365–70.

80. Provins L, Christophe B, Danhaive P, et al. First dual M_3 antagonists-PDE4 inhibitors: synthesis and SAR of 4,6-diaminopyrimidine derivatives. Bioorg Med Chem Lett 2006; 16:1834–9.

81. Giembycz MA. Re-inventing the wheel: non-selective phosphodiesterase inhibitors for chronic inflammatory diseases. In: Beavo JA, Francis SH, Houslay MD, eds. Cyclic Nucleotide Phosphodiesterases in Health and Disease. Boca Raton: CRC Press, 2007:649–65.

82. Rogers DF. The role of airway secretions in COPD: pathophysiology, epidemiology and pharmacotherapeutic options. COPD 2005; 2:341–53.

83. Rogers DF, Barnes PJ. Treatment of airway mucus hyper-secretion. Ann Med 2006; 38:116–25.

84. http://goldcopd.com/Guidelineitem.asp?l1=2&l2=1&intId=996 (last accessed September 4, 2007).

85. Rogers DF. Mucoactive drugs for asthma and COPD: any place in therapy? Expert Opin Investig Drugs 2002; 11:15–35.

86. National Institute for Clinical Excellence (NICE). Chronic obstructive pulmonary disease. National clinical guideline on management of chronic obstructive pulmonary disease in adults in primary and secondary care—Managing stable COPD. Thorax 2004; 59:i39–130.

87. Poole PJ, Black PN. Mucolytic agents for chronic bronchitis or chronic obstructive pulmonary disease. Cochrane Database Syst Rev 2003; CD001287.

88. Poole PJ, Black PN. Mucolytic agents for chronic bronchitis or chronic obstructive pulmonary disease. Cochrane Database Syst Rev 2000; CD001287.

89. Poole PJ, Black PN. Oral mucolytic drugs for exacerbations of chronic obstructive pulmonary disease: systematic review. Br Med J 2001; 322:1271–4.

90. Grandjean EM, Berthet P, Ruffmann R, et al. Efficacy of oral long-term N-acetylcysteine in chronic bronchopulmonary disease: a meta-analysis of published double-blind, placebo-controlled clinical trials. Clin Ther 2000; 22:209–21.

91. Stey C, Steurer J, Bachmann S, et al. The effect of oral N-acetylcysteine in chronic bronchitis: a quantitative systematic review. Eur Respir J 2000; 16:253–62.

92. Poole PJ, Black PN. Mucolytic agents for chronic bronchitis or chronic obstructive pulmonary disease. Cochrane Database Syst Rev 2006; 3:CD001287.

93. Gerrits CM, Herings RM, Leufkens HG, et al. N-acetylcysteine reduces the risk of re-hospitalisation among patients with chronic obstructive pulmonary disease. Eur Respir J 2003; 21:795–8.

94. Dechant KL, Noble S. Erdosteine. Drugs 1996; 52:875–81.

95. Moretti M, Marchioni CF. An overview of erdosteine antioxidant activity in experimental research. Pharmacol Res 2007; 55:249–54 (epub—ahead of print).

96. Moretti M, Bottrighi P, Dallari R, et al. The effect of long-term treatment with erdosteine on chronic obstructive pulmonary disease: the EQUALIFE Study. Drugs Exp Clin Res 2004; 30:143–52.

97. Panina P, Mariani M, D'Ambrosio D. Chemokine receptors in chronic obstructive pulmonary disease (COPD). Curr Drug Targets 2006; 7:669–74.

98. Traves SL, Culpitt SV, Russell RE, et al. Increased levels of the chemokines GROα and MCP-1 in sputum samples from patients with COPD. Thorax 2002; 57:590–5.

99. Keatings VM, Collins PD, Scott DM, et al. Differences in interleukin-8 and tumor necrosis factor-α in induced sputum from patients with chronic obstructive pulmonary disease or asthma. Am J Respir Crit Care Med 1996; 153:530–4.

100. Donnelly LE, Barnes PJ. Chemokine receptors as therapeutic targets in chronic obstructive pulmonary disease. Trends Pharmacol Sci 2006; 27:546–53.

101. Traves SL, Smith SJ, Barnes PJ, et al. Specific CXC but not CC chemokines cause elevated monocyte migration in COPD: a role for $CXCR_2$. J Leukoc Biol 2004; 76:441–50.

102. Wagstaff AJ, Goa KL. Rosiglitazone: a review of its use in the management of type 2 diabetes mellitus. Drugs 2002; 62:1805–37.

103. Spears M, McSharry C, Thomson NC. Peroxisome proliferator-activated receptor-γ agonists as potential anti-inflammatory agents in asthma and chronic obstructive pulmonary disease. Clin Exp Allergy 2006; 36:1494–504.

104. Belvisi MG, Hele DJ, Birrell MA. Peroxisome proliferator-activated receptor-γ agonists as therapy for chronic airway inflammation. Eur J Pharmacol 2006; 533:101–9.

105. Halbert RJ, Natoli JL, Gano A, et al. Global burden of COPD: systematic review and meta-analysis. Eur Respir J 2006; 28:523–32.

17

Managing Exacerbations: An Overview

J. J. SOLER-CATALUÑA
Unidad de Neumología, Servicio de Medicina Interna, Hospital General de Requena, Requena, Valencia, Spain

ROBERTO RODRÍGUEZ-ROISIN
Servei de Pneumologia, Hospital Clínic, Universitat de Barcelona, Barcelona, Spain

I. Introduction

The clinical course of chronic obstructive pulmonary disease (COPD) includes frequent episodes of increased severity of symptoms, commonly referred to as exacerbations. At first glance, such episodes of clinical instability were considered mere epiphenomena in the natural history of COPD. However, recent emerging evidence indicates that, quite to the contrary, exacerbations greatly contribute to the decline of health-related quality of life (HRQoL) (1), have a negative impact on disease progression (2,3), and increase the risk of mortality (4). In addition, exacerbations cause enormous socioeconomic costs including utilization of health care resources (5). This challenge to the traditional point of view corresponds to a shift in how we currently conceive the natural history of COPD, now seen not simply as chronic airflow limitation, but rather as a complex and multidimensional disease in which lung and systemic inflammation play a significant etiopathogenic role.

Recent studies suggest that frequent exacerbations produce a faster decline in pulmonary function (2,3), thereby contributing to disease progression. However, these effects that account approximately for 25% of forced expiratory volume in one second (FEV_1) annual decline (6) are not enough to explain the overall impact of exacerbation on symptoms, HRQoL, and prognosis. Other domains of COPD can also deteriorate as a result of exacerbations, which in turn produce even worse consequences. During exacerbations, there is an amplification of the basal airway inflammation (7,8) resulting in further airflow limitation, acute-on-chronic lung hyperinflation, and pulmonary gas exchange defects along with worsening of any coexisting cardiovascular disturbances (9,10). Furthermore, exacerbations are associated with systemic inflammation, which may lead to systemic manifestations (7,11). After exacerbations, the recovery is sometimes incomplete (12). However, there are conflicting data as to whether exacerbations are associated with a step-like decline in physiology or whether patients generally return to their pre-exacerbation status. In one study, lung function and symptoms had not returned to baseline values after five weeks following the onset of the acute events in approximately 25% of exacerbations; and by three months there was still a significant level of non-recovery following exacerbation (12). If inflammatory markers do not return to pre-exacerbation levels, it is likely that the increased ongoing airway inflammation would influence the subsequent decline in lung function. Persistent systemic inflammation also can influence the systemic component of the disease. Therefore, reducing exacerbations and decreasing their severity may have a positive impact on the natural history of COPD. This chapter reviews the evidence for management of COPD exacerbation while focusing on prevention and treatment, both requiring a multidisciplinary approach due to the pathophysiologic heterogeneity of exacerbations.

II. Pathophysiology

Expiratory flow limitation (EFL), as a consequence of airway inflammation, is the pathophysiologic hallmark of COPD (13). It is reasonable to assume that worsening airway inflammation is the primary inciting event of COPD exacerbations and may be caused by bacteria, viruses, and/or environmental pollutants, including cigarette smoke. However, relationships between airway inflammation, etiology, and frequency and severity in COPD exacerbations have not been sufficiently well established as yet. Increased airway inflammation induces many pathologic changes on the airway, namely increased mucus production, airway wall thickening, airway wall edema, and bronchoconstriction, which altogether cause airway narrowing acutely leading to EFL together with lung hyperinflation (Fig. 1) (13,14). The latter increases the work of the respiratory muscles and oxygen consumption resulting in decreased mixed venous oxygen tension (9). Airway narrowing also increases ventilation-perfusion (V_A/Q) inequalities, and a greater proportion of pulmonary blood flow is diverted to alveolar units with a low V_A/Q ratio (9,10). The combination of the latter mechanisms worsens pulmonary gas exchange more intensely in patients with severe COPD exacerbations. The acutely worsened lung hyperinflation superimposed on that chronically present may also reduce right ventricular preload as a result of impaired venous return. Consistent with this, pulmonary artery pressures are generally higher at any cardiac output in patients with COPD than in healthy subjects (13), particularly during exacerbations.

During exacerbations there is also an increase in systemic inflammation (11), although there is limited information regarding the persistence of these effects. Recently, a study has been completed showing changes in inflammatory markers and in exacerbation frequency over a seven-year period (15). Patients with frequent exacerbations had a faster rise in plasma fibrinogen over time, suggesting that this patient population may be at greater risk of further cardiovascular morbidity.

Although increased pulmonary inflammation is thought to be central to the pathogenesis of COPD, not all exacerbations are associated with increased inflammation (16). The mechanisms of acute worsening of EFL in the absence of airway inflammation are less well understood. There are common clinical conditions often associated with COPD which easily mimic and/or amplify the impact of exacerbations, including pulmonary (pneumonia, pneumothorax, pleural effusion, lung cancer, upper airway obstruction, rib fracture), cardiovascular (pulmonary embolism, right/left heart failure), and drug-related (sedatives, narcotics) conditions (17). Some of these are difficult to differentiate from COPD exacerbation. A French study (18) has shown that 25% of COPD exacerbation of unknown etiology is associated with pulmonary embolism, while approximately 31% of severe exacerbations admitted to an intensive care unit (ICU) are associated with left-heart dysfunction (19). The first finding has to be contrasted,

Pathophysiologic events during COPD exacerbations

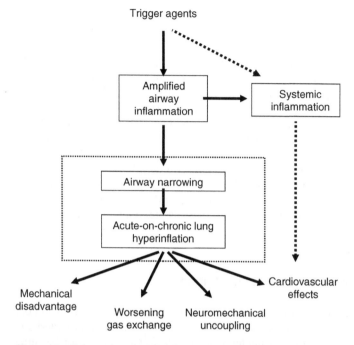

Figure 1 Schematic of pathophysiologic events in COPD exacerbation. The triggering event(s), which may be varied, lead to airway and systemic inflammation, airway narrowing, and dynamic hyperinflation. This, in turn, results in several additional consequences that can lead to symptoms.

however, with a more recent report of a modest 6% prevalence of pulmonary embolism in COPD exacerbations requiring hospitalization (20).

III. Prevention of Exacerbations

Exacerbation frequency is an important determinant of COPD-related economic cost, health status, lung function, and prognosis (1–5). Thus, prevention of exacerbations is a major therapeutic goal. Recently, in an observational prospective cohort study of over 304 male patients, we showed that exacerbation frequency increased the risk of death (4). Patients who had one or two severe exacerbations attending the hospital, either as an emergency visit or an admission to hospital, increased the risk of death by a twofold [95% confidence interval (CI): 1.01–3.98] and those who were frequent exacerbators (three or more exacerbations) who had a fourfold risk (95% CI: 1.80–9.45) of death compared with patients who did not exacerbate. Severity of exacerbation was also important, because hospitalized patients had a higher risk of death than those who were attended in the emergency room and were not eventually admitted (4). Frequency of COPD exacerbations is also a determinant of HRQoL. Seemungal et al. (1) have shown that patients who had frequent exacerbations had lower scores on the St. George

Respiratory Questionnaire, i.e., worse HRQoL, an effect that was independent of severity of disease. Andersson and colleagues have calculated that the cost of treating COPD exacerbations averages 35% to 45% of the entire costs of managing COPD as a disease (21). Severe COPD exacerbations requiring a visit to the emergency room or resulting in a hospitalization were on average 10 times more expensive than those that were moderate, defined as requiring a visit to a primary care physician or to a hospital outpatient clinic. Severe exacerbations were 60 times more expensive than mild-to-moderate exacerbations that involved telephone contact with a health care center and/or treatment with antibiotics and/or systemic corticosteroids. Accordingly, prevention strategies should reduce not only the number of exacerbations but also decrease their severity. Several approaches can be suggested to minimize the impact of exacerbations, including: (*i*) prevention of some of the triggers (i.e., infectious agents); (*ii*) minimizing the inflammatory response (anti-inflammatory therapy); (*iii*) improvement of lung mechanics through the use of long-acting inhaled bronchodilators; and/or (*iv*) improvement of the patient's ability to withstand the effects of an acute infective/inflammatory insult that has precipitated the exacerbation (i.e., nonpharmacologic treatment).

IV. Prevention of Infective Exacerbations

Many exacerbations occur as a consequence of bacterial and/or viral lower respiratory tract infections (22), the latter being especially important when there is underlying chronic bronchial colonization (see Chapter 15). Therefore, vaccination for bacterial and viral infections or eradication treatment for bacterial colonization could have important beneficial consequences.

A. Benefits of Vaccination

The most common viruses identified in COPD exacerbations are rhinoviruses and respiratory syncytial virus. However, we presently lack effective methods of preventing viral infections. Together, influenza A and B account for 5.4% of exacerbations (23), but there is reasonable evidence showing that immunization with an appropriate polyvalent vaccine can be effective (24,25). A recent Cochrane's review (25) only selected six randomized controlled trials (RCTs) performed in COPD patients. Inactive vaccine resulted in a significant reduction in the total number of exacerbations per vaccinated subjects compared with those who received placebo (weighted mean difference, -0.37; 95% CI: -0.64 to -0.11; $p=0.006$). This was due to the reduction in "late" exacerbations occurring after three or four weeks. The studies were too small though to have detected any effect on mortality. By contrast, community studies show that patients who are vaccinated have fewer admissions and that mortality is reduced, the effects being greater as age increases (26).

The use of pneumococcal vaccination is more controversial. *Streptococcus pneumoniae* is one of the most frequently identified bacterial pathogens in COPD exacerbations (22). A Cochrane's analysis concluded that case-control studies show a significant effect in reducing invasive pneumococcal disease in adults [odds ratio (OR), 0.47; 95% CI: 0.37–0.39]. The earlier randomized studies showed a greater effect than the more recent ones. Altogether, however, neither the reduction in death

(OR, 0.9; 95% CI: 0.76–1.07) nor in pneumonia (OR, 0.77; 95% CI: 0.58–1.02) was statistically significant (27). Alfageme et al. (28) have shown in a recent RCT that the protective efficacy for the prevention of pneumonia is linked to two factors: age of the patient and severity of EFL. The vaccine had an efficacy of 76% (95% CI: 20–93) in patients younger than 65 years, and 91% (95% CI: 35–99) in those who also had severe airflow obstruction. The effect of pneumococcal vaccination over COPD exacerbation rate was not assessed in this study.

B. Benefits of Bacterial Eradication

A pooled analysis of data from studies that used the protected specimen brush (PSB) method has shown that approximately one quarter of the patients with COPD are colonized (10^2 CFU/mL or greater) by potentially pathogenic microorganisms during stable COPD (29). This lower airway bacterial load (i.e., bronchial colonization) has been associated with increased airway inflammation and accelerated FEV_1 decline (30,31). Stimulation of inflammation is likely to be dependent on the nature of the organism and, perhaps more importantly, their number (32). *Haemophilus influenzae* has also been shown to produce higher levels of airway inflammation than other bacteria (33). Therefore, reducing sputum bacterial load or eradicating carriage, especially *H. influenzae* could be associated with better short- and long-term benefits. Likewise, bacterial eradication has been associated with a reduction in bronchial inflammation (34) and also prolongs the time between exacerbations (35). The MOSAIC study (a multi-center, multinational, prospective, randomized, double-blind study to compare the effectiveness of Moxifloxacin Oral tablets to Standard oral Antibiotics regimen given as a first-line therapy in outpatients with acute Infective exacerbations of Chronic bronchitis) compared moxifloxacin with three standard antibiotic regimens given as first-line therapy in a prospective, randomized, double-blinded manner in patients with exacerbations of chronic bronchitis. Many of these subjects likely would have qualified for COPD. The principal results of this study were that moxifloxacin achieved significantly superior bacteriologic eradication, which was largely due to *H. influenzae* persistence in the control group. The time until next exacerbation was significantly more prolonged after moxifloxacin treatment, and this difference in exacerbation-free interval was larger in patients with risk factors for a poor outcome (35).

V. Anti-inflammatory Treatment

A. Inhaled Corticosteroids

There is now emerging evidence that inhaled corticosteroids (ICs) reduce the exacerbation rate in patients with COPD. Using a meta-analysis approach, Alsaedi et al. (36) showed in over nine RCTs (3976 patients) that the use of ICs reduces the rate of exacerbations by about a third [risk ratio (RR), 0.70; 95% CI: 0.58–0.84]. These beneficial effects are most evident in patients with spirometry-defined COPD severity in the moderate-to-severe range of the disease (37). Consistent with this, the Global Initiative on Obstructive Lung Disease (GOLD) guidelines have recommended ICs, preferably in combination with a long-acting inhaled beta-agonist, in patients with post-bronchodilator FEV_1 values lower than 50% predicted and a history of repeated exacerbations, preferably three or more during the last year. It is of note that withdrawing ICs can lead to worsening symptoms and increased exacerbations. For example, in one study, in patients with moderate-to-severe COPD, exacerbations were more frequent in those randomized to corticosteroid withdrawal (57% vs. 47%) (38). In the COSMIC study (COPD and Seretide: a Multicenter Intervention and Characterization), which was a placebo-controlled trial where ICs were withdrawn but salmeterol was continued in both limbs of the trial, similar findings were shown with an annual incidence of moderate-to-severe exacerbation rate of the order of 1.6 without IC compared to 1.3 in those treated with IC (39).

ICs are considered generally to be safe. However, two recent trials have shown an increase in physician-reported risk for pneumonia in patients who received this treatment (40,41). The results of the toward a revolution in COPD health (TORCH) trial show that the arms of the study containing fluticasone (alone or combined with a long-acting β-agonist bronchodilator) showed a higher number of pneumonias versus the placebo or salmeterol groups [salmeterol/fluticasone (SFC) group, 7.1%; fluticasone, 6.9%; salmeterol, 4.2%; placebo, 4.2%; $p < 0.001$] (40). Similarly, Kardos et al. (41) in a study comparing salmeterol versus SFC treatment showed seven cases of suspected pneumonia in the salmeterol group, whereas 23 cases were observed in the SFC limb. In both studies, it was not mandatory to confirm a suspected pneumonia by chest X ray. It is unclear if this increase in physician-reported pneumonia, which occurred despite decreasing overall incidence of exacerbations, is due to an increase in pneumonic infiltrates or merely a different clinical presentation of exacerbations after ICs treatment. It is worth mentioning that, in the SFC group, a higher proportion of antibiotics per exacerbation were deemed necessary by the investigators (67.7% vs. 54.7%) (41). Clearly, more research is needed to investigate the issues raised by these observations.

B. Phosphodiesterase Inhibitors

These new agents have many attractive pharmacologic properties that might potentially reduce the patient's likelihood of exacerbation (42,43). However, there are so far few published data to support this contention. Roflumilast has been shown to induce sustained improvements in FEV_1 over 24 weeks of treatment compared with placebo (44). This was accompanied by a reduction in the overall exacerbation rate from 1.13 (placebo) to 1.03 and 0.75 (roflumilast 250 and 500 μg daily) events. More recently, Calverley et al. (45) have assessed in a one-year double-blinded controlled trial the effects of roflumilast on exacerbations. In this study, the overall rate of exacerbations was low in both study groups (exacerbations per patient per year: 0.86 for roflumilast vs. 0.92 for placebo). In a subset of patients with very severe COPD characterized by a high exacerbation rate (1.6 exacerbations per patient per year), roflumilast treatment resulted in a lower rate of exacerbations with an estimated reduction of 36%.

VI. Long-Acting Inhaled Bronchodilators

A. Long-Acting Inhaled β₂-Agonists

Several studies have shown that long-acting inhaled β_2-agonists (LABAs) reduce exacerbation rates. Original data with salmeterol and formoterol suggested that exacerbations rates were unaffected over a three-month study period (46), although the time to first exacerbation was significantly lengthened (47). More recently, the salmeterol treatment limb of the Trial of Inhaled Steroids and Long-Acting β-agonist Study (TRISTAN trial) was associated with a reduction in exacerbations of approximately 20% compared with those randomized to placebo (48). Likewise, inhaled formoterol was effective in reducing the number of "bad days" (equivalent to mild exacerbations) in some studies (49) but did not change the overall rate of moderate-to-severe exacerbations in two studies with more severely affected COPD patients (50,51).

Several mechanisms have been proposed to explain the ability of LABA monotherapy to reduce exacerbations, including sustained bronchodilation (47) and improved mucociliary clearance (52), although neither mechanism has been demonstrated as yet.

B. Long-Acting Antimuscarinic (Tiotropium)

The impact of tiotropium on exacerbations and associated health care utilization resources has been assessed in a meta-analysis including more than 8000 randomized patients (53). Tiotropium reduced COPD exacerbations compared with placebo and also compared with ipratropium, but there were no significant differences when compared with salmeterol. The corresponding number needed to treat (NNT) for tiotropium to prevent one exacerbation per year was 13 (95% CI: 10–21). Tiotropium also reduced the risk of hospitalization for COPD exacerbations compared with placebo without showing differences with ipratropium or salmeterol. The corresponding NNT for tiotropium to prevent one exacerbation-related hospitalization per year was 38 (95% CI: 26–76) (53). Table 1 includes several studies (54–59) that assess the effects of tiotropium on COPD exacerbations.

The mechanisms by which tiotropium reduce exacerbations remain to be elucidated. The most likely explanation for the reduction in exacerbations with this agent is the improvement in lung mechanics due to reduced lung hyperinflation and air trapping including a reduction of the tone of bronchial smooth muscle, so that patients may be less vulnerable to triggers of exacerbations. In earlier phases of the disease, this

Table 1 The Effect of Tiotropium on Exacerbations and Related Hospitalizations

	No. of patients	Duration (week)	Baseline FEV_1 (L)	Comparator	Exacerbations	Hospitali-zations
Casaburi (54)	921	52	1.02	Placebo	↓ (20%)	↓ (47%)
Vincken (55)	535	52	1.25	Ipratropium	↓ (24%)	↓ (38%)
Brusasco (56)	1207	26	1.12	Placebo	↓	NS
Brusasco (56)	1207	26	1.12	Salmeterol	NS	NS
Niewoehner (57)	1829	26	1.04	Placebo	↓ (19%)	↓ (28%)
Dusser (58)	1010	52	1.37	Placebo	↓	NS
Aaron (59)	449	52	1.08	Tio + SAL	NS	NS
Aaron (59)	449	52	1.08	Tio + SFC	NS	↓ (47%)[a]

[a] Decrease of hospitalizations a favor of tiotropium plus salmeterol/fluticasone.
Abbreviations: ↓, significant reduction in exacerbation or associated hospitalization versus comparator; NS, no significant reduction in exacerbation or associated hospitalization versus comparator; SAL, salmeterol; SFC, salmeterol/fluticasone; Tio, tiotropium.

beneficial effect is unlikely to be noticed by the patient, but it may become critically important in patients with more advanced disease. Tiotropium also may have a direct anti-inflammatory effect (60). A third, not proven hypothesis as yet, could be an improved alveolar ventilation to pulmonary blood flow balance associated with a better cardiovascular performance, namely increased cardiac output, which results from the reduction of lung hyperinflation discussed above.

VII. Combination Therapy (LABAs Plus ICs)

Table 2 shows the effectiveness of therapy in terms of the reduction of COPD exacerbations compared with placebo, both as total exacerbations and those exacerbations that are treated by short courses of oral corticosteroids (40,41,48,50,51). A Cochrane's review showed a significant effect on exacerbations in favor of ICs/ LABA (SFC) combination therapy over placebo. However, there was conflicting evidence for an additive effect of ICs treatment over LABAs alone with regard to exacerbations (61). Kardos et al. (41) have compared, in patients with severe COPD, SFC against salmeterol alone. The study showed a 35% reduction in moderate-to-severe exacerbations in the SFC arm compared with the salmeterol arm such that the number of patients treated with SFC to prevent one moderate-to-severe exacerbation per year was 2.08. Along these lines, the TORCH study showed a reduction of 25% in the number of exacerbations over a three-year period in the combination treat-ment arm (40). This effect was significantly superior to the placebo and also to the individual components alone, either salmeterol or fluticasone. The primary outcome in this study was mortality, the results showing a relative decrease of 17.5% (95% CI: 0.681–1.002) in the risk of death that just failed to reach statistical significance ($p = 0.052$) (40).

VIII. Triple Combination Therapy (Tiotropium Plus LABA Plus ICs)

A recent Canadian trial, performed in 449 patients with moderate-to-severe COPD, has been performed to determine whether or not tiotropium alone compared to the combination with either salmeterol or SFC could improve a number of clinical outcomes, more importantly the number of exacerbations (59). Unfortunately, the proportion of patients in the tiotropium plus placebo limb who experienced an exacerbation (62.8%) did not differ from that in the tiotropium plus salmeterol arm (60.8%) or in the triple combination (tiotropium plus SFC) arm. However, the triple combination did reduce the number of hospitalizations for COPD exacerbation (incidence rate ratio, 0.53; 95% CI: 0.33–0.86) compared with tiotropium alone. Both lung function and HRQoL were also significantly improved with the triple combination therapy. In contrast, tiotropium plus salmeterol did not significantly improve lung function or hospitalization rates compared with tiotropium plus placebo. One of the major limitations of this study was that more than 40% of patients who received tiotropium alone and tiotropium plus salmeterol discontinued therapy prematurely, such that many crossed over to treatment with open-label inhaled steroids or LABAs.

Table 2 Representative Studies of the Effect of Combination of Long-Acting Bronchodilators and Inhaled Steroids in COPD Exacerbations

	No. of patients	Duration (year)	Mean FEV$_1$ (% predicted)	Exacerbations per year (placebo group)[a]	Comparator	% Reduction all	% Reduction moderate-severe exacerbations
TRISTAN (48)	719	1	44	1.30 (0.76)	SFC vs. placebo	25	39.5
Calverley et al. (51)	510	1	36	1.80 (1.07)	BDF vs. placebo	24	42
Szafranski et al. (50)	413	1	36	1.80 (1.14)	BDF vs. placebo	24	30.5
Kardos et al. (41)	998	1	32	(1.92)[b]	SFC vs. SAL		35
TORCH (40)	3058	3	44	(1.13)	SFC vs. placebo		25

[a] The mean number of moderate-to-severe exacerbations of COPD is given in parentheses.

[b] In the study of Kardos et al., the exacerbations per year correspond to salmeterol group.

Abbreviations: BDF, budesonide/formoterol; Combination, inhaled corticosteroids maintenance treatment plus long-acting inhaled β-agonist in the same inhaler; SAL, salmeterol; SFC, salmeterol/fluticasone; TORCH, toward a revolution in COPD health; TRISTAN, trial of inhaled steroids and long-acting β-agonist.

IX. Mucolytics and Antioxidants

Exacerbations are more common in patients with COPD with chronic phlegm (62). This raises the possibility of sputum modification as a therapeutic target. A Cochrane's analysis has shown a reduction in exacerbations from 2.7 to 1.9 per year in a range of RCTs using mucolytic agents (63). Most of the positive results involved the exclusive use of *N*-acetylcysteine (NAC), which has also been shown in in vivo conditions to have significant antioxidant effects. Notwithstanding, the large Bronchitis Randomized on *N*-acetylcysteine Cost-Utility Study trial (BRONCUS) using NAC (600 mg/day) was unable to reproduce these findings (64). It is of note that, in this trial, the analysis of a subset of patients who were not receiving concomitant ICs showed significantly fewer exacerbations (0.76 vs. 1.11 moderate-to-severe exacerbations per year) with NAC, a finding that needs further prospective confirmation.

X. Nonpharmacological Treatment

A. Pulmonary Rehabilitation and Physical Activity

Few RCTs have examined the effectiveness of pulmonary rehabilitation programs on the use of health care resources. Griffiths and coworkers reported that patients with COPD spent fewer days hospitalized during a one-year follow-up period (65). Several uncontrolled studies also support the effects of pulmonary rehabilitation as an effective therapeutic approach to reduce hospital days (66). After suffering from an exacerbation of COPD, pulmonary rehabilitation has also been shown to reduce readmissions (RR, 0.26; 95% CI: 0.12–0.54) and mortality (RR, 0.45; 95% CI: 0.22–0.91), in a recent meta-analysis of six clinical studies (67).

A decrease in hospitalization has been reported with moderate-to-high levels of physical activity. In a study conducted in a cohort of 346 patients with moderate-to-severe COPD followed up to one year in Barcelona, patients with COPD who reported physical activity equivalent to walking at least 1 hr/day had a lower risk of admission for a COPD exacerbation than those who had exhibited a degree of physical activity equivalent to walking only 20 min/day or less (68). Recently, the same group of investigators has shown in an observational study using the Copenhagen Heart City Study database that levels of physical activity equivalent to walking or cycling 2 hr/wk or more were associated with a 30% to 40% reduction in the risk of hospital admission due to COPD and also with a reduction in respiratory mortality (69).

The mechanisms underlying the potential beneficial effects of regular physical activity or rehabilitation programs in COPD remain unsettled, although some evidence regarding the beneficial effects of muscle function, exercise capacity, and/or lung inflammation may give support to its biologic plausibility (70). Important anti-inflammatory and antioxidant effects have been reported in COPD patients participating in rehabilitation programs (71,72).

B. Domiciliary Oxygen

Retrospective observational data suggest that there is a significant reduction of days spent in hospital after long-term supplementary oxygen is started, although other factors related to patient care could influence these results (73). More recently, the effect of home oxygen therapy on hospitalization rates in moderate hypoxemic COPD patients (PaO$_2$ on room air and at rest, 55–71 mmHg) were prospectively studied. By contrast, the admission rate, number of days spent in hospital, and number of patients with at least one hospitalization were not reduced (74).

C. Educational Programs

The role of educational interventions in COPD has, for some years, been a source of some debate. A Cochrane's review of eight RCTs concluded that there is currently insufficient evidence to draw firm conclusions or make solid recommendations in this area (75). Variations in the patients studied and use of different outcome measures in each individual study are invoked as the most plausible factors to explain this lack of consistency, which is further complicated by the selection of participants. Bourbeau et al. (76) in a study of 191 patients with severe COPD and a clinical history of at least one hospitalization for exacerbation during the previous year reported a 40% reduction in hospital admissions and a significant decline in visits to both the emergency department and to primary care physicians. Similarly, one of our groups studied, in a single-controlled fashion, 32 patients with frequent exacerbations who were allocated to conventional treatment or a specific educational program, while optimizing preventive measures and frequent clinical assessments (77). In the subset of patients who participated in the specific interventional program, the number of exacerbations decreased significantly resulting in a reduction in hospitalizations by 73% and in inpatient bed-days by 77%; by contrast, inpatient bed-days almost doubled in the control group. Other investigators, however, have failed to show any effect in less selected COPD populations (78,79).

XI. Management of Exacerbations

The management of exacerbations may occur in the home or in the hospital depending on factors and aspects considered in the diagnostic assessment section (Table 3). Nevertheless, with the exception of ventilatory support most of the therapeutic approaches alluded to are available at home and can be used safely in that setting. Accordingly, hospital at home (HaH) and supported discharge programs are likely to become more common and extensively applied in the future. Two schemes of

Table 3 Indications for Hospital Assessment or Admission for Exacerbations of COPD

Marked increase in intensity of symptoms, such as sudden development of resting dyspnea
Severe underlying COPD
Onset of new physical sign (e.g., cyanosis, peripheral edema)
Failure of exacerbations to respond to initial medical management
Significant comorbidities
Frequent exacerbations
Newly occurring arrhythmias
Diagnostic uncertainty
Older age
Insufficient home support

Local resources need to be considered.
Source: From Ref. 80.

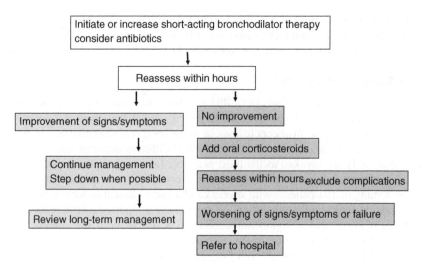

Figure 2 Schematic of a decision tree for the management of mild-to-moderate exacerbations of chronic obstructive pulmonary disease. *Source*: From Ref. 81.

management for mild-to-moderate (Fig. 2) and moderate-to-severe (Fig. 3) COPD exacerbations (82) are recommended and approached in greater detail by the GOLD (83) and the American Thoracic Society/European Respiratory Society (ATS/ERS) guidelines (84). Both are based on the clinical presentation of the patient. Notwithstanding, grading severity of mild-to-moderate exacerbations remains contentious (80), since exacerbations can be categorized either on clinical presentation (symptom driven) (85) or health care utilization (action or event driven) (17). In the

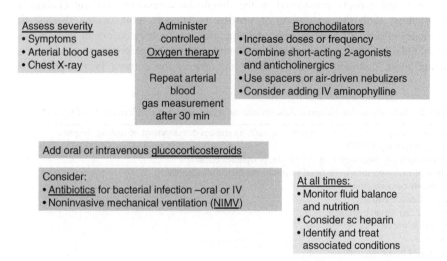

Figure 3 Key steps for the management of moderate-to-severe exacerbations of chronic obstructive pulmonary disease. *Source*: From Ref. 81.

case of the latter, definitions of severity that depend on treatments do little to assist the clinician faced with treating a newly presenting patient.

XII. Treatment of Exacerbations

A. Pharmacological Therapy

Bronchodilators

Short-Acting Inhaled Bronchodilators

Both short-acting inhaled β_2-agonists and anticholinergics bronchodilators [or short-acting inhaled bronchodilators (SABDs)] remain, as a class, the mainstay of treatment to alleviate symptoms and improve airflow obstruction during COPD exacerbations. The efficacy of these agents on lung function as a class, using FEV_1 as the outcome, is not questioned despite the absence of proper placebo-controlled trials (86,87). There is no detectable evidence between the different classes of SABDs on the level of induced bronchodilation at 90 minutes after inhalation (88–90). When inhaled, short-acting β_2-agonists (SABAs) such as salbutamol (albuterol in the United States) and terbutaline induce bronchodilation within five minutes with maximum airflow peaking at 30 minutes; ipratropium effects start over 10 to 15 minutes with a peak at 30 to 60 minutes. The effects of the two classes of SADBs decline after two to three hours and can last as long as four to six hours depending on their individual properties (91). Inspiratory capacity also increases significantly at 30 and 90 minutes after nebulized salbutamol by approximately 12% (92), suggesting a complementary benefit on acute-on-chronic air trapping and static lung hyperinflation (93). In contrast, there is no detrimental effect on the pulmonary gas exchange status when given at therapeutic doses.

By contrast, the efficacy of combinations of SABDs remains unsettled. Unlike in stable COPD, where the simultaneous concurrent administration of two SABDs is more efficacious over either agent given alone (94), the combination of two SABDs given sequentially in exacerbations does not provide additional benefit (88,95,96). A systematic review on the modes of delivery of SABDs (97) concluded that there were no significant FEV_1 differences when SABDs were administered by handheld metered dose inhalers with a good inhaler technique, with or without a spacer device, and nebulizers. However, the latter devices, which are independent of inspiratory airflow rate and require little patient effort and coordination, should be more appropriate for the sickest patients to facilitate better delivery and penetration of the particles. Increasing the dose and/or the frequency of existing SABDs therapy with SABAs is the strategy recommended by the ATS/ERS (84) and the GOLD (83) guidelines. The addition of a short-acting inhaled anticholinergic (ipratropium or oxitropium bromide) if the clinical response is not immediately favorable is also recommended, despite the uncertainties about SABDs combinations (97). While without evidence generated by RTCs, it is currently common practice to nebulize two different classes of SABDs as initial therapy during exacerbations.

Long-Acting Inhaled Bronchodilators

Formoterol, a fast-onset LABA, previously used as an as-needed reliever in both stable and acute asthma (98) and in exacerbations of COPD without major adverse effects (99), has also been proposed in a cumulative manner for exacerbations (100). While evidence suggests that high doses of formoterol are well tolerated, it remains uncertain whether this dosing of formoterol can be used as an alternative, or even complementarily, to SABDs during COPD exacerbations (101). A recent pilot study to assess the effects of formoterol, tiotropium, and their combination in patients with exacerbation of COPD has been completed. Twenty-one patients with mild-to-moderate exacerbations were enrolled. Both formoterol and tiotropium significantly improved the area under curves for FEV_1, forced vital capacity, and IC over a 12- and 24-hour period. The results were significantly superior for the combination showing a complementary effect (102).

Methylxanthines (Theophylline)

In the face of an inadequate or insufficient response to the use of SABDs, theophylline has been currently relegated to second-line intravenous therapy for the management of exacerbations. However, a meta-analysis shows that methylxanthines do not confer significant benefits for lung function, clinical outcomes, or symptoms in patients with exacerbations of COPD, but significantly increase nausea and vomiting (103).

Systemic Corticosteroids

Exacerbations are associated with increased airway inflammation (7,8), which therefore provides a rationale for the use of anti-inflammatory systemic corticosteroid treatment. Six RCTs (104–110) and three systematic reviews (86,111,112) of the efficacy of systemic corticosteroids for exacerbations of COPD support the conclusion that a short course of these agents improve spirometry and decrease relapse rate in patients with exacerbation of COPD. However, the optimal dose and duration of treatment remains uncertain, as the studies conducted have varied greatly in dosage, length of treatment, administration, and setting.

In 1980, Albert at al. (104) provided the first evidence for the routine use of systemic steroids during the care of hospitalized patients with COPD exacerbations. Forty-four patients with COPD and acute respiratory failure were randomized to placebo or methylprednisolone, 0.5 mg/kg intravenously every six hours for three days. Those treated with steroids were significantly more likely to achieve a 40% or greater increase in FEV_1 over their baseline. Almost two decades after, in the largest study of systemic glucocorticoids in COPD exacerbations so far conducted, the Systemic Corticosteroids in Chronic Obstructive Pulmonary Disease Exacerbations trial (105), two groups of patients received i.v. methylprednisolone (125 mg q.i.d. for three days) followed by two or eight weeks of a tapering dose of oral prednisone (starting with 60 mg q.d.) while a third group received placebo throughout. Compared with placebo, treatment failure rate was significantly reduced in the combined steroid groups on days 30 (33% vs. 23%) and 90 (48% and 37%) but not at six months. Length of hospital stay was shorter by one day and FEV_1 improved at a faster rate in the steroid groups (by approximately 100 mL) from day 1, although there was no difference at two weeks. Adverse events, however, were more prevalent in the steroid-treated groups. Manifestations of diabetes were common (67%), including hyperglycemia requiring treatment (15%). The steroid group treated for eight weeks had a higher proportion of secondary infections. While increasing the duration of the steroid regime increased side effects, it was not associated with increased efficacy. While these studies used relatively high doses of parenteral corticosteroids, Davis et al. (106) showed that oral prednisolone (30 mg q.d.) produced similar benefits in severe patients hospitalized for a nonacidotic exacerbation.

The fourth RCT in inpatients (107) had the novelty of comparing nebulized budesonide (0.5 mg/mL; 2 mg q.i.d. for three days) followed by 2 mg/day of budesonide for seven days, with oral prednisolone (30 mg b.i.d. for three days) followed by 40 mg q.d. for a week, and with placebo in patients with severe COPD hospitalized for moderate-to-severe nonacidotic exacerbations. Compared with the placebo group, post-BD FEV_1 changes within the first three days of therapy were greater with both active treatment groups (budesonide, by 100 mL; prednisolone, by 160 mL, without differences between them), although this difference was not present after two weeks.

Superiority compared with placebo was also observed for both active treatments in pre-BD FEV_1 (significant in the prednisolone group only), in PaO_2 (significant only in the prednisolone group), and in $PaCO_2$. Length of hospital stay, dyspnea, and corticosteroid-related adverse events were similar in the three arms, with disease deterioration as the most serious event in the prednisolone group. Hyperglycemia was more common in the systemic steroid group. A very recent study in 158 patients hospitalized for severe COPD exacerbations (108), using similar doses of budesonide and prednisolone to the former trial, has also shown that nebulized budesonide may be an effective and safe alternative to systemic corticosteroids in the treatment of exacerbations of COPD.

Two studies were carried out in the outpatient setting (109,110). In both, oral prednisone (40–60 mg for less than 10 days) showed a more rapid improvement in FEV_1 and a decrease in the failure of treatment rate.

Antibiotics

The use of antibiotics in exacerbations of COPD remains controversial. Nevertheless, a recent survey in the United States showed that 85% of all patients hospitalized for exacerbations of COPD were given antibiotics (113). The most frequent etiologies of a COPD exacerbation is infection of the lower airways with bacteria or virus and/or air pollution, even though the cause of one-third of exacerbations is still unknown (22). The predominant bacterial microorganisms recovered in the airways of patients with mild exacerbations are *H. influenzae, S. pneumoniae,* and *Moraxella catarrhalis* (114), while in patients with severe COPD acute episodes (115) both enteric gram-negative bacilli and *Pseudomonas aeruginosa* may become more common. Viral infections (rhinoviruses, influenza A, and respiratory syncytial virus) are more likely to play a role during severe COPD exacerbations (116,117). The presence of a coinfection with both viruses and bacteria was found in 25% of exacerbations in hospitalized patients and is most common in severe exacerbations (118).

Antoine et al. (85) showed evidence of benefit from antibiotics in COPD exacerbations characterized by at least two of the following three symptoms: increased dyspnea, sputum purulence, and/or sputum volume. However, of the three symptoms, the most important criterion to predict bacterial infection is sputum purulence. Along these lines, Shockley et al. (119) showed that sputum purulence should be expected when bacteria are causing infection as the activation of host defenses leads to Europhile recruitment to the airway. In contrast, mucous sputum rarely reflects bacterial airway infection. Soler et al. (120), using quantitative culture of PSB samples in patients with severe COPD, have recently shown that a self-reported presence of purulence in the sputum predicts the presence of bacteria at high concentrations in the airway with a positive predictive value of 77% and a negative predictive value of 89%. Also, being hospitalized previously, suffering from more than four COPD exacerbations per year and an $FEV_1 < 50\%$ increases the probability of having high bacterial counts in the distal airways. Notwithstanding, the value of clinical inspection of the purulence of sputum remains an unsettled area with many uncertainties. Thus, all three systematic reviews (86,121,122) of antibiotic therapy advocate their use for COPD exacerbations in the presence of purulent sputum., The most recent review (122) observed a reduction in the risk of mortality (RR, 0.23; 95% CI: 0.10–0.52 with NNT of 8; 95% CI: 6–17), treatment failure (RR, 0.75; 95% CI: 0.63–0.90 with NNT of 3; 95% CI: 3–5) and sputum purulence (RR, 0.51; 95% CI: 0.41–0.77 with NNT of 8; 95% CI: 6–17). These results need, however, to be tempered, given the differences in patient selection, antibiotic choice, the small number of trials, and the lack of control for other therapeutic interventions that influence outcome. In addition, antibiotics did not improve arterial blood gases or peak flow. Finally, there was a small increase in risk of diarrhea with antibiotics (RR, 2.86; 95% CI: 1.06–7.76).

Serum levels of procalcitonin increase rapidly in the presence of infection (123,124), induced either by microbial toxins (i.e., endotoxin) and/or indirectly by humoral factors or the cell-mediated host response (125,126). This induction is rather attenuated by cytokines released during viral infections (126). Therefore, circulating levels of procalcitonin are markedly elevated in patients with bacterial infections compared to those with viral infections or other inflammatory conditions (123,124). Stolz et al. (127) have shown that procalcitonin guidance during exacerbations of COPD offers an advantage. Procalcitonin guidance reduced antibiotic prescriptions (40% vs. 72%, $p < 0.001$) and antibiotic exposure (RR, 0.56; 95% CI: 0.43–073) compared with standard therapy during exacerbations. Clinical outcomes, such as exacerbations rate, rehospitalization rate and mean time to next rehospitalization rate, were similar in both groups within six months. Over a six-month interval, the use of procalcitonin reduced achieved reduction in antibiotic exposure with an NNT of 3. Procalcitonin cannot guide the choice of antibiotic, which should be based on the clinical history and patterns of local bacterial resistance (83).

B. Nonpharmacological Therapy

Controlled Oxygen Therapy

Hypoxia during exacerbation of COPD is primarily the consequence of V_A/Q imbalance and may be life threatening (128). Likewise, oxygen therapy is of great beneficial value in acute respiratory failure during COPD exacerbations. However, a recent Cochrane's review (81) concluded that there is an urgent need for robust, well-designed RCTs to investigate the effect of oxygen therapy in patients with exacerbations of COPD since no relevant trials have been published to date. The primary objective of oxygen therapy is to raise PaO_2 to prevent life-threatening hypoxemia and to optimize oxygen delivery to peripheral tissues. In clinical practice, physicians administrate controlled low inspired oxygen concentrations, either 24% or 28%, delivered through high flow (Venturi) masks or by nasal oxygen at limited flow rates of 2 to 4 L/min, which approximates these concentrations. This strategy provides modest but effective increases in PaO_2 (of the order of 10–20 mmHg) with the goal of keeping PaO_2 values >60 mmHg and thus providing adequate SaO_2 levels ($\geq 90\%$), without risking detrimental carbon dioxide retention and respiratory or mixed acidosis. The low flow devices, such as nasal prongs or cannulae, are less accurate. Since, which is relatively rare, oxygen therapy can result in suppression of respiratory drive, carbon dioxide narcosis, and eventually respiratory arrest, all patients treated with oxygen should be closely monitored (129). Ideally, arterial blood gas analysis from radial stabs (or from another peripheral artery) provides the most accurate assessment, including acid-base status. Pulse oximetry, which provides information on SaO_2 alone, is a noninvasive alternative useful for trending and/or adjusting oxygen therapy settings, but will not monitor carbon dioxide retention. During moderate-to-severe exacerbations, arterial pH and blood gases should be always measured before and one hour after starting oxygen therapy. Around 20% of patients with an exacerbation present to hospital with acidemia (130).

Assisted Mechanical Support

The primary therapeutic goal of ventilatory support in patients with exacerbations with acute respiratory failure is to decrease both mortality and morbidity and relieve symptoms that are present despite optimal medical therapy (24,83,84). Mechanical ventilation can be delivered noninvasively or invasively (conventionally) using different modes. All are, in essence, positive pressure devices (negative ventilation is currently not recommended) whether used for noninvasive ventilation (NIV) with either a nasal or facial mask or used for invasive ventilation with an endotracheal tube or a tracheostomy.

Noninvasive Ventilation

This modality has become one of the most robust and widely used therapeutic tools to provide mechanical support for exacerbations of COPD, and with straightforward inclusion criteria have been established. A systematic review (131) based on several RCTs (132–138) provided evidence that NIV, as an adjunct approach to standard medical care, decreased mortality, need for endotracheal intubation (for every five patients treated with NIV one patient would avoid intubation) and treatment failure. Moreover, NIV increased pH, reduced hypercapnia, and respiratory rate within one hour of its institution; shortened length of hospital stay by more than three days irrespective of environment [high dependency/ICU vs. medical ward]; and decreased complications associated with therapy. Likewise, NIV is cost-effective compared with usual therapeutic care alone (139,140).

Invasive Ventilation

The most life-threatening episodes of acute respiratory failure during very severe COPD exacerbations may require intubation and mechanical ventilation. Despite the need for invasive ventilation, relatively good survival is observed with mortality around 20% (141). These figures, however, are considerably lower than those observed in patients with respiratory failure from other etiologies treated in general intensive care settings (141). Compared with acute respiratory distress syndrome, mean duration of ventilation in acute COPD was significantly shorter (9 vs. 5 days) (141) as was length of intensive care stay (14 vs. 11 days) (141). A subsequent study found even shorter duration of mechanical ventilation in COPD patients (142).

NIV has also been used to effectively shorten the period of invasive ventilation in the presence of difficult weaning and may reduce extended stays in the ICU (143,144). However, an RCT found no evidence for the utility of NIV compared with medical therapy in COPD; 221 patients developed signs of respiratory failure within 48 hours following extubation from mechanical ventilation (145).

XIII. HaH and Supported Discharge Services

HaH services represent a new health care model, potentially appealing, for the management of selected nonacidotic patients with exacerbations of COPD presenting to emergency departments (146). At first glance, patients with altered mental status or confusion, acute electrocardiographic or radiographic changes, serious comorbidities, and/or poor social conditions should not be eligible for these innovative health care schemes. The objectives for these exacerbated patients who are provided cared at home are: immediate or early discharge from the hospital to avoid or shorten length of hospital stay, provision of a tailored individualized management, and patient home support by a skilled specialized respiratory team. The major finding of the most recent meta-analysis of HaH (147) including several robust RCTs (148–154) concluded that HaH services could be used as safely as hospital care. Compared with inpatient care, HaH-assigned patients generated substantial financial savings mostly due to a shorter length of hospital stay.

References

1. Seemungal TAR, Donaldson GC, Paul EA, Bestall JC, Jeffries DJ, Wedzicha JA. Effect of exacerbation on quality of life in patients with chronic obstructive pulmonary disease. Am J Respir Crit Care Med 1998; 157:1418–22.
2. Donaldson GC, Seemungal TAR, Bhowmik A, et al. Relationship between exacerbation frequency and lung function decline in chronic obstructive pulmonary disease. Thorax 2002; 57:847–52.
3. Kanner RE, Anthonisen NR, Connett JE. Lower respiratory illnesses promote FEV(1) decline in current smokers but not exsmokers with mild chronic obstructive pulmonary disease. Am J Respir Crit Care Med 2001; 164:358–64.
4. Soler-Cataluña JJ, Martínez-Garcia MA, Román Sánchez P, et al. Severe acute exacerbations and mortality in patients with chronic obstructive pulmonary disease. Thorax 2005; 60:925–31.
5. Wouters EF. Economic analysis of the confronting COPD surven: an overview of results. Respir Med 2003; 97:S3–4.
6. Wedzicha JA, Donaldson GC. Exacerbations of chronic obstructive pulmonary disease. Respir Care 2003; 48:1204–13.
7. Aaron SD, Angel JB, Lunau M, et al. Granulocyte inflammatory markers and airway infection during acute exacerbation of chronic obstructive pulmonary disease. Am J Respir Crit Care Med 2001; 163:349–55.
8. Bhowmik A, Seemungal TA, Sapsford RJ, Wedzicha JA. Relation of sputum inflammatory markers to symptoms and lung function changes in COPD exacerbations. Thorax 2000; 55:114–20.
9. Barbera JA, Roca J, Ferrer A, et al. Mechanisms of worsening gas exchange during acute exacerbations of chronic obstructive pulmonary disease. Eur Respir J 1997; 10:1285–91.
10. Rodriguez-Roisin R, MacNee W. Pathophysiology of chronic obstructive pulmonary disease. Eur Respir Mon 2006; 38:177–200.
11. Hurst JR, Perera W, Wilkinson TM, Donaldson GC, Wedzicha JA. Systemic and upper and lower airway inflammation at exacerbation of chronic obstructive pulmonary disease. Am J Respir Crit Care Med 2006; 173:71–8.

12. Seemungal TAR, Donaldson GC, Bhowmik A, Jeffries DJ, Wedzicha JA. Time course and recovery of exacerbations in patients with chronic obstructive pulmonary disease. Am J Respir Crit Care Med 2000; 161:1608–18.
13. O'Donnell DE, Parker CM. COPD exacerbations. Pathophysiology. Thorax 2006; 61:354–61.
14. Tsoumakidou M, Siafakas NM. Novel insights into the aetiology and pathophysiology of increased airway inflammation during COPD exacerbations. Respir Res 2006; 7:80.
15. Donaldson GC, Seemungal TAR, Patel IS, et al. Airway and systemic inflammation and decline in lung function, in chronic obstructive pulmonary disease. Chest 2005; 128:1995–2004.
16. Gompertz S, O'Brien CO, Bayley DL, Hill SL, Stockley RA. Changes in bronchial inflammation during acute exacerbations of chronic bronchitis. Eur Respir J 2001; 17:1112–9.
17. Rodríguez-Roisin R. Toward a consensus definition for COPD exacerbation. Chest 2000; 117:398s–401.
18. Tille-Leblond I, Marquette CH, Perez T, et al. Pulmonary embolism in patients with unexplained exacerbation of chronic obstructive pulmonary disease: prevalence and risk factors. Ann Intern Med 2006; 144:390–6.
19. Abroug F, Quanes-Besbes L, Nciri N, et al. Association of left-heart dysfunction with severe exacerbation of chronic obstructive pulmonary disease. Diagnostic performance of cardiac biomarkers. Am J Respir Crit Care Med 2006; 174:990–6.
20. Rutschmann OT, Cornuz J, Poletti PA, et al. Should pulmonary embolism be suspected in exacerbations of chronic obstructive pulmonary disease? Thorax 2007; 62:121–5.
21. Andersson F, Borg S, Jansson SA, et al. The costs of exacerbatons in chronic obstructive pulmonary disease (COPD). Respir Med 2002; 96:700–8.
22. Sapey E, Stockley A. COPD exacerbations: aetiology. Thorax 2006; 61:250–8.
23. Seemungal T, Harper-Owen R, Bhowmik A, et al. Respiratory viruses, symptoms, and inflammatory markers in acute exacerbations and stable chronic obstructive pulmonary disease. Am J Respir Crit Care Med 2001; 164:1618–23.
24. National Institute for Clinical Excellence (NICE). Chronic obstructive pulmonary disease. National clinical guideline on management of chronic obstructive pulmonary disease in adults in primary and secondary care. Thorax 2004; 59(Suppl. 1):1–232.
25. Poole PJ, Chacko E, Wood-Baker RW, Cates CJ. Influenza vaccine for patients with chronic obstructive pulmonary disease. Cochrane Database Syst Rev 2006; 25(1):CD002733.
26. Nichol KL, Margolis KL, Wuorenmma J, Von Sternberg T. The efficacy and cost effectiveness of vaccination against influenza among elderly persons living in the community. N Engl J Med 1994; 331:778–84.
27. Dear KBG, Andrews RR, Holden J, Tatham DP. Vaccines for preventing pneumococcal infections in adults. Cochrane Database Syst Rev 2003; 4:CD000422.
28. Alfageme I, Vazquez R, Reyes N, et al. Clinical efficacy of anti-pneumococcal vaccination in patients with COPD. Thorax 2006; 61:189–95.
29. Rosell A, Monsó E, Soler N, et al. Microbiologic determinants of exacerbation in chronic obstructive pulmonary disease. Arch Intern Med 2005; 165:891–7.
30. Patel IS, Seemungal TAR, Wiks M, et al. Relationship between bacterial colonisation and the frequency, character, and severity of COPD exacerbations. Thorax 2002; 57:759–64.
31. Wilkinson TA, Patel IS, Wiks M, et al. Airway bacterial load and FEV1 decline in patients with chronic obstructive pulmonary disease. Am J Respir Crit Care Med 2003; 167:1090–5.
32. Murphy TF, Sethi S, Klingman KL, et al. Simultaneous respiratory tract colonisation by multiple strains of nontypeable *Haemophilus influenzae* in chronic obstructive pulmonary disease: implications for antibiotic therapy. J Infect Dis 1999; 189:404–9.
33. Chin CL, Manzel LJ, Lehman EE, Humlicek AL, Shi L, Starner TD. *Haemophilus influenzae* from patients with chronic obstructive pulmonary disease exacerbation induce more inflammation than colonizers. Am J Respir Crit Care Med 2005; 172:85–91.
34. White AJ, Gompertz S, Bayley DL, et al. Resolution of bronchial inflammation is related to bacterial eradication following treatment of exacerbations of chronic bronchitis. Thorax 2003; 58:680–5.
35. Wilson R, Allegar L, Huchon G, et al. Shor-term and long-term outcomes of moxifloxacin compared to standard antibiotic treatment in acute exacerbations of chronic bronchitis. Chest 2004; 125:953–64.
36. Alsaeedi A, Sin DD, McAlister FA. The effects of inhaled corticosteroids in chronic obstructive pulmonary disease: a systematic review of randomised placebo-controlled trials. Am J Med 2002; 113:59–65.

37. Jones PW, Willits LR, Burge PS, et al. Disease severity and the effect of fluticasone propionate on chronic obstructive pulmonary disease exacerbations. Eur Respir J 2003; 21:68–73.
38. Van der Valk P, Monninkhof E, van derl Polen J, et al. Effect of discontinuation of inhaled corticosteroids in patients with chronic obstructive pulmonary disease. The COPE study. Am J Respir Crit Care Med 2002; 166:1358–63.
39. Wouters EF, Postma DS, Fokkens B, et al. Withdrawal of fluticasone propionate from combined salmeterol/fluticasone treatment in patients with COPD causes inmediate and susstained disease deterioration: a randomised controlled trial. Thorax 2005; 60:480–7.
40. Calverley PM, Anderson JA, Celli B, et al. Salmeterol and fluticasone propionate and survival in chronic obstructive pulmonary disease. N Engl J Med 2007; 356:775–89.
41. Kardos P, Wencher M, Glaab T, Vogelmeier C. Impact of salmeterol/fluticasone propionate versus salmeterol on exacerbations in severe chronic obstructive pulmonary disease. Am J Respir Crit Care Med 2007; 175:144–9.
42. Profita M, Chiappara G, Mirabella F, et al. Effect of cilomilast (Ariflo) on TNF-alpha, IL-8, and GM-CSF release by airway cells of patient with COPD. Thorax 2003; 58:573–9.
43. Gamble E, Grotendorst DC, Brightling CE, et al. Antiinflammatory effects of the phosphodiesterase-4 inhibitor cilomilast (Ariflo) in chronic obstructive pulmonary disease. Am J Respir Crit Care Med 2003; 168:976–82.
44. Rabe KF, Bateman ED, O'Donnell D, et al. Roflumilast—an oral antiinflammatory treatment for chronic obstructive pulmonary disease: a randomised controlled trial. Lancet 2005; 366:563–71.
45. Calverley PM, Sanchez-Toril F, McIvor RA, Teichmann P, Bredenbroeker D, Fabbri LM. Effect of one year treatment with roflumilast in severe chronic obstructive pulmonary disease. Am J Respir Crit Care Med 2007; 176:154–61 (Epub ahead of print).
46. Rennard SI, Anderson W, ZuWallack R, et al. Use of long-acting inhaled beta2-adrenergic agonist, salmeterol xinofoate, in patients with chronic obstructive pulmonary disease. Am J Respir Crit Care Med 2001; 163:1087–92.
47. Mahler DA, Donohue JF, Barbee RA, et al. Efficacy of salmeterol xinofoate in the treatment of COPD. Chest 1999; 115:957–65.
48. Calverley P, Pauwels R, Vestbo J, et al. Combined salmeterol and fluticasone in the treatment of chronic obstructive pulmonary disease: a randomised controlled trial. Lancet 2003; 361:449–56.
49. Aalbers R, Ayres J, Backer V, et al. Formoterol in patients with chronic obstructive pulmonary disease: a randomized, controlled, 3-months trial. Eur Respir J 2002; 19:936–43.
50. Szafransky W, Cukier A, Ramirez A, et al. Efficacy and safety of budesonide/formoterol and formoterol in chronic obstructive pulmonary diseases. Eur Respir J 2003; 22:912–8.
51. Calverley PM, Boonsawat W, Cseke Z, Zhong N, Peterson S, Olsson H. Maintenance therapy with budesonide and formoterol in chronic obstructive pulmonary disease. Eur Respir J 2003; 22:912–9.
52. Piatti G, Ambrosetti U, Santus P, Allegra L. Effects of salmeterol on cilia and mucus in COPD and pneumonia patients. Pharmacol Res 2005; 51:165–8.
53. Barr RG, Bourbeau J, Camargo CA, Ram FSF. Tiotropium for stable chronic obstructive pulmonary disease: a meta-analysis. Thorax 2006; 61:854–62.
54. Casaburi R, Mahler DA, Jones PW, et al. A long-term evaluation of once-daily inhaled tiotropium in chronic obstructive pulmonary disease. Eur Respir J 2002; 19:217–24.
55. Vincken W, van Noord JA, Greefhorst APM, et al. Improved health outcomes in patients with COPD during 1 yr's treatment with tiotropium. Eur Respir J 2002; 19:209–16.
56. Brusasco V, Hodder R, Miravitlles M, et al. Health outcomes following treatment for six months with once daily tiotropium compared with twice daily salmeterol in patients with COPD. Thorax 2003; 58:399–404.
57. Niewoehner DE, Rice K, Cote C, et al. Prevention of exacerbations of chronic obstructive pulmonary disease with tiotropium, a once-daily inhaled anticholinergic bronchodilator: a randomized trial. Ann Intern Med 2005; 143:317–26.
58. Dusser D, Bravo ML, Iacono P. The effect of tiotropium on exacerbations and airflow in patients with COPD. Eur Respir J 2006; 27:547–55.
59. Aaron SD, Vandemheen KL, Fergusson D, et al. Tiotropium in combination with palcebo, salmeterol or fluticasone–salmeterol for treatment of chronic obstructive pulmonary disease. Ann Intern Med 2007; 146:545–55.
60. Disse B. Antimuscarinic treatment for lung disease from research to clinical practice. Life Sci 2001; 68:2257–64.

61. Nannini L, Cates CJ, Lasserson TJ, Poole P. Combined corticosteroid and long acting beta-agonist in one inhaler for chronic obstructive pulmonary disease. Cochrane Database Syst Rev 2004; 3:CD003784.

62. Vestbo J, Prescott E, Lange P, Copenhagen City Heart Study Group. Association of chronic mucus hypersecretion with FEV1 decline and COPD morbidity. Am J Respir Crit Care Med 1996; 153: 1530–5.

63. Poole PJ, Black PN. Mucolytic agents for chronic bronchitis or chronic obstructive pulmonary disease. The Cocharne Library. Chichester, UK: Willey, 2004.

64. Decramer M, Rutten-van-Molken M, Dekhuijzen PN, et al. Effects of *N*-acetylcysteine on outcomes in chronic obstructive pulmonary disease (Bronchitis Randomised on NAV Cost-Utility Study, BRONCHUS): a randomised placebo-controlled study. Lancet 2005; 365:1552–60.

65. Griffiths TL, Burr ML, Cambell IA, et al. Results at 1 year of multidisciplinary pulmonary rehabilitation: a randomised controlled trial. Lancet 2000; 355:362–8.

66. Troosters T, Casaburi R, Gosseslink R, Decramer M. Pulmonary rehabilitation in chronic obstructive pulmonary disease. State of the art. Am J Respir Crit Care Med 2005; 172:19–38.

67. Puhan MA, Scharplatz M, Troosters T, Steurer J. Respiratory rehabilitation after acute exacerbation of COPD may reduce risk for readmission and mortality: a systematic review. Respir Res 2005; 6:54.

68. Garcia-Aymerich J, Farrero E, Felez MA, et al. Risk factors of readmission to hospital for a COPD exacerbation: a prospective study. Thorax 2003; 58:100–5.

69. García-Aymerich J, Lange P, Benet M, Schnohr P, Antó JM. Regular physical activity reduces hospital admission and mortality in chronic obstructive pulmonary disease: a population-based cohort study. Thorax 2006; 61:772–8.

70. Casaburi R. Skeletal muscle dysfunction in chronic obstructive pulmonary disease. Med Sci Sports Exerc 2001; 33(Suppl. 7):S662–70 (Review).

71. Casaburi R, Porszasz J, Burns MR, et al. Physiologic benefits of exercise training in rehabilitation of patients with severe chronic obstructive pulmonary disease. Am J Respir Crit Care Med 1997; 155:1541–51.

72. Rabinovich RA, Ardite E, Troosters T, et al. Reduced muscle redox capacity after endurance training in patients with chronic obstructive pulmonary disease. Am J Respir Crit Care Med 2001; 164:1114–8.

73. Ringbaek TJ, Viskum K, Lange P. Does long-term oxygen therapy reduce hospitalizations in hypoxaemic chronic obstructive pulmonary disease? Eur Respir J 2002; 20:38–42.

74. Ringbaek TJ, Fabricius P, Lange P. The effect of home oxygen therapy on hospitalization in moderate hypoxaemic COPD. Chron Respir Dis 2005; 2:107–8.

75. Monninkhof E, Van der Valk P, Van der Palen J, Van Herwaarden C, Partridge MR, Ziehlhuis G. Self-management education for patients with chronic obstructive pulmonary disease: a systematic review. Thorax 2003; 58:394–8.

76. Bourbeau J, Julien M, Maltais F, et al. Reduction of hospital utilization in patients with chronic obstructive pulmonary disease. Arch Intern Med 2003; 163:585–91.

77. Soler JJ, Martínez MA, Román P, Orero R, Terrazas S, Martínez-Pechuan A. Eficacia de un programa específico para pacientes con EPOC que presentan frecuentes exacerbaciones. Arch Bronconeumol 2006; 42(10):501–8.

78. Monninkhof E, van der Valk P, van der Palen J, van Herwaarden C, Ziehluis G. Effects of comprehensive self-management programme in patients with chronic obstructive pulmonary disease. Eur Respir J 2003; 22:815–20.

79. Gallefoss F, Bakke PS, Rsgaard PK. Quality of life assessment after patient education in a randomized controlled study on asthma and chronic obstructive pulmonary disease. Am J Respir Crit Care Med 1999; 159:812–7.

80. Burge S, Wedzicha JA. COPD exacerbations: definitions and classifications. Eur Respir J Suppl 2003; 21(Suppl. 41):46s–53.

81. Rodriguez-Roisin R, Lloyd-Owen S, Wedzicha JA, Koff PB. Exacerbations of COPD, 2003. www.tmed.com/respiratory (last accessed August 31, 2007).

82. Rabe KF, Hurd S, Anzueto A, et al. Global strategy for the diagnosis, management, and prevention of COPD—2006 update. Am J Respir Crit Care Med 2007 (Epub ahead of print).

83. Celli BR, MacNee W. Standards for the diagnosis and treatment of patients with COPD: a summary of the ATS/ERS position paper. Eur Respir J 2004; 23:932–46.

84. Anthonisen NR, Manfreda J, Warren CP, Hershfield ES, Harding GK, Nelson NA. Antibiotic therapy in exacerbations of chronic obstructive pulmonary disease. Ann Intern Med 1987; 106:196–204.

85. McCrory DC, Brown CD. Anti-cholinergic bronchodilators versus beta2-sympathomimetic agents for acute exacerbations of chronic obstructive pulmonary disease. Cochrane Database Syst Rev 2002; 4:CD003900.

86. McCrory DC, Brown C, Gelfand SE, Bach PB. Management of acute exacerbations of COPD: a summary and appraisal of published evidence. Chest 2001; 119:1190–209.

87. Karpel JP, Pesin J, Greenberg D, Gentry E. A comparison of the effects of ipratropium bromide and metaproterenol sulfate in acute exacerbations of COPD. Chest 1990; 98:835–9.

88. Rebuck AS, Chapman KR, Abboud R, et al. Nebulized anticholinergic and sympathomimetic treatment of asthma and chronic obstructive airways disease in the emergency room. Am J Med 1987; 82:59–64.

89. Johnson MK, Stevenson RD. Management of an acute exacerbation of COPD: are we ignoring the evidence? Thorax 2002; 57(Suppl. 2):II15–23.

90. Rennard SI. Treatment of stable chronic obstructive pulmonary disease. Lancet 2004; 364:791–802.

91. Polverino E, Gomez FP, Manrique H, et al. Gas exchange response to short-acting beta2-agonists in COPD severe exacerbations. Am J Respir Crit Care Med 2007; 176:350–5.

92. Parker CM, Voduc N, Aaron SD, Webb KA, O'Donnell DE. Physiologic changes during symptom recovery from moderate exacerbation of COPD. Eur Respir J 2005; 26:420–8.

93. COMBIVENT Inhalation Solution Study Group. Routine nebulized ipratropium and albuterol together are better than either alone in COPD. Chest 1997; 112:1514–21.

94. Patrick DM, Dales RE, Stark RM, Laliberte G, Dickinson G. Severe exacerbations of COPD and asthma. Incremental benefit of adding ipratropium to usual therapy. Chest 1990; 98:295–7.

95. Moayyedi P, Congleton J, Page RL, Pearson SB, Muers MF. Comparison of nebulised salbutamol and ipratropium bromide with salbutamol alone in the treatment of chronic obstructive pulmonary disease. Thorax 1995; 50:834–7.

96. Turner MO, Patel A, Ginsburg S, FitzGerald JM. Bronchodilator delivery in acute airflow obstruction. A meta-analysis. Arch Intern Med 1997; 157:1736–44.

97. Tattersfield AE, Lofdahl CG, Postma DS, et al. Comparison of formoterol and terbutaline for as-needed treatment of asthma: a randomised trial. Lancet 2001; 357:257–61.

98. Malolepszy J, Boszormenyi NG, Selroos O, Larsso P, Brander R. Safety of formoterol Turbuhaler at cumulative dose of 90 µg in patients with acute bronchial obstruction. Eur Respir J 2001; 18:928–34.

99. Cazzola M, Di Marco F, Santus P, et al. The pharmacodynamic effects of single inhaled doses of formoterol, tiotropium and their combination in patients with COPD. Pulm Pharmacol Ther 2004; 17:35–9.

100. Barnes PJ, Stockley RA. COPD: current therapeutic interventions and future approaches. Eur Respir J 2005; 25:1084–106.

101. Di Marco F, Verga M, Santus P, Morelli N, Cazzola M, Centanni S. Effect of formoterol, tiotropium, and their combination in patients with acute exacerbations of chronic obstructive pulmonary disease: a pilot study. Respir Med 2006; 100:1925–32.

102. Barr RG, Rowe BH, Camargo CA, Jr. Methylxanthines for exacerbations of chronic obstructive pulmonary disease: meta-analysis of randomised trials. Br Med J 2003; 327:643.

103. Albert RK, Martin TR, Lewis SW. Controlled clinical trial of methylprednisolone in patients with chronic bronchitis and acute respiratory insufficiency. Ann Intern Med 1980; 92:753–8.

104. Niewoehner DE, Erbland ML, Deupree RH, et al. Effect of systemic glucocorticoids on exacerbations of chronic obstructive pulmonary disease. Department of Veterans Affairs Cooperative Study Group. N Engl J Med 1999; 340:1941–7.

105. Davies L, Angus RM, Calverley PM. Oral corticosteroids in patients admitted to hospital with exacerbations of chronic obstructive pulmonary disease: a prospective randomised controlled trial. Lancet 1999; 354:456–60.

106. Maltais F, Ostinelli J, Bourbeau J, et al. Comparison of nebulized budesonide and oral prednisolone with placebo in the treatment of acute exacerbations of chronic obstructive pulmonary disease: a randomized controlled trial. Am J Respir Crit Care Med 2002; 165:698–703.

107. Gunen H, Hacievliyagil SS, Yetkin O, Gulban G, Mutly LC, In E. The role of neublized budesonide in the treatment of exacerbations of COPD. Eur Respir J 2007; 29:660–7.

108. Aaron SD, Vandemheen KL, Hebert P, et al. Outpatient oral prednisone after emergency treatment of chronic obstructive pulmonary disease. N Engl J Med 2003; 348:2618–25.

109. Thompson WH, Nielson CP, Carvalho P, Charan NB, Crowley JJ. Controlled trial of oral prednisone in outpatients with acute COPD exacerbation. Am J Respir Crit Care Med 1996; 154:407–12.

110. Singh JM, Palda VA, Stanbrook MB, Chapman KR. Corticosteroid therapy for patients with acute exacerbations of chronic obstructive pulmonary disease: a systematic review. Arch Intern Med 2002; 162:2527–36.

111. Wood-Baker RR, Gibson PG, Hannay M, Walters EH, Walters JA. Systemic corticosteroids for acute exacerbations of chronic obstructive pulmonary disease. Cochrane Database Syst Rev 2005; 1:CD001288.

112. Lindenauer PK, Pekow P, Gao S, et al. Quality of care for patients hospitalized for acute exacerbations of chronic obstructive pulmonary disease. Ann Intern Med 2006; 144:894–903.

113. Monso E, Ruiz J, Rosell A, et al. Bacterial infection in chronic obstructive pulmonary disease. A study of stable and exacerbated outpatients using the protected specimen brush. Am J Respir Crit Care Med 1995; 152:1316–20.

114. Soler N, Torres A, Ewig S, et al. Bronchial microbial patterns in severe exacerbations of chronic obstructive pulmonary disease (COPD) requiring mechanical ventilation. Am J Respir Crit Care Med 1998; 157:1498–505.

115. Rohde G, Wiethege A, Borg I, et al. Respiratory viruses in exacerbations of chronic obstructive pulmonary disease requiring hospitalisation: a case-control study. Thorax 2003; 58:37–42.

116. Fagon JY, Chastre J, Trouillet JL, et al. Characterization of distal bronchial microflora during acute exacerbation of chronic bronchitis. Use of the protected specimen brush technique in 54 mechanically ventilated patients. Am Rev Respir Dis 1990; 142:1004–8.

117. Papi A, Bellettato CM, Braccioni F, et al. Infections of airway inflammation in chronic obstructive pulmonary disease severe exacerbations. Am J Respir Crit Care Med 2006; 173:1114–21.

118. Stockley RA, O'Brien C, Pye A, Hill SL. Relationship of sputum color to nature and outpatient management of acute exacerbations of COPD. Chest 2000; 117:1638–45.

119. Soler N, Agustí C, Angrill J, Puig de la Bellacasa J, Torres A. Bronchoscopic validation of the significance of sputum purulence in severe exacerbations of chronic obstructive pulmonary disease. Thorax 2007; 62:29–35.

120. Saint S, Bent S, Vittinghoff E, Grady D. Antibiotics in chronic obstructive pulmonary disease exacerbations. A meta-analysis. J Am Med Assoc 1995; 273:957–60.

121. Ram FS, Rodriguez-Roisin R, Garcia-Aymerich J, Granados AN, Barnes NC. Antibiotics for exacerbations of chronic obstructive pulmonary disease. Cochrane Database Syst Rev 2006; 19(2):CD004403.

122. Christ-Crain M, Müller B. Procalcitonin in bacterial infections: hype, hope, more or less? Swiss Med Wkly 2005; 125:451–60.

123. Muller B, Becker KL, Schachinger H, et al. Calcitonin precursors are reliable markers of sepsis in a medical intensive care unit. Crit Care Med 2000; 28:977–83.

124. Muller B, White JC, Nylen ES, et al. Ubiquitous expression of the calcitonin-I gene in multiple tissues in response to sepsis. J Clin Endocrinol Metab 2001; 86:396–404.

125. Linscheid P, Seboek D, Schaer DJ, et al. Expression and secretion of procalcitonin and calcitonin gene-related peptide by adherent monocytes and by macrophage-activated adipocytes. Crit Care Med 2004; 32:1715–21.

126. Stolz D, Christ-Crain M, Bingisser R, et al. Antibiotic treatment of exacerbations of COPD. A randomized, controlled trial comparing procalcitonin-guidance with standard therapy. Chest 2007; 131:9–19.

127. Rodríguez-Roisin R. COPD exacerbations. 5: management. Thorax 2006; 61:535–44.

128. Agusti AG, Carrera M, Barbe F, Muñoz A, Togores B. Oxygen therapy during exacerbations of chronic obstructive pulmonary disease. Eur Respir J 1999; 14:934–9.

129. Austin M, Wood-Baker R. Oxygen therapy in the pre-hospital setting for acute exacerbations of chronic obstructive pulmonare disease. Cochrane Database Syst Rev 2006; 19(3):CD005534.

130. Plant PK, Owen J, Elliot MW. One year period prevalence study of respiratory acidosis in acute exacerbations of COPD: implications for the provision of non-invasive ventilation and oxygen administration. Thorax 2000; 55:550–4.

131. Lightowler JV, Wedzicha JA, Elliott MW, Ram FS. Non-invasive positive pressure ventilation to treat respiratory failure resulting from exacerbations of chronic obstructive pulmonary disease: cochrane systematic review and meta-analysis. Br Med J 2003; 326:185–7.

132. Brochard L, Mancebo J, Wysocki M, et al. Noninvasive ventilation for acute exacerbations of chronic obstructive pulmonary disease. N Engl J Med 1995; 333:817–22.

133. Bott J, Carroll MP, Conway JH, et al. Randomised controlled trial of nasal ventilation in acute ventilatory failure due to chronic obstructive airways disease. Lancet 1993; 341:1555–7.

134. Celikel T, Sungur M, Ceyhan B, Karakurt S. Comparison of noninvasive positive pressure ventilation with standard medical therapy in hypercapnic acute respiratory failure. Chest 1998; 114:1636–42.
135. Plant PK, Owen JL, Elliott MW. Early use of non-invasive ventilation for acute exacerbations of chronic obstructive pulmonary disease on general respiratory wards: a multicentre randomised controlled trial. Lancet 2000; 355:1931–5.
136. Barbe F, Quera-Salva MA, de Lattre J, Gajdos P, Agusti AG. Long-term effects of nasal intermittent positive-pressure ventilation on pulmonary function and sleep architecture in patients with neuromuscular diseases. Chest 1996; 110:1179–83.
137. Avdeev SN, Tretiakov AV, Grigoriants RA, Kutsenko MA, Chuchalin AG. Study of the use of noninvasive ventilation of the lungs in acute respiratory insufficiency due exacerbation of chronic obstructive pulmonary disease. Anesteziol Reanimatol 1998; 3:45–51.
138. Dikensoy O, Ikidag B, Filiz A, Bayram N. Comparison of non-invasive ventilation and standard medical therapy in acute hypercapnic respiratory failure: a randomised controlled study at a tertiary health centre in SE Turkey. Int J Clin Pract 2002; 56:85–8.
139. Keenan SP, Gregor J, Sibbald WJ, Cook D, Gafni A. Noninvasive positive pressure ventilation in the setting of severe, acute exacerbations of chronic obstructive pulmonary disease: more effective and less expensive. Crit Care Med 2000; 28:2094–102.
140. Plant PK, Owen JL, Parrott S, Elliott MW. Cost effectiveness of ward based non-invasive ventilation for acute exacerbations of chronic obstructive pulmonary disease: economic analysis of randomised controlled trial. Br Med J 2003; 326:956.
141. Esteban A, Anzueto A, Frutos F, et al. Characteristics and outcomes in adult patients receiving mechanical ventilation: a 28-day international study. J Am Med Assoc 2002; 287:345–55.
142. Breen D, Churches T, Hawker F, Torzillo PJ. Acute respiratory failure secondary to chronic obstructive pulmonary disease treated in the intensive care unit: a long term follow up study. Thorax 2002; 57:29–33.
143. Nava S, Ambrosino N, Clini E, et al. Noninvasive mechanical ventilation in the weaning of patients with respiratory failure due to chronic obstructive pulmonary disease. A randomized, controlled trial. Ann Intern Med 1998; 128:721–8.
144. Ferrer M, Esquinas A, Arancibia F, et al. Noninvasive ventilation during persistent weaning failure: a randomized controlled trial. Am J Respir Crit Care Med 2003; 168:70–6.
145. Esteban A, Frutos-Vivar F, Ferguson ND, et al. Noninvasive positive-pressure ventilation for respiratory failure after extubation. N Engl J Med 2004; 350:2452–60.
146. Gravil JH, Al Rawas OA, Cotton MM, Flanigan U, Irwin A, Stevenson RD. Home treatment of exacerbations of chronic obstructive pulmonary disease by an acute respiratory assessment service. Lancet 1998; 351:1853–5.
147. Ram FS, Wedzicha JA, Wright J, Greenstone M. Hospital at home for patients with acute exacerbations of chronic obstructive pulmonary disease: systematic review of evidence. Br Med J 2004; 329:315.
148. Shepperd S, Harwood D, Gray A, Vessey M, Morgan P. Randomised controlled trial comparing hospital at home care with inpatient hospital care II: cost minimisation analysis. Br Med J 1998; 316:1791–6.
149. Cotton MM, Bucknall CE, Dagg KD, et al. Early discharge for patients with exacerbations of chronic obstructive pulmonary disease: a randomized controlled trial. Thorax 2000; 55:902–6.
150. Nicholson C, Bowler S, Jackson C, Schollay D, Tweeddale M, O'Rourke P. Cost comparison of hospital- and home-based treatment models for acute chronic obstructive pulmonary disease. Aust Health Rev 2001; 24:181–7.
151. Davies L, Wilkinson M, Bonner S, Calverley PM, Angus RM. "Hospital at home" versus hospital care in patients with exacerbations of chronic obstructive pulmonary disease: prospective randomised controlled trial. Br Med J 2000; 321:1265–8.
152. Skwarska E, Cohen T, Skwarski KM, et al. Randomized controlled trial of supported discharge in patients with exacerbations of chronic obstructive pulmonary disease. Thorax 2002; 55:907–12.
153. Ojoo JC, Moon T, McGlone S, et al. Patients' and carers' preferences in two models of care for acute exacerbations of COPD: results of a randomised controlled trial. Thorax 2002; 57:167–9.
154. Hernandez C, Casas A, Escarrabill J, et al. Home hospitalisation of exacerbated chronic obstructive pulmonary disease patients. Eur Respir J 2003; 21:58–67.

18

Exercise Training in COPD

THIERRY TROOSTERS
Respiratory Rehabilitation and Respiratory Division, University Hospitals, and Faculty of Kinesiology and Rehabilitation Sciences, Katholieke Universiteit Leuven, Leuven, Belgium, and Postdoctoral Fellow of the Research Foundation–Flanders, Brussels, Belgium

RIK GOSSELINK, CHRIS BURTIN, and MARC DECRAMER
Respiratory Rehabilitation and Respiratory Division, University Hospitals, and Faculty of Kinesiology and Rehabilitation Sciences, Katholieke Universiteit Leuven, Leuven, Belgium

I. Introduction

The World Health Organization defines rehabilitation as "The use of all means to aim at reducing the impact of disabling and handicapping conditions and at enabling people with disabilities to achieve optimal social integration." Rehabilitation, hence, is not confined to a specific organ or structure, but rather to the functioning and interaction of persons in their environment. Pulmonary rehabilitation is a form of rehabilitation dealing with patients suffering primarily from respiratory disorders and limited participation in daily life. The rehabilitation process, however, is not oriented at improving lung function, but rather improves the functioning of patients by improving the long-term systemic consequences patients with lung diseases may suffer from. These so-called "systemic consequences" include, but are not limited to, muscle weakness, nutritional depletion and exercise intolerance, symptoms that are often out of proportion of the lung function abnormality, and impaired mental state.

The goals of pulmonary rehabilitation are patient and society centered in the sense that rehabilitation aims at improving symptoms, exercise tolerance, patient participation in daily life, and health-related quality of life as well as at reducing the overall cost of care in these patients by reducing or postponing utilization of health-care recourses (1–5). In order to be efficient, rehabilitation programs should be an integral part of the overall care plan. Ideally, they facilitate communication between health-care providers across lines of health care. In a recent document of the American Thoracic Society and the European Respiratory Society (6), pulmonary rehabilitation was explicitly put within the context of integrated care and was defined as "an evidence-based, multidisciplinary, and comprehensive intervention for patients with chronic respiratory diseases who are symptomatic and often have decreased daily life activities. Integrated into the individualized treatment of the patient, pulmonary rehabilitation is designed to reduce symptoms, optimize functional status, increase participation, and reduce health care costs through stabilizing or reversing systemic manifestations of the disease."

This definition acknowledges the significant evidence base for rehabilitation programs and recognizes that its primary aim is not to enhance lung function. The definition, however, is rather comprehensive and follows that a thorough discussion of all components of pulmonary rehabilitation is outside the scope of this chapter, which focuses on one intervention, often referred to as the cornerstone of rehabilitation programs for patients suffering from respiratory diseases: exercise training. In addition, most of the discussion pertains to patients with chronic obstructive pulmonary disease (COPD). Indeed, most of the research has been conducted in this large patient population. Finally, most of the discussed techniques can be transposed to patients with other lung diseases. In fact, many of these techniques are also used in diseases other than lung diseases, such as frailty, osteoporosis, congestive heart failure, etc.

II. Exercise Limitation in Lung Disease

Exercise capacity is severely reduced in patients with COPD. Exercise tolerance is conventionally assessed using incremental ergometry exercise testing. Alternatively, field tests, such as timed walking tests or incremental walking tests (shuttle walking tests), can be used to assess exercise tolerance. From these tests, the exercise limitations of patients can be evaluated. In Figure 1, it is observed that exercise capacity is severely reduced in patients with COPD, but that timed walking tests and incremental exercise tests do not provide similar information regarding exercise limitations of patients. Indeed, it has been shown that timed walking tests result in near maximal oxygen uptake (7), but provide an index of maximal sustainable exercise tolerance (8). In contrast, incremental ergometer tests provide information on the maximal exercise tolerance and the factors that contribute to the exercise limitation in patients (9).

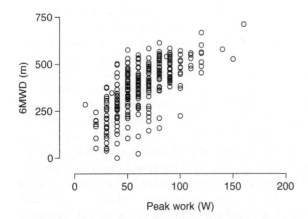

Figure 1 Relation between peak work rate obtained in an incremental cycle test [expressed in watts (W)] and the six-minute walking distance [6MWD; expressed in meters (m)] in a cohort of 289 chronic obstructive pulmonary disease patients referred for pulmonary rehabilitation. Although there is a significant link ($R=0.67$, $p<0.001$), it can be appreciated that for a given peak work rate the scatter on the 6MWD in individual patients is large.

Intuitively, exercise tolerance is thought to be limited by lung function impairment in patients. Consequently, exercise tolerance should be reduced proportional to lung function impairment. The relation between lung function and maximal exercise tolerance is rather weak (10). Hence, it should be concluded that exercise limitation in patients with COPD is multifactorial and factors limiting exercise capacity may vary between subjects. Several factors were identified to contribute to exercise intolerance and recently reviewed in detail (6). Identification of one factor limiting exercise tolerance in a patient is often difficult as several factors may be intimately related. However, from an incremental cardiopulmonary exercise test, it is possible to gain insight in the factors contributing directly or indirectly to the exercise limitation. Factors directly associated with lung function impairment include airflow obstruction, resulting in a reduction maximal ventilatory capacity. Flow limitation results in dynamic hyperinflation during exercise, which in turn increases the work of breathing and is the best correlate of symptoms of exertional dyspnea. Gas exchange abnormalities including ventilation/perfusion inadequacies may contribute to the exercise intolerance of patients. Pulmonary gas exchange abnormalities are likely to contribute indirectly to the exercise intolerance as it increases ventilatory requirements for a given exercise. Potential cardiac limitations in COPD are poorly investigated. Obviously, pulmonary hypertension during exercise may contribute to exercise intolerance and perceived symptoms of exertional dyspnea (11). The role of dynamic hyperinflation on cardiac output, and particularly on ventricular filling and stroke volume, is clearly a focus for further research (12). In healthy subjects, breathing against a fixed expiratory load of 10 cm H_2O did impair cardiac output, whereas voluntary hyperinflation did alleviate these negative effects (13). It remains to be studied whether the impact of flow limitation (increased expiratory load) and dynamic hyperinflation are of clinical relevance in COPD.

Skeletal muscle dysfunction has recently been unrevealed as a factor directly limiting exercise tolerance in a good fraction of COPD patients (14). Saey and coworkers found that in patients presenting with skeletal muscle fatigue after exercise, the administration of a short-acting bronchodilator did not enhance exercise tolerance, whereas exercise endurance time was almost doubled in patients not presenting with skeletal muscle fatigue after a single exercise bout. This study for the first time demonstrated that muscle fatigue does contribute directly to exercise tolerance. Other studies already suggested that skeletal muscle weakness was related to exercise intolerance in COPD. Deconditioning may also lead to exercise limitation. Early lactate release, a typical consequence of deconditioning (15,16), does lead to increased ventilatory requirements. Casaburi et al. calculated that 1 mmol lactate reduction resulted in 2.5 L/min pulmonary ventilation reduction (17). Conversely, lactate release is likely to be associated with rise in pulmonary ventilation or rise in $PaCO_2$ (when patients are reaching the boundaries of the ventilatory system).

In the context of understanding the effects of exercise training, it is important to know the exercise limitation of the patient. Many patients may be ventilatory limited, but the ventilatory limitation—often estimated from the maximum voluntary ventilation—is reached prematurely due to enhanced ventilatory requirements during exercise. This can be attributed to a high dead space ventilation, hypoxia, or deconditioning-induced lactic acidosis. In patients reaching the ventilatory boundaries prematurely, the challenge is to elucidate why the patient has increased ventilatory demands. The design of the training program should ideally take the exercise limitation of patients maximally into account (see below).

III. Exercise Tolerance and Health-Related Quality of Life After Exercise Training

The success of achieving the goals of rehabilitation can be assessed through physiological, psychosocial, and economical outcome measures. In a recent meta-analysis, the effects of pulmonary rehabilitation programs on exercise tolerance were systematically reviewed (18). In incremental tests, peak work rate improved on the average by 18% compared to baseline [weighted mean of studies (18–21), reporting maximal exercise tolerance in a parallel group design]. Peak oxygen uptake improved by 11% when the rehabilitation groups are compared with their respective controls. The effect of pulmonary rehabilitation on whole body constant work rate exercise tolerance is much larger. As a weighted average of five randomized controlled studies (21–25), whole body endurance exercise time improved by an average of 87%. Exertional dyspnea is consistently reported to be reduced after pulmonary rehabilitation (26).

The clinical relevance of the benefit of pulmonary rehabilitation is illustrated by the improved functional capacity, as measured by the six-minute walking test (6MWT). The pooled effect size of all randomized controlled studies of the results of pulmonary rehabilitation is 48 m, with a 95% confidence interval (CI) of 32 to 65 m (18). The minimal clinically important difference (MCID) of the 6MWT has been estimated to be 54 m (27). From a randomized controlled study conducted in the authors' center (30), the number needed to treat, in order to have one patient with a clinically significant benefit, was 3 (95% CI: 1.7–6.4). Others found similar results (29), even if sustained improvement over a 24-month follow-up period was used as a criterion.

A review of the published literature shows that the improvement in health-related quality of life after pulmonary rehabilitation clearly exceeds the MCID. When disease-specific instruments were used, the lower limit of the 95% CI exceeded the MCID (14). To improve health-related quality of life, the effects of adding pulmonary rehabilitation to the treatment of a patient with COPD may be greater than adding another drug (30).

Improved health-related quality of life is observed even in the absence of clinically significant improvements in exercise capacity (31,32). Hence, the enhanced health-related quality of life is surely not influenced by the physiological benefits alone. Improved mental state, enhanced self-efficacy, enhanced symptom control, and ameliorated perception of symptoms are among the non-physiological pathways likely to contribute to an enhanced health-related quality of life. Long-term follow-up has shown that quality of life benefits are maintained above control levels if rehabilitation yields clinically significant effects on exercise tolerance (28,29,33).

IV. The Exercise Training Intervention

A. Rationale

From the definition of pulmonary rehabilitation, it follows that "reversing the systemic consequences" of the lung disease renders the benefits of rehabilitation programs.

As expected, exercise training may impact on the cardiovascular function. At isowork, heart rate is reduced after high-intensity exercise training (17,34), and it has also been suggested that baroreflex sensitivity is altered favorably after exercise training (35). Whether exercise training has also favorable effects on vascular function, as in patients with heart failure (36), or cardiac structure, has not been investigated in COPD. Exercise training aims at reversing the skeletal muscle abnormalities. Clinically, skeletal muscle strength has been reported reduced, in proportion to skeletal muscle mass (37). Local endurance is even more impaired than skeletal muscle strength. The skeletal muscle of patients with COPD is also more rapidly fatigued during exercise (38), compared to healthy muscle. Several authors also reported deranged muscle bioenergetics (39). At the microscopic level, generalized skeletal muscle atrophy has been reported with a predominance of glycolytic fibers (40). This pattern is slightly different from that observed with aging, where typically type II fibers atrophy is present. In addition, the number of capillary to fiber contacts is reduced in COPD (40). In the context of pulmonary rehabilitation, two important findings at the molecular level deserve to be mentioned. First, the activity of two important enzymes, citrate synthase and 3-hydroxyacyl-coenzyme A dehydrogenase (HADH), has been reported to be consistently reduced in patients with COPD (41). These enzymes play an important role in the oxidative energy processes in the skeletal muscle. As a result, the skeletal muscle has to rely on anaerobic glycolysis at abnormally low work rates. The produced lactate poses a burden on the compromised ventilatory system and leads to early ventilatory limitation. Secondly, the skeletal muscle seems to be more vulnerable to oxidative stress. In a subset of patients with low body mass index, this may compromise the benefits of exercise training (42).

Most, if not all, skeletal muscle consequences of COPD are also seen after severe deconditioning. It appears, hence, likely that inactivity is the main driver of the skeletal muscle abnormalities seen in most patients. However, in subgroups of patients, other mechanisms may further impair skeletal muscle function. Such subgroups of patients include those (*i*) with hypoxemia or hypercapnia, (*ii*) rapidly loosing body weight, or (*iii*) treated with high doses of oral corticosteroids. These are discussed in detail elsewhere (43). Most of the deconditioning-induced abnormalities are at least partially reversible. After exercise training, skeletal muscle force is increased (28), and the limb muscles are less prone to exercise-induced contractile fatigue (44). At the molecular and fiber level, oxidative enzyme capacity is enhanced (45), skeletal muscle fibers do hypertrophy, and there are more capillary contacts per fiber (40).

B. Exercise Training: Practical Aspects

In general, exercise training in patients with COPD follows the principles of exercise training in the healthy elderly. Programs generally consist of a warm-up, a core program in which at least 30 minutes of active exercise is included, and a cooling down. Close supervision and proper monitoring ensure safety during the program. In fact, very few exercise-related events and, as far as the authors are aware, no fatal events have been reported after pulmonary rehabilitation in the published literature. Table 1A–C summarizes a suggested training schedule for patients with COPD used in the authors' center.

Table 1 Training Scheme for the Treadmill Exercises Used in the Authors' Institute

(A) Endurance training on the treadmill

Week	Duration (min)	Training load (% 6MWT)
1	10	75
2	12	75
3	12	80
4	14	80
5	14	85
6	14	90
7	16	90
8	16	95
9	16	100
10	16	105
11	16	110
12	16	110

(B) Interval training on a bicycle

Week	Duration (min)	Number of blocks	Training load (% W_{max})
1	2	5×	60
2	2	6×	60
3	2	6×	65
4	2	7×	65
5	2	7×	70
6	2	7×	70
7	2	7×	75
8	2	8×	75
9	2	8×	80
10	2	8×	80
11	2	8×	85
12	2	8×	85

(C) Resistance training program

Week	Load (% 1 RM)	Reps
1	70	3×8
2	70	3×8
3	76	3×8
4	82	3×8
5	88	3×8
6	94	3×8
7	100	3×8
8	106	3×8
9	112	3×8
10	115	3×8
11	118	3×8
12	121	3×8

Examples of training programs: (A) Proposed endurance training on a treadmill based on the speed obtained during a 6MWT. Week is displayed along with the duration of the block of exercise and the intensity, relative to the speed during a 6MWT. (B) Proposed interval training schedule on a cycle ergometer. The intensity is given relative to the peak workload obtained during a maximal incremental cycle test. In between the different blocks, patients are allowed to rest or they can continue cycling at reduced work rate. (C) Resistance training. The training load is expressed as percentage of 1 RM, the maximal weight a patient can lift once over the whole range of motion without compensatory movements. The Reps remains identical throughout the training: three series of eight repetitions.

Abbreviations: 6MWT, six-minute walking test; RM, repetition maximum; Reps, number of repetitions.

Whole Body Exercise

Exercise training has been included in virtually all studies investigating the benefits of pulmonary rehabilitation. In order to successfully increase skeletal muscle properties and render measurable physiological benefits, it is important that patients do exercise at relative high workloads. In order to do so, the exercise training intervention can be adapted to the individual exercise limitations of the patient (see above). The conventionally used form to deliver exercise training to COPD patients is endurance training. In COPD patients with primarily moderate disease, exercise training conducted at $\approx 75\%$ of the peak work rate (60% of the difference between the lactate threshold and peak oxygen uptake) resulted in significant physiological effects (17). A similar training strategy was shown to be effective in patients with more severe disease (46).

Others have confirmed that high training intensity is required to elicit physiologic training effects (34,47). Interval exercise training has been used and showed to result in physiological benefits, comparable to those of endurance training (48–51). The advantage of interval training is that the ventilatory requirements remain relatively limited (52). Alternatively, exercises can be limited to single leg exercise (53), but from a clinical perspective this may be less practical. In our center, interval training is used in patients with severe ventilatory limitation or those not able to sustain long exercise bouts (i.e., more than 10 minutes). It is important to adjust and increase the training load in every session. Trained personnel should be available to ensure close supervision on the training intensity. Training intensity can be monitored using Borg symptom scales. A score of 4 to 6 is generally advised as an appropriate training intensity, provided the patients are familiar with the 10-point scale. Interestingly, a given Borg symptom score is generally chosen by a patient at a fixed relative work rate. Hence, as patients improve during training, the same Borg rating will be achieved at higher absolute work rates (54). Since most patients are not limited by the cardiovascular system, using heart frequency to guide exercise training is not advised.

Interventions to minimize the ventilatory burden during exercise training are the use of (*i*) supplemental oxygen, (*ii*) non-invasive ventilation, and (*iii*) low-density gas mixtures (helium–oxygen). Oxygen dose dependently reduces the ventilation for a given exercise intensity (55,56). Application of oxygen supplements hence allows training at higher training intensity (57). Non-invasive mechanical ventilation reduces the work of breathing and has been used successfully in severe COPD as an adjunct to exercise training (58–60). In less severe COPD, the impact of using non-invasive mechanical ventilation was not significant (61). Lastly, the required ventilation can be reduced simply by reducing the amount of muscles put at work. If exercise is confined to one leg, ventilation is considerably reduced, allowing a significant increase in training load on the targeted muscle (53). Along the same lines, during cycling less muscles are recruited compared to walking exercises; it is hence not surprising that for a given level of whole body oxygen consumption, cycling is more fatiguing (62). It would be interesting to conduct a head-to-head comparison study on the physiologic effects of cycling versus walking exercises, when applied in a rehabilitation program to check whether, on the basis of the larger potential to elicit muscle fatigue, cycling would be a form of exercise training that results in larger physiological effects, compared to walking. Such a study is currently unavailable.

Obviously, optimal bronchodilator therapy does also allow for larger pulmonary ventilation during exercise. This may be of particular benefit during walking exercises

(62). In one study, a potent long-term anticholinergic drug showed to enhance exercise training effects compared to the use of short-acting bronchodilators alone (63).

Resistance Training

Another form of conventional training is resistance training. This form of exercise, generally consisting of weight lifting, can be used as the only form of training (23,64,65), or in combination with whole body exercises (65–67). In all the latter studies, muscle strength was significantly more increased when resistance training was added to the exercise regimen. Increase in muscle strength is an important treatment objective in patients with COPD suffering from muscle weakness, as activities of daily life do require strength on top of muscle endurance. As mentioned above, muscle weakness is an important factor related to morbidity and even mortality in COPD. It follows that patients suffering from muscle weakness may be particularly good candidates to a resistance training program.

Resistance training is easy to apply in clinical practice. Patients are instructed to lift weights. Generally, this is done on a multigym device. Lifting free weights is a valid option, but range of motion is less controlled. Whether this may elicit high risk for injury has not been investigated. The weight imposed and the number of repetitions ensure overload of the skeletal muscle. In patients with COPD and several other chronic diseases, resistance training is started with approximately 70% of the weight a patient can lift once (i.e., the 1 repetition maximum). The effects of resistance training programs may be enhanced in male hypogonadal patients by testosterone replacement therapy. A combination of resistance training and weekly intramuscular injections with testosterone, aiming at restoring testosterone levels to normal values in initially hypogonadal men, tended to enhance skeletal muscle force more than either of the interventions alone (68). Further studies are required to investigate the long-term safety of this intervention. However, since skeletal muscle dysfunction is in itself a negative prognostic factor, short-term use of testosterone may be beneficial to result in a rapid restoration of skeletal muscle force.

Another intervention used to specifically stimulate the peripheral muscles is neuromuscular electrical stimulation. Four studies have investigated successfully the effects of this intervention (69–72). Studies showed that there was more strength gain in the skeletal muscles treated with electrical stimulation, both as monotherapy and in combination with general exercise training (72). This intervention may prove to be attractive in patients who have difficulties to take part in regular rehabilitation.

In summary, exercise training programs can be adjusted to the individual exercise limitations of patients with COPD. In individual patients, endurance training, interval training, or resistance training can be offered to keep the training stimulus attractive and with acceptable symptoms. Several interventions can be considered to further alleviate the ventilatory burden or specifically stimulate the peripheral muscle. An empirical flow chart that may guide the clinician to design the exercise intervention is given in Figure 2. It should be recognized that this flow chart is not directly validated, but rather compiles the available knowledge and clinical expertise.

Specific Respiratory Muscle Training

The respiratory muscles have been specifically targeted for training in COPD. Inspiratory muscle training programs can be conducted at home using resistive breathing with target inspiratory pressures or target inspiratory flows or with threshold loading devices. Normocapnic hyperpnea has also been applied, albeit less frequently, in COPD (73). When training load is appropriate (controlled and more than 40% of PI_{max}), inspiratory muscle training leads consistently to reductions in dyspnea and improved measures of inspiratory muscle performance (74). Programs are relatively inexpensive, but require regular supervision. Training intensity can be gradually increased, particularly during the first weeks of a training program (75). Whether inspiratory muscle training translates to increased exercise tolerance and quality of life is much less clear (74,75). Therefore, there has been some debate as to whether inspiratory muscle training should be part of rehabilitation programs in COPD, with evidence-based guidelines concluding that it should not be a routine component (1,3,76).

In patients with inspiratory muscle weakness, it can be speculated that increasing respiratory muscle function may transform into functional benefits. This has indeed been confirmed, to some extent, by a systematic literature review (74). Therefore, in

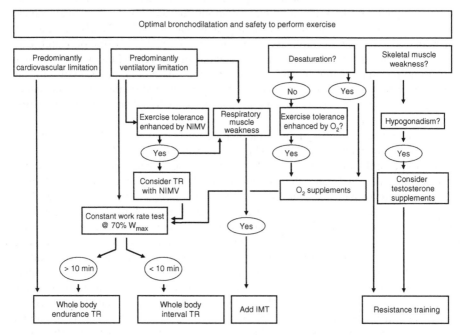

Figure 2 Empirical algorithm that could help the clinician to prescribe exercise therapy to individual patients. Based on the exercise limitation of the patient (investigated in an incremental exercise test) and further clinical findings, different training strategies or combinations can be prescribed. Typical cutoffs are: (*i*) respiratory muscle weakness: $PI_{max} <$ 60% predicted (74); (*ii*) hypogonadism: total serum testosterone: <400 ng/dL (68); and (*iii*) desaturation: saturation upon exercise $<85\%$. Constant work rate test @ 70% W_{max} is an exercise performed at 70% of the peak work rate from the incremental test. *Abbreviations*: W_{max}, maximum work-rate during progressive cycle ergometry; PI_{max}, maximum inspiratory pressure; TR, training; NIMV, non-invasive mechanical ventilation; IMT, inspiratory muscle training.

patients with inspiratory muscle weakness, the prescription of strictly standardized inspiratory muscle training may be justified as an adjunct to exercise training (73,77,78), with the aim of improving exercise-induced symptoms of dyspnea. It should be noted however that whole body exercise training, by itself, has improved inspiratory muscle force in some studies (28,79). Inspiratory muscle training as a stand-alone treatment is clearly inferior to general exercise training in COPD if the goal is to improve function or health-related quality of life.

V. Pulmonary Rehabilitation: More Than Exercise Training

Exercise training is considered the cornerstone of a pulmonary rehabilitation program. Nevertheless, COPD is a complex disease. Its impact on the psychological function, nutritional status, and participation in everyday life may require interventions other than exercise training. Typically, rehabilitation programs offer nutritional interventions, social support, occupational therapy, and psychological counseling to selected patients. In patients who suffer from exacerbations, the addition of a self-management program may be an essential cost-saving intervention (80). Clearly, pulmonary rehabilitation is a multidisciplinary intervention offered by a team of health-care providers. Typically, for each patient the content of the rehabilitation program and the disciplines intervening is individually tailored based on the severity of the limitation of activities of daily life, the psychological morbidity, the nutritional status, the perceived and received social support, and the knowledge and appropriate action regarding the disease condition.

In summary, pulmonary rehabilitation programs are clearly an "evidence-based" intervention in patients with COPD. This is reflected in the most recent guideline on pulmonary rehabilitation and in a regularly updated meta-analysis (26). It has become clear over the last few decades that pulmonary rehabilitation is an essential cornerstone in the treatment of patients with reduced physical activity levels or with unresolved symptoms despite medical treatment. Based on the exercise limitation of the patient and taking into account the factors contributing to the exercise limitation, an exercise training program can be designed. This chapter elaborated on the exercise training intervention, but it should be emphasized that rehabilitation involves by definition multiple disciplines of health-care providers. Two comprehensive review papers give more insight in what can be expected from interventions such as learning self-management strategies, psychological counseling, occupational therapy, social counseling, nutritional advice, and optimal medical treatment (6,30). It is important to recognize the value of a multidisciplinary team which places the patient in the center of the care and assembles the required health-care providers around a patient in order to provide optimal and individualized care.

References

1. Pulmonary rehabilitation: joint ACCP/AACVPR evidence-based guidelines. ACCP/AACVPR Pulmonary Rehabilitation Guidelines Panel. American College of Chest Physicians. American Association of Cardiovascular and Pulmonary Rehabilitation. Chest 1997; 112:1363–96.

2. Pulmonary rehabilitation-1999. American Thoracic Society. Am J Respir Crit Care Med 1999; 159:1666–82.
3. British Thoracic Society Standards of Care Subcommittee on Pulmonary Rehabilitation. Pulmonary rehabilitation. Thorax 2001; 56:827–34.
4. Donner CF, Decramer M. Pulmonary rehabilitation. Eur Respir Monogr 2000; 13:1–200.
5. Donner CF, Muir JF. Selection criteria and programmes for pulmonary rehabilitation in COPD patients. Rehabilitation and chronic care scientific group of the European Respiratory Society. Eur Respir J 1997; 10:744–57.
6. Nici L, Donner C, Wouters E, ZuWallack R, Ambrosino N, Bourbeau J, Carone M, Celli B, Engelen M, Fahy B, et al. American thoracic society/European respiratory society statement on pulmonary rehabilitation. Am J Respir Crit Care Med 2006; 173:1390–413.
7. Troosters T, Vilaro J, Rabinovich RA, et al. Physiological responses to six minute walking test in COPD patients. Eur Respir J 2002; 20:564–9.
8. Casas A, Vilaro J, Rabinovich R, et al. Encouraged 6-min walking test indicates maximum sustainable exercise in COPD patients. Chest 2005; 128:55–61.
9. Wasserman K, Hansen JE, Sue DJ, Whipp BJ, Casaburi R. Principles of Exercise Testing and Interpretation. 2nd ed. Philadelphia: Williams & Wilkins, 1994:479.
10. Gosselink R, Troosters T, Decramer M. Peripheral muscle weakness contributes to exercise limitation in COPD. Am J Respir Crit Care Med 1996; 153:976–80.
11. Chaouat A, Bugnet AS, Kadaoui N, et al. Severe pulmonary hypertension and chronic obstructive pulmonary disease. Am J Respir Crit Care Med 2005; 172:189–94.
12. Baril J, de SM, Leroy D, et al. Does dynamic hyperinflation impair submaximal exercise cardiac output in chronic obstructive pulmonary disease? Clin Invest Med 2006; 29:104–9.
13. Stark-Leyva KN, Beck KC, Johnson BD. Influence of expiratory loading and hyperinflation on cardiac output during exercise. J Appl Physiol 2004; 96:1920–7.
14. Saey D, Debigare R, LeBlanc P, et al. Contractile leg fatigue after cycle exercise. A factor limiting exercise in patients with COPD. Am J Respir Crit Care Med 2003; 168:425–30.
15. Hamilton AL, Killian KJ, Summers E, Jones NL. Muscle strength, symptom intensity, and exercise capacity in patients with cardiorespiratory disorders. Am J Respir Crit Care Med 1995; 152:2021–31.
16. Saey D, Michaud A, Couillard A, et al. Contractile fatigue, muscle morphometry, and blood lactate in chronic obstructive pulmonary disease. Am J Respir Crit Care Med 2005; 171:1109–15.
17. Casaburi R, Patessio A, Ioli F, Zanaboni S, Donner CF, Wasserman K. Reductions in exercise lactic acidosis and ventilation as a result of exercise training in patients with obstructive lung disease. Am Rev Respir Dis 1991; 143:9–18.
18. Lacasse Y, Goldstein R, Lasserson TJ, et al. Pulmonary rehabilitation for chronic obstructive pulmonary disease. Cochrane Database Syst Rev 2006;CD003793.
19. O'Donnell DE, McGuire M, Samis L, Webb KA. The impact of exercise reconditioning on breathlessness in severe chronic airflow limitation. Am J Respir Crit Care Med 1995; 152:2005–13.
20. Reardon J, Awad E, Normandin E, Vale F, Clark B, ZuWallack RL. The effect of comprehensive outpatient pulmonary rehabilitation on dyspnea. Chest 1994; 105:1046–52.
21. Ries AL, Kaplan RM, Limberg TM, Prewitt LM. Effects of pulmonary rehabilitation on physiologic and psychosocial outcomes in patients with chronic obstructive pulmonary disease. Ann Intern Med 1995; 122:823–32.
22. Weiner P, Azgad Y, Ganam R. Inspiratory muscle training combined with general exercise reconditioning in patients with COPD. Chest 1992; 102:1351–6.
23. Simpson K, Killian K, McCartney N, Stubbing DG, Jones NL. Randomised controlled trial of weightlifting exercise in patients with chronic airflow limitation. Thorax 1992; 47:70–5.
24. Hernandez MT, Rubio TM, Ruiz FO, Riera HS, Gil RS, Gomez JC. Results of a home-based training program for patients with COPD. Chest 2000; 118:106–14.
25. Cambach W, Chadwick-Straver RV, Wagenaar RC, van Keimpema AR, Kemper HC. The effects of a community-based pulmonary rehabilitation programme on exercise tolerance and quality of life: a randomized controlled trial. Eur Respir J 1997; 10:104–13.
26. Gigliotti F, Coli C, Bianchi R, et al. Exercise training improves exertional dyspnea in patients with COPD: evidence of the role of mechanical factors. Chest 2003; 123:1794–802.
27. Redelmeier DA, Bayoumi AM, Goldstein RS, Guyatt GH. Interpreting small differences in functional status: the six minute walk test in chronic lung disease patients. Am J Respir Crit Care Med 1997; 155:1278–82.

28. Troosters T, Gosselink R, Decramer M. Short- and long-term effects of outpatient rehabilitation in patients with chronic obstructive pulmonary disease: a randomized trial. Am J Med 2000; 109:207–12.
29. Guell R, Casan P, Belda J, et al. Long-term effects of outpatient rehabilitation of COPD: a randomized trial. Chest 2000; 117:976–83.
30. Troosters T, Casaburi R, Gosselink R, Decramer M. Pulmonary rehabilitation in chronic obstructive pulmonary disease. Am J Respir Crit Care Med 2005; 172:19–38.
31. Normandin EA, McCusker C, Connors M, Vale F, Gerardi D, ZuWallack RL. An evaluation of two approaches to exercise conditioning in pulmonary rehabilitation. Chest 2002; 121:1085–91.
32. Puente-Maestu L, Sanz ML, Sanz P, Cubillo JM, Mayol J, Casaburi R. Comparison of effects of supervised versus self-monitored training programmes in patients with chronic obstructive pulmonary disease. Eur Respir J 2000; 15:517–25.
33. Strijbos JH, Postma DS, van Altena R, Gimeno F, Koeter GH. A comparison between an outpatient hospital-based pulmonary rehabilitation program and a home-care pulmonary rehabilitation program in patients with COPD. A follow-up of 18 months. Chest 1996; 109:366–72.
34. Puente-Maestu L, Sanz ML, Sanz P, Ruiz de Ona JM, Rodriguez-Hermosa JL, Whipp BJ. Effects of two types of training on pulmonary and cardiac responses to moderate exercise in patients with COPD. Eur Respir J 2000; 15:1026–32.
35. Costes F, Roche F, Pichot V, Vergnon JM, Garet M, Barthelemy JC. Influence of exercise training on cardiac baroreflex sensitivity in patients with COPD. Eur Respir J 2004; 23:396–401.
36. Hambrecht R, Gielen S, Linke A, et al. Effects of exercise training on left ventricular function and peripheral resistance in patients with chronic heart failure: a randomized trial. J Am Med Assoc 2000; 283:3095–101.
37. Bernard S, LeBlanc P, Whittom F, et al. Peripheral muscle weakness in patients with chronic obstructive pulmonary disease. Am J Respir Crit Care Med 1998; 158:629–34.
38. Mador MJ, Deniz O, Aggarwal A, Kufel TJ. Quadriceps fatigability after single muscle exercise in patients with chronic obstructive pulmonary disease. Am J Respir Crit Care Med 2003; 168:102–8.
39. Sala E, Roca J, Marrades RM, et al. Effects of endurance training on skeletal muscle bioenergetics in chronic obstructive pulmonary disease. Am J Respir Crit Care Med 1999; 159:1726–34.
40. Whittom F, Jobin J, Simard PM, et al. Histochemical and morphological characteristics of the vastus lateralis muscle in patients with chronic obstructive pulmonary disease. Med Sci Sports Exerc 1998; 30:1467–74.
41. Maltais F, LeBlanc P, Whittom F, et al. Oxidative enzyme activities of the vastus lateralis muscle and the functional status in patients with COPD. Thorax 2000; 55:848–53.
42. Rabinovich RA, Ardite E, Mayer AM, et al. Training depletes muscle glutathione in patients with chronic obstructive pulmonary disease and low body mass index. Respiration 2006; 73:757–61.
43. Debigare R, Cote CH, Maltais F. Peripheral muscle wasting in chronic obstructive pulmonary disease. Clinical relevance and mechanisms. Am J Respir Crit Care Med 2001; 164:1712–7.
44. Mador MJ, Kufel TJ, Pineda LA, et al. Effect of pulmonary rehabilitation on quadriceps fatiguability during exercise. Am J Respir Crit Care Med 2001; 163:930–5.
45. Maltais F, LeBlanc P, Simard C, et al. Skeletal muscle adaptation to endurance training in patients with chronic obstructive pulmonary disease. Am J Respir Crit Care Med 1996; 154:442–7.
46. Casaburi R, Porszasz J, Burns MR, Carithers ER, Chang RS, Cooper CB. Physiologic benefits of exercise training in rehabilitation of patients with severe chronic obstructive pulmonary disease. Am J Respir Crit Care Med 1997; 155:1541–51.
47. Gimenez M, Servera E, Vergara P, Bach JR, Polu JM. Endurance training in patients with chronic obstructive pulmonary disease: a comparison of high versus moderate intensity. Arch Phys Med Rehabil 2000; 81:102–9.
48. Vogiatzis I, Nanas S, Roussos C. Interval training as an alternative modality to continuous exercise in patients with COPD. Eur Respir J 2002; 20:12–9.
49. Vogiatzis I, Terzis G, Nanas S, et al. Skeletal muscle adaptations to interval training in patients with advanced COPD. Chest 2005; 128:3838–45.
50. Coppoolse R, Schols AM, Baarends EM, et al. Interval versus continuous training in patients with severe COPD: a randomized clinical trial. Eur Respir J 1999; 14:258–63.
51. Puhan MA, Busching G, Schunemann HJ, VanOort E, Zaugg C, Frey M. Interval versus continuous high-intensity exercise in chronic obstructive pulmonary disease: a randomized trial. Ann Intern Med 2006; 145:816–25.
52. Sabapathy S, Kingsley RA, Schneider DA, Adams L, Morris NR. Continuous and intermittent exercise responses in individuals with chronic obstructive pulmonary disease. Thorax 2004; 59:1026–31.

53. Dolmage TE, Goldstein RS. Response to one-legged cycling in patients with COPD. Chest 2006; 129:325–32.

54. Mahler DA, Ward J, Mejia-Alfaro R. Stability of dyspnea ratings after exercise training in patients with COPD. Med Sci Sports Exerc 2003; 35:1083–7.

55. Porszasz J, Emtner M, Goto S, Somfay A, Whipp BJ, Casaburi R. Exercise training decreases ventilatory requirements and exercise-induced hyperinflation at submaximal intensities in patients with COPD. Chest 2005; 128:2025–34.

56. Somfay A, Porszasz J, Lee SM, Casaburi R. Dose-response effect of oxygen on hyperinflation and exercise endurance in nonhypoxaemic COPD patients. Eur Respir J 2001; 18:77–84.

57. Emtner M, Porszasz J, Burns M, Somfay A, Casaburi R. Benefits of supplemental oxygen in exercise training in non-hypoxemic COPD patients. Am J Respir Crit Care Med 2003; 168:1034–42.

58. Hawkins P, Johnson LC, Nikoletou D, et al. Proportional assist ventilation as an aid to exercise training in severe chronic obstructive pulmonary disease. Thorax 2002; 57:853–9.

59. Costes F, Agresti A, Court-Fortune I, Roche F, Vergnon JM, Barthelemy JC. Noninvasive ventilation during exercise training improves exercise tolerance in patients with chronic obstructive pulmonary disease. J Cardiopulm Rehabil 2003; 23:307–13.

60. van't HA, Gosselink R, Hollander P, Postmus P, Kwakkel G. Training with inspiratory pressure support in patients with severe COPD. Eur Respir J 2006; 27:65–72.

61. Bianchi L, Foglio K, Porta R, Baiardi R, Vitacca M, Ambrosino N. Lack of additional effect of adjunct of assisted ventilation to pulmonary rehabilitation in mild COPD patients. Respir Med 2002; 96:359–67.

62. Pepin V, Saey D, Whittom F, LeBlanc P, Maltais F. Walking versus cycling: sensitivity to bronchodilation in chronic obstructive pulmonary disease. Am J Respir Crit Care Med 2005; 172:1517–22.

63. Casaburi R, Kukafka D, Cooper CB, Witek TJ, Jr., Kesten S. Improvement in exercise tolerance with the combination of tiotropium and pulmonary rehabilitation in patients with COPD. Chest 2005; 127:809–17.

64. Spruit MA, Gosselink R, Troosters T, De Paepe C, Decramer M. Resistance versus endurance training in patients with COPD and skeletal muscle weakness. Eur Respir J 2002; 19:1072–8.

65. Ortega F, Toral J, Cejudo P, et al. Comparison of effects of strength and endurance training in patients with chronic obstructive pulmonary disease. Am J Respir Crit Care Med 2002; 166:669–74.

66. Bernard S, Whittom F, LeBlanc P, et al. Aerobic and strength training in patients with chronic obstructive pulmonary disease. Am J Respir Crit Care Med 1999; 159:896–901.

67. Mador MJ, Bozkanat E, Aggarwal A, Shaffer M, Kufel TJ. Endurance and strength training in patients with COPD. Chest 2004; 125:2036–45.

68. Casaburi R, Bhasin S, Cosentino L, et al. Anabolic effects of testosterone replacement and strength training in men with COPD. Am J Respir Crit Care Med 2004; 170:870–8.

69. Neder JA, Sword D, Ward SA, Mackay E, Cochrane LM, Clark CJ. Home based neuromuscular electrical stimulation as a new rehabilitative strategy for severely disabled patients with chronic obstructive pulmonary disease (COPD). Thorax 2002; 57:333–7.

70. Bourjeily-Habr G, Rochester C, Palermo F, Snyder P, Mohsenin V. Randomised controlled trial of transcutaneous electrical muscle stimulation of the lower extremities in patients with chronic obstructive pulmonary disease. Thorax 2002; 57:1045–9.

71. Zanotti E, Felicetti G, Maini M, Fracchia C. Peripheral muscle strength training in bed-bound patients with COPD receiving mechanical ventilation: effect of electrical stimulation. Chest 2003; 124:292–6.

72. Vivodtzev I, Pepin JL, Vottero G, et al. Improvement in quadriceps strength and dyspnea in daily tasks after 1 month of electrical stimulation in severely deconditioned and malnourished COPD. Chest 2006; 129:1540–8.

73. Scherer TA, Spengler CM, Owassapian D, Imhof E, Boutellier U. Respiratory muscle endurance training in chronic obstructive pulmonary disease: impact on exercise capacity, dyspnea, and quality of life. Am J Respir Crit Care Med 2000; 162:1709–14.

74. Lotters F, Van Tol B, Kwakkel G, Gosselink R. Effects of controlled inspiratory muscle training in patients with COPD: a meta-analysis. Eur Respir J 2002; 20:570–6.

75. Hill K, Jenkins SC, Philippe DL, et al. High-intensity inspiratory muscle training in COPD. Eur Respir J 2006; 27:1119–28.

76. Lacasse Y, Guyatt GH, Goldstein RS. The components of a respiratory rehabilitation program: a systematic overview. Chest 1997; 111:1077–88.

77. Wanke T, Formanek D, Lahrmann H, et al. Effects of combined inspiratory muscle and cycle ergometer training on exercise performance in patients with COPD. Eur Respir J 1994; 7:2205–11.

78. Dekhuijzen PN, Beek MML, Folgering HT, van Herwaarden CL. Psychological changes during pulmonary rehabilitation and target-flow inspiratory muscle training in COPD patients with a ventilatory limitation during exercise. Int J Rehabil Res 1990; 13:109–17.
79. O'Donnell DE, McGuire M, Samis L, Webb KA. General exercise training improves ventilatory and peripheral muscle strength and endurance in chronic airflow limitation. Am J Respir Crit Care Med 1998; 157:1489–97.
80. Gadoury MA, Schwartzman K, Rouleau M, et al. Self-management reduces both short- and long-term hospitalisation in COPD. Eur Respir J 2005; 26:853–7.

19

New Components of Pulmonary Rehabilitation in COPD

EMIEL F. M. WOUTERS
Center for Integrated Rehabilitation of Organ Failure, Horn, The Netherlands, and Department of Respiratory Medicine, University Hospital Maastricht, Maastricht, The Netherlands

MARTIJN A. SPRUIT
Department of Research, Development, and Education, Center for Integrated Rehabilitation of Organ Failure, Horn, The Netherlands

I. Introduction

Chronic obstructive pulmonary disease (COPD) is a disease state characterized by a progressive airflow limitation that is partly reversible after optimal pharmacological treatment (1). Although the pulmonary dysfunction may explain to a certain extent the degree of severity of each day's symptoms of dyspnea and fatigue (2), it does not appear to be the foremost determining factor of exercise tolerance (3), survival (4–7), disease-specific quality of life (8), hospital readmission rate (9), and daily physical activity level (10) in COPD patients. Indeed, abnormal loss of body weight and fat-free mass, physical deconditioning, and the level of dyspnea during everyday life appear to be stronger determinants of the aforementioned clinically relevant outcomes (4–7,11). These observations provide a clear rationale to start a comprehensive interdisciplinary pulmonary rehabilitation in patients with COPD, irrespective of the degree of airway obstruction (12,13). In fact, it validates the worldwide attention that pulmonary rehabilitation has received in the past 15 years.

Pulmonary rehabilitation is a very important part in the management of patients with moderate-to-severe COPD (14), which should probably be combined with a continuum of self-management (15). In fact, the World Health Organization advocates adding pulmonary rehabilitation programs to the chronic disease management of patients with moderate-to-very severe COPD (1). The present chapter will discuss the advantages and disadvantages of new modalities in pulmonary rehabilitation of patients with moderate-to-very severe COPD.

II. New Modalities of Pulmonary Rehabilitation

A. Resistance Training

Whole-body endurance training (i.e., treadmill walking and ergometry cycling) has frequently been used to improve functional and peak exercise capacity in patients with COPD (16). Nevertheless, a clear loss of fat-free mass (17) and skeletal muscle dysfunction (18) have been shown to be related to a decreased exercise capacity in COPD, irrespective of the degree of severity of the pulmonary impairment (3,19). It therefore seems reasonable to add resistance training to pulmonary rehabilitation of COPD. Resistance training is an exercise modality in which small muscle groups are trained by repetitive lifting (three series of eight repetitions) of relatively heavy weights ($\sim 75\%$ of the one-repetition maximum = the maximum load that can be moved only once over the full range of motion without compensatory movements).

Resistance training has shown to be a very effective exercise intervention to improve peak force of large muscle groups of the upper and lower extremities COPD patients (16). Indeed, changes in functional exercise capacity and disease-specific quality of life have been found to be similar in COPD patients following 12 weeks of resistance or endurance training (20,21). Unfortunately, no studies have been performed to investigate intramuscular changes following resistance training in COPD patients. Then again, Jubrias and colleagues have recently shown large increases in oxidative capacity ($+57\%$) in healthy elderly following six months of resistance training, accompanied by a rise in mitochondrial volume density and quadriceps femoris muscle size (22).

The low demand on the respiratory system and, in turn, a lower sensation of dyspnea are most probably major advantages of resistance training compared with whole-body endurance training (23). In fact, the moderate load on the impaired respiratory system remained stable over time while the training intensity of the resistance training increased during pulmonary rehabilitation in patients with moderate-to-severe COPD (23).

B. Endurance Training

Endurance training has shown to be effective to improve disease-specific quality of life and endurance exercise capacity in patients with moderate-to-severe COPD, as reviewed by Lacasse and colleagues (24). Nevertheless, heterogeneous results have been found among patients with moderate-to-severe COPD (20,25–27). Therefore, recent studies have focussed on enhancing the effects of endurance training in COPD by combining it with other treatment modalities, such as resistance training, respiratory muscle endurance training, inspiratory pressure support (IPS), long-acting broncho-dilators, or supplemental oxygen.

C. Endurance Training and Resistance Training

Recently, the effects of endurance training in combination with resistance training have been studied in patients with moderate-to-severe COPD. The combination of a 12-week endurance and resistance training augmented the increase in peak strength of quadriceps femoris muscles, pectoralis major muscles, and latissimus dorsi muscles compared with endurance training alone (28). Additionally, the combination of endurance and resistance training has been shown to result in a significant increase in thigh muscle cross-sectional area. This change was lacking following endurance training alone and, in turn, was significantly better compared with endurance training alone (28). Then again, the aforementioned changes in skeletal muscle mass and function did not result in a significantly higher increase of functional exercise capacity, quadriceps muscle fatigability, or disease-specific quality of life (28,29). These somewhat contradictory findings warrant further investigation.

D. Endurance Training and IPS

Exercise capacity of patients with COPD may, at least in part, be limited by a misbalance between respiratory muscle load and its capacity (30). Consequently, exercise capacity may improve by reducing the respiratory load and/or improving the respiratory muscle endurance. Indeed, unloading the overworked weak inspiratory muscles using IPS of 10 cm H_2O has shown to result directly into a better cycling endurance in COPD patients compared with cycling without IPS or cycling with IPS of 5 cm H_2O (31). Therefore, it is reasonable to hypothesize that performing endurance training while receiving 10 cm H_2O IPS will enhance the magnitude of endurance training. Indeed, normocapnic patients with COPD who had IPS (10 cm H_2O) during high-intensity endurance cycling training had significantly better improvements in exercise endurance capacity than COPD patients who underwent sham IPS (5 cm H_2O) during endurance training. This, however, did not translate in significant differences in change in scores on a disease-specific quality of life questionnaire (32). It can therefore be questioned whether and to what extent if IPS may be an important adjunct during endurance training in normocapnic patients with severe COPD. Moreover, IPS has two important practical disadvantages: (*i*) discomfort of the mouthpiece or mask can be the foremost reason of dropout from pulmonary rehabilitation (33) and (*ii*) IPS is labor intensive, which will make the pulmonary rehabilitation more expensive (32).

Noninvasive ventilation may still be meaningful to consider during endurance training in stable hypercapnic COPD patients. Firstly, chronic alveolar hypoventilation is likely to develop in COPD patients who have a combination of high inspiratory loads and inspiratory muscle weakness (34). Secondly, COPD patients with severe baseline hypercapnia ($PaCO_2 \geq 54$ mmHg) have been shown to have a lower mean improvement in six-minute walking distance ($+79.6$ m) following pulmonary rehabilitation than COPD patients with moderate hypercapnia ($PaCO_2$ 45–54 mmHg, $+101.0$ m) or normocapnia at baseline ($PaCO_2 < 45$ mmHg, $+124.0$ m) (35). Thirdly, diurnal short-term intermittent noninvasive mechanical ventilation (3 hr/day, 5 day/wk for three weeks) alone has already shown to result in clear improvements in symptom perception (e.g., dyspnea) and functional exercise capacity in clinically stable hypercapnic COPD patients compared with those patients receiving sham (36). Finally, Dreher and colleagues recently have shown that noninvasive positive pressure ventilation in combination with supplemental oxygen improved the six-minute walking distance in hypercapnic COPD patients compared with walking with only supplemental oxygen, accompanied with a decrease in the dyspnea sensation and an increase in arterial oxygen tension (37).

E. Endurance Training and Inspiratory Muscle Training

The effects of inspiratory muscle training alone on exercise capacity have been shown to be limited and only to be effective in patients with explicit inspiratory muscle weakness (baseline maximal inspiratory mouth pressure <60% of the reference values) (38). Additionally, inspiratory muscle training did also not augment the effects of endurance training on COPD patients (38).

Recently, inspiratory muscle isocapnic hyperpnea endurance training during an eight-week outpatient pulmonary rehabilitation program (consisting of endurance training, muscle endurance training, and weekly one-hour group education) has been shown to result in significantly greater improvement in inspiratory muscle endurance than rehabilitation alone (39). Nevertheless, improvements in inspiratory muscle endurance did not translate into more improvements in disease-specific quality of life or functional exercise capacity (39). Unfortunately, Mador and colleagues mostly included normocapnic COPD patients who did not have apparent baseline respiratory muscle dysfunction (39), while inspiratory muscle isocapnic hyperpnea endurance training may be meaningful in weak and hypercapnic patients with COPD (34,38).

F. Endurance Training and Long-Acting Bronchodilators

Patients with clinically stable COPD should have an optimal pharmacological treatment consisting of long-acting inhaled bronchodilators and, in more severe disease, inhaled corticosteroids (40,41). Indeed, several long-acting inhaled bronchodilators have shown to improve pulmonary function (42–44), reduce static and dynamic lung hyperinflation (45–48), reduce exertional dyspnea (45,47,49), improve disease-specific quality of life (48–51), and improve symptom-limited exercise tolerance in COPD patients (45,47,52). Long-acting inhaled bronchodilators therefore seem to be an important addition to the optimal management of COPD. In fact, tiotropium, a once-daily inhaled anticholinergic bronchodilator, in combination with an eight-week treadmill walking endurance program improved treadmill walking endurance time and produced clinically meaningful improvements in disease-specific quality of life and perception of dyspnea compared with an eight-week treadmill walking endurance program alone (53). These differences between groups were also observed three months after conclusion of the pulmonary rehabilitation (53). Regrettably, long-acting β-agonists were not permitted during the study in the control group, which weakens the findings of the latter study. Nevertheless, long-acting inhaled bronchodilators should be part of an optimal pharmacological treatment before the start of and during the course of a comprehensive pulmonary rehabilitation program.

G. Endurance Training and Supplemental Oxygen

The impaired oxygen transport from the lung (e.g., impaired transfer factor for carbon monoxide) to the muscle [e.g., anemia (54), lower capillary density (55), and reduced oxidative enzyme activity in skeletal muscle (56,57)] will result in an early lactate production and an increased dyspnea sensation (58). Indeed, patients with COPD have been shown to have a higher lactate production for a similar amount of oxygen consumption than healthy age-matched control subjects (59). Buffering the extra lactate by plasma bicarbonate will result in an extra carbon dioxide production during exercise, which will result in an extra burden on the ventilatory drive (58).

Supplemental oxygen has shown to improve exercise capacity and to decrease dyspnea sensation in COPD patients who were hypoxemic or nonhypoxemic at rest (60–62). For example, Somfay and colleagues have shown a dose-dependent improvement in cycling endurance time in nonhypoxemic COPD patients up to 50% inspired oxygen fraction (FiO_2) (63). This improved exercise performance was partly related to a lower ventilatory requirement through direct chemoreceptor inhibition (64) and, in turn, a slower breathing pattern (64) and a decreased dynamic lung hyperinflation (63). Whether and to what extent an increased FiO_2 may improve the amount of oxygen at the level of the muscle and, in turn, can result in an increased exercise capacity in patients with COPD remains currently unknown. Nevertheless, it is still reasonable to hypothesize that supplemental oxygen provided during high-intensity cycle endurance training may yield higher training intensities and greater gains in exercise tolerance in nonhypoxemic patients with moderate-to-severe COPD. Indeed, in a double-blinded randomized controlled trial, Emtner and colleagues found a favorable effect of supplemental oxygen during a seven-week high-intensity cycling endurance training program in nonhypoxemic COPD patients compared with patients who were receiving compressed air during endurance training (65). The training intensity in the oxygen-trained group increased faster over time than the compressed air-trained group. In addition, the symptom-limited constant work rate cycle endurance tests (with and without oxygen) increased significantly more in the oxygen-trained patients than in the compressed air-trained patients (65). Supplemental oxygen during exercise training appears to be promising even in nonhypoxemic patients with COPD. Then again, additional studies are warranted since contentious results have been reported (66,67). In addition, it remains currently unknown whether and to what extent exercise training at higher intensities (due to supplemental oxygen) may result in greater improvements in disease-specific quality of life and energy metabolism of skeletal muscles.

H. Interval Training

Not all patients with moderate-to-severe COPD achieve the quantity and quality of endurance training as recommended by the American College of Sports Medicine to develop exercise endurance capacity (13,68). Therefore, other training modalities have to be considered to achieve significant improvements in exercise capacity and health-related quality of life.

Interval training may be a clinically useful alternative. Several studies have shown comparable changes in health-related quality of life and exercise capacity in patients with moderate-to-severe COPD following interval training or whole-body endurance training (69–71). In addition, changes at the level of the muscle were comparable following interval or endurance type of training (70). In fact, patients with COPD were able to complete a greater amount of work during intermittent cycling (at 70% of baseline peak power output, one minute of exercise interspersed with one minute of rest) than during continuous cycling (at 70% of baseline peak power output), while changes from rest to end of exercise in plasma lactate and end-expiratory lung volumes were significantly lower following the former type of exercise (72). These findings most probably explain the lower change from rest to end of exercise in ratings of self-perceived dyspnea following intermittent cycling (72). Interval treadmill walking and interval ergometry cycling should therefore be considered in a pulmonary rehabilitation program of patients with severe COPD. Especially, in those patients with an early dynamic hyperinflation during a peak cycling test (73).

I. Neuromuscular Electrical Stimulation

Unfortunately, active participation in pulmonary rehabilitation programs does not appear to be feasible in COPD patients with prolonged respiratory failure or with very severe daily complaints of dyspnea (74,75). Therefore, other interventions should be considered to prepare these patients for active participation in an inpatient or outpatient pulmonary rehabilitation program. Neuromuscular electrical stimulation might be an interesting option. It can be used for skeletal muscle strengthening; maintenance of skeletal muscle mass and strength during prolonged periods of immobilization; and for selective muscle retraining, without pain (76), muscle lesions, or other adverse effects (77). Indeed, in COPD patients with prolonged respiratory failure, it has shown to improve skeletal muscle function and to reduce the number of days needed to make a transfer from bed to chair (from 14 to 11 days) (74). Moreover, neuromuscular electrical stimulation has also shown to be a powerful home-based intervention to improve skeletal muscle force, peak oxygen consumption, and symptoms of fatigue in COPD patients with high baseline scores on the dyspnea scale of the Medical Research Council (75). In fact, patients were able to continue the neuromuscular electrical stimulation at home during acute exacerbations of COPD and all patients were able to complete the intervention (75). The positive effects of neuromuscular electrical stimulation appear to be limited to weak and deconditioned COPD patients. Indeed, the effects of six-week neuromuscular electrical stimulation of the quadriceps femoris muscles on skeletal muscle function and structure were rather modest in COPD patients with well-preserved functional exercise capacity, skeletal muscle strength, and skeletal muscle mass (78).

III. Supplements During Exercise Training

Reduced daily physical activity is a major contributing factor to the existence of fat-free mass depletion and skeletal muscle weakness (10,79). Nevertheless, other underlying factors are to be considered (14,80–83). Consequently, exercise training in combination with hormonal, nutritional, antioxidant, and/or anti-inflammatory supplements appears to be indicated in highly selected patients with moderate-to-severe COPD.

A. Anabolic Steroids

Endocrinological disturbances have been observed in patients with COPD which may influence skeletal muscle mass and function (82,84). For example, hypogonadism has been shown to be present in male patients with COPD and has been shown to be related to quadriceps muscle weakness (85). Anabolic steroids may therefore be a promising adjunct to pulmonary rehabilitation. Schols and colleagues studied the effects of nandrolone decanoate treatment and nutritional support during pulmonary rehabilitation in a prospective double-blind placebo-controlled randomized trial (86). After stratification for body weight and fat-free mass, patients were randomly assigned to receive placebo nandrolone decanoate treatment, placebo nandrolone decanoate treatment and supplemental nutrition, or nandrolone decanoate treatment and supplemental nutrition during an eight-week inpatient pulmonary rehabilitation program.

Nandrolone decanoate as well as nutritional supplements in combination with exercise training resulted in comparable significant gains in body weight in the depleted patients, but different changes in body composition (86). Weight gain in the group of patients receiving placebo nandrolone decanoate treatment and supplemental nutrition was predominantly due to an expansion of fat mass, while the relative changes in fat-free mass were more favorable in the patients who received nandrolone decanoate treatment and supplemental nutrition. Of interest, no side effects were found following nandrolone decanoate treatment (86). Moreover, patients with COPD who were receiving a maintenance low-dose of oral glucocorticosteroids during pulmonary rehabilitation did not show improvements in body composition or respiratory muscle function following eight weeks of inpatient rehabilitation, unless they received a nandrolone decanoate treatment during pulmonary rehabilitation (87).

Effects of testosterone enanthate with and without progressive resistance training on body composition, skeletal muscle force, skeletal muscle endurance, and exercise capacity have recently been studied in hypogonadal male COPD patients (88). Patients were randomly assigned to 10 weeks of placebo injections without resistance training, weekly testosterone enanthate injections without resistance training, placebo injections and resistance training, or testosterone enanthate injections and resistance training.

Only weekly injections of testosterone enanthate have shown to result in significant increases in body weight, lean body mass, and quadriceps muscle function, but not in respiratory muscle function or exercise capacity. Moreover, improvements in skeletal muscle force were amplified by concomitant progressive resistance training. However, the changes in skeletal muscle function following progressive resistance training were not significantly different from those observed following progressive resistance training with testosterone enanthate (88). Therefore, it remains questionable whether and to what extent testosterone enanthate should be used in hypogonadal male COPD patients. Especially, because the long-term safety and the optimal doses have not been established (89).

B. Exercise Training and Polyunsaturated Fatty Acids

Recently, effects of pulmonary rehabilitation with polyunsaturated fatty acids (PUFA), long-chain fatty acids containing two or more double bonds, on body composition, systemic inflammation, and exercise capacity have been studied in a double-blind placebo-controlled randomized trial in patients with moderate-to-severe COPD (90).

All patients received nine capsules daily during an eight-week inpatient pulmonary rehabilitation program. Each capsule contained 1 g of either a blend of PUFA or placebo. All capsules were enriched with 3.5 mg/g vitamin E to stabilize the oil and to serve as an antioxidant. In addition, depleted patients also received daily liquid nutritional supplements containing 2.85 g linoleic acid and 0.6 g α-linolenic acid.

Fat-free mass and skeletal muscle function improved significantly within both groups. Nevertheless, PUFA modulation in combination with pulmonary rehabilitation has shown to enhance the increase in exercise capacity in COPD compared with only pulmonary rehabilitation (90). This difference cannot be attributed to changes in fat-free mass, skeletal muscle force, or systemic inflammatory response. Consequently, the differences in changes in exercise capacity are most probably due to intrinsic changes at the level of the skeletal muscles. Unfortunately, Broekhuizen and colleagues did not take skeletal muscle biopsies in their study.

C. Oral Creatine Supplements

Oral creatine supplementation has been used as ergogenic aid to enhance gains in skeletal muscle function and skeletal muscle mass during exercise training. Indeed, exercise training combined with oral creatine supplements resulted in greater improvements in peak muscle force and muscle endurance when compared with exercise training and placebo in young and elderly healthy subjects (91,92). Oral creatine supplementation has also been shown to stimulate skeletal muscle hypertrophy and maximal knee extension power during rehabilitative resistance training following two weeks of knee immobilization in healthy university students (93). As a matter of fact, muscle function and local exercise capacity improved in other chronic diseases after only ingestion of 6 g creatine per day for 14 days without exercise training (94–98).

Recently, the effects of oral creatine supplementation and resistance training have been studied in patients with moderate-to-severe COPD in a double-blind randomized controlled trial (99). After stratification by body weight and fat-free mass, patients were randomly assigned to receive 5 g of creatine with 35 g of glucose per dose or placebo. Supplements were taken three times daily for 14 days (loading phase), followed by once-daily administration for 10 weeks (maintenance phase) during which patients attended pulmonary rehabilitation.

Resistance training and creatine with a glucose polymer led to significantly higher increases in fat-free mass, skeletal muscle strength and endurance, and health status compared with resistance training with a glucose polymer (99). Nevertheless, the improved body composition and skeletal muscle function did not translate in greater gains in exercise capacity. The latter finding is not really a surprise considering the fact that intake of oral creatine supplements increases muscle creatine content and thereby enhances muscular performance during short maximal exercise over repeated bouts (93).

IV. Conclusions

Pulmonary rehabilitation has been shown to be an important part of the management of patients with COPD. Future trials should focus on new adjuncts to conventional pulmonary rehabilitation programs to optimize its effects on health-related quality of life, exercise capacity, body composition, and muscle function in patients with moderate-to-very severe COPD. Therefore, a patient-tailored approach is inevitable. Based on well-defined baseline characteristics, patients should be individually selected. At present, new modalities of pulmonary rehabilitation have shown to improve body composition, skeletal muscle function, and sometimes also exercise capacity. However, the translation to a better disease-specific quality of life is currently lacking. Moreover, long-term effects and cost-effectiveness of these new modalities have not been properly assessed.

References

1. Pauwels RA, Buist AS, Calverley PM, Jenkins CR, Hurd SS. Global strategy for the diagnosis, management, and prevention of chronic obstructive pulmonary disease. NHLBI/WHO Global Initiative for Chronic Obstructive Lung Disease (GOLD) Workshop summary. Am J Respir Crit Care Med 2001; 163(5):1256–76.
2. Breslin E, van der Schans C, Breukink S, et al. Perception of fatigue and quality of life in patients with COPD. Chest 1998; 114(4):958–64.
3. Baarends EM, Schols AM, Mostert R, Wouters EF. Peak exercise response in relation to tissue depletion in patients with chronic obstructive pulmonary disease. Eur Respir J 1997; 10(12):2807–13.
4. Pinto-Plata VM, Cote C, Cabral H, Taylor J, Celli BR. The 6-min walk distance: change over time and value as a predictor of survival in severe COPD. Eur Respir J 2004; 23(1):28–33.

5. Schols AM, Broekhuizen R, Weling-Scheepers CA, Wouters EF. Body composition and mortality in chronic obstructive pulmonary disease. Am J Clin Nutr 2005; 82(1):53–9.
6. Vestbo J, Prescott E, Almdal T, et al. Body mass, fat-free body mass, and prognosis in patients with chronic obstructive pulmonary disease from a random population sample: findings from the Copenhagen City Heart Study. Am J Respir Crit Care Med 2006; 173(1):79–83.
7. Marquis K, Debigare R, Lacasse Y, et al. Midthigh muscle cross-sectional area is a better predictor of mortality than body mass index in patients with chronic obstructive pulmonary disease. Am J Respir Crit Care Med 2002; 166(6):809–13.
8. Oga T, Nishimura K, Tsukino M, et al. Longitudinal changes in health status using the chronic respiratory disease questionnaire and pulmonary function in patients with stable chronic obstructive pulmonary disease. Qual Life Res 2004; 13(6):1109–16.
9. Garcia-Aymerich J, Farrero E, Felez MA, Izquierdo J, Marrades RM, Anto JM. Risk factors of readmission to hospital for a COPD exacerbation: a prospective study. Thorax 2003; 58(2):100–5.
10. Pitta F, Troosters T, Spruit MA, Probst VS, Decramer M, Gosselink R. Characteristics of physical activities in daily life in chronic obstructive pulmonary disease. Am J Respir Crit Care Med 2005; 171(9):972–7.
11. Nishimura K, Izumi T, Tsukino M, Oga T. Dyspnea is a better predictor of 5-year survival than airway obstruction in patients with COPD. Chest 2002; 121(5):1434–40.
12. Vogiatzis I, Williamson AF, Miles J, Taylor IK. Physiological response to moderate exercise workloads in a pulmonary rehabilitation program in patients with varying degrees of airflow obstruction. Chest 1999; 116(5):1200–7.
13. Maltais F, LeBlanc P, Jobin J, et al. Intensity of training and physiologic adaptation in patients with chronic obstructive pulmonary disease. Am J Respir Crit Care Med 1997; 155(2):555–61.
14. Wouters EF. Management of severe COPD. Lancet 2004; 364(9437):883–95.
15. Bourbeau J, Julien M, Maltais F, et al. Reduction of hospital utilization in patients with chronic obstructive pulmonary disease: a disease-specific self-management intervention. Arch Intern Med 2003; 163(5):585–91.
16. Spruit MA, Troosters T, Trappenburg JC, Decramer M, Gosselink R. Exercise training during rehabilitation of patients with COPD: a current perspective. Patient Educ Couns 2004; 52(3):243–8.
17. Schols AM, Soeters PB, Dingemans AM, Mostert R, Frantzen PJ, Wouters EF. Prevalence and characteristics of nutritional depletion in patients with stable COPD eligible for pulmonary rehabilitation. Am Rev Respir Dis 1993; 147(5):1151–6.
18. Gosker HR, Lencer NH, Franssen FM, van der Vusse GJ, Wouters EF, Schols AM. Striking similarities in systemic factors contributing to decreased exercise capacity in patients with severe chronic heart failure or COPD. Chest 2003; 123(5):1416–24.
19. Gosselink R, Troosters T, Decramer M. Peripheral muscle weakness contributes to exercise limitation in COPD. Am J Respir Crit Care Med 1996; 153(3):976–80.
20. Spruit MA, Gosselink R, Troosters T, De Paepe K, Decramer M. Resistance versus endurance training in patients with COPD and peripheral muscle weakness. Eur Respir J 2002; 19(6):1072–8.
21. Ortega F, Toral J, Cejudo P, et al. Comparison of effects of strength and endurance training in patients with chronic obstructive pulmonary disease. Am J Respir Crit Care Med 2002; 166(5):669–74.
22. Jubrias SA, Esselman PC, Price LB, Cress ME, Conley KE. Large energetic adaptations of elderly muscle to resistance and endurance training. J Appl Physiol 2001; 90(5):1663–70.
23. Probst VS, Troosters T, Pitta F, Decramer M, Gosselink R. Cardiopulmonary stress during exercise training in patients with COPD. Eur Respir J 2006; 27(6):1110–8.
24. Lacasse Y, Brosseau L, Milne S, et al. Pulmonary rehabilitation for chronic obstructive pulmonary disease. Cochrane Database Syst Rev 2002; (3):CD003793.
25. Goldstein RS, Gort EH, Stubbing D, Avendano MA, Guyatt GH. Randomised controlled trial of respiratory rehabilitation. Lancet 1994; 344(8934):1394–7.
26. Spruit MA, Gosselink R, Troosters T, Kasran A, Van Vliet M, Decramer M. Low-grade systemic inflammation and the response to exercise training in patients with advanced COPD. Chest 2005; 128(5):3183–90.
27. Troosters T, Gosselink R, Decramer M. Short- and long-term effects of outpatient rehabilitation in patients with chronic obstructive pulmonary disease: a randomized trial. Am J Med 2000; 109(3):207–12.
28. Bernard S, Whittom F, Leblanc P, et al. Aerobic and strength training in patients with chronic obstructive pulmonary disease. Am J Respir Crit Care Med 1999; 159(3):896–901.

29. Mador MJ, Bozkanat E, Aggarwal A, Shaffer M, Kufel TJ. Endurance and strength training in patients with COPD. Chest 2004; 125(6):2036–45.
30. Laghi F, Tobin MJ. Disorders of the respiratory muscles. Am J Respir Crit Care Med 2003; 168(1):10–48.
31. van 't Hul A, Gosselink R, Hollander P, Postmus P, Kwakkel G. Acute effects of inspiratory pressure support during exercise in patients with COPD. Eur Respir J 2004; 23(1):34–40.
32. van 't Hul A, Gosselink R, Hollander P, Postmus P, Kwakkel G. Training with inspiratory pressure support in patients with severe COPD. Eur Respir J 2006; 27(1):65–72.
33. Bianchi L, Foglio K, Porta R, Baiardi R, Vitacca M, Ambrosino N. Lack of additional effect of adjunct of assisted ventilation to pulmonary rehabilitation in mild COPD patients. Respir Med 2002; 96(5):359–67.
34. Begin P, Grassino A. Inspiratory muscle dysfunction and chronic hypercapnia in chronic obstructive pulmonary disease. Am Rev Respir Dis 1991; 143(5 Pt 1):905–12.
35. Foster S, Lopez D, Thomas HM, III. Pulmonary rehabilitation in COPD patients with elevated PCO_2. Am Rev Respir Dis 1988; 138(6):1519–23.
36. Diaz O, Begin P, Andresen M, et al. Physiological and clinical effects of diurnal noninvasive ventilation in hypercapnic COPD. Eur Respir J 2005; 26(6):1016–23.
37. Dreher M, Storre JH, Windisch W. Noninvasive ventilation during walking in patients with severe COPD: a randomised cross-over trial. Eur Respir J 2007; 29(5):930–6.
38. Lotters F, van Tol B, Kwakkel G, Gosselink R. Effects of controlled inspiratory muscle training in patients with COPD: a meta-analysis. Eur Respir J 2002; 20(3):570–6.
39. Mador MJ, Deniz O, Aggarwal A, Shaffer M, Kufel TJ, Spengler CM. Effect of respiratory muscle endurance training in patients with COPD undergoing pulmonary rehabilitation. Chest 2005; 128(3):1216–24.
40. Calverley PM, Walker P. Chronic obstructive pulmonary disease. Lancet 2003; 362(9389):1053–61.
41. Wouters EF, Postma DS, Fokkens B, et al. Withdrawal of fluticasone propionate from combined salmeterol/fluticasone treatment in patients with COPD causes immediate and sustained disease deterioration: a randomised controlled trial. Thorax 2005; 60(6):480–7.
42. Ulrik CS. Efficacy of inhaled salmeterol in the management of smokers with chronic obstructive pulmonary disease: a single centre randomised, double blind, placebo controlled, crossover study. Thorax 1995; 50(7):750–4.
43. van Noord JA, Aumann JL, Janssens E, et al. Comparison of tiotropium once daily, formoterol twice daily and both combined once daily in patients with COPD. Eur Respir J 2005; 26(2):214–22.
44. Vincken W, van Noord JA, Greefhorst AP, et al. Improved health outcomes in patients with COPD during 1 yr's treatment with tiotropium. Eur Respir J 2002; 19(2):209–16.
45. Man WD, Mustfa N, Nikoletou D, et al. Effect of salmeterol on respiratory muscle activity during exercise in poorly reversible COPD. Thorax 2004; 59(6):471–6.
46. O'Donnell DE, Voduc N, Fitzpatrick M, Webb KA. Effect of salmeterol on the ventilatory response to exercise in chronic obstructive pulmonary disease. Eur Respir J 2004; 24(1):86–94.
47. O'Donnell DE, Fluge T, Gerken F, et al. Effects of tiotropium on lung hyperinflation, dyspnoea and exercise tolerance in COPD. Eur Respir J 2004; 23(6):832–40.
48. Stockley RA, Chopra N, Rice L. Addition of salmeterol to existing treatment in patients with COPD: a 12 month study. Thorax 2006; 61(2):122–8.
49. Casaburi R, Mahler DA, Jones PW, et al. A long-term evaluation of once-daily inhaled tiotropium in chronic obstructive pulmonary disease. Eur Respir J 2002; 19(2):217–24.
50. Donohue JF, van Noord JA, Bateman ED, et al. A 6-month, placebo-controlled study comparing lung function and health status changes in COPD patients treated with tiotropium or salmeterol. Chest 2002; 122(1):47–55.
51. Jones PW, Bosh TK. Quality of life changes in COPD patients treated with salmeterol. Am J Respir Crit Care Med 1997; 155(4):1283–9.
52. Maltais F, Hamilton A, Marciniuk D, et al. Improvements in symptom-limited exercise performance over 8 h with once-daily tiotropium in patients with COPD. Chest 2005; 128(3):1168–78.
53. Casaburi R, Kukafka D, Cooper CB, Witek TJ, Jr., Kesten S. Improvement in exercise tolerance with the combination of tiotropium and pulmonary rehabilitation in patients with COPD. Chest 2005; 127(3):809–17.
54. John M, Lange A, Hoernig S, Witt C, Anker SD. Prevalence of anemia in chronic obstructive pulmonary disease: comparison to other chronic diseases. Int J Cardiol 2006; 111(3):365–70.
55. Saey D, Michaud A, Couillard A, et al. Contractile fatigue, muscle morphometry, and blood lactate in chronic obstructive pulmonary disease. Am J Respir Crit Care Med 2005; 171(10):1109–15.

56. Allaire J, Maltais F, Doyon JF, et al. Peripheral muscle endurance and the oxidative profile of the quadriceps in patients with COPD. Thorax 2004; 59(8):673–8.
57. Maltais F, LeBlanc P, Whittom F, et al. Oxidative enzyme activities of the vastus lateralis muscle and the functional status in patients with COPD. Thorax 2000; 55(10):848–53.
58. Tardif C, Bonmarchand G, Gibon JF, et al. Respiratory response to CO_2 in patients with chronic obstructive pulmonary disease in acute respiratory failure. Eur Respir J 1993; 6(5):619–24.
59. Maltais F, Simard AA, Simard C, Jobin J, Desgagnes P, LeBlanc P. Oxidative capacity of the skeletal muscle and lactic acid kinetics during exercise in normal subjects and in patients with COPD. Am J Respir Crit Care Med 1996; 153(1):288–93.
60. O'Donnell DE, Bain DJ, Webb KA. Factors contributing to relief of exertional breathlessness during hyperoxia in chronic airflow limitation. Am J Respir Crit Care Med 1997; 155(2):530–5.
61. Woodcock AA, Gross ER, Geddes DM. Oxygen relieves breathlessness in "pink puffers". Lancet 1981; 1(8226):907–9.
62. Dean NC, Brown JK, Himelman RB, Doherty JJ, Gold WM, Stulbarg MS. Oxygen may improve dyspnea and endurance in patients with chronic obstructive pulmonary disease and only mild hypoxemia. Am Rev Respir Dis 1992; 146(4):941–5.
63. Somfay A, Porszasz J, Lee SM, Casaburi R. Dose–response effect of oxygen on hyperinflation and exercise endurance in nonhypoxaemic COPD patients. Eur Respir J 2001; 18(1):77–84.
64. Somfay A, Porszasz J, Lee SM, Casaburi R. Effect of hyperoxia on gas exchange and lactate kinetics following exercise onset in nonhypoxemic COPD patients. Chest 2002; 121(2):393–400.
65. Emtner M, Porszasz J, Burns M, Somfay A, Casaburi R. Benefits of supplemental oxygen in exercise training in nonhypoxemic chronic obstructive pulmonary disease patients. Am J Respir Crit Care Med 2003; 168(9):1034–42.
66. Wadell K, Henriksson-Larsen K, Lundgren R. Physical training with and without oxygen in patients with chronic obstructive pulmonary disease and exercise-induced hypoxaemia. J Rehabil Med 2001; 33(5):200–5.
67. Garrod R, Paul EA, Wedzicha JA. Supplemental oxygen during pulmonary rehabilitation in patients with COPD with exercise hypoxaemia. Thorax 2000; 55(7):539–43.
68. American College of Sports Medicine Position Stand. The recommended quantity and quality of exercise for developing and maintaining cardiorespiratory and muscular fitness, and flexibility in healthy adults. Med Sci Sports Exerc 1998; 30(6):975–91.
69. Coppoolse R, Barstow TJ, Stringer WW, Carithers E, Casaburi R. Effect of acute bicarbonate administration on exercise responses of COPD patients. Med Sci Sports Exerc 1997; 29(6):725–32.
70. Vogiatzis I, Terzis G, Nanas S, et al. Skeletal muscle adaptations to interval training in patients with advanced COPD. Chest 2005; 128(6):3838–45.
71. Vogiatzis I, Nanas S, Roussos C. Interval training as an alternative modality to continuous exercise in patients with COPD. Eur Respir J 2002; 20(1):12–9.
72. Sabapathy S, Kingsley RA, Schneider DA, Adams L, Morris NR. Continuous and intermittent exercise responses in individuals with chronic obstructive pulmonary disease. Thorax 2004; 59(12):1026–31.
73. Vogiatzis I, Georgiadou O, Golemati S, et al. Patterns of dynamic hyperinflation during exercise and recovery in patients with severe chronic obstructive pulmonary disease. Thorax 2005; 60(9):723–9.
74. Zanotti E, Felicetti G, Maini M, Fracchia C. Peripheral muscle strength training in bed-bound patients with COPD receiving mechanical ventilation: effect of electrical stimulation. Chest 2003; 124(1):292–6.
75. Neder JA, Sword D, Ward SA, Mackay E, Cochrane LM, Clark CJ. Home based neuromuscular electrical stimulation as a new rehabilitative strategy for severely disabled patients with chronic obstructive pulmonary disease (COPD). Thorax 2002; 57(4):333–7.
76. Lake DA. Neuromuscular electrical stimulation. An overview and its application in the treatment of sports injuries. Sports Med 1992; 13(5):320–36.
77. McMiken DF, Todd-Smith M, Thompson C. Strengthening of human quadriceps muscles by cutaneous electrical stimulation. Scand J Rehabil Med 1983; 15(1):25–8.
78. Dal Corso S, Napolis L, Malaguti C, et al. Skeletal muscle structure and function in response to electrical stimulation in moderately impaired COPD patients. Respir Med 2007; 101(6):1236–43.
79. Serres I, Gautier V, Varray A, Prefaut C. Impaired skeletal muscle endurance related to physical inactivity and altered lung function in COPD patients. Chest 1998; 113(4):900–5.
80. Broekhuizen R, Wouters EF, Creutzberg EC, Schols AM. Raised CRP levels mark metabolic and functional impairment in advanced COPD. Thorax 2006; 61(1):17–22.

81. American Thoracic Society/European Respiratory Society. Skeletal muscle dysfunction in chronic obstructive pulmonary disease. A statement of the American Thoracic Society and European Respiratory Society. Am J Respir Crit Care Med 1999; 159(4 Pt 2):S1–40.

82. Spruit MA, Gosselink R, Troosters T, et al. Muscle force during an acute exacerbation in hospitalised patients with COPD and its relationship with CXCL8 and IGF-I. Thorax 2003; 58(9):752–6.

83. Wouters EF, Creutzberg EC, Schols AM. Systemic effects in COPD. Chest 2002; 121(Suppl. 5):127S–30.

84. Creutzberg EC, Casaburi R. Endocrinological disturbances in chronic obstructive pulmonary disease. Eur Respir J Suppl 2003; 46:76s–80.

85. Van Vliet M, Spruit MA, Verleden G, et al. Hypogonadism, quadriceps weakness and exercise intolerance in chronic obstructive pulmonary disease. Am J Respir Crit Care Med 2005; 172:1105–11.

86. Schols AM, Soeters PB, Mostert R, Pluymers RJ, Wouters EF. Physiologic effects of nutritional support and anabolic steroids in patients with chronic obstructive pulmonary disease. A placebo-controlled randomized trial. Am J Respir Crit Care Med 1995; 152(4 Pt 1):1268–74.

87. Creutzberg EC, Wouters EF, Mostert R, Pluymers RJ, Schols AM. A role for anabolic steroids in the rehabilitation of patients with COPD? A double-blind, placebo-controlled, randomized trial Chest 2003; 124(5):1733–42.

88. Casaburi R, Bhasin S, Cosentino L, et al. Effects of testosterone and resistance training in men with chronic obstructive pulmonary disease. Am J Respir Crit Care Med 2004; 170(8):870–8.

89. Gruenewald DA, Matsumoto AM. Testosterone supplementation therapy for older men: potential benefits and risks. J Am Geriatr Soc 2003; 51(1):101–15 (discussion 115).

90. Broekhuizen R, Wouters EF, Creutzberg EC, Weling-Scheepers CA, Schols AM. Polyunsaturated fatty acids improve exercise capacity in chronic obstructive pulmonary disease. Thorax 2005; 60(5):376–82.

91. Vandenberghe K, Goris M, Van Hecke P, Van Leemputte M, Vangerven L, Hespel P. Long-term creatine intake is beneficial to muscle performance during resistance training. J Appl Physiol 1997; 83(6):2055–63.

92. Chrusch MJ, Chilibeck PD, Chad KE, Davison KS, Burke DG. Creatine supplementation combined with resistance training in older men. Med Sci Sports Exerc 2001; 33(12):2111–7.

93. Hespel P, Op't Eijnde B, Van Leemputte M, et al. Oral creatine supplementation facilitates the rehabilitation of disuse atrophy and alters the expression of muscle myogenic factors in humans. J Physiol 2001; 536(Pt 2):625–33.

94. Vorgerd M, Grehl T, Jager M, et al. Creatine therapy in myophosphorylase deficiency (McArdle disease): a placebo-controlled crossover trial. Arch Neurol 2000; 57(7):956–63.

95. Mazzini L, Balzarini C, Colombo R, et al. Effects of creatine supplementation on exercise performance and muscular strength in amyotrophic lateral sclerosis: preliminary results. J Neurol Sci 2001; 191(1-2):139–44.

96. Jacobs PL, Mahoney ET, Cohn KA, Sheradsky LF, Green BA. Oral creatine supplementation enhances upper extremity work capacity in persons with cervical-level spinal cord injury. Arch Phys Med Rehabil 2002; 83(1):19–23.

97. Gordon A, Hultman E, Kaijser L, et al. Creatine supplementation in chronic heart failure increases skeletal muscle creatine phosphate and muscle performance. Cardiovasc Res 1995; 30(3):413–8.

98. Felber S, Skladal D, Wyss M, Kremser C, Koller A, Sperl W. Oral creatine supplementation in Duchenne muscular dystrophy: a clinical and ^{31}P magnetic resonance spectroscopy study. Neurol Res 2000; 22(2):145–50.

99. Fuld JP, Kilduff LP, Neder JA, et al. Creatine supplementation during pulmonary rehabilitation in chronic obstructive pulmonary disease. Thorax 2005; 60(7):531–7.

20

Long-Term Oxygen Therapy for the Patient with COPD

EMMANUEL WEITZENBLUM and MATTHIEU CANUET
Service de Pneumologie, Hôpital Universitaire de Strasbourg, Strasbourg, France

ARI CHAOUAT
Service de Pathologie, Respiratoire, et Réanimation Respiratoire, Hôpital Universitaire de Nancy, Nancy, France

ROMAIN KESSLER
Service de Pneumologie, Hôpital Universitaire de Strasbourg, Strasbourg, France

I. Introduction

Long-term oxygen therapy (LTOT) is the only treatment which has been shown to improve significantly life expectancy in patients with severe chronic obstructive pulmonary disease (COPD) exhibiting marked hypoxemia. There has been a considerable development of LTOT in the last two decades and it is estimated that more than 800,000 people, including a large majority of COPD patients, receive home oxygen therapy in the United States. In France, about 80,000 COPD patients are treated with home oxygen therapy.

In this chapter, we first review the scientific rationale for the use of LTOT in stable COPD patients with chronic hypoxemia. We then discuss the indications of LTOT in advanced COPD. Finally, we consider the practical aspects of LTOT including the general rules of prescription and the oxygen delivery systems.

II. Beneficial Effects of LTOT in Hypoxemic COPD

While severe chronic hypoxemia has well-known deleterious effects, LTOT has been shown to improve survival, ameliorate quality of life, and have favorable physiological effects in patients with severe COPD and marked hypoxemia (Table 1).

A. LTOT Improves Survival

In patients with advanced COPD, life expectancy is poor. Forced expiratory volume in one second (FEV_1) is known to be the best prognostic index (1–4) and the prognosis is particularly poor when FEV_1 falls below 1 L; in these patients, survival is about 50% after five years. Marked hypoxemia, hypercapnia, and the presence of pulmonary hypertension also have a high prognostic value (1–7). The recent study by Celli et al. (8) has shown that a composite index including FEV_1, body mass index, degree of dyspnea, and exercise capacity (BODE index) is better than FEV_1 alone in predicting the risk of death in COPD patients.

397

Table 1 Deleterious Effects of Chronic Hypoxemia Compared to Beneficial Effects of Long-Term Oxygen Therapy in Chronic Obstructive Pulmonary Disease Patients

Deleterious effects of severe chronic hypoxemia (PaO$_2$ ≤ 55 mmHg)	Beneficial effects of long-term oxygen therapy given during ≥ 18 hr/day
Life expectancy	
Poor survival	Improved survival
Quality of life	
Poor quality of life	Improved quality of life
Poor exercise tolerance	Improved exercise tolerance
Increased hospital demand	Reduced hospitalization
Neuropsychological disturbance	Improved neuropsychological status
Physiological effects	
Reduced oxygen transport and delivery	Improved oxygen transport and delivery
Development of polycythemia	Reduction (but rarely correction) of polycythemia
Cardiac arrhythmias during sleep	Marked improvement of cardiac arrhythmias during sleep
Pulmonary circulation	
Development and worsening of pulmonary hypertension	Progression of pulmonary hypertension is reversed or stabilized or attenuated

The Medical Research Council (MRC) trial (9) has clearly indicated that LTOT administered during 15 hr/day significantly improves survival in patients with hypoxemic COPD (PaO$_2$ < 60 mmHg; average PaO$_2$ of about 50 mmHg). The survival difference between the two groups became apparent at 500 days and was statistically significant after third, fourth, and fifth years. These data relate to the 66 male patients included in the study. In the 21 female patients, the improved survival in the treated group was observed from the start of LTOT but the number of patients was small.

In the North American Nocturnal Oxygen Therapy Trial (NOTT) study (10), nocturnal oxygen therapy (NOT) during 10 to 12 hr/day was compared to continuous or nearly continuous oxygen therapy (COT) (> 18 hr/day and 20.5 hr/day as a mean). Survival was better from the start of O$_2$ therapy in COT patients when compared to NOT patients. After two years, the mortality rates were 40.8% and 22.4% in NOT and COT patients respectively and the difference between the survival curves was significant ($p < 0.01$). When combining the results of the NOTT and MRC studies, which included patients with a similar degree of severity (mean PaO$_2$ at inclusion of 50–52 mmHg in both studies), it appears that the poorest survival was observed in the MRC control group (no oxygen) and the best survival in the COT group. It can be concluded that some oxygen is better than no oxygen, but nearly continuous oxygen (> 18 hr/day) is better than 12 to 15 hr/day (11).

The follow-up of patients included in the NOTT and MRC studies was limited to three to five years. In the noncontrolled study by Cooper et al. (12), where the follow-up was longer, the survival rate at five years was 62%, which can be compared to the 16% survival rate at five years in the control group (no O$_2$) of the MRC trial; the 10-year survival rate was 26% (12). Whereas the improved survival of patients on LTOT is well established, its explanation is uncertain. The NOTT study has found no correlation between improvement of pulmonary hemodynamics and that of life expectancy.

The prognostic factors in patients under LTOT have been extensively investigated. The following variables predict a poor prognosis: lower FEV$_1$ (12–15), lower PaO$_2$ (14–16), higher mean pulmonary artery pressure (13,16), lower CO transfer factor (15), and advanced age (15,17,18). The prognostic significance of hypercapnia is debated (15,16,18,19) and according to several studies it is not a predictor of poor prognosis in patients under LTOT (15,16,19). In the large Swedish study (18) byStrom, which included 403 patients with LTOT, women ($n=202$) had a lower mortality than men, and oral steroid medication was associated with an increased mortality rate in women. Recent studies have emphasized the negative prognostic value of denutrition estimated from the body mass index (20), of comorbidity (20), and of a low hematocrit (21).

It must be emphasized that the beneficial effects of LTOT have been demonstrated in patients with severe COPD, marked hypoxemia, and pulmonary hypertension. They cannot be applied to patients with modest hypoxemia. A Polish study by Gorecka et al. (13) has compared 68 COPD patients on LTOT to 67 control patients. Hypoxemia was mild to moderate (PaO$_2$ in the range 56–65 mmHg), whereas bronchial obstruction was severe. The cumulative survival rates at first, second, and third years were identical in patients treated with LTOT and controls (Fig. 1). Thus, LTOT is probably not justified in patients with mild-to-moderate hypoxemia, at least when PaO$_2$ is >60 mmHg.

B. LTOT Improves Quality of Life

Quality of Life Assessed by Disease-Specific Health Measures

When the NOTT and MRC studies (9,10) were performed, questionnaires about quality of life were not available. A study in the United Kingdom using the St. George's Respiratory Questionnaire (22) included 23 hypoxemic COPD patients, starting LTOT,

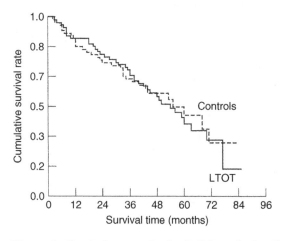

Figure 1 Survival curves in the Polish study by Gorecka et al. Sixty-seven chronic obstructive pulmonary disease (COPD) patients with severe airway obstruction and moderate hypoxemia (PaO$_2$ in the range 56–65 mmHg) served as controls and were compared to 68 similar COPD patients who received oxygen therapy [long-term oxygen therapy (LTOT)] during 13.5 ± 4.4 hr/day. It can be seen that there is no difference in survival ($p=0.89$) between the two groups. *Source*: From Ref. 13.

who were compared to 18 COPD patients less severely hypoxemic but not given LTOT. The initial quality of life was lower in the LTOT group. No change in quality of life was detected on LTOT over six months. A more recent study (23) compared 43 COPD patients fulfilling criteria and commenced on LTOT and 25 patients not fulfilling criteria and continued on standard care. Health-related quality of life (HRQL) was measured with the Chronic Respiratory Questionnaire. Significant improvements in HRQL were noted after six months in the LTOT group, while the non-LTOT group demonstrated a progressive decline in HRQL.

Neuropsychological Status

The NOTT study (10) included a neuropsychological study before the onset of oxygen therapy and after 6 and 12 months of treatment. Prior to LTOT, COPD patients had an impaired neuropsychological functioning when compared to age-matched controls. The most characteristic disturbances concerned the distracting ability, the motor skills, and the perceptual motor abilities (24). PaO_2 was significantly but modestly correlated with the neuropsychological deficit.

At six months, there was no significant difference in the rate of neuropsychological improvement between patients on COT and patients on NOT (24). However, at 12 months, the follow-up of a small subgroup of 37 patients showed that the results were better in patients on COT than in those on NOT. IQ and brain-age quotient were higher in the former.

Improved Exercise Capacity

The walking distance is increased in COPD patients receiving portable liquid oxygen, compared to liquid air, as first demonstrated by Lilker et al. (25). These results have been confirmed by Leggett and Flenley (26). An increased walking distance when breathing O_2 has also been observed in a French multicenter trial which included 159 COPD patients (27): the distance walked increased by about 17%. The exact mechanism by which supplemental O_2 improves exercise capacity is not totally elucidated but it has been shown that decreased ventilatory demand and hyperinflation, improved respiratory muscle function, and decreased perception of dyspnea are important mechanisms.

Reduced Hospitalization

Hospital needs are reduced in COPD patients receiving LTOT (11). In the NOTT study (10), patients on COT had fewer hospitalizations than those on NOT, but the difference was not statistically significant (NS).

C. Favorable Physiological Effects of LTOT

Oxygen Transport and Delivery

Oxygen therapy improves oxygen transport, which is the product of cardiac output and O_2 content of arterial blood ($\dot{Q} \times CaO_2$). In case of severe chronic hypoxemia with $PaO_2 < 50$ mmHg and $SaO_2 < 85\%$, CaO_2 decreases, which could lead to a decreased O_2 transport. In fact, the fall in SaO_2 is often counterbalanced by the increased hemoglobin concentration (secondary polycythemia). Therefore, O_2 transport is rarely compromised except during acute exacerbations of the disease. The extraction of O_2 by tissues (oxygen uptake), which is essential to life, is maintained even during episodes of acute respiratory failure.

In stable COPD patients receiving supplemental O_2, an increased oxygen transport has been observed by MacNee et al. (28), whereas Morrison et al. (29) reported that the coefficient of oxygen delivery, which is the ratio of O_2 transport to O_2 uptake, increased only in those patients in whom cardiac output increased after one month of COT.

Reduction of Secondary Polycythemia

Polycythemia is beneficial with regard to O_2 transport. However, it also has deleterious effects, the most important being hyperviscosity. It is generally accepted that increased blood viscosity contributes to pulmonary hypertension, but the classical study by Segel and Bishop (30) has shown that the effects of polycythemia-related hypervolemia on pulmonary hemodynamics were more important than those of hyperviscosity.

A significant decrease in the red cell mass under LTOT was observed in the NOTT patients receiving O_2 for > 18 hr/day (10). In this COT group, hematocrit fell by 9% as a mean after 18 months of therapy, but this improvement was not observed in patients receiving only NOT or in the patients included in the MRC study (9) who were given 15 hr O_2/day. These discrepancies are probably explained by the daily duration of LTOT which varies from one study to another, the best results being observed when O_2 is given for ≥ 18 hr/day (10). One must also consider that some patients continue to smoke. Calverley et al. (31) observed that, in patients under LTOT who do not discontinue smoking, the red cell mass does not decrease.

Whereas permanent (daytime) hypoxemia is a well-known cause of polycythemia, isolated nocturnal hypoxemia does not appear to be associated with an increased red blood cell mass (32,33), which is in agreement with a study on erythropoietin production in COPD patients (34).

Cardiac Arrhythmias During Sleep

Some COPD patients exhibit tachycardia and other arrhythmias during sleep (35,36). Shepard et al. (36) observed that premature ventricular contractions occurred during sleep in more than 60% of patients in a series of 42 stable COPD patients; they were frequent in those subjects who had marked nocturnal O_2 desaturation (nocturnal $SaO_2 < 80\%$). These arrhythmias, which are mainly observed during rapid eye movement (REM) sleep, are improved by NOT (35).

Effects of Oxygen Therapy on Pulmonary Hypertension

One of the aims of LTOT is the reduction of pulmonary hypertension induced by chronic alveolar hypoxia; can this be achieved? We know that hypoxic pulmonary hypertension observed in high-altitude residents disappears when these (healthy) subjects stay at sea level for several months (37). We also know that the precapillary pulmonary hypertension observed in these healthy highlanders (38) is rather similar to that observed in COPD (modest level of pulmonary hypertension, comparable pulmonary vascular "remodeling"). Furthermore, experimental studies in rats (39,40) have shown that continuous normoxia could reverse pulmonary artery hypertension and right ventricular hypertrophy induced by continuous inhalation of a hypoxic mixture during a few weeks; intermittent normoxia for 16 hr/day had no effect. All these data have raised the hope that a reversibility of pulmonary vascular changes could occur in COPD patients under LTOT.

However, we do not know whether the structural changes of the small pulmonary vessels, which are observed in these advanced COPD patients, are potentially reversible on LTOT. We do not know either whether these structural changes are fully accounted for by chronic alveolar hypoxia. Even if there are some similarities, the morphological changes in the pulmonary vasculature are not identical in hypoxemic (healthy) high-altitude residents and hypoxemic COPD patients (41).

During 1967 to 1968, studies performed in Denver (42) and Birmingham (43) have shown that continuous (24 hr/day) oxygen therapy given during four to eight weeks improved markedly pulmonary hypertension; however, a normalization (<20 mmHg) of pulmonary artery mean pressure (PAP) was not observed in individual cases. These studies concerned small groups of patients ($n = 6$ in both studies) and there was no control group.

In addition, these promising results have not been confirmed by the well-known NOTT and MRC studies (9,10). These multicentric controlled studies were not mainly devoted to evaluate pulmonary hemodynamics under LTOT, but rather to assess the effect of this treatment on life expectancy. Nevertheless, pulmonary hemodynamic data were available at the onset in all patients and follow-up right heart catheterizations were performed in a relatively large number of patients.

In the MRC study (9), 42 patients who survived >500 days from the onset of the study were catheterized again after at least one year of follow-up. PAP was stable (rate of change/yr ~ 0) in the subgroup of 21 patients given LTOT (15 hr/day), whereas it increased significantly ($+2.8$ mmHg/yr) in the control group of 21 patients. Thus, LTOT did not improve pulmonary hypertension, but its stabilization was a rather good result when compared to its worsening in patients not receiving LTOT.

In the NOTT study (10,44), hemodynamic data at the onset and after six months of LTOT were available in 117 patients whose initial resting and exercising PAP were 29 ± 10 and 50 ± 16 mmHg respectively. In both conditions, COT decreased slightly but PAP (resting PAP: -3 mmHg as a mean; exercising PAP: -6 mmHg as a mean) and pulmonary vascular resistance decreased significantly, whereas NOT (10–12 hr/day) did not.

Another way of investigating the effects of LTOT is to compare the course of pulmonary hemodynamics before and after the onset of O_2 therapy, the patients being their own controls. This has been done in our department (45). In 16 patients, we observed a reversal of the progression of pulmonary hypertension with LTOT since PAP increased from 23.3 ± 6.8 to 28.0 ± 7.4 mmHg ($p < 0.005$) before the initiation of LTOT (average length of this period $= 48$ months), and decreased back to 23.9 ± 6.6 mmHg during LTOT [17–18 hr/day as a mean; average length of the period $= 31$ months compared to six months in the NOTT trial (44)]. Thus, PAP was not normalized but returned to its baseline level. The evolution of PAP paralleled that of pulmonary vascular resistance. When changes in PAP were expressed as changes per year, the difference was also statistically significant: an increase of 1.5 mmHg/yr before the onset of LTOT versus a decrease of 2.1 mmHg/yr after the initiation of LTOT ($p < 0.01$) (45). An improvement of pulmonary hypertension during oxygen therapy was observed in 12/16 patients.

More recently, Zielinski et al. (46) investigated 95 patients under LTOT (14–15 hr/day), among whom 39 could be catheterized again after two years: PAP fell from 25 ± 8 to 23 ± 6 mmHg (NS). In the 12 patients who completed six years of LTOT, PAP fell from 25 ± 7 to 21 ± 4 mmHg after two years but increased to 26 ± 6 mmHg after six years ($p < 0.01$ for two vs. six years). Thus, as a mean there was a long-term stabilization of pulmonary hypertension under LTOT.

The differences between the results of some studies are probably explained by the daily duration of O_2 therapy which varies from 14 to 15 hr/day (9,46) to > 18 hr/day (10,44). The best results have been obtained in the continuous O_2 group of the NOTT study (> 18 hr/day) and in our own study (17–18 hr/day) (45), whereas the results were less favorable in the MRC study (15 hr/day) (9) and in the study by Zielinski et al. (14–15 hr/day) (46). It has been demonstrated that, in these patients, removing O_2 for not more than three hours had marked hemodynamic consequences (47). Accordingly, one should recommend COT.

Finally, even in long-term responders to O_2, a normalization of PAP is rarely observed, which could be explained by the nonreversibility of the pulmonary vascular remodeling under LTOT (41). In fact, Calverley et al. (48) found opposed results.

In summary, LTOT stabilizes or at least attenuates, and sometimes reverses the progression of pulmonary hypertension, but PAP seldom returns to normal. It is clear that the longer the daily duration of LTOT, the better the pulmonary hemodynamic results.

Effects of Oxygen Therapy on Sleep-Related Pulmonary Hypertension

Sleep-related episodes of nocturnal hypoxemia, particularly frequent during REM sleep, can induce an episodic worsening of pulmonary hypertension (49–52). Fletcher and Levin (52) have shown that these peaks of pulmonary hypertension are prevented by NOT with conventional flows (1.5–3 L/min). When oxygen therapy is discontinued, sleep-related peaks of pulmonary hypertension rapidly reappear (52).

Pulmonary hypertension is generally observed in COPD patients with marked daytime hypoxemia ($PaO_2 < 55$–60 mmHg). Two studies suggested that sleep-related hypoxemia could favor the development of pulmonary hypertension in patients whose diurnal PaO_2 is > 60 mmHg (33,53). However, a more recent multicenter trial (54), including more patients ($n = 94$) than these two studies taken together, has shown that, among COPD patients with mild daytime hypoxemia (diurnal PaO_2 in the range 56–69 mmHg), nocturnal desaturators did not exhibit a higher diurnal PAP than nondesaturators. In addition, PAP was not correlated with the degree and duration of nocturnal hypoxemia. These results do not support the hypothesis that sleep-related hypoxemia favors the development of permanent pulmonary hypertension.

A study by Fletcher et al. (55) indicated that supplemental oxygen during sleep to reverse episodic desaturation in COPD patients with a daytime > 60 mmHg had a beneficial effect in reducing PAP, but only nine control subjects and seven subjects given NOT could complete the study. The recent European multicentric trial quoted above (54,56) has included 76 nocturnal desaturators, of whom 46 could complete the two-year follow-up: in the 24 patients given NOT and in the 22 control patients, the pulmonary hemodynamic changes were similar and rather small after two years (Table2). This study (56) showed that NOT does not modify the evolution of pulmonary hemodynamics in COPD patients with significant sleep-related O_2 desaturation but without marked daytime hypoxemia.

Table 2 Evolution of Arterial Blood Gases and Pulmonary Hemodynamics in COPD Patients with Mild-to-Moderate Daytime Hypoxemia ($PaO_2 = 56$–69 mmHg), Exhibiting Nocturnal Desaturation [Patients are Given or Not Nocturnal Oxygen Therapy (NOT)]

	NOT group Patients ($n = 24$)		Control group Patients ($n = 22$)		
	T0	T2	T0	T2	
PaO_2 (mmHg)	63.0 ± 3.3	62.2 ± 7.4	63.1 ± 2.8	64.5 ± 5.7	NS
$PaCO_2$ (mmHg)	45.0 ± 5.6	46.3 ± 5.9	44.3 ± 4.2	44.9 ± 5.6	NS
PAP rest (mmHg)	18.3 ± 4.7	19.5 ± 5.3	19.8 ± 5.6	20.5 ± 6.5	NS
PAP exercise (mmHg)	35.2 ± 7.2	38.3 ± 10.3	36.2 ± 11.7	37.1 ± 11.3	NS
PWP (mmHg)	7.8 ± 3.1	8.8 ± 4.5	10.1 ± 4.0	9.5 ± 4.2	NS
Cardiac output ($L/min/m^2$)	2.86 ± 0.51	3.16 ± 0.51	3.01 ± 0.74	3.14 ± 0.64	NS
Mean nocturnal SaO_2 (%)	87.9 ± 2.7	87.9 ± 4.2	88.6 ± 2.0	89.3 ± 2.9	NS
$tSaO_2 < 90\%$ (%)	62.5 ± 25.3	57.9 ± 31.9	64.7 ± 24.8	51.2 ± 36.2	NS

It can be seen that the evolution of PAP is identical in patients given NOT and in the control group. NOT does not modify the evolution of pulmonary hemodynamics in patients with significant sleep-related O_2 desaturation but without marked daytime hypoxemia.
Abbreviations: T0, onset of the study; T2, end of the study (two years); NS, not statistically significant; COPD, chronic obstructive pulmonary disease; PAP, pulmonary artery mean pressure; PWP, pulmonary capillary wedge pressure; $tSaO_2 < 90\%$, percent of sleep time with a SaO_2 90%.
Source: From Ref. 56.

III. Indications of LTOT in COPD

Widely accepted as well as debated indications of LTOT are summarized in Table 3.

Table 3 Indications for Long-Term Oxygen Therapy

Accepted indications
  PaO_2 in a stable clinical state (2 measurements separated by at least 3 weeks) ≤ 55 mmHg (which is equivalent to $SaO_2 \leq 88\%$)
  PaO_2 in the range 55–59 mmHg in the presence of
    Polycythemia (hematocrit $> 55\%$)
    Pulmonary hypertension ($PAP \geq 25$ mmHg)
    EKG signs of right ventricular hypertrophy
    Edema resulting from right heart failure
    Significant worsening of hypoxemia during sleep (mean nocturnal $SaO_2 \leq 88\%$)
Discussed indications
  If the patient is normoxemic or slightly hypoxemic at rest ($PaO_2 > 60$ mmHg) but desaturates during exercise ($PaO_2 \leq 55$ mmHg) oxygen, appropriately titrated, can be given solely during exercise
  If the patient is normoxemic or slightly hypoxemic during daytime ($PaO_2 > 60$ mmHg) but desaturates during sleep (mean nocturnal $SaO_2 \leq 88\%$), oxygen can be given during sleep, but the benefits of isolated nocturnal O_2 therapy have not so far been demonstrated

Abbreviations: EKG, electrocardiographic; PAP, pulmonary artery mean pressure.

A. Widely Accepted Indications

Guidelines from scientific societies (57–61) are largely based on inclusion criteria in the MRC (9) and NOTT (10) studies. Stable COPD patients whose PaO_2 is persistently <55 mmHg (which corresponds to a $SaO_2 < 88\%$) must be prescribed LTOT. This threshold value of 55 mmHg indicates the presence of significant hypoxemia and subsequently increased risk of impaired oxygen transport, pulmonary hemodynamics, brain function, etc.

When PaO_2 is in the range 55 to 59 mmHg (59 mmHg corresponds to an SaO_2 of 89–90%), LTOT is also justified in case of polycythemia (hematocrit $> 55\%$), pulmonary hypertension ($PAP \geq 25$ mmHg), electrocardiographic (EKG) signs of right ventricular hypertrophy, edema resulting from right heart failure, and when hypoxemia significantly worsens during sleep with a mean nocturnal $SaO_2 \leq 88\%$.

Before initiating LTOT, the patient must be on an optimum medical regimen including bronchodilators and physiotherapy. Hypoxemia must be persistent, which means that arterial blood gases should be measured when the patient is clinically stable on at least two occasions, three to four weeks apart. In our opinion, when hypoxemia is not very severe ($PaO_2 > 50$ mmHg), a two- to three-month follow-up period is preferable since a multicentric French study (62) clearly indicated that among a group of clinically stable COPD patients whose initial PaO_2 was <55 mmHg, 30% had progressive improvement, the PaO_2 exceeding 60 mmHg after a three-month follow-up period (Fig. 2). In this regard, LTOT must not be confounded with short-term oxygen therapy. A recent study (63) concluded that reassessment of applicants for domiciliary

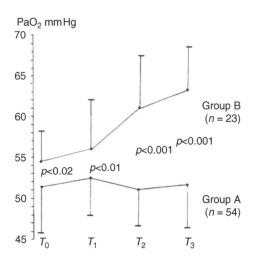

Figure 2 Evolution of PaO_2 over three months in chronic obstructive pulmonary disease patients candidates for long-term oxygen therapy (LTOT) and clinically stable at T_0. It can be seen that PaO_2 is stable in the majority of the patients (Group A, $n = 54$). However, in Group B, which represents 30% of the patients ($n = 23$), PaO_2 increases regularly from T_0 to T_3. Consequently, these patients do no fulfill the usual criteria for LTOT at T_3. *Abbreviations*: T_0, onset of the study; T_1, after one month; T_2, after two months; T_3, after three months. *Source*: From Ref. 62.

oxygen after several months of stability identifies an appreciable portion of initially eligible patients who no longer fulfill the required criteria.

Many COPD patients may require hospitalization because of an exacerbation of their disease. Some of these patients may be clinically unstable and significantly hypoxemic ($PaO_2 < 55$ mmHg) when they leave the hospital. Oxygen therapy which has been started in the hospital can be continued at home, but arterial blood gases must be retested during the next two to three months (63) which is mandatory in the United States for all Medicare patients (64). If hypoxemia is persistent, short-term oxygen therapy becomes LTOT. If PaO_2 is repeatedly over 60 mmHg, home oxygen therapy can be discontinued.

B. Debated Indications

Oxygen Therapy for Exercise-Induced Hypoxemia

In advanced COPD, hypoxemia most often worsens during exercise, particularly in patients of the emphysematous type. Exercise induces a transient but marked elevation of PAP, which can increase by as much as 20 to 30 mmHg during a steady-state 40-W exercise (65). Breathing oxygen during exercise produces a small but significant fall of PAP and pulmonary vascular resistance (65,66). Accordingly, if a COPD patient meets LTOT criteria at rest, it is clear that appropriately titrated O_2 should also be given during exercise (57). But what about patients who develop significant hypoxemia only during exertion? In that case, supplemental oxygen is recommended by scientific societies (57) even though studies designed to determine the long-term benefit of oxygen given solely during exercise are lacking.

An objective improvement with supplemental oxygen has also been observed even in COPD patients who were not hypoxemic either at rest or during exercise (67), but it is generally accepted that oxygen should not be prescribed as a treatment for dyspnea when hypoxemia is not present.

NOT for Sleep-Related Hypoxemia

Patients who are hypoxemic while awake will be hypoxemic during sleep as well. In most COPD patients, hypoxemia does in fact worsen during sleep and especially during REM sleep, which is characterized by a reduced ventilation (68). Thus, it appears particularly important to oxygenate these patients during sleep. It is often recommended to add 1 L/min of oxygen flow to the daytime resting prescription (57).

Some COPD patients have no significant hypoxemia when awake ($PaO_2 > 60$ mmHg), but are hypoxemic during sleep (32,33) with a mean nocturnal transcutaneous $SaO_2 < 90\%$. Is it necessary to give supplemental oxygen during sleep to these COPD patients in whom significant hypoxemia is limited to nighttime? Current guidelines are ambiguous (57), probably due to the lack of demonstrative studies in this field. In the ATS Statement (57), it is written that "research should be undertaken to determine if treatment with supplemental oxygen of isolated falls in nocturnal SaO_2, in the absence of severe daytime hypoxemia, prevents morbidity and mortality in patients with COPD."

As mentioned above, there are only two controlled studies which have investigated the effects of NOT given to COPD patients exhibiting sleep-related hypoxemia (without significant daytime hypoxemia): the study by Fletcher et al. (55)

and the more recent multicentric European study (56,69). Fletcher et al. (55) investigated 38 patients, 19 receiving NOT (3 L/min) and 19 receiving room air (3 L/min). There was no difference in mortality between the two groups (five deaths in the NOT group vs. six in the control group), but the very high attrition rate of the study (11/38 patients being dropped) precluded any firm conclusion. The European study (56,69) compared 41 patients treated with NOT to 35 controls: there were nine deaths in the NOT group versus seven in the control group; the difference was not significant, but again the small numbers of patients and deaths precluded a firm conclusion. Interestingly, the European study showed that NOT did not allow to delay the prescription of LTOT, similar numbers of patients in the NOT group and in the control group requiring LTOT during follow-up.

Finally, whereas Fletcher et al. (55) observed an improvement of pulmonary hypertension after three years in their seven NOT patients compared to their nine control patients ($p<0.02$), the European study (56) observed no difference in pulmonary hemodynamic changes after two years between the 24 NOT patients and the 22 control patients (Table 2).

At present, the beneficial effects of isolated NOT have not been demonstrated in COPD patients with sleep-related hypoxemia. Accordingly, this treatment is probably not justified in COPD patients.

LTOT in Patients with Borderline Hypoxemia (60–65 mmHg)

Although 55 mmHg is universally accepted as the level of PaO_2 under which LTOT is required, many patients with $PaO_2 \geq 60$ mmHg are currently being prescribed LTOT. In the United States and the Canadian State of Ontario, the prevalence of home oxygen therapy largely exceeds that of countries like France or the United Kingdom (70). But, even in France, a study (71) has shown that 18.5% of a large series ($n=7700$) of COPD patients who were prescribed LTOT via the Association Nationale pour le Traitement A Domicile des Insuffisants Respiratoires (ANTADIR) French network had a stable $PaO_2 \geq 60$ mmHg when LTOT was initiated. The Polish study by Gorecka et al. (13), which included 135 COPD patients, has clearly shown that LTOT did not improve survival in patients with moderate hypoxemia (PaO_2 in the range 56–65 mmHg, mean value = 60.5 mmHg; Fig. 1). However, aspects other than survival, such as quality of life, have not been investigated in this study (13,72).

Thus, beneficial effects of LTOT in patients with a stable PaO_2 over 60 mmHg have not been demonstrated so far. Accordingly, home oxygen therapy is probably not warranted in these patients.

C. Contraindications to LTOT

There is no express contraindication to LTOT. In the past, there has been overemphasis on the fear that oxygen therapy might lead to respiratory drive depression, which could result in worsening of hypercapnia and respiratory acidosis. CO_2 retention may indeed occur in some patients (73), but it is rarely severe in stable COPD patients when O_2 therapy is given at low flow (1–3 L/min) with a resulting PaO_2 in the range 60 to 70 mmHg. It was suspected that the elevation of $PaCO_2$ under O_2 therapy could be more pronounced during sleep, due to the reduction of the respiratory chemical drive (decreased sensitivity to hypoxia and hypercapnia). However, the study by Goldstein et al. (74) showed that transcutaneous $PaCO_2$ did not increase more in sleeping than in awake patients: this increase was generally <6 mmHg, occurred early during sleep and $PaCO_2$ rapidly stabilized.

Consequently, the presence of marked hypercapnia is not a contraindication to LTOT. It should be reminded that the first patients given LTOT in Denver and Birmingham (42,43) had severe hypercapnia but oxygen therapy was particularly well tolerated. The situation may be different during acute exacerbations of the disease, as well as in patients who have both COPD and obstructive sleep apneas; hypercapnia may increase markedly during sleep in these patients (74).

Some authors do not prescribe LTOT to patients who continue to smoke because they presume that these patients will not be compliant enough. Furthermore, it has been demonstrated that some deleterious effects of chronic hypoxemia, like polycythemia, are not corrected under LTOT when the blood level of CO remains abnormally high, due to tobacco smoking (31). Finally, one of the major physical hazards with oxygen therapy in patients who smoke is fire or explosions. Most fires have been caused by patients lighting cigarettes as oxygen flows in their noses (75). Patients and family must be warned not to smoke.

IV. Home Oxygen Therapy

A. General Rules for LTOT

The most important rule concerns the daily duration of LTOT, which should be ≥18 hr/day. The best results, with regard to survival and pulmonary hemodynamics, have been observed in patients who were on COT (in fact >18 hr/day and 20.5 hr/day as a mean) (10,44). The more continuously oxygen is administered, the greater the benefit (57). Consequently, it is recommended that patients be given oxygen continuously, which implies that they can be provided an ambulatory source of oxygen.

LTOT includes the sleep period, which is often characterized by a worsening of hypoxemia, particularly during REM sleep (68). Oxygen therapy must be given during exercise (e.g., walking) and other activities (e.g., eating) which lead to more severe hypoxemia, but its delivery may be difficult in some circumstances (e.g., washing). A recent Canadian study (76) concluded that a widespread provision of ambulatory oxygen to COPD patients necessitating LTOT was not justified; however, this study mainly investigated quality of life and it is certainly difficult to refuse ambulatory oxygen to patients who are already markedly hypoxemic at rest.

PaO_2 under LTOT must be at least 60 to 65 mmHg and, if possible, closer to 70 to 75 mmHg. This level of PaO_2 is generally easy to achieve in most COPD patients with O_2 flows in the range 1.5 to 3 L/min. The resting flow rate can be adjusted by monitoring pulse oxymetry to obtain an SaO_2 >90% and, whenever possible, ≥92%. Thirty minutes of oxygen are required for this test. It is recommended to measure arterial blood gases at the end of the test in order to validate the oxymetric results and assess the change in $PaCO_2$.

In the NOTT trial (10), oxygen flow rates were arbitrarily increased by 1 L/min above the resting level, during exercise and sleep. Is this justified? It appears more appropriate to monitor continuously SaO_2 with pulse oxymetry during sleep and exercise, using if possible the patient's own oxygen delivery system. SaO_2 must be kept ≥90%. Then, in some patients it is not necessary to increase the O_2 flow during sleep, in good agreement with previous studies (74) which have shown that usual O_2 flows

(2—3 L/min) are usually sufficient to correct sleep-related hypoxemia, even in patients who desaturate markedly during sleep. If nocturnal SaO_2 is <90%, the O_2 flow is increased by steps of 0.5 L/min. Exercise testing can be easily accomplished with a six-minute walk, SaO_2 being measured by pulse oxymetry, but it must be reminded that pulse oxymetry is less reliable in exercise studies that at rest (57). Most often, it is necessary to increase the O_2 flow by 1 to 2 L/min during walking.

The treatment must not be too constraining and should be compatible with a good quality of life. The best solution is certainly to give the patient an equipment for ambulatory oxygen therapy, but some patients refuse to have supplemental O_2 outside their home. The prescribing physician must be aware that compliance to LTOT is poor in some patients (see below) with an actual daily duration of oxygen therapy for three to four hours less than what is prescribed. This is a supplemental reason for prescribing at least 18 hr/day.

B. Oxygen Delivery Systems

Three basic delivery systems are currently available for LTOT in the home: compressed-oxygen cylinders, liquid oxygen, and oxygen concentrators. Outside the home, liquid oxygen and compressed-oxygen cylinders can be used.

The respective advantages and drawbacks of the three sources of oxygen are listed in Table 4. At present, oxygen concentrators represent the most practical and less costly method for providing oxygen therapy at home. These devices concentrate oxygen from air by extracting nitrogen. Most concentrators use a molecular sieve device and can deliver a concentration of $O_2 \geq 90\%$ at flows up to 3 to 4 L/min. The maximal flow delivered by a concentrator is generally 5 to 6 L/min, but it is possible

Table 4 Advantages and Drawbacks of the Three Sources of Oxygen

	Advantages	Drawbacks
Concentrators	No limitation of O_2 volume	$FiO_2 < 100\%$, particularly for high flows
	High flows can be provided by a combination of 2 concentrators	Do not allow ambulatory O_2 therapy
	Low maintenance	
	Relatively cheap	
	Available almost everywhere (in developed countries)	
Gaseous oxygen	Provide the highest flows	Limited quantity of O_2 available
	Can be used for deambulation (small cylinders)	Cylinders are heavy and of great size
	Available everywhere	Risk of explosion
		High maintenance
		Relatively high cost
Liquid oxygen	Important quantity of O_2 available	Risk of thermal burns
	Can provide moderate to high flows	Not available everywhere
	The most convenient portable system	High maintenance
		High cost (the most expensive system)

to associate two concentrators. Periodic assessment of delivered FiO_2 as well as regular checking of the filters located at the entrance of ambient air are required.

The major drawback of the concentrator is that it is a stationary source of oxygen. The concentrator weighs 35 lb (and up to 50 lb for some devices) and is not portable. It is most often located in one room but can be easily moved from a room to another. Light-weight, portable concentrators, powered by an external battery, are presently available but their cost is very high.

Gaseous (compressed) oxygen cylinders have been historically the first source for LTOT. In some countries where concentrators are not readily available, they are still the primary source of oxygen at home. They can provide very high flows of oxygen. They need a high maintenance and must be secured to prevent injury. Their major drawbacks are their volume and weight. The quantity of oxygen provided by a given cylinder is limited, most often ranging between 3000 and 5000 L, which represents a duration of use of 24 to 36 hours for a 2 to 3 L/min flow. Small cylinders can be used for deambulation, delivering from 150 to 600 L of O_2, which represents an autonomy of one to four hours at a flow of 2.5 to 3 L/min.

Liquid oxygen has two major advantages: firstly, the volume of oxygen available is much larger than with compressed cylinders, and secondly, oxygen can be transfilled from the large stationary source to portable systems, which are particularly adapted to ambulatory oxygen therapy (Fig. 3) since they are relatively light, weighing from 5 to 12 lb and have a large autonomy when compared to portable compressed cylinders. One liter of liquid oxygen contains 860 L of gaseous oxygen (autonomy of near five hours for 3 L/min flow) and weighs only 1.1 kg. The stationary source has an autonomy of 3.5 to 12 days for a flow of 2 L/min. The major drawback of liquid oxygen is its cost since it is the most expensive system. Furthermore, availability is limited, it requires a high maintenance, and the risk of thermal burns must be underlined. Liquid oxygen allows the delivery of O_2 flows as high as 8 L/min. Some devices allow even higher flows up to 12 L/min. Liquid oxygen provides the most convenient portable system and is particularly adapted to patients who often deambulate outside their home.

C. Oxygen Delivery Methods

Oxygen is most often given via a dual-prong nasal cannula which is simple, reliable, and well tolerated by most patients. The use of face masks, such as Venturi masks, is uncommon at home. This device gives fixed oxygen concentration but requires relatively high flows. With the nasal cannula each liter/min of O_2 flow adds about 3% to 4% to the ambient FiO_2 (20.9%). For instance, an O_2 flow of 2 L/min increases the FiO_2 to 28%. In fact, the actual FiO_2 is dependent on several factors including the respiratory rate, which is inversely related to FiO_2 (a higher respiratory rate reduces FiO_2).

In most COPD patients, O_2 flows in the range 1.5 to 3 L/min are sufficient to achieve a $PaO_2 > 60$ mmHg. In some patients with very advanced COPD, high flows (> 6 L/min) are needed and transtracheal catheters may be of interest. They permit lower flows of O_2 by reducing the anatomical dead space. With transtracheal oxygen (TTO), patients use 50% less oxygen than with nasal oxygen (77–79). But TTO is not free of inconvenients, the most important being the obstruction of the catheter by mucous secretions. Some patients choose TTO for cosmetic reasons, but it must be emphasized that TTO needs an active participation by the patient who has to learn the required maintenance.

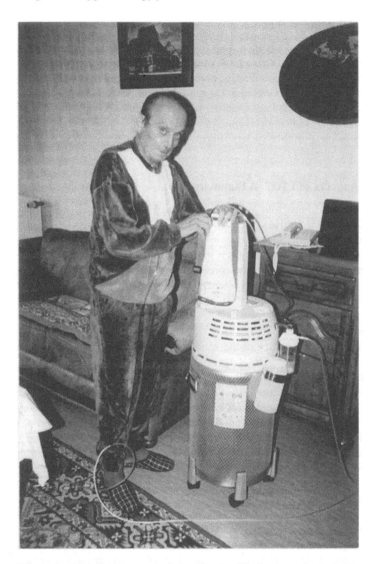

Figure 3 With liquid oxygen, O_2 can be transfilled at home from the large stationary source to portable systems which are particularly adapted to ambulatory oxygen therapy.

Besides TTO, oxygen-conserving devices also aim to improve mobility and comfort. They can reduce the cost of oxygen therapy in the home. These devices deliver all of the oxygen during early inhalation. Reservoir cannulas (80,81) operate by storing oxygen in a small chamber during exhalation for subsequent delivery during early inhalation. Demand pulse oxygen devices (82,83) deliver a small bolus of pure oxygen at the onset of inhalation. They are interposed between the patient and the oxygen source.

Humidification is generally not necessary when oxygen is given by nasal cannula at relatively low flows ($\leq$5–6 L/min).

D. Hazards of Oxygen at Home

The major physical hazards of oxygen therapy are fires and explosions (57). As mentioned earlier, most accidents have been observed in patients lighting cigarettes while they inhale oxygen (75). Accordingly, patients and their relatives should be warned and educated not to smoke. Containers of gaseous (compressed) oxygen and of liquid oxygen should not be installed near sources of heat or flames. Freeze burns have been observed if the patient is not cautious enough when transfilling liquid oxygen from the stationary source to the portable system. Fortunately, major accidents associated with LTOT at home are rare (57).

E. Practical Aspects of LTOT: A Summary

A probationary period of at least four weeks is necessary for assessing the stability of hypoxemia ($PaO_2 < 55$–60 mmHg), thereby confirming the indication of LTOT. One single determination of arterial blood gases is insufficient, particularly after an acute exacerbation of the disease. When PaO_2 is in the range 55 to 60 mmHg in a stable patient, LTOT can be prescribed in the presence of polycythemia, pulmonary hypertension (or right ventricular enlargement), and when there is a significant worsening of hypoxemia during sleep (57). Accordingly, investigations such as nocturnal oximetry, polysomnography, or echocardiographic estimation of PAP may be indicated in some patients.

   One important point is the choice of the source of oxygen. This choice depends on several variables including the patient's age, the daily duration of oxygen therapy, the required oxygen flow, the patient's activity, the need for deambulation, and the patient's personal wishes. In the majority of patients, LTOT is provided by a concentrator, which is the simplest and most economical method of oxygen delivery (84). In that case, ambulatory oxygen can be supplied by small compressed-gas cylinders with an autonomy of one to four hours. When the patient is relatively young, active, and walks outside their home every day, liquid oxygen should be considered. It must be remembered that the cost of each delivery system is not the same (Table 4), liquid oxygen being the most expensive. In our experience, liquid oxygen is required in about 25% of patients in whom LTOT is needed.

   As indicated above, the adequate O_2 flow is assessed by arterial blood gases measurements or by oxymetry, the target PaO_2 being in the range 60 to 75 mmHg, corresponding to a target transcutaneous SaO_2 greater than 90%. The assessment of the adequate flow is generally performed using a piped hospital oxygen (wall-oxygen) as supply source, and the oxygen flow required to achieve an identical PaO_2 from a concentrator may be greater as shown in a recent study (85). Accordingly, it is important to check, at home, oximetry while the patient is on their concentrator.

   It is easier for the patient to have the same flow during day and night, but it is useful to check, by nocturnal oxymetry, the efficiency of supplemental oxygen on sleep-related hypoxemia. During walking and other activities, the O_2 flow must be adequately increased. Usual O_2 flows at rest range between 1.5 and 3 L/min. The flow necessary to correct hypoxemia may vary with time and it is recommended to check it at least once per year.

   The oxygen delivery system must be regularly checked at the patient's home by a technician. A high level of maintenance is necessary for compressed oxygen as well as for liquid oxygen and concentrators. In the case of liquid oxygen, there is generally a weekly refilling of the stationary source. A periodic validation of the delivered flow is necessary. In the case of concentrators, the FiO_2 delivered by the device must be regularly assessed. The maintenance is provided by home care companies or by non-profit organizations such as the ANTADIR network, regularly operating in France.

Reimbursement criteria and their documentation will not be developed in this chapter because they vary from one country to another. However, in most countries the physician who prescribes LTOT must provide appropriate documentation that oxygen is necessary and that the patient meets the usual physiological criteria.

F. Compliance with Oxygen Therapy at Home

One of the major problems with oxygen therapy is compliance with the treatment. LTOT is undoubtedly a constraining therapy, and this probably explains why compliance is often poor, as indicated in several reports (86–90). Howard et al. (89) observed that, in patients to whom LTOT was prescribed for 15 or more hours per day ($n = 339$), the actual usage of concentrators (13.4 hours as a mean) was markedly lower than the prescribed usage (17.9 hours as a mean). Pepin et al. (90) observed that the mean duration of effective oxygen therapy was of 14.5 ± 5 hr/day in a large population of 930 COPD patients, but the mean duration of oxygen prescribed was only 16 ± 3 hr/day. These observations and other studies of the literature (27,91) suggest that efforts to improve the observance of LTOT should be focused on three major targets: better education for prescribing physicians, better education for patients, and improving the quality of life under LTOT.

The prescribing physicians must be aware of the minimal daily duration of an efficient LTOT, which is probably 18 hours or more per day rather than 16 hours. They should be convinced that the longer the daily duration of LTOT is, the better the results (improved survival, pulmonary hemodynamics, etc.) will be. They must also be aware that stopping oxygen for more than 3 to 6 hr/day may have deleterious effects.

The education of patients must not be limited to home education given by a nurse or a physiotherapist, even if this kind of education is of great importance. Physicians should also be involved in the education of patients. A Swiss study (91) has demonstrated that compliance to LTOT can be improved by an education program given by both physicians and physiotherapists during short (48 hours) hospital stays.

Finally, it must be kept in mind that LTOT is a constraining therapy that may deteriorate the quality of life of some patients. Accordingly, all efforts must be made to supply possibilities of ambulatory oxygen to those patients who remain active. Liquid oxygen may represent the best solution. A multicenter study (27) of 169 patients clearly showed that those patients who used portable oxygen had a significantly longer daily duration of oxygen therapy and this was particularly true when the patients used liquid oxygen.

References

1. Burrows B, Earle RH. Course and prognosis of chronic obstructive lung disease. A prospective study of 200 patients. N Engl J Med 1969; 280:397–404.
2. Boushy SF, Thompson HKJ, North LB, Beale AR, Snow TR. Prognosis in chronic obstructive pulmonary disease. Am Rev Respir Dis 1973; 108:1373–83.

3. Postma DS, Burema J, Gimeno F, et al. Prognosis in severe chronic obstructive pulmonary disease. Am Rev Respir Dis 1979; 119:357–67.

4. Traver GA, Cline MG, Burrows B. Predictors of mortality in chronic obstructive pulmonary disease. A 15-year follow-up study. Am Rev Respir Dis 1979; 119:895–902.

5. Ourednik A, Susa Z. How long does the pulmonary hypertension last in chronic obstructive pulmonary disease?. In: Widimsky J, ed. Pulmonary Hypertension. Basel: Karger, 1975:24–8.

6. Weitzenblum E, Hirth C, Ducolone A, Mirhom R, Rasaholinjanahary J, Ehrhart M. Prognostic value of pulmonary artery pressure in chronic obstructive pulmonary disease. Thorax 1981; 36:752–8.

7. Bishop JM, Cross KW. Physiological variables and mortality in patients with various categories of chronic respiratory disease. Bull Eur Physiopathol Respir 1984; 20:495–500.

8. Celli BR, Cote CG, Marin JM, et al. The body-mass index, airflow obstruction dyspnéea, and exercise capacity index in chronic obstructive pulmonary disease. N Engl J Med 2004; 350:1005–12.

9. Medical Research Council Working Party. Report of long term domiciliary oxygen therapy in chronic hypoxic cor pulmonale complicating chronic bronchitis and emphysema. Lancet 1981; 1:681–5.

10. Nocturnal Oxygen Therapy Trial Group. Continuous or nocturnal oxygen therapy in hypoxemic chronic obstructive lung disease. Ann Intern Med 1980; 93:391–8.

11. Petty TL. Long-term outpatient oxygen therapy. In: Petty TL, ed. Chronic Obstructive Pulmonary Disease. New York: Marcel Dekker, 1985:375–88.

12. Cooper CB, Waterhouse J, Howard P. Twelve year clinical study of patients with hypoxic cor pulmonale given long term domiciliary oxygen therapy. Thorax 1987; 42:105–10.

13. Gorecka D, Gorzelak K, Sliwinski P, Tobiasz M, Zielinski J. Effect of long-term oxygen therapy on survival in patients with chronic obstructive pulmonary disease with moderate hypoxaemia. Thorax 1997; 52:674–9.

14. Skwarski K, MacNee W, Wraith PK, Sliwinski P, Zielinski J. Predictors of survival in patients with chronic obstructive pulmonary disease treated with long-term oxygen therapy. Chest 1991; 100:1522–7.

15. Chailleux E, Fauroux B, Binet F, Dautzenberg B, Polu JM. Predictors of survival in patients receiving domiciliary oxygen therapy or mechanical ventilation. A 10-year analysis of ANTADIR Observatory. Chest 1996; 109:741–9.

16. Dubois P, Jamart J, Machiels J, Smeets F, Lulling J. Prognosis of severely hypoxemic patients receiving long-term oxygen therapy. Chest 1994; 105:469–74.

17. Oswald-Mammosser M, Weitzenblum E, Quoix E, Moser G, Chaouat A, Kessler R. Prognostic factors in COPD patients receiving long-term oxygen therapy. Importance of pulmonary artery pressure. Chest 1995; 107:1193–8.

18. Strom K. Survival of patients with chronic obstructive pulmonary disease receiving long-term domiciliary oxygen therapy. Am Rev Respir Dis 1993; 147:585–91.

19. Aida A, Miyamoto K, Nishimura M, Aiba M, Kira S, Kawakami Y. Prognostic value of hypercapnia in patients with chronic respiratory failure during long-term oxygen therapy. Am J Respir Crit Care Med 1998; 158:188–93.

20. Marti S, Munoz X, Rios J, Morell F, Ferrer J. Body weight and comorbidity predict mortality in COPD patients treated with oxygen therapy. Eur Respir J 2006; 27:689–96.

21. Chambellan A, Chailleux E, Similowski T. Prognostic value of the hematocrit in patients with severe COPD receiving long-term oxygen therapy and the ANTADIR Observatory Group. Chest 2005; 128:1201–8.

22. Okubadejo AA, Paul EA, Jones PW, Wedzicha JA. Does long-term oxygen therapy affect quality of life in patients with chronic obstructive pulmonary disease and severe hypoxaemia? Eur Respir J 1996; 9:2335–9.

23. Eaton T, Lewis C, Young P, Kennedy Y, Garret JE, Kolbe J. Long-term oxygen therapy improves health-related quality of life. Respir Med 2004; 98:285–93.

24. Heaton RK, Grant I, McSweeny AJ, Adams KM, Petty TL. Psychologic effects of continuous and nocturnal oxygen therapy in hypoxemic chronic obstructive pulmonary disease. Arch Intern Med 1983; 143:1941–7.

25. Lilker ES, Karnick A, Lerner L. Portable oxygen in chronic obstructive lung disease with hypoxemia and cor pulmonale. A controlled double-blind crossover study. Chest 1975; 68:236–41.

26. Leggett RJ, Flenley DC. Portable oxygen and exercise tolerance in patients with chronic hypoxic cor pulmonale. Br Med J 1977; 2:84–6.

27. Vergeret J, Brambilla C, Mounier L. Portable oxygen therapy: use and benefit in hypoxaemic COPD patients on long-term oxygen therapy. Eur Respir J 1989; 2:20–5.

28. MacNee W, Wathen CG, Flenley DC, Muir AD. The effects of controlled oxygen therapy on ventricular function in patients with stable and decompensated cor pulmonale. Am Rev Respir Dis 1988; 137:1289–95.

29. Morrison DA, Henry R, Goldman S. Preliminary study of the effects of low flow oxygen on oxygen delivery and right ventricular function in chronic lung disease. Am Rev Respir Dis 1986; 133:390–5.

30. Segel N, Bishop JM. The pulmonary circulation in patients with chronic bronchitis and emphysema at rest and during exercise, with special reference to the influence of changes in blood viscosity and blood volume on the pulmonary circulation. J Clin Invest 1966; 45:1555–68.

31. Calverley PM, Leggett RJ, McElderry L, Flenley DC. Cigarette smoking and secondary polycythemia in hypoxic cor pulmonale. Am Rev Respir Dis 1982; 125:507–10.

32. Fletcher EC, Miller J, Divine GW, Fletcher JG, Miller T. Nocturnal oxyhemoglobin desaturation in COPD patients with arterial oxygen tensions above 60 mmHg. Chest 1987; 92:604–8.

33. Levi-Valensi P, Weitzenblum E, Rida Z, et al. Sleep-related oxygen desaturation and daytime pulmonary haemodynamics in COPD patients. Eur Respir J 1992; 5:301–7.

34. Fitzpatrick MF, Mackay T, Whyte KF, et al. Nocturnal desaturation and serum erythropoietin: a study in patients with chronic obstructive pulmonary disease and in normal subjects. Clin Sci (Lond) 1993; 84:319–24.

35. Tirlapur VG, Mir MA. Nocturnal hypoxemia and associated electrocardiographic changes in patients with chronic obstructive airways disease. N Engl J Med 1982; 306:125–30.

36. Shepard JWJ, Garrison MW, Grither DA, Evans R, Schweitzer PK. Relationship of ventricular ectopy to nocturnal oxygen desaturation in patients with chronic obstructive pulmonary disease. Am J Med 1985; 78:28–34.

37. Harris P, Heath D. The Human Pulmonary Circulation. Edinburgh: Churchill Livingstone, 1986.

38. Penaloza D, Sime F, Branchero N, Gamboa P. Pulmonary hypertension in healthy man born and living at high altitudes. Med Thoracalis 1962; 19:449–60.

39. Kay JM. Effect of intermittent normoxia on chronic hypoxic pulmonary hypertension, right ventricular hypertrophy, and polycythemia in rats. Am Rev Respir Dis 1980; 121:993–1001.

40. Kay JM, Suyama KL, Keane PM. Effect of intermittent normoxia on muscularization of pulmonary arterioles induced by chronic hypoxia in rats. Am Rev Respir Dis 1981; 123:454–8.

41. Wilkinson M, Langhorne CA, Heath D, Barer GR, Howard P. A pathophysiological study of 10 cases of hypoxic cor pulmonale. Q J Med 1988; 66:65–85.

42. Levine BE, Bigelow DB, Hamstra RD, et al. The role of long-term continuous oxygen administration in patients with chronic airway obstruction with hypoxemia. Ann Intern Med 1967; 66:639–50.

43. Abraham AS, Cole RB, Bishop JM. Reversal of pulmonary hypertension by prolonged oxygen administration to patients with chronic bronchitis. Circ Res 1968; 23:147–57.

44. Timms RM, Khaja FU, Williams GW. Hemodynamic response to oxygen therapy in chronic obstructive pulmonary disease. Ann Intern Med 1985; 102:29–36.

45. Weitzenblum E, Sautegeau A, Ehrhart M, Mammosser M, Pelletier A. Long-term oxygen therapy can reverse the progression of pulmonary hypertension in patients with chronic obstructive pulmonary disease. Am Rev Respir Dis 1985; 131:493–8.

46. Zielinski J, Tobiasz M, Hawrylkiewicz I, Sliwinski P, Palasiewicz G. Effects of long-term oxygen therapy on pulmonary hemodynamics in COPD patients: a 6-year prospective study. Chest 1998; 113:65–70.

47. Selinger SR, Kennedy TP, Buescher P, et al. Effects of removing oxygen from patients with chronic obstructive pulmonary disease. Am Rev Respir Dis 1987; 136:85–91.

48. Calverley PM, Howatson R, Flenley DC, Lamb D. Clinicopathological correlations in cor pulmonale. Thorax 1992; 47:494–8.

49. Coccagna G, Lugaresi E. Arterial blood gases and pulmonary and systemic arterial pressure during sleep in chronic obstructive pulmonary disease. Sleep 1978; 1:117–24.

50. Boysen PG, Block AJ, Wynne JW, Hunt LA, Flick MR. Nocturnal pulmonary hypertension in patients with chronic obstructive pulmonary disease. Chest 1979; 76:536–42.

51. Weitzenblum E, Muzet A, Ehrhart M, Ehrhart J, Sautegeau A, Weber L. Variations nocturnes des gaz du sang et de la pression arterielle pulmonaire chez les bronchitiques chroniques insuffisants respiratoires. Nouv Presse Med 1982; 11:1119–22.

52. Fletcher EC, Levin DC. Cardiopulmonary hemodynamics during sleep in subjects with chronic obstructive pulmonary disease. The effect of short- and long-term oxygen. Chest 1984; 85:6–14.

53. Fletcher EC, Luckett RA, Miller T, Costarangos C, Kutka N, Fletcher JG. Pulmonary vascular hemodynamics in chronic lung disease patients with and without oxyhemoglobin desaturation during sleep. Chest 1989; 95:757–64.

54. Chaouat A, Weitzenblum E, Kessler R, et al. Sleep-related O_2 desaturation and daytime pulmonary haemodynamics in COPD patients with mild hypoxaemia. Eur Respir J 1997; 10:1730–5.

55. Fletcher EC, Luckett RA, Goodnight-White S, Miller CC, Qian W, Costarangos-Galarza C. A double-blind trial of nocturnal supplemental oxygen for sleep desaturation in patients with chronic obstructive pulmonary disease and a daytime PaO_2 above 60 mmHg. Am Rev Respir Dis 1992; 145:1070–6.

56. Chaouat A, Weitzenblum E, Kessler R, et al. A randomized trial of nocturnal oxygen therapy in chronic obstructive pulmonary disease patients. Eur Respir J 1999; 14:1002–8.

57. American Thoracic Society. Standards for the diagnosis and care of patients with chronic obstructive pulmonary disease. Am J Respir Crit Care Med 1995; 152:S77–120.

58. Siafakas NM, Vermeire P, Pride NB, et al. Optimal assessment and management of chronic obstructive pulmonary disease (COPD). Eur Respir J 1995; 8:1398–420.

59. BTS guidelines for the management of chronic obstructive pulmonary disease. The COPD Guidelines Group of the Standards of Care Committee of the BTS. Thorax 1997; 52:S1–28.

60. Pauwels RA, Buist AS, Calverley PMA, Jenkins CR, Hurd SS. Global strategy for the diagnosis, management, and prevention of chronic obstructive pulmonary disease. Am J Respir Crit Care Med 2001; 163:1256–76.

61. Fabbri L, Pauwels RA, Hurd SS. Global strategy for the diagnosis, management, and prevention of chronic obstructive pulmonary disease: GOLD executie summary updated 2003. COPD 2004; 1:105–41.

62. Levi-Valensi P, Weitzenblum E, Pedinielli JL, Racineux JL, Duwoos H. Three-month follow-up of arterial blood gas determinations in candidates for long-term oxygen therapy. A multicentric study. Am Rev Respir Dis 1986; 133:547–51.

63. Guyatt GH, Nonoyama M, Lacchetti C, et al. A randomized trial of strategies for assessing eligibility for long-term domiciliary oxygen therapy. Am J Respir Crit Care Med 2005; 172:573–80.

64. Conference Report. New problems in supply, reimbursement and certification of medical necessity for long-term oxygen therapy. Am Rev Respir Dis 1990; 142:721–4.

65. Weitzenblum E, Vandevenne A, Hirth C, Parini JP, Roeslin N, Oudet P. L'hemodynamique pulmonaire au cours de l'exercice musculaire chez les bronchiteux chroniques. Effets de l'oxygénation et de la repetition de l'exercice. Respiration 1973; 30:64–88.

66. Horsfield K, Segel N, Bishop JM. The pulmonary circulation in chronic bronchitis at rest and during exercise breathing air and 80 per cent oxygen. Clin Sci 1968; 34:473–83.

67. Woodcock AA, Gross ER, Geddes DM. Oxygen relieves breathlessness in "pink puffers". Lancet 1981; 1:907–9.

68. Catterall JR, Douglas NJ, Calverley PMA, et al. Transient hypoxemia during sleep in chronic obstructive pulmonary disease is not a sleep apnea syndrome. Am Rev Respir Dis 1983; 128:24–9.

69. Chaouat A, Weitzenblum E, Kessler R, et al. Outcome of COPD patients with mild daytime hypoxaemia with or without sleep-related oxygen desaturation. Eur Resipr J 2001; 17:848–55.

70. O'Donohue WJJ, Plummer AL. Magnitude of usage and cost of home oxygen therapy in the United States. Chest 1995; 107:301–2 (Editorial).

71. Veale D, Chailleux E, Taytard A, Cardinaud JP. Characteristics and survival of patients prescribed long-term oxygen therapy outside prescription guidelines. Eur Respir J 1998; 12:780–4.

72. Zielinski J. Long-term oxygen therapy in COPD patients with moderate hypoxaemia: does it add years to life? Eur Respir J 1998; 12:756–8.

73. Dunn WF, Nelson SB, Hubmayr RD. Oxygen-induced hypercarbia in obstructive pulmonary disease. Am Rev Respir Dis 1991; 144:526–30.

74. Goldstein RS, Ramcharan V, Bowes G, McNicholas WT, Bradley D, Phillipson EA. Effect of supplemental nocturnal oxygen on gas exchange in patients with severe obstructive lung disease. N Engl J Med 1984; 310:425–9.

75. West GA, Primeau P. Nonmedical hazards of long-term oxygen therapy. Respir Care 1983; 28:906–12.

76. Lacasse Y, Lecours R, Pelletier C, Bégin R, Maltais F. Randomised trial of ambulatory oxygen in oxygen-dependent COPD. Eur Respir J 2005; 25:1032–8.

77. Heimlich HJ. Respiratory rehabilitation with transtracheal oxygen system. Ann Otol Rhinol Laryngol 1982; 91:643–7.

78. Christopher KL, Spofford BT, Petrun MD, McCarty DC, Goodman JR, Petty TL. A program for transtracheal oxygen delivery. Assessment of safety and efficacy. Ann Intern Med 1987; 107:802–8.

79. Hoffman LA, Wesmiller SW, Sciurba FC, Johnson JT, Ferson F, Dauber JH. Nasal cannula and transtracheal oxygen delivery. A comparison of patient response after 6 months of each technique. Am Rev Respir Dis 1992; 145:827–31.
80. Soffer M, Tashkin DP, Shapiro BJ, Littner M, Harvey E, Farr S. Conservation of oxygen supply using a reservoir nasal cannula in hypoxemic patients at rest and during exercise. Chest 1985; 88:663–8.
81. Carter R, Williams JS, Berry J, Peavler M, Griner D, Tiep B. Evaluation of the pendant oxygen-conserving nasal cannula during exercise. Chest 1986; 89:806–10.
82. Bower JS, Brook CJ, Zimmer K, Davis D. Performance of a demand oxygen saver system during rest, exercise, and sleep in hypoxemic patients. Chest 1988; 94:77–80.
83. Tiep BL, Christopher KL, Spofford BT, Goodman JR, Worley PD, Macy SL. Pulsed nasal and transtracheal oxygen delivery. Chest 1990; 97:364–8.
84. Kacmarek RM. Oxygen delivery systems for long-term oxygen therapy. In: O'Donohue WJJ, ed. Long-Term Oxygen Therapy. New York: Marcel Dekker, 1995:219–34.
85. Dheda K, Lim K, Ollivere B, et al. Assessments for oxygen therapy in COPD: are we under correcting arterial oxygen tensions? Eur Respir J 2004; 24:954–7.
86. Evans TW, Waterhouse J, Howard P. Clinical experience with the oxygen concentrator. Br Med J 1983; 287:459–61.
87. Vergeret J, Tunon de Lara M, Douvier JJ, et al. Compliance of COPD patients with long term oxygen therapy. Eur J Respir Dis 1986; 69:421–5.
88. Walshaw MJ, Lim R, Evans CC, Hind CR. Factors influencing the compliance of patients using oxygen concentrators for long-term home oxygen therapy. Respir Med 1990; 84:331–3.
89. Howard P, Waterhouse JC, Billings CG. Compliance with long-term oxygen therapy by concentrator. Eur Respir J 1992; 5:128–9.
90. Pepin JL, Barjhoux CE, Deschaux C, Brambilla C. ANTADIR Working Group on Oxygen Therapy. Long-term oxygen therapy at home. Compliance with medical prescription and effective use of therapy. Chest 1996; 109:1144–50.
91. Frey JG, Kaelin RM, De Werra M, Jordan B, Tschopp JM. Oxygenotherapie continue a domicile. Etude de l'observance des extracteurs d'oxygene apres un programme d'enseignement. Rev Mal Respir 1992; 9:301–5.

21

Noninvasive Ventilation in COPD

M. W. ELLIOTT

Department of Respiratory Medicine, St. James's University Hospital, Leeds, U.K.

I. Introduction

Over the last few years noninvasive positive pressure ventilation has established itself as having a major role in the management of patients with severe chronic obstructive airway disease (COPD). Although its use was first evaluated in chronic stable patients with ventilatory failure due to COPD, where it has really made a major mark is in the acute situation.

II. Noninvasive Positive Pressure Ventilation in Exacerbations of COPD

An exacerbation of COPD of sufficient severity to necessitate hospital admission indicates a poor prognosis, carrying a 6% to 26% mortality (1–3). The outcome of invasive mechanical ventilation (IMV) in patients with COPD is disappointing, with reported survivals of between 20% and 50% (4). Patients who are intubated may subsequently prove difficult to wean from ventilation (5). Endotracheal intubation (ETI) is associated with a range of complications of which the most important is ventilator associated pneumonia (VAP). For every day intubated there is a 1% risk of developing VAP, which results in a high morbidity and mortality (6,7).

Noninvasive positive pressure ventilation (NPPV) now has a major role in the management of exacerbations of COPD (8,9). It has a number of potential advantages compared with IMV. Physiologically NPPV is little different from IMV, but because of difficulties in getting a perfect seal with the mask it is theoretically less efficient than invasive ventilation. However, this may also be to its advantage. Barotrauma, such as pneumothorax, is not uncommon with ventilation after intubation but it has not been reported in any of the major studies of NPPV, perhaps because the lack of a complete seal between the mask and the face acts as a safety valve, preventing high pressures being transmitted to the lungs. NPPV decreases inspiratory muscle effort and respiratory rate and increases tidal volumes (10). Arterial PO_2 increases and $PaCO_2$ decreases (11,12).

The obvious attraction of NPPV is the avoidance of intubation and its attendant complications. Its use opens up new opportunities in the management of patients with ventilatory failure, particularly with regard to location and the timing of intervention. With NPPV paralysis and sedation are not needed and ventilation outside the intensive care unit (ICU) is an option; given the considerable pressure on ICU beds in some countries, the high costs, and that for some patients admission to ICU is a distressing experience (13) this is an attractive option. With NPPV ventilatory support can be introduced at an earlier stage in the evolution of ventilatory failure than would be usual when a patient is intubated and it is possible with NPPV to give very short periods of ventilatory support, which in some cases may be sufficient to reverse the downward spiral into life threatening ventilatory failure. Patients can cooperate with physiotherapy and eat normally (14). Intermittent ventilatory support is possible, patients can start mobilizing at an early stage and can communicate with medical and nursing staff and with their family; this is likely to reduce feelings of powerlessness and anxiety associated with ventilatory support (15). A reduction in complications, particularly infections, is a consistent and important finding (16–18). However NPPV does have limitations. Concerns have been voiced that it may delay ETI and mechanical ventilation (MV), resulting in a worse outcome (19–21). NPPV may be time consuming for medical and nursing staff (22) though in part this may represent a learning effect. Some patients find the mask claustrophobic and unpleasant. Facial pressure sores occur in 2% of patients (Table 1) (16).

There have now been a number of prospective randomized controlled trials (RCTs) of the use of NPPV in acute exacerbations of COPD. They have been performed in a variety of different locations, in different health care systems, and in patients with exacerbations of varying severity. A reduction in the need for ETI is a consistent finding and in the larger studies this translated into an improvement in survival. It was the studies performed in the ICU, particularly the landmark study of Brochard et al. (16) that showed that NPPV was both feasible and could be effective. They showed that NPPV reduced the intubation (11/43 vs. 31/42, $p < 0.001$) and mortality rates (4/43 vs. 12/42, $p = 0.02$) compared to conventional medical therapy. NPPV also improved pH, PaO_2, respiratory rate and encephalopathy score at one hour and was associated with a shorter hospital stay (23 vs. 35 days, $p = 0.005$) and a lower complication rate (16% vs. 48%, $p = 0.001$). Most of the excess mortality and complications, particularly pneumonia, were attributed to ETI. In a smaller study ($n = 31$) in two North American ICUs, Kramer et al. (23) showed a marked reduction in intubation rate, particularly in the subgroup with COPD ($n = 23$) (67% vs. 9% $p < 0.05$). However, mortality, hospital stay, and charges were unaffected. Those enrolled had a severe exacerbation, as evidenced by a mean pH of 7.28. In another ICU study Celikel (24) showed a more rapid improvement in various physiological parameters and a trend

Table 1 Advantages and Disadvantages of NPPV

Advantages	Disadvantages
Intermittent ventilation possible	May be less efficient
"Early" ventilatory support an option	Uncomfortable/claustrophobic
Ventilation outside the ICU possible	May be time consuming
Patients can cooperate with physiotherapy	Facial pressure sores
Patients can eat and drink normally	Airway not protected
Communication easier	No direct access to bronchial tree for suctioning

Abbreviations: ICU, intensive care unit; NPPV, noninvasive positive pressure ventilation.

toward a reduction in the need for ventilatory support, but there was no difference in intubation rate or survival. Martin et al. (25) reported a prospective RCT comparing NPPV with usual medical care in 61 patients including 23 with COPD. In common with other studies there was a significant reduction in intubation rate (6.4 vs. 21.3 intubations per 100 ICU days, $p=0.002$) but no difference in mortality (2.4 vs. 4.3 deaths per 100 ICU days, $p=0.21$). Although the intubation rate was lower in the COPD subgroup (5.3 vs. 15.6 intubations per 100 ICU days, $p=0.12$) this did not reach statistical significance; this may simply reflect the small sample size.

A number of studies have suggested that NPPV is less likely to be successful in more severely affected patients (16,19,26); all these studies excluded patients who required immediate ETI and MV. The concern has been voiced therefore that, particularly in the more severely ill, NPPV may be harmful by delaying the institution of the "gold" standard therapy, namely ETI and MV (21). However Conti et al. (27) reported a prospective RCT of NPPV versus immediate ETI and MV in patients with an exacerbation of COPD. Not surprisingly their patients were sicker than those reported in previous studies, as evidenced by the mean pH of 7.2, compared with 7.27 in the study of Brochard et al. (16). There were two important messages from this study. Firstly, in these sicker patients they showed that NPPV was no worse than ETI and MV. Secondly, in those who could be managed successfully with NPPV there was an advantage both in the short term (reduced duration of ICU stay) but also in the year after hospital discharge [fewer readmissions and patients needing de novo long-term oxygen therapy (LTOT)]. The intubation rate of 52% in the NPPV group was higher than in other RCTs, which is not surprising given that these were a sicker group of patients. It is important however to recognize that if you work in a critical care unit dealing only with the very severely ill end of the spectrum the results from NPPV will not be as good as those published in the literature, usually obtained in the less severely ill. In common with other studies some patients were still excluded, in particular those intubated prior to transfer to the ICU or those with respiratory arrest or pauses, psychomotor agitation requiring sedation, heart rate below 60 or systolic blood pressure below 80 mmHg.

A recent study has extended the use of NPPV to another group previously deemed unsuitable for NPPV, namely those with coma (28). In a prospective, uncontrolled study of 958 patients receiving NPPV for acute respiratory failure (ARF) 95 (10.1%) had Glasgow coma score (GCS) on ICU admission < 8. In the subgroup of patients with COPD, the success rate in those with severe encephalopathy was 86%. Variables related to the success of NPPV were GCS score at one hour and higher levels of multi organ dysfunction (28). Despite these studies NPPV remains primarily a complimentary technique to invasive ventilation.

There have been four prospective RCTs of NPPV outside the ICU (21,29–31). In the largest ($n=236$), in which NPPV was delivered on general respiratory wards in 13 centers (31) NPPV was applied by the usual ward staff according to a simple protocol. "Treatment failure," a surrogate for the need for intubation, defined by a priori criteria was reduced from 27% to 15% by NPPV ($p<0.05$). In hospital mortality was also reduced from 20% to 10% ($p<0.05$). Subgroup analysis suggested that the outcome in patients with pH < 7.30 after initial treatment was inferior to that in the studies performed in the ICU; these patients are probably best managed in a higher dependency setting with individually tailored ventilation. Staff training and support are crucial wherever NPPV is performed and operator expertise more than any other factor is likely to determine the success or otherwise of NPPV. This study did however confirm that "early" NPPV is advantageous. In patients with a pH > 7.30, 80% of patients will get better with conventional therapy alone but only 10 patients need to receive NPPV to avoid one intubation. Once the pH drops below 7.30 approaching 50% of patients met intubation criteria, confirming the findings of earlier studies of the significance of pH in prognosis in exacerbations of COPD (3). These observations are of important practical significance in day-to-day management. A period of observation is not unreasonable in a patient with a pH > 7.30 who is poorly tolerant of NPPV as most will improve anyway. Once the pH drops below 7.30 however the patient should be encouraged strongly to continue with NPPV as the risks without it are substantial for intubation and death.

If NPPV is started on the ward is advantageous it is logical to consider initiation even earlier, on presentation to the emergency department. However, studies in which NPPV has been instituted in the Accident and Emergency Department (21,30) have failed to show any advantage to NPPV. The numbers of patients have been small and at the level of severity seen, the majority of patients would have been expected to get better anyway. In another study (32), which also included a sham arm, in patients with more severe respiratory failure, there was 100% success in the NPPV treated patients and 100% failure in those treated with sham ventilation. However, patients with cardiogenic pulmonary edema were included and the speed of response was much quicker than would usually be the case in patients with COPD. Most were showing improvements in the physiological variables within a few minutes and all were better within 90 minutes. This speed of improvement is usually only seen in patients receiving NPPV for cardiogenic pulmonary edema. There is therefore no convincing evidence that early NPPV delivered in the emergency room is advantageous.

In a one-year period prevalence study Plant et al. (33) found that 20% of patients admitted to hospital with an exacerbation of COPD were acidotic on arrival in the Accident and Emergency Department and that 20% of these corrected their pH into the normal range over the next few hours without any need for ventilatory support. This was not related to the severity of the acidosis and there was a relationship with the PaO_2 on the initial arterial blood gasses; the authors hypothesized that hypercapnia had been precipitated by oxygen therapy during transfer to hospital. The usual focus of therapy in the first hour or so of admission to hospital should be on instituting standard medical therapy, particularly properly controlled oxygen therapy. This will usually mean a 24% or 28% Venturi mask or the use of nasal cannulae targeting an oxygen saturation of 88% to 92% (34,35).

III. The Role of NPPV After IMV

Some patients require intubation from the outset and others after a failed trial of NPPV. Patients with COPD may be difficult to wean from IMV (36) and NPPV has been used successfully in weaning (17,37–39). A Cochrane review (40) involving 171 participants with predominantly COPD showed that, compared to IMV, NPPV decreased mortality, the incidence of VAP, ICU, and hospital length of stay, total duration of mechanical support and the duration of endotracheal MV. Subgroup analyses suggested fewer weaning failures and a greater survival benefit with NPPV, although differences were nonsignificant.

A proportion of patients weaned from invasive ventilation subsequently deteriorates and requires further ventilatory support. An early study using historical controls (41) reported 30 patients with COPD who developed hypercapnic respiratory distress within 72 hours of extubation. They showed a reduction in the need for re-intubation, in the total duration of ventilatory support. However, two multicenter prospective RCTs of NPPV to treat post-extubation respiratory failure in heterogeneous patient populations have failed to show any benefit from NPPV (42,43). In the first, ($n=81$) there was no difference in the rate of re-intubation or hospital mortality in the patients receiving NPPV compared to conventional therapy. However, importantly one year after the study was started, because of the emerging literature of the benefit of NPPV in acute exacerbations of COPD, no more patients with a primary diagnosis of COPD were recruited. In total, only three patients randomized to NPPV had COPD.

In the second study patients in 37 centers in eight countries who were electively extubated after at least 48 hours of MV and who had respiratory failure within the subsequent 48 hours were randomly assigned to either NPPV by face mask or standard medical therapy. A total of 221 patients with similar baseline characteristics had been randomly assigned to either NPPV or standard medical therapy when the trial was stopped early after an interim analysis. There was no difference in the primary end point, the need for reintubation. The rate of death in the ICU was higher in the NPPV group than in the standard-therapy group (25% vs. 14%; relative risk, 1.78; 95% confidence interval, 1.03 to 3.20; $p=0.048$), and the median time from respiratory failure to reintubation was longer in the NPPV group (12 hours vs. 2 hours 30 minutes, $p=0.02$). However, a number of patients 28/107 crossed over to NPPV and of these 21 did not require re-intubation. If these are included with the other NPPV patients there was actually an advantage to NPPV. Secondly, some centers recruited very few patients raising concerns that they were relatively inexperienced at NPPV or had insufficient patients passing through their Unit to maintain skills. Finally, only 14 patients randomized to NPPV and nine to standard therapy had COPD. These data cannot therefore be taken as evidence that NPPV is inappropriate to treat post-extubation respiratory failure in patients with COPD.

IV. Longer Term Effects of NPPV in Exacerbations of COPD

A number of studies have shown longer term benefit for patients treated with NPPV compared to those invasively ventilated (44–46). In the study of Conti et al. (27) for those patients who could be managed successfully with NPPV there was also an advantage in the year after hospital discharge with a lower readmission rate and fewer patients requiring de novo oxygen supplementation. If ICU care has been prolonged and weaning difficult, there may be reluctance on the part of either medical staff or the patients themselves to consider IMV for a subsequent exacerbation. Second, it is possible that IMV has adverse effects which may be significant later; electrophysiological and biopsy evidence of muscle dysfunction has been shown after as little as one week of invasive ventilation (47,48). Such dysfunction of the respiratory muscles will reduce the capacity of the respiratory muscle pump, which may increase the risk of ventilatory failure in subsequent exacerbation. These observations however are speculative.

V. When Should NPPV be Discontinued?

While there are clear criteria as to when NPPV or should be started, when it should be stopped has not been studied in any systematic way (Table 2). In practice patients often decide for themselves that they have had enough and opt to discontinue NPPV. The studies of Wood et al. (21), and Esteban et al. (43) however raised important caveats about the danger of continuing NPPV for too long. It is sensible when starting NPPV to have a clear plan in place as to what is going to be done if the patient fails with NPPV and to have criteria so that this can be recognized. The decision as to when to abandon NPPV will depend in part upon the severity of the physiological disturbance at the time of presentation. In the less severely affected there is more time to try to optimize the interface, adjust the ventilator settings etc. Change in pH and respiratory rate within the first hour or two have been shown to be good predictors of outcome in a number of studies (16,19,26,50). Patients with high APACHE II scores, inability to minimize the amount of mouth leak (because of lack of teeth, secretions, or breathing pattern) or inability to coordinate with NPPV are less likely to improve with NPPV (51). Comorbidities may also be important (19,52).

Confalonieri et al. (53) in a multicenter series of 1033 patients receiving NPPV developed a "traffic light" chart to predict the likely outcome from NPPV at the time it was initiated and also after two hours. Variables that impacted upon this were pH, respiratory rate, APACHE II score, and GCS; the more physiologically disturbed the less likely was success.

One problem with all these studies is that failure criteria are likely to be self-fulfilling. If it is decided that the patient will be intubated if arterial blood gas tensions do not improve after 30 minutes or if there is severe acidosis that the patient will only be given a very limited trial of NPPV these will then become failure criteria, even though with persistence, adjustment of settings change of interface etc. a different outcome might have been achieved. Coma or confusion, upper gastrointestinal bleeding, high risk of aspiration, hemodynamic instability or uncontrolled arrhythmia have been suggested as contraindications to NPPV (54). This is primarily for theoretical reasons and because these patients have been excluded from previous studies and not because there is any evidence that IMV is superior in these situations. As the study of Diaz et al. (28) has shown coma should no longer be considered a contraindication to NPPV.

Table 2 NPPV Is Less Likely to Be Successful Acutely if...

pH and respiratory rate do not improve within the first 30 minutes (49)
  to two hours of NPPV (16,19,50)
High APACHE II scores (19,51)
Inability to minimize leak (51)
Excessive secretions (51)
Inability to coordinate with NPPV (19,51)
Pneumonia (19)
Patient underweight (19)
Greater level of neurological compromise (19)
Low pH prior to starting NPPV (19)

Abbreviation: NPPV, noninvasive positive pressure ventilation.

VI.   Where Should NPPV be Performed?

The issue of where NPPV should be performed will depend upon a number of different factors including local expertise, the severity of respiratory failure and what will be done if NPPV fails (Table 3). As stated above, NPPV should not usually be initiated on presentation to hospital with the main focus being upon optimization of oxygen therapy and the delivery of bronchodilators and so on. There will however be a proportion of patients who present in extremis and the studies of Conti et al. (27) and Diaz et al. (28) suggest that there is nothing to be lost by a short trial of NPPV. One danger of this approach is that emergency room staff will only treat the sickest patients and will not have the opportunity to learn the skills, and develop the confidence that comes with treating the less severely ill. The main debate is as to whether NPPV should be delivered on an ICU or whether it is acceptable to provide it on a general ward. The RCT evidence supports the use of NPPV in both locations though generally sicker patients should be treated on the ICU. Data from Italy however has shown that with the passage of time outcomes for sicker patients improve, the location in which NPPV is delivered can switch from the ICU to a general ward and more severely ill patients can be cared for in the lower dependency setting (55). It is also likely to be the case that in a hospital with well-established NPPV service outcomes even in the sicker patients are likely to be better on the general ward, which is doing a lot of NPPV, compared to the ICU which only does it rarely. One major attraction of NPPV or outside the ICU is of major potential cost savings. Plant et al. showed that such a service was highly cost-effective delivering a better outcome at less cost, primarily through the avoidance of ICU utilization (56).

The best location for an NPPV service will depend critically upon local factors, particularly the skill levels of doctors, nurses, and therapists in looking after patients receiving NPPV. Patient throughput is an important factor which impacts upon the development, and retention, of the particular skills needed for NPPV. A proportion of patients will fail with NPPV, requiring intubation, and invasive ventilation; it is important that personnel and the facility for intubation be rapidly available if needed, if the trend to increased mortality with NPPV, as reported by Wood et al. is to be avoided (21). It could be argued that for patients with a high likelihood of failing NPPV should be initiated on the ICU and once stabilized the patient could be transferred to the ward normally providing NPPV. In any discussion about location of an NPPV service it is important to note that the model of hospital care differs from country to country and that

Table 3   Factors to be Considered in Deciding Location for NPPV for Patients with Exacerbations of COPD

Staff with relevant training and expertise

Adequate staff numbers available throughout 24-hour period (will also depend upon nursing needs of other patients—for instance one nurse responsible for two very ill patients may have less time than one nurse responsible for four less severely ill patients)

Likelihood of a successful outcome from NPPV

Rapid access to ETI and IMV

Severity of respiratory failure

Abbreviations: COPD, chronic obstructive airway disease; ETI, endotracheal intubation; IMV, invasive mechanical ventilation; NPPV, noninvasive positive pressure ventilation.

"ICU," "high dependency unit (HDU)" and "general ward" will have different levels of staffing, facilities for monitoring etc. Care must therefore be taken in the extrapolation of results obtained in one environment to other hospitals and countries.

In summary staff training and experience are more important than location, and adequate numbers of staff, skilled in NPPV, must be available throughout the 24-hour period. Because of the demands of looking after these acutely ill patients, and to aid training and skill retention, NPPV is usually best carried out in one single sex location with one nurse, experienced in noninvasive ventilation, responsible for no more than three to four patients in total. Whether this is called an ICU, a HDU, or is part of a General Ward is largely irrelevant.

VII. Long-Term Domiciliary NPPV for Stable COPD

The concept of mechanically assisted ventilation in stable COPD is not new. It has been delivered by day using intermittent positive pressure breathing through a mouthpiece (57), but without evidence of benefit. Various trials of inhospital assisted ventilation, using negative pressure devices, in patients with COPD during wakefulness have been reported but use at home and during sleep has been largely unsuccessful (58–60). Patients were generally unable to sleep during negative pressure ventilation and most either failed to complete the protocol, because of lack of improvement or discomfort associated with the use of the equipment (60). In the largest study Shapiro et al. (61) studied 184 patients randomized to active or sham negative pressure ventilation at home using a poncho wrap ventilator. They did not show any significant difference between the two groups, but compliance with treatment was much less than anticipated, with most patients unable to sleep during negative pressure ventilation. The mean $PaCO_2$ of the patients studied was only 44 mmHg and a review of the literature suggests that it is hypercapnic patients who are most likely to benefit from noninvasive ventilation. The conclusions from these studies are that negative pressure ventilation at home of patients with COPD is poorly tolerated, cannot usually be used during sleep and results in little benefit.

In 1983 Sullivan et al. (62) described the delivery of continuous positive pressure to the upper airway using a well-fitting nasal mask for patients with obstructive sleep apnoea. Although NPPV had been described before this (63) the technique really took off as it became clear that patients could tolerate, and benefit from, facial interfaces and because industry has developed increasingly sophisticated interfaces. NPPV is now very well-accepted therapy for patients with chronic respiratory failure, due to chest wall deformity neuromuscular disease. Although its use is not underpinned by RCT evidence for most diseases it would not be considered ethical to deny treatment to patients with symptoms of nocturnal hyperventilation due to these disorders. NPPV has also been used at home during sleep in patients with COPD with some success (64–66). Case series of NPPV for patients with COPD (67,68) suggest survival comparable to that seen in the oxygen treated patients in the Medical Research Council and Nocturnal Oxygen Therapy Trial studies (69–71). Although direct comparison cannot be made with historical controls from 30 years ago it is important to note that the patients with COPD selected for home ventilation were often those who had "failed" (not rigorously defined) on oxygen therapy and were usually hypercapnic. A number of studies suggest that hypercapnia is a poor prognostic sign in COPD (69,72).

There have been a number of short-term RCTs, involving small numbers of patients, and two longer term studies. Strumpf et al. (73) performed a randomized controlled cross over study in 19 patients with COPD. There were considerable problems with acceptance and in the seven who did complete the study, there were significant differences only in neuropsychologic testing. Lin (74) studied 12 patients in a prospective randomized cross over study of oxygen alone, NPPV alone and oxygen plus NPPV each for two weeks. There were no differences in any measured variable. Sleep efficiency was worse during NPPV than with oxygen alone. Gay et al. (75) randomized 13 clinically stable patients with severe COPD and daytime hypercapnia ($PaCO_2 > 45$ mmHg) to NPPV or sham treatment, consisting of nightly use of a bi-level positive airway pressure device set to deliver an inspiratory positive airway pressure (IPAP) either 10 or 0 cm of H_2O. The device was used in the spontaneous or timed mode and set to an expiratory positive airway pressure (EPAP) of 2 cm H_2O. Patients underwent extensive physiologic testing including polysomnography and were introduced to NPPV during a 2.5-day hospital stay. However, only four patients in the NPPV group were still using it at the completion of the three-month trial, as opposed to all six patients in the sham group. Only one patient had a significant reduction in diurnal $PaCO_2$. The level of IPAP in this study was modest and during overnight polysomnography $TcCO_2$ was not measured and there was no change in mean or nadir SaO_2. Importantly, two patients in the sham group reported that their breathing improved despite unchanged results of the objective measures, suggesting a significant placebo effect. In the only positive study Meecham Jones et al. (76) in a randomized cross over study of the use of NPPV and oxygen with oxygen alone showed improved daytime arterial blood gas tensions, better quality sleep, and improved quality of life during the pressure support limb of the study. The authors used higher inflation pressures than those seen in the other studies and the improvement in daytime $PaCO_2$ correlated with a reduction in overnight transcutaneous CO_2.

The reasons for these predominantly negative results include poor acclimatization to the technique, inadequate inflation pressures, failure to confirm any effect of noninvasive ventilation overnight and the fact that in some studies patients were not particularly hypercapnic. It is also important to note that these studies were performed fairly soon after NPPV had become widely available at which time the range of interfaces was much more limited than it is now and there have also been considerable advances in ventilator technology as the understanding of what is needed from a ventilator for effective noninvasive ventilation has evolved.

There have been two longer term controlled trials. In a one-year trial Casanova et al. (77) randomized 52 patients with severe stable COPD to either NPPV plus "standard care" or to standard care alone. The adequacy of ventilation was determined by close observation of the patient, during the day and night, but was not confirmed objectively. The level of support was modest, mean IPAP $12 + 2$ cm H_2O. One-year survival was similar in both groups (78%) as was the number of exacerbations. The number of hospital admissions was less at three months in the NPPV group (5% vs. 15%, $p < 0.05$), but this difference was not seen at six months (18% vs. 19%, respectively). There was either no or little difference between the groups in dyspnea scales, gas exchange, hematocrit, pulmonary function, cardiac function, and neuropsychological performance. However, the number of patients was too small to avoid a type II error and the period of follow-up too short to evaluate fully the effect upon outcome.

Clini et al. (78) reported a prospective RCT of NPPV during sleep in stable COPD patients with a significant number of patients, followed for a reasonable period of time. Ninety patients with stable chronic hypercapnia who had been on LTOT for at least six months were randomized to continuing LTOT or LTOT and the addition of NPPV. Compliance with LTOT was excellent as was that with NPPV, patients using it for an average of nine hours per night. Overall the results were disappointing. There were small improvements in resting $PaCO_2$, dyspnea scores and health related quality of life in the NPPV group. There was no improvement in survival or hospitalization rates. When the year before randomization was compared with the first year of the study there was a trend toward a lesser time in hospital in the NPPV group compared to an increase in the LTOT group. Comparing the same time periods ICU stay was reduced in both groups, but more in the NPPV than in the LTOT group. There are a number of criticisms of this study. In common with most other studies there was inadequate confirmation that effective ventilation had been delivered. NPPV was deemed to be adequate when the $PaCO_2$ was reduced by 5% during wakefulness; this reduction in CO_2 during NPPV when awake is modest. Monitoring during sleep was based upon achieving an adequate saturation but when oxygen is also being delivered nothing can be inferred from this about adequacy of ventilation. The changes in diurnal $PaCO_2$, which was the primary end point that informed the power calculation, were small and it remains to be seen whether more aggressive ventilation would have resulted in a bigger change in this and other end points. The average IPAP was 14 ± 3 and EPAP 2 ± 1 cm H_2O, suggesting that there was room to increase the pressures, at least, to levels closer to those seen in the study of Meecham Jones et al. (76). The fact that the effectiveness of ventilation during sleep was not confirmed is an important limitation of the study and it is possible that there was in fact no change in $PaCO_2$ overnight, given that the pressures used were comparable to those used in the study of Lin (74), in which no effect of NPPV was seen upon nocturnal hypoventilation. If this is correct the question arises as to why patients reported less dyspnea and an improved quality of life. Firstly this could have been a placebo effect, as was seen in the study of Gay et al. (75). A significant placebo effect has been seen with sham continuous positive airway pressure (79) and the placebo effect of a "breathing machine" should not be underestimated. Secondly exacerbations have been shown to have a detrimental effect upon quality of life (80) in patients with COPD. NPPV offloads the respiratory muscles (81) and reduces the sensation of dyspnea (29,31) associated with an acute exacerbation at ventilator settings similar to those used in this study. It is possible that NPPV therefore reduced the impact of exacerbations upon the patient; this may also have contributed to the trend toward reduced hospitalization. The mean daily use of 9 ± 2 hr/day suggests that at least some patients were using the ventilator during wakefulness, which lends some support to this hypothesis. Thirdly no data are given about input from health care givers; this may impact upon quality of life and dyspnea (82). It is possible that patients receiving NPPV, which requires considerable staff input at least initially, had greater contact with medical and paramedical staff than those on LTOT alone.

In most patients with chest wall deformity and neuromuscular disease NPPV is usually delivered overnight, firstly because hypoventilation is more marked during sleep, secondly correction of the sleep related abnormalities of breathing brings about daytime improvement and finally it is much more convenient for the patient as they are free to lead a more normal life by day. However, it does not have to be delivered during sleep to improve both daytime and sleep parameters. Diaz et al. (83) also showed significant increases in daytime PaO_2 (mean increase 8.6 mmHg) and $PaCO_2$ (mean decrease -8.4 mmHg) when patients with COPD were ventilated for three hours per day five days per week for three weeks. Although the effect upon sleep was not evaluated they found that the improvement in $PaCO_2$ correlated with changes in dynamic hyperinflation, intrinsic positive end-expiratory pressure ($PEEP_i$), inspiratory lung impedance, tidal volume, and functional residual capacity. There was no demonstrable effect upon tests of respiratory muscle function. They concluded that the primary effect of NPPV was upon respiratory system load. In a subsequent, similarly designed study, the same authors showed an improvement in exercise capacity, as measured by a six-minute walking test, and a reduction in dyspnea (84). Daytime ventilation may be an option in patients who cannot tolerate NPPV during sleep, but this strategy warrants more detailed evaluation.

Patients who have been admitted to hospital with an exacerbation and hypercapnia are at high risk of readmission and death (2) and this is even greater if they have received NPPV acutely (85). In a small group of highly selected patients admitted to hospital recurrently with exacerbations of COPD requiring NPPV Tuggey et al. (86) showed a reduction in the need for hospital and ICU admission in the year following the introduction of home NPPV compared to the year before. This was associated with a reduction in costs even when that of the ventilator, masks etc. was taken into account. However, this study was uncontrolled and the quality of life of the patients was not measured. A placebo effect of NPPV cannot be discounted.

There are three potential roles for long-term domiciliary NPPV in patients with stable severe COPD. Firstly patients who are genuinely intolerant of LTOT because of severe symptomatic hypercapnia may benefit from NPPV if hypercapnia is controlled. Secondly NPPV may improve survival and quality of life in patients already established on LTOT, but who are also hypercapnic; the published evidence to date does not support this role. However, the existing RCTs can be criticized. A multicenter German study which aims to randomize a total of 300 patients to NPPV or standard medical therapy with all cause mortality as the primary end point may help to answer this question (87). Thirdly, NPPV may have a role in patients who have required noninvasive ventilation acutely because of a severe exacerbation. Most studies suggest that it is the patients with more severe hypercapnia who are likely to benefit and there is no place for nocturnal NPPV, at present, in those without sustained daytime hypercapnia. Adequate control of nocturnal hypoventilation should be confirmed as this has been a feature of the studies in which benefit has been seen (64,76).

VIII. Practical Problems Specific to Patients with COPD

COPD patients may have $PEEP_i$ because of premature airway closure and air trapping (88), particularly during an acute exacerbation. The presence of $PEEP_i$ increases the work of breathing during spontaneous or triggered ventilation by adding an inspiratory threshold load. In addition it decreases the effective trigger sensitivity because $PEEP_i$ must first be overcome before pressure change, flow occur and can be sensed at the nose (89). This may result in asynchrony between the patient's inspiratory efforts and machine breaths, which is inefficient and uncomfortable for the patient, and can be improved by counterbalancing $PEEP_i$ with extrinsic PEEP. Some patients with COPD prefer to mouth breathe. As well as promoting leaks, this effectively bypasses the ventilator, which is therefore not triggered in response to patient efforts and marked asynchrony occurs. The primary aim when starting NPPV is the effective capture of ventilation, such that there is complete synchrony between patient and ventilator. In such circumstances full face mask ventilation may be successful. One area of controversy is what inflation pressures should be used. Some authors (90,91) have favored higher pressures aimed at reducing carbon dioxide tensions whereas others have favored lower pressures both for reasons of patient tolerance but also because of increased asynchrony with ineffective efforts during pressure support ventilation (81,92,93). It is significant that the advocates of higher pressures tend to use assist control modes of ventilation. It has been suggested that high levels of ventilation may just result in increased leak, possibly by inducing glottic closure (94), without increasing ventilation. The studies in which glottic closure was demonstrated were in normal subjects ventilated to very low levels of $PaCO_2$ which are extremely unlikely to be achieved in patients with COPD. Tuggey and Ellliott (95) in a study in which pressures were titrated upwards and effects on ventilation and leak measured, showed that although leak did tend to increase with higher pressures there were still worthwhile increases in ventilation overall, with marked intra patient variability. There did seem to be a threshold at 20 cm H_2O with pressures above this causing more leaks.

IX. Conclusion

There is now a robust evidence base for the use of NPPV in acute exacerbations of COPD. NPPV should be considered primarily as a means of preventing, rather than a direct alternative to, ETI and MV but the study of Conti et al. (27) suggests that there is little to be lost except in a few situations by a short trial of NPPV. When ETI is deemed necessary, or NPPV fails, a strategy of early extubation onto NPPV should be considered. The reduction in complications, particularly pneumonia, is a consistent and important finding. The location in which NPPV is performed depends critically upon local factors, particularly staff training and expertise. In many institutions all NPPV should be performed on the ICU/HDU, but in others the General Ward is a realistic alternative for some patients. The role of NPPV in chronic stable patients is much less clear-cut and indeed the published evidence does not support its use. Although it cannot currently be recommended as first line treatment for hypercapnic patients with COPD a trial of NPPV should be considered in those cases deteriorating despite, or intolerant of, long-term oxygen therapy. The option of short periods of ventilation during the day is interesting and warrants further study. Perhaps the group who has the most to gain is that of those patients who have been admitted with an exacerbation of COPD requiring NPPV. This is an important area of future research.

References

1. Martin TR, Lewis SW, Albert RK. The prognosis of patients with chronic obstructive pulmonary disease after hospitalization for acute respiratory failure. Chest 1982; 82(3):310–4.
2. Connors AF, Jr., Dawson NV, Thomas C, et al. Outcomes following acute exacerbation of severe chronic obstructive lung disease. The SUPPORT investigators (Study to Understand Prognoses and Preferences for Outcomes and Risks of Treatments). Am J Respir Crit Care Med 1996; 154:959–67.

3. Jeffrey AA, Warren PM, Flenley DC. Acute hypercapnic respiratory failure in patients with chronic obstructive lung disease: risk factors and use of guidelines for management. Thorax 1992; 47:34–40.
4. Hudson LD. Survival data in patients with acute and chronic lung disease requiring mechanical ventilation. Am Rev Respir Dis 1989; 140:S19–24.
5. Brochard L, Rauss A, Benito S, et al. Comparison of three methods of gradual withdrawal from ventilatory support during weaning from mechanical ventilation. Am J Respir Crit Care Med 1994; 150:896–903.
6. Torres A, Aznar R, Gatell JM, et al. Incidence, risk, and prognosis factors of nosocomial pneumonia in mechanically ventilated patients. Am Rev Respir Dis 1990; 142(3):523–8.
7. Fagon JY, Chastre J, Hance A, Montravers P, Novara A, Gibert C. Nosocomial pneumonia in ventilated patients: a cohort study evaluating attributable mortality and hospital stay. Am J Med 1993; 94:281–7.
8. Brochard L. Non-invasive ventilation for acute exacerbations of COPD: a new standard of care. Thorax 2000; 55:817–8.
9. Elliott MW. Non-invasive ventilation in acute exacerbations of chronic obstructive pulmonary disease: a new gold standard? Intensive Care Med 2002; 28(12):1691–4.
10. Girault C, Richard J, Chevron V, et al. Comparative physiological effects of noninvasive assist-control and pressure support ventilation in acute hypercapnic respiratory failure. Chest 1997; 111:1639–48.
11. Brochard L, Isabey D, Piquet J, et al. Reversal of acute exacerbations of chronic obstructive lung disease by inspiratory assistance with a face mask. N Engl J Med 1990; 323:1523–30.
12. Diaz O, Iglesia R, Ferrer M, et al. Effects of noninvasive ventilation on pulmonary gas exchange and hemodynamics during acute hypercapnic exacerbations of chronic obstructive pulmonary disease. Am J Respir Crit Care Med 1997; 156:1840–5.
13. Easton C, MacKenzie F. Sensory-perceptual alterations: delirium in the intensive care unit. Heart Lung 1988; 17:229–37.
14. Pingleton SK. Complications of acute respiratory failure. Am Rev Respir Dis 1988; 137:1463–93.
15. Seneff MG, Wagner DP, Wagner RP, Zimmerman JE, Knaus WA. Hospital and 1-year survival of patients admitted to intensive care units with acute exacerbation of chronic obstructive pulmonary disease. J Am Med Assoc 1995; 274:1852–7.
16. Brochard L, Mancebo J, Wysocki M, et al. Noninvasive ventilation for acute exacerbations of chronic obstructive pulmonary disease. N Engl J Med 1995; 333:817–22.
17. Nava S, Ambrosino N, Cini E, et al. Non invasive mechanical ventilation in the weaning of patients with respiratory failure due to chronic obstructive pulmonary disease: a randomized study. Ann Intern Med 1998; 128(9):721–8.
18. Girou E, Brun-Buisson C, Taille S, Lemaire F, Brochard L. Secular trends in nosocomial infections and mortality associated with noninvasive ventilation in patients with exacerbation of COPD and pulmonary edema. J Am Med Assoc 2003; 290(22):2985–91.
19. Ambrosino N, Foglio K, Rubini F, Clini E, Nava S, Vitacca M. Non-invasive mechanical ventilation in acute respiratory failure due to chronic obstructive airways disease: correlates for success. Thorax 1995; 50:755–7.
20. Ambrosino N. Noninvasive mechanical ventilation in acute respiratory failure. Eur Respir J 1996; 9:795–807.
21. Wood KA, Lewis L, Von Harz B, Kollef MH. The use of noninvasive positive pressure ventilation in the emergency department. Chest 1998; 113:1339–46.
22. Chevrolet JC, Jolliet P, Abajo B, Toussi A, Louis M. Nasal positive pressure ventilation in patients with acute respiratory failure. Chest 1991; 100:775–82.
23. Kramer N, Meyer TJ, Meharg J, Cece RD, Hill NS. Randomized, prospective trial of noninvasive positive pressure ventilation in acute respiratory failure. Am J Respir Crit Care Med 1995; 151:1799–806.
24. Celikel T, Sungur M, Ceyhan B, Karakurt S. Comparison of noninvasive positive pressure ventilation with standard medical therapy in hypercapnic acute respiratory failure. Chest 1998; 114:1636–42.
25. Martin TJ, Hovis JD, Costantino JP, et al. A randomized, prospective evaluation of noninvasive ventilation for acute respiratory failure. Am J Respir Crit Care Med 2000; 161:807–13.
26. Plant PK, Owen JL, Elliott MW. Non-invasive ventilation in acute exacerbations of chronic obstructive pulmonary disease: long term survival and predictors of in-hospital outcome. Thorax 2001; 56:708–12.
27. Conti G, Antonelli M, Navalesi P, et al. Noninvasive vs. conventional mechanical ventilation in patients with chronic obstructive pulmonary disease after failure of medical treatment in the ward: a randomized trial. Intensive Care Med 2002; 28(12):1701–7.

28. Diaz GG, Alcaraz AC, Talavera JCP, et al. Noninvasive positive-pressure ventilation to treat hypercapnic coma secondary to respiratory failure. Chest 2005; 127(3):952–60.

29. Bott J, Carroll MP, Conway JH, et al. Randomised controlled trial of nasal ventilation in acute ventilatory failure due to chronic obstructive airways disease. Lancet 1993; 341:1555–7.

30. Barbe F, Togores B, Rubi M, Pons S, Maimo A, Agusti AGN. Noninvasive ventilatory support does not facilitate recovery from acute respiratory failure in chronic obstructive pulmonary disease. Eur Respir J 1996; 9:1240–5.

31. Plant PK, Owen JL, Elliott MW. Early use of non-invasive ventilation for acute exacerbations of chronic obstructive pulmonary disease on general respiratory wards: a multicentre randomised controlled trial. Lancet 2000; 355:1931–5.

32. Thys F, Roeseler J, Reynaert M, Liistro G, Rodenstein D. Noninvasive ventilation for acute respiratory failure: a prospective randomised placebo-controlled trial. Eur Respir J 2002; 20:545–55.

33. Plant PK, Owen J, Elliott MW. One year period prevalance study of respiratory acidosis in acute exacerbation of COPD; implications for the provision of non-invasive ventilation and oxygen administration. Thorax 2000; 55:550–4.

34. Moloney ED, Kiely JL, McNicholas WT. Controlled oxygen therapy and carbon dioxide retention during exacerbations of chronic obstructive pulmonary disease. Lancet 2001; 357(9255):526–8.

35. Jubran A, Tobin MJ. Reliability of pulse oximetry in titrating supplemental oxygen therapy in ventilator-dependent patients. Chest 1990; 97:1420–5.

36. Grassino A, Comtois N, Galdiz HJ, Sinderby C. The unweanable patient. Monaldi Arch Chest Dis 1994; 49(6):522–6.

37. Udwadia ZF, Santis GK, Steven MH, Simonds AK. Nasal ventilation to facilitate weaning in patients with chronic respiratory insufficiency. Thorax 1992; 47:715–8.

38. Restrick LJ, Scott AD, Ward EM, Feneck RO, Cornwell WE, Wedzicha JA. Nasal intermittent positive-pressure ventilation in weaning intubated patients with chronic respiratory disease from assisted positive-pressure ventilation. Respir Med 1993; 87:199–204.

39. Ferrer M, Esquinas A, Arancibia F, et al. Non-invasive ventilation during persistent weaning failure. A randomized controlled trial. Am J Respir Crit Care Med 2003; 168:70–6.

40. Burns KE, Adhikari NK, Meade MO. Noninvasive positive pressure ventilation as a weaning strategy for intubated adults with respiratory failure. Cochrane Database Syst Rev 2003; (4):CD004127.

41. Hilbert G, Gruson D, Porel L, Gbikpi-Benissan G, Cardinaud JP. Noninvasive pressure support ventilation in COPD patients with post extubation hypercapnic respiratory insufficiency. Eur Respir J 1998; 11:1349–53.

42. Keenan SP, Powers C, McCormack DG, Block G. Noninvasive positive-pressure ventilation for postextubation respiratory distress: a randomized controlled trial. J Am Med Assoc 2002; 287(24):3238–44.

43. Esteban A, Frutos-Vivar F, Ferguson ND, et al. Noninvasive positive-pressure ventilation for respiratory failure after extubation. N Engl J Med 2004; 350(24):2452–60.

44. Confalonieri M, Parigi P, Scartabellati A, et al. Noninvasive mechanical ventilation improves the immediate and long-term outcome of COPD patients with acute respiratory failure. Eur Respir J 1996; 9:422–30.

45. Vitacca M, Clini E, Rubini F, Nava S, Foglio K, Ambrosino N. Non-invasive mechanical ventilation in severe chronic obstructive lung disease and acute respiratory failure: short- and long-term prognosis. Intensive Care Med 1996; 22:94–100.

46. Bardi G, Pierotello R, Desideri M, Valdisseri L, Bottai M, Palla A. Nasal ventilation in COPD exacerbations: early and late results of a prospective, controlled study. Eur Respir J 2000; 15:98–104.

47. Coakley JH, Nagendran K, Honavar M, Hinds CJ. Preliminary observations on the neuromuscular abnormalities in patients with organ failure and sepsis. Intensive Care Med 1993; 19:323–8.

48. Coakley JH, Nagendran K, Ormerod IE, Ferguson CN, Hinds CJ. Prolonged neurogenic weakness in patients requiring mechanical ventilation for acute airflow limitation. Chest 1992; 101:1413–6.

49. Poponick JM, Renston JP, Bennett RP, Emerman CL. Use of a ventilatory support system (BiPAP) for acute respiratory failure in the emergency department. Chest 1999; 116:166–71.

50. Meduri GU, Turner RE, Abou-Shala N, Wunderink R, Tolley E. Noninvasive positive pressure ventilation via face mask. First-line intervention in patients with acute hypercapnic and hypoxemic respiratory failure. Chest 1996; 109:179–93.

51. Soo Hoo GW, Santiago S, Williams AJ. Nasal mechanical ventilation for hypercapnic respiratory failure in chronic obstructive pulmonary disease: determinants of success and failure. Crit Care Med 1994; 22:1253–61.

52. Scala R, Bartolucci S, Naldi M, Rossi M, Elliott MW. Comorbidity and acute decompensations of COPD requiring non-invasive positive-pressure ventilation. Intensive Care Med 2004; 30(9):1747–54.
53. Confalonieri M, Garuti G, Cattaruzza MS, et al. A chart of failure risk for noninvasive ventilation in patients with COPD exacerbation. Eur Respir J 2005; 25(2):348–55.
54. Ambrosino N. Noninvasive mechanical ventilation in acute on chronic respiratory failure: determinants of success and failure. Monaldi Arch Chest Dis 1997; 52:73–5.
55. Carlucci A, Delmastro M, Rubini F, Fracchia C, Nava S. Changes in the practice of non-invasive ventilation in treating COPD patients over 8 years. Intensive Care Med 2003; 29(3):419–25.
56. Plant PK, Owen JL, Parrott S, Elliott MW. Cost effectiveness of ward based non-invasive ventilation for acute exacerbations of chronic obstructive pulmonary disease: economic analysis of randomised controlled trial. Br Med J 2003; 326:956–61.
57. The Intermittent Positive Pressure Breathing Trial Group. Intermittent positive pressure breathing therapy of chronic obstructive pulmonary disease. Ann Intern Med 1983; 99:612–20.
58. Ambrosino N, Montagna T, Nava S, et al. Short term effect of intermittent negative pressure ventilation in COPD patients with respiratory failure. Eur Respir J 1990; 3:502–8.
59. Celli B, Lee H, Criner G, et al. Controlled trial of external negative pressure ventilation in patients with severe chronic airflow limitation. Am Rev Respir Dis 1989; 140:1251–6.
60. Zibrak JD, Hill NS, Federman EC, Kwa SL, O'Donnell C. Evaluation of intermittent long term negative-pressure ventilation in patients with severe COPD. Am Rev Respir Dis 1988; 138:1515–8.
61. Shapiro SH, Ernst P, Gray-Donald K, et al. Effect of negative pressure ventilation in severe chronic obstructive pulmonary disease. Lancet 1992; 340:1425–9.
62. Sullivan CE, Berthon-Jones M, Issa FG. Reversal of obstructive sleep apnoea by continuous positive airway pressure applied through the nares. Lancet 1983; 1:862–5.
63. Sadoul P, Aug M, Gay R. Traitement par ventilation instrumentale de 100 cas d'insuffisants respiratoires chroniques. Bull Eur Physiopathol Respir 1965; 1:519–49.
64. Elliott MW, Simonds AK, Carroll MP, Wedzicha JA, Branthwaite MA. Domiciliary nocturnal nasal intermittent positive pressure ventilation in hypercapnic respiratory failure due to chronic obstructive lung disease: effects on sleep and quality of life. Thorax 1992; 47:342–8.
65. Sivasothy P, Smith IE, Shneerson JM. Mask intermittent positive pressure ventilation in chronic hypercapnic respiratory failure due to chronic obstructive pulmonary disease. Eur Respir J 1998; 11:34–40.
66. Jones SE, Packham S, Hebden M, Smith AP. Domiciliary nocturnal intermittent positive pressure ventilation in patients with respiratory failure due to severe COPD; long term follow up and effect on survival. Thorax 1998; 53(6):495–8.
67. Simonds AK, Elliott MW. Outcome of domiciliary nasal intermittent positive pressure ventilation in restrictive and obstructive disorders. Thorax 1995; 50:604–9.
68. Leger P, Bedicam JM, Cornette A, et al. Nasal intermittent positive pressure ventilation. Long-term follow-up in patients with severe chronic respiratory insufficiency. Chest 1994; 105:100–5.
69. Medical Research Council Working Party Report. Long term domiciliary oxygen therapy in chronic hypoxic cor pulmonale complicating chronic bronchitis and emphysema. Lancet 1981; 1:681–5.
70. Nocturnal Oxygen Therapy Trial Group. Continuous or nocturnal oxygen therapy in hypoxemic chronic obstructive lung disease, a clinical trial. Ann Intern Med 1980; 93:391–8.
71. Hamnegard CH, Wragg SD, Mills GH, et al. Clinical assessment of diaphragm strength by cervical magnetic stimulation of the phrenic nerves. Thorax 1996; 51:1239–42.
72. Cooper CB, Waterhouse J, Howard P. Twelve year clinical study of patients with hypoxic cor pulmonale given long term domiciliary oxygen therapy. Thorax 1987; 42:105–10.
73. Strumpf DA, Millman RP, Carlisle CC, et al. Nocturnal positive-pressure ventilation via nasal mask in patients with severe chronic obstructive pulmonary disease. Am Rev Respir Dis 1991; 144:1234–9.
74. Lin CC. Comparison between nocturnal nasal positive pressure ventilation combined with oxygen therapy and oxygen monotherapy in patients with severe COPD. Am J Respir Crit Care Med 1996; 154:353–8.
75. Gay PC, Hubmayr RD, Stroetz RW. Efficacy of nocturnal nasal ventilation in stable, severe chronic obstructive pulmonary disease during a 3-month controlled trial. Mayo Clin Proc 1996; 71(6):533–42.
76. Meecham Jones DJ, Paul EA, Jones PW, Wedzicha JA. Nasal pressure support ventilation plus oxygen compared with oxygen therapy alone in hypercapnic COPD. Am J Respir Crit Care Med 1995; 152:538–44.
77. Casanova C, Celli BR, Tost L, et al. Long-term controlled trial of nocturnal nasal positive pressure ventilation in patients with severe COPD. Chest 2000; 118(6):1582–90.

78. Clini E, Sturani C, Rossi A, et al. The Italian multicentre study on noninvasive ventilation in chronic obstructive pulmonary disease patients. Eur Respir J 2002; 20(3):529–38.
79. Jenkinson C, Davies RJ, Mullins R, Stradling JR. Comparison of therapeutic and subtherapeutic nasal continuous positive airway pressure for obstructive sleep apnoea: a randomised prospective parallel trial. Lancet 1999; 353(9170):2100–5.
80. Seemungal TA, Donaldson GC, Paul EA, Bestall JC, Jeffries DJ, Wedzicha JA. Effect of exacerbation on quality of life in patients with chronic obstructive pulmonary disease. Am J Respir Crit Care Med 1998; 157(5 Pt 1):1418–22.
81. Appendini L, Patessio A, Zanaboni S, et al. Physiologic effects of positive end-expiratory pressure and mask pressure support during exacerbations of chronic obstructive pulmonary disease. Am J Respir Crit Care Med 1994; 149:1069–76.
82. Cockcroft A, Bagnall P, Heslop A, et al. Controlled trial of respiratory health worker visiting patients with chronic respiratory disability. Br Med J (Clin Res Ed) 1987; 294(6566):225–8.
83. Diaz O, Begin P, Torrealba B, Jover E, Lisboa C. Effects of noninvasive ventilation on lung hyperinflation in stable hypercapnic COPD. Eur Respir J 2002; 20(6):1490–8.
84. Diaz O, Begin P, Andresen M, et al. Physiological and clinical effects of diurnal noninvasive ventilation in hypercapnic COPD. Eur Respir J 2005; 26(6):1016–23.
85. Chu CM, Chan VL, Lin AWN, Wong IWY, Leung WS, Lai CKW. Readmission rates and life threatening events in COPD survivors treated with non-invasive ventilation for acute hypercapnic respiratory failure. Thorax 2004; 59(12):1020–5.
86. Tuggey JM, Plant PK, Elliott MW. Domiciliary non-invasive ventilation for recurrent acidotic exacerbations of COPD: an economic analysis. Thorax 2003; 58(10):867–71.
87. Kohnlein T, Criee C-P, Kohler D, Laier-Groeneveld G. Multicenter study on "non-invasive ventilation in patients with severe chronic obstructive pulmonary disease and emphysema (COPD)". Pneumologie 2004; 58:566–9.
88. Pepe PE, Marini JJ. Occult positive end expiratory pressure in mechanically ventilated patients with airflow limitation. Am Rev Respir Dis 1982; 126:166–70.
89. Smith TC, Marini JJ. Impact of PEEP on lung mechanics and work of breathing in severe airflow obstruction. J Appl Physiol 1988; 65:1488–99.
90. Windisch W, Vogel M, Sorichter S, et al. Normocapnia during nIPPV in chronic hypercapnic COPD reduces subsequent spontaneous $PaCO_2$. Respir Med 2002; 96(8):572–9.
91. Elliott MW. Noninvasive ventilation in chronic ventilatory failure due to chronic obstructive pulmonary disease. Eur Respir J 2002; 20(3):511–4.
92. Fanfulla F, Delmastro M, Berardinelli A, Lupo ND, Nava S. Effects of different ventilator settings on sleep and inspiratory effort in patients with neuromuscular disease. Am J Respir Crit Care Med 2005; 172(5):619–24.
93. Rossi A, Ganassini A, Polese G, Grassi V. Pulmonary hyperinflation and ventilator-dependent patients. Eur Respir J 1997; 10:1663–74 (Review-90 Refs.).
94. Jounieaux V, Aubert G, Dury M, Delguste P, Rodenstein DO. Effects of nasal positive-pressure hyperventilation on the glottis in normal sleeping subjects. J Appl Physiol 1995; 79:186–93.
95. Tuggey JM, Elliott MW. Titration of non-invasive positive pressure ventilation in chronic respiratory failure. Respir Med 2006; 100(7):1262–9.

22

Surgical Therapy for COPD

FERNANDO J. MARTINEZ
Division of Pulmonary and Critical Care Medicine, Department of Internal Medicine,
University of Michigan Health System, Ann Arbor, Michigan, U.S.A.

ANDREW C. CHANG
Section of Thoracic Surgery, Department of Surgery, University of Michigan Health System,
Ann Arbor, Michigan, U.S.A.

KEVIN M. CHAN
Division of Pulmonary and Critical Care Medicine, Department of Internal Medicine,
University of Michigan Health System, Ann Arbor, Michigan, U.S.A.

I. Introduction

Chronic obstructive pulmonary disease (COPD) is a category of diseases with a varying pathophysiological basis but with chronic airflow obstruction and hyperinflation (1). Over the past 50 years, many advances have been made in the management of COPD. The Global Initiative on Obstructive Lung Disease (GOLD) committee (2) and the American Thoracic Society/European Respiratory Society (3) have published detailed, evidence-based reviews of management, providing stepped-care algorithms for pharmacologic and nonpharmacologic therapy. Despite these advances, many patients continue to experience incapacitating breathlessness and exercise limitation. Over the past several decades, this has led to numerous surgical approaches to ameliorate symptoms in these patients.

II. History of Surgical Therapy for Emphysema

Detailed discussions of the surgical history of emphysema management have been provided by numerous authors (4–7). These surgical approaches reflected the state of knowledge for their era. Early investigators attempted to improve thoracic mobility, with procedures including costochondrectomy and transverse sternotomy (4,6); results were unpredictable. Subsequently, surgeons advocated techniques to decrease the size of the thoracic cage, including thoracoplasty and phrenicectomy, or to improve diaphragmatic architecture and function (4,6). Although transient relief could be obtained, practical considerations limited widespread use of these techniques (4,6). Denervation was used to treat the airway component of chronic airflow obstruction, while others supported the membranous trachea using various prosthetic devices (6). Significant morbidity and unpredictable results dampened widespread enthusiasm.

To reduce hyperinflation, Brantigan and colleagues hypothesized that by surgically reducing lung volume one could restore radial traction on the terminal bronchioles, thereby improving airflow obstruction and improving diaphragmatic position and function (8,9). Although symptomatic improvement was reported in most patients, significant operative mortality (6 of 33–18%) (8) limited widespread application. Over the subsequent 40 years, various groups applied similar principles in small case series using various surgical techniques (10–15).

The current era of surgical lung volume reduction was ushered by Cooper and colleagues who reported dramatic improvement following bilateral lung volume reduction surgery (LVRS) performed via median sternotomy (MS) (16). Subsequently multiple investigators reported more limited improvement as reviewed by others (17–19). The results of the National Emphysema Treatment Trial (NETT) (20,21) and other randomized trials (22–24) have provided much more definitive recommendations regarding the role of LVRS in patients with advanced emphysema.

Lung transplantation dates to the early 1960s with 36 transplants performed between 1963 and 1974; 14 were performed for patients with emphysema (25). Uniformly poor results were noted with only three patients living more than 1 month and the longest living 10 months. The major causes of death among the COPD patients were respiratory failure due to rejection, infection, or bronchial disruption (26–28). The first successful lung transplantation occurred as part of a transplanted heart–lung block for treatment of pulmonary vascular disease in 1981 (29). The first successful single lung transplants (SLT) were two cases reported in 1986 in patients with idiopathic pulmonary fibrosis (30). Because of differences in lung compliance, SLT was felt inappropriate for COPD patients with early reports supporting these concerns (31,32). Patterson et al. reported successful double lung transplantation (DLT) in COPD patients (33–35), while Mal et al. reported successful SLT in COPD patients (36). SLT has become the predominant surgical therapy for advanced COPD (7,25) which remains the main indication for lung transplantation (38%) (37).

III. Surgical Techniques

Exhaustive descriptions of the surgical techniques are outside the scope of this article. The important concepts will be briefly reviewed in this manuscript.

A. Bullectomy

Multiple techniques have been utilized to achieve resection of localized bullae, including standard lateral thoracotomy (4), bilateral resection via MS (38), and video-assisted thoracoscopy (VATS) with stapling (39) or VATS with endoloop ligation (40).

B. LVRS Without Giant Bullae

The approach to LVRS has included MS (41), standard thoracotomy, and VATS (42). Laser ablation has fallen out of favor as postoperative improvements were similar to stapled, unilateral LVRS but with a higher complication rate (43). Comparative studies have suggested greater improvement with bilateral procedures (44,45), although not all authors agree (46). Results from the recently completed NETT prospectively compared bilateral VATS with MS (21). Similar morbidity and mortality were noted with both surgical techniques although the overall length of stay was longer for MS (10 days vs.

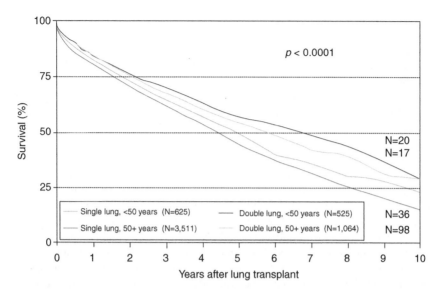

Figure 1 Kaplan–Meier survival after lung transplantation for recipients with chronic obstructive pulmonary disease (COPD) for transplantations performed between January 1990 and June 2004, stratified by age range and procedure type. *Source*: From Ref. 37.

9 days, $p = 0.01$). By 30 days after surgery, 70.5% of MS patients and 80.9% of VATS patients were living independently.

C. Lung Transplantation

Much controversy continues to revolve around the optimal transplant procedure in patients with COPD (47). The current surgical approaches and principles of postoperative management are outside the scope of this chapter (25,48–50). Interestingly, recent data suggest improved long-term outcomes in COPD patients treated with DLT versus SLT (37,51–57). Data from the Registry of the International Society of Heart and Lung Transplantation reveal significantly better survival after DLT for COPD even when stratified by age (Fig. 1). In fact, in 2004, bilateral lung transplantations accounted for 56% of all lung transplant procedures (58). Despite these findings, this information is limited by the lack of prospective data collection, adjustment for influencing variables, and randomization to ensure comparable treatment groups. As such, clear recommendations require further study.

IV. What Are the Results of Surgery?

A. Bullectomy

Bullectomy appears to be of short-term benefit in highly selected patients (59–65). Snider provided an elegant review of case series published from 1950 to the early 1990s (66). None of the 22 studies included a control group and the most were retrospective in nature, such that firm conclusions were difficult to reach. Improvements in hypoxemia and hypercapnia were most frequently reported; improvement in airflow was more heterogeneous. When measured total lung capacity (TLC), residual volume (RV), and trapped gas (measured as the difference between plethysmographic and dilutional lung volumes) generally decreased. In highly selected patients, cor pulmonale reversed if hypoxemia and hypercapnia were present. Most authors described improvement in dyspnea. A recent series confirms significant improvement in spirometry, RV, and six-minute walk distance (67).

Little long-term follow-up data have been reported. Fitzgerald et al. reported results in 84 patients who underwent 95 surgical procedures performed over a greater than 20-year period. The mean follow-up was 7.3 years (60). Long-term follow-up was available in 47 patients. Inconsistent maintenance of improvement was generally noted, although some patients demonstrated improvement for three to five years. Pearson and Ogilvie noted short-term improvement in 11 patients during a mean follow-up of 7.3 years (68); a gradual decrement in physiological improvement was noted in most patients. Although not quantified, the authors stated that dyspnea returned, with four of nine patients back to their preoperative level at last follow-up. During a mean follow-up of 4.5 years in 43 patients who underwent bullectomy, Schipper and colleagues noted initial improvement in spirometry, RV, and six-minute walk distance, although a gradual worsening was noted over the years (67). In general, one-third to one-half of patients maintained benefits for about five years. Palla and colleagues noted a decrease in dyspnea which lasted about four years; by the fifth year dyspnea progressed but remained below that recorded before surgery (69). Importantly, physiological improvement was maintained throughout five years of follow-up in the 36 of 41 patients who completed long-term follow-up. Most recently, Neviere and colleagues reported detailed physiological follow-up in 12 patients treated with bullectomy (70). Over four years of follow-up, hyperinflation improved as did exercise capacity and dyspnea.

B. LVRS Without Giant Bullae

Since the early report of Cooper and colleagues in 1995 (16) numerous reports of outcomes following LVRS have appeared in the literature. Summaries of these studies have been reviewed (18,19). Although several of these studies likely reported duplicate patient data, several methodological problems were noted consistently in these studies, including (*i*) variable surgical techniques and selection criteria (*ii*), short and often incomplete follow-up (*iii*), retrospective data collection, and (*iv*) the absence of a control group in all but a few published reports. The results of several randomized, controlled trials have clarified results of LVRS (22–24,71–74). In particular, the NETT was a large prospective, randomized, multicenter study comparing optimum medical therapy with optimum therapy plus LVRS (20). Of 3777 patients considered for entry, 1218 progressed through screening evaluation, formal pulmonary rehabilitation, repeat physiological and radiological testing, and randomization to treatment. Of the 608 patients randomized to surgical therapy, 580 (95.4%) underwent LVRS either by using a MS approach (406 patients) or by means of VATS (174 patients). The remaining 28 patients declined surgery after randomization or were felt to be unfit for operation. Long-term follow-up of patients enrolled in the NETT was reported recently (75). Most notably, LVRS was associated with an improvement in long-term mortality compared with medically treated patients (Fig. 2).

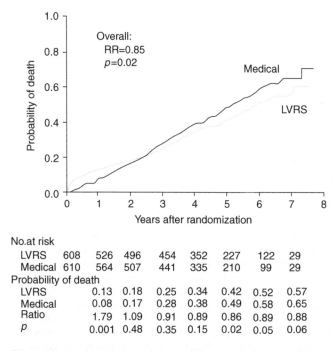

No.at risk

LVRS	608	526	496	454	352	227	122	29
Medical	610	564	507	441	335	210	99	29

Probability of death

LVRS	0.13	0.18	0.25	0.34	0.42	0.52	0.57
Medical	0.08	0.17	0.28	0.38	0.49	0.58	0.65
Ratio	1.79	1.09	0.91	0.89	0.86	0.89	0.88
p	0.001	0.48	0.35	0.15	0.02	0.05	0.06

Figure 2 Kaplan–Meier estimates of the cumulative probability of death as a function of years after randomization to LVRS (*gray line*) or medical treatment (*black line*) in the National Emphysema Treatment Trial. The *p* value is for the Fisher's exact test for the difference in the proportions of patients who died during the 4.3 years (median) follow-up in all patients randomized. *Abbreviation*: LVRS, lung volume reduction surgery. *Source*: From Ref. 75.

Pulmonary Function

Although the initial report of Cooper and colleagues documented an 82% improvement in forced expiratory volume in one second (FEV_1) approximately six months after bilateral LVRS via MS (16), subsequent studies by this group and those of subsequent case series by others confirmed significant mean improvements in spirometry although to a lesser extent than initially suggested (18). Reported changes in pulmonary function clearly indicated a short-term improvement in spirometry favoring surgery over medical therapy. This was exemplified by the results of two randomized trials (Fig. 3A,B).

In general, bilateral LVRS resulted in greater short-term improvement, although there were few direct comparisons between unilateral and bilateral procedures (44–46,76–80). One multicenter prospective study compared unilateral VATS LVRS with bilateral VATS LVRS noted that pulmonary function improvement favored the bilateral approach (80). The results of laser procedures appeared to be worse than stapling techniques. McKenna and colleagues reported greater short-term improvement in FEV_1 (32.9%) for those patients treated with staple resection than those undergoing laser reduction (13.4%) (43). In addition, Keenan et al. (81) noted a much higher

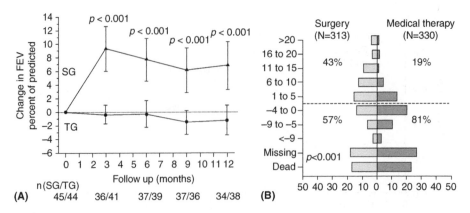

Figure 3 (**A**) Absolute change in FEV$_1$ % predicted in patients treated with SG compared to those treated with continued TG. (**B**) Histograms of changes from baseline in FEV$_1$ after 24 months of follow-up. Baseline measurements were performed after pulmonary rehabilitation. Patients previously identified as high risk were excluded. Patients who were too ill to complete the procedure or who declined to complete the procedure but did not explain why were included in the "missing" category. p values were determined by the Wilcoxon rank-sum test. The degree to which the bars are shifted to the upper left of the chart indicates the degree of relative benefit of lung volume reduction surgery over medical treatment. The percentage shown in each quadrant is the percentage of patients in the specified treatment group with a change in the outcome falling into that quadrant. This was an intention-to-treat analysis. *Abbreviations*: FEV$_1$, forced expiratory volume in one second; SG, surgery; TG, training. *Source*: From Refs. 20,74.

morbidity in a limited number of patients undergoing unilateral laser reduction ($n = 10$) compared with a group undergoing predominantly stapled resections ($n = 57$).

Several groups have compared the short-term physiological results of bilateral LVRS performed by VATS or MS. Kotloff and colleagues (77) noted no difference in short-term spirometric outcomes although the total in-hospital mortality was significantly higher in the MS group (13.8% vs. 2.5%). Wisser et al. (82) noted little difference in all outcomes, including spirometry, between 15 patients treated with bilateral LVRS via MS compared with 15 undergoing bilateral VATS LVRS. These data support the retrospective findings of other investigators (78,83). In contrast, Ko and Waters noted a much higher total mortality (25%) in 19 patients undergoing bilateral LVRS via MS compared with 23 patients treated thoracoscopically (8%) (84). Furthermore, the improvement in FEV$_1$ was higher in the VATS group (62% vs. 28%). Data from the NETT have confirmed similar functional benefits between bilateral LVRS performed using MS or VATS (21).

The variance around the mean improvement in FEV$_1$ is demonstrated in remarkably few studies (77,85,86). Figure 3B illustrates the heterogeneous spirometric response for the NETT subjects 24 months after randomization to surgery or medical therapy. A significant proportion of patients experienced little improvement in FEV$_1$, even in the short term. Interestingly, many of the patients experiencing limited spirometric improvement demonstrate significant improvement in breathlessness, highlighting the limitation of FEV$_1$ as a sole measure of improvement (87).

Although data are limited, lung volumes have generally decreased during short-term follow-up while changes in DL_{CO} have been modest (18). Changes in resting arterial blood gases have ranged from significant improvements in PaO_2 and decreases in $PaCO_2$ to little change (18,88).

Data regarding long-term functional follow-up are limited. Roue and colleagues reported the results in 13 patients treated with varying surgical techniques (unilateral in 11) (89). Symptomatic improvement was noted in 12 of 13 patients at six months while FEV_1 improved in the same 12 patients. Four of six patients with available data maintained a greater than 20% improvement in FEV_1 at two years but neither of two patients maintained improvement at four years. Brenner et al. reported the rate of FEV_1 change greater than six months after LVRS (90). They noted a greater decrease in FEV_1 (0.255 ± 0.057 L/yr) in those patients experiencing the greatest improvement in the initial six months after surgery. The lowest rate of drop in FEV_1 appeared in those with the least initial improvement. Flaherty et al. documented a gradual decrement in FEV_1 over the course of three years after bilateral LVRS (91), while another group presented a median of four years of follow-up in 200 patients treated with bilateral LVRS (92). Although data collection were not complete, a majority of patients still exhibited spirometric improvement three and five years after surgery.

Exercise Capacity

Most available data have described simple measures of exercise capacity such as timed measures of walk distance. Consistent improvements in walk distance have been reported (18). The NETT investigators confirmed a modest improvement in six-minute walk distance for surgically treated patients with a consistent decrease in medically treated patients (20).

Several groups have reported consistent, short term, increases in maximal workload, VO_2 and V_E (18). Keller and colleagues confirmed increases in workload, VO_2 and V_E before and after unilateral LVRS (85). The improved maximal ventilation was achieved through increased tidal volume, V_T, with a modest change in respiratory rate, f_b. Benditt et al. reported an improved exercise capacity but decreased heart rate at similar workloads after bilateral LVRS (93). Martinez and colleagues reported that improved dyspnea at isowork correlated best with decreased dynamic hyperinflation (87). In addition, Tschernko et al. noted a significant decrease in the work of breathing during exercise after LVRS (94). Ferguson and colleagues reported an improved V_T at submaximal workloads during steady-state testing while physiological dead space improved (95). Criner et al. noted a significant improvement in maximal VO_2 in patients undergoing bilateral LVRS (96). The NETT investigators confirmed an increase in maximal achieved wattage during oxygen supplemented cycle ergometry in surgically patients; lesser improvement was noted in patients that continued aggressive medical management (20). Dolmage and colleagues (97) reported results from a randomized controlled trial of LVRS of 39 patients, including 19 randomized to operation. These investigators documented improved peak VO_2 and power with a greater minute ventilation and tidal volume. Importantly, this study confirmed an improvement in operational lung volumes among patients undergoing operation (Fig. 4).

The short-term effects of LVRS on the pulmonary vasculature during exercise has been described by several groups (98–100). These studies described little change in

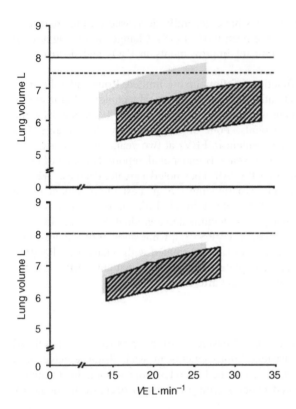

Figure 4   The baseline reference tidal volume (V_T;□) and V_T at six months (■) during incremental exercise for the treatment (upper panel) and control (lower panel) groups. end-inspiratory lung volumes (EILV) (top border of areas) and end-expiratory lung volumes (EELV) (bottom border of areas). The positive slope of the EELV indicates the presence of dynamic hyperinflation; total lung capacity (TLC) at baseline; — TLC post-surgery; --- TLC baseline and post-randomization. *Source*: From Ref. 97.

pulmonary hemodynamics at rest or during exercise, although improvement in right heart function during exercise has been reported (101). Weg et al. (102) reported an elevation of resting pulmonary artery pressures in nine patients three months after bilateral LVRS. Further data are required to define better these changes and their clinical significance.

Limited data are available regarding long-term maintenance of improvements in exercise capacity. Cordova et al. noted a higher six-minute walk distance in six patients 18 months after surgery compared with preoperative values (103). In this study, improvements in cardiopulmonary performance tended to be maintained 12 months after surgery (103). Flaherty et al. also described maintenance of improvement in six-minute walk distance despite spirometric decrement over three years after bilateral surgery (91). NETT investigators noted that surgical patients, in contrast to medically treated patients, were more likely to maintain improved maximal wattage during oxygen supplemented cardiopulmonary exercise testing during long-term follow-up (Fig. 5) (75).

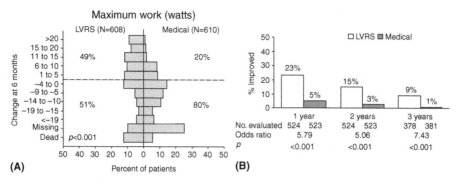

Figure 5 (A) Histograms of changes from postrehabilitation baseline in exercise capacity (maximum work) for all patients. The change from baseline for each survivor completing the procedure was scored 2–11, with higher scores indicating more improvement. Patients who were too ill to complete the procedure, who declined to complete the procedure, or who could pedal only with the ergometer set at 0 W were included in the missing category and scored 1. Patients who died were scored 0. The *p* values were determined from the Wilcoxon rank-sum test. The degree to which the bars are shifted to the upper left of the chart indicates the degree of relative benefit of LVRS over medical treatment. The percentage shown in each quadrant is the percentage of patients with a change in the outcome falling into that quadrant. This is an intention-to-treat analysis. (B) Improvement in exercise capacity (increase in maximum work of > 10 W above the patient's postrehabilitation baseline) at one, two, and three years after randomization to LVRS (*open box*) or medical treatment (*filled box*) for all patients. Shown below each graph are the number of patients evaluated, the odds ratio for improvement (LVRS:Medical), and the Fisher's exact *p* value for difference in proportion improved. Patients who died or who did not complete the assessment were considered not improved. This is an intention-to-treat analysis. *Abbreviation*: LVRS, lung volume reduction surgery. *Source*: From Ref. 75.

Medication and Oxygen Requirements

Numerous groups have described improvements in oxygen requirement after surgery (18). Keenan and colleagues reported an elimination of O_2 requirement in 17% and a decrease in O_2 requirement in 25% of patients three months after unilateral LVRS (81). Naunheim et al. reported that 48% of patients had discontinued O_2 three months after unilateral LVRS (104). These results are similar to those reported by others (43,76, 105–107). Cooper and colleagues noted that of the 52% of patients using O_2 continuously before surgery only 16% were using O_2 continuously six months after bilateral LVRS (108). Similar data have been reported by others (82–84,107,109–112). In the Canadian controlled trial, oxygen was required by 37% of patients before LVRS; this percentage was reduced by 28% postoperatively (73). Several investigative groups have reported significant discontinuation of oral steroid after LVRS (16,41,76,83,104,105,113,114). Unfortunately, the majority of studies provided limited detail regarding specific steroid reduction protocols which markedly limits the ability to adequately interpret the data.

Health Status

Several groups have demonstrated short-term improvement in the Medical Research Council dyspnea scores (16,41,43,45,76,112,115–119). Others have confirmed varying

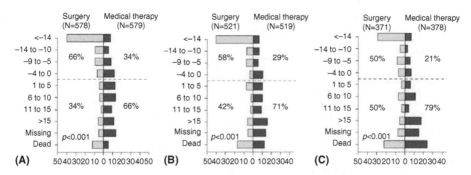

Figure 6 Histograms of changes from baseline in the UCSD SOBQ after (**A**) 6, (**B**) 12, and (**C**) 24 months of follow-up. Baseline measurements were performed after pulmonary rehabilitation. Patients previously identified as high risk were excluded. Patients who were too ill to complete the procedure or who declined to complete the procedure but did not explain why were included in the "missing" category. *p* Values were determined by the Wilcoxon rank-sum test. The degree to which the bars are shifted to the upper left of the chart indicates the degree of relative benefit of lung volume reduction surgery over medical treatment. The percentage shown in each quadrant is the percentage of patients in the specified treatment group with a change in the outcome falling into that quadrant. This was an intention-to-treat analysis. *Source*: From Ref. 20.

findings using the transitional dyspnea index (16,41,81,85,87,91,104,106,111,114, 120,121). NETT investigators have presented detailed assessment of breathlessness using the University of California Shortness of Breath Questionnaire (Fig. 6); a heterogeneous response was noted, although a clear benefit is noted in the surgically treated group compared with medically managed patients.

Results of formal health status measurement have been reviewed (122). Cooper et al. (16,41) reported short-term improvements using the Medical Outcomes Survey (MOS)—Short Form 36 (SF-36) and the Nottingham Health Profile (NHP), both generic instruments, which have been validated in patients with COPD (123–125). The improvement after LVRS was noted in measures of vitality, social functioning, physical functioning, general health, and in an increased ability to perform various roles. Similar results have been reported by others (74,83,95,126). Moy and colleagues reported SF-36 values before and after comprehensive pulmonary rehabilitation and again after bilateral LVRS via VATS in 19 patients (127). They noted no significant change in any of the domains after pulmonary rehabilitation although significant improvement was noted in vitality after LVRS. When compared to the baseline scoring, the combination of rehabilitation and bilateral LVRS resulted in significant improvement in four of the eight domains. Importantly, pulmonary rehabilitation accounted for most of the improvement in role limitations while LVRS accounted for most of the improvement in physical functioning, vitality, and social functioning.

Several groups have reported health status using disease-specific instruments. Bagley and colleagues described improvement in the Chronic Respiratory Questionnaire (CRQ) (107), while Norman et al. reported disease-specific measurement of health-related quality of life (HRQL) using the St. George's Respiratory Questionnaire (SGRQ) (128). The Canadian controlled trial reported clear improvement in health

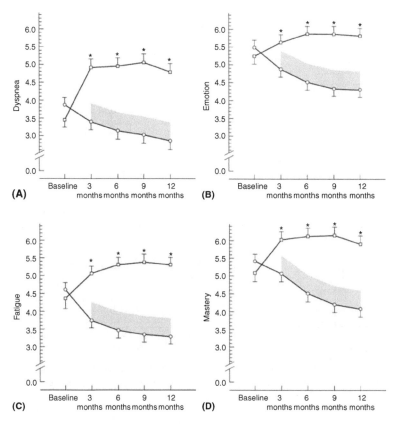

Figure 7 Panels (**A–D**) reflect the effect of surgery (*open box*) and medical control treatment (*open circle*) on each of the four domains of the Chronic Respiratory Questionnaire (dyspnea, emotional function, fatigue, and mastery) at baseline and 3, 6, 9, and 12 months after randomization. Values at follow-up are adjusted least square mean (SE). The shaded area shows the minimum clinically important difference for each measure. *Source*: From Ref. 23.

status measured with the CRQ in patients treated surgically compared with a matched group randomized to medical therapy (Fig. 7) (23). The NETT investigators noted significant improvement in the SGRQ of surgically treated patients, while clinically significant improvement in SGRQ scores was seen in a minority of medically treated patients (20). Long-term SGRQ follow-up from this sentinel study has been reported (Fig. 8) (75). A beneficial response favoring the surgically treated patients was seen out to four years of follow-up.

C. Lung Transplantation

Long-term results of lung transplantation are limited by significant complications which impair survival. Data from the Registry of the International Society for Heart and Lung Transplantation suggest 82% 1 year, 49% 5 years and 19% 10 years survival for emphysema patients (37). While emphysema patients enjoy the greatest survival advantage in the first year after lung transplantation, they have the lowest survival rate

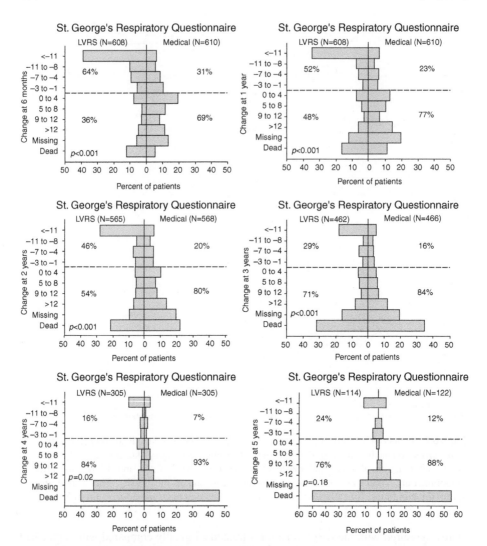

Figure 8 Histograms of changes from postrehabilitation baseline in health-related quality of life (St. George's Respiratory Questionnaire) scores for all patients in the National Emphysema Treatment Trial (NETT). The change from baseline for each survivor completing the procedure was scored 2–9, with higher scores indicating more improvement. Patients who were too ill to complete the procedure or who declined to complete the procedure were included in the missing category and were scored 1. Patients who died were scored 0. The *p* values were determined from the Wilcoxon rank-sum test. The degree to which the bars are shifted to the upper left of the chart indicates the degree of relative benefit of LVRS over medical treatment. The percentage shown in each quadrant is the percentage of patients with a change in the outcome falling into that quadrant. This is an intention-to-treat analysis. *Abbreviation*: LVRS, lung volume reduction surgery. *Source*: From Ref. 75.

at 10 years (37). Low perioperative complication rates and the advanced age of many COPD patients may contribute to this finding. The most frequent causes of late death include chronic allograft rejection (obliterative bronchiolitis, OB), infection, and malignancy (37,129).

Pulmonary Function

The published literature has consistently demonstrated spirometric improvement after both SLT and DLT with lesser improvement generally reported for SLT compared with DLT (52,110,130–139). Levine et al. described functional results in 28 patients undergoing 29 SLT. In their report, FEV_1 increased from a baseline of 16% predicted to 57% predicted at three months and to 60% predicted at six months after SLT (130). Several groups have examined determinants affecting postoperative spirometry after SLT. Brunsting et al. (139) suggested that recipient chest wall factors determined postoperative pulmonary function. Cheriyan et al. (140) confirmed the importance of recipient factors by noting that pulmonary function after SLT reflected restriction of the transplanted lung and obstruction in the native lung with a decreased transpulmonary pressure. In an elegant study, Estenne et al. (141) confirmed hyperinflation of the native lung in all patients with a lower, yet stable, TLC in the allograft. Importantly, the graft exhibited a normal functional residual capacity (FRC) suggesting that expansion of the rib cage allows preservation of the FRC in the transplanted lung. In contrast, patients undergoing DLT experience a significantly higher FEV_1 with most series reporting near normal values. For example, Gaissert et al. (110) described functional results in 33 patients undergoing bilateral LVRS (mean age 57 years), 39 patients undergoing SLT for COPD (mean age 55 years), and 27 undergoing DLT for COPD (mean age 49 years). A greater improvement was noted after DLT compared with SLT and LVRS. These data are qualitatively similar to those published by others (132–134).

Documentation of long-term results of pulmonary function is scarce. In general, early reports noted that some patients demonstrated stability in FEV_1 improvement while others experienced a decline in pulmonary function after several months (135). Levine et al. (130) noted an increase in FEV_1 from 16% predicted before SLT to 57% predicted at three months, 60% predicted at six months, 54% predicted at 12 months, and 52% predicted at 24 months after transplantation. The importance of OB on this loss of lung function has been recently reviewed (142,143). In fact, given the difficulty in histological confirmation of OB, the bronchiolitis obliterans syndrome (BOS) has been defined physiologically as a persistent 20% or greater drop in postoperative FEV_1, in the absence of other acute conditions (airway complications, infection, congestive heart failure, reversible airway reactivity, and systemic disease) (144). Furthermore, BOS can be staged according to the drop in FEV_1 from the peak, post-transplant value.

Bjortuft et al. (137) contrasted pulmonary function in stable recipients of SLT for COPD to recipients who developed histological OB or BOS. Several groups have suggested that a decrease in pulmonary function with BOS is particularly likely in SLT recipients (52,145,146). Gerbase and colleagues (147) corroborated this hypothesis describing seven-year outcomes in 10 SLT and 14 DLT recipients with native emphysema. FEV_1 improved from 21% predicted to 59% predicted at one year in SLT recipients then fell to 50% predicted by year 7. Greater improvement in FEV_1 from 28% predicted to 88% predicted was noted in DLT patients with a reduction in mean values between year 5 and 7 to 79% predicted (147). The relative risk for the development of BOS was 2.86 in SLT patients compared with DLT recipients (147).

Exercise Capacity

Numerous investigators have reported improved six-minute walk distance after both SLT and DLT. Kaiser and colleagues described rising walk distance during the first 24 weeks after SLT in 11 patients with emphysema (131); similar results have been reported by others (135). Early comparisons suggested a greater improvement in walking distance in emphysema patients undergoing SLT than DLT (52,132,138). In contrast, others described similar six-minute walk distances in patients undergoing SLT or DLT for COPD (110,133).

Exercise after SLT or DLT appears to be limited by aerobic capacity and not by ventilatory limitation. Early reports noted persistent aerobic limitation in DLT (148) and SLT for COPD (149). Short-term data reported by other investigators have been consistent (150,151). Orens et al. extended these findings by contrasting maximal exercise response 3, 6, and 9 to 12 months after SLT for COPD (152); maximal achieved VO_2 rose from 3 to 6 months after transplantation but tended to fall by 12 months. Schwaiblmair and colleagues demonstrated a severe aerobic limitation before transplantation which improved significantly after surgery (153). Importantly, no evidence of ventilatory limitation was noted after transplantation with a significant decrease in physiological dead space and $P(A–a)O_2$ at peak exercise.

Most reports support peripheral muscle dysfunction as the predominant cause of exercise limitation after lung transplantation (154–156). Reinsma and associates (155) recently described exercise limitation in 25 patient (11 with COPD) one year following lung transplantation. VO_2 peak was only 57% predicted despite near normal lung function and a low lactate threshold of $<40\%$ predicted was common in all patients (155). These data, together with less than predicted improvement in peripheral muscle forces after transplantation, support muscle dysfunction as a cause of exercise limitation in this patient population. Lands and colleagues confirmed limited exercise capacity in 10 SLT and 9 DLT recipients 37.5 months after transplantation (157); the investigators postulated that most of the peripheral muscle dysfunction was attributable to detraining. Pantoja and colleagues examined nine lung transplant recipients (eight SLT, one DLT) 5 to 102 months after transplantation (158). In a subset of six patients, maximal voluntary contraction of the tibialis anterior muscle was decreased. Although maximal inspiratory pressures did not differ from control values, the maximal expiratory pressures were diminished by 30% relative to control ($p<0.05$). The authors concluded that peripheral and expiratory muscle weakness, atrophy, and reduction in muscular function with exercise were present in patients up to three years post-transplant (158). Evans and colleagues noted that quadriceps muscle intracellular pH was more acidic at rest and fell during exercise at a lower metabolic rate in transplant recipients versus the healthy controls (159); the persistent decrease in VO_{2max} correlated closely with the metabolic rate at which muscle pH fell. Using a noninvasive optical technique for the analysis of oxygen delivery and utilization in exercising muscle, Tirdel and colleagues reported that six post-lung transplant patients had a reduced maximum oxygen consumption and an earlier onset of anaerobic threshold compared with six-matched healthy controls, suggesting an alteration in peripheral oxygen utilization by the myocyte (160). Wang and colleagues extended these findings by analyzing vastus lateralis muscle biopsies in post-lung transplant patients following exercise (161). These biopsies demonstrated a lower mitochondrial adenosine triphosphate (ATP) production rate, a lower activity of mitochondrial enzymes, a lower proportion of type 1 fibers, and a higher lactate and inosine monophosphate content in the transplant recipients versus controls. Furthermore, a higher lactate and inosine monophosphate and lower ATP content at rest were noted, suggesting greater reliance on anaerobic metabolism. These findings are concordant with previous reports from this investigative group that reduced muscle calcium regulation and impaired potassium regulation after lung transplantation contribute to impaired muscle performance during exercise (162,163). The cause of this peripheral muscle dysfunction post-transplantation remains unclear, although chronic disease, drug therapy, disuse, and poor nutrition have all been invoked (164–166).

Reports of long-term exercise data after lung transplantation are few. Sundaresan and colleagues noted persistent improvement in six-minute walk distance after both SLT and DLT for COPD up to four years after transplantation (52). The same group has recently published a 13-year experience with lung transplantation in COPD (167). These authors noted a mild decrease in six-minute walk distance five years after transplantation although continued stability up to seven years after surgery in DLT recipients has been described (147). Maximal achieved VO_2 has been documented to change little in SLT or DLT recipients from three months to one to two years after transplantation in the report of Williams et al. (150). The most detailed report of long-term cardiopulmonary exercise response after SLT for COPD was presented by Levine et al. (130). These investigators reported remarkably little change in maximal achieved VO_2 3 (43% predicted), 6 (43% predicted), 12 (48% predicted), and 24 months (55% predicted) after transplantation. As such, a significant limitation to exercise remains for patients after lung transplantation, although the effect of long-term aerobic training has not been described in this patient population.

Health Status

Limited data are available detailing changes in health status after lung transplantation. Gross et al. administered lung transplant candidates and recipients the Medical Outcome Study Health Survey (MOS 20), the Index of Well-Being, the Karnofsky Performance Status Index, and questions assessing work history (168). Lung transplant candidates, most of whom had obstructive disease, demonstrated significant impairment in health status. In those with sequential measurement, significant improvement was noted 6 to 12 months after transplantation. In a rare longitudinal study, TenVergert and colleagues noted improvement in the NHP one month after transplantation (13 of 24 patients with emphysema) (169). Further improvement was noted during the first four postoperative months such that NHP scores were comparable to those of the general population. Cohen et al. extended these findings by noting that pre-transplant anxiety and psychopathology predicted post-transplant adjustment with greater anxiety predicting worse post-transplant quality of life (170). Gross et al. noted a similar result on the MOS 20 questionnaire in 17 recipients tested 19 to 36 months and 16 recipients tested greater than 36 months after transplantation when compared with responses 11 months after surgery (168). Importantly, recipients with BOS showed decrements in health status, particularly in the physical and social functioning and bodily pain. Similar results have been demonstrated by others (169,171,172).

Long-term data evaluating HRQL are now available. Seven-year follow-up of SLT and DLT COPD patients using the SGRQ revealed persistent improvement from pre-transplant values (147). However, the mean absolute values of the SGRQ were greater in DLT patients, especially four years after transplantation (147). In addition, while all three domains of the SGRQ improved in DLT recipients, the respiratory symptom domain lacked significant change in SLT patients. Improved long-term HRQL after DLT compared to SLT for COPD was implied (146,147). Rodrigue et al. administered both the SF-36 and the Transplant Specific Frequency Questionnaire to lung transplant recipients; the majority (34 of 66) having an underlying diagnosis of COPD (173). After a mean follow-up of two years, significant improvement in seven of eight subscales of the SF-36 were noted but remained below that of the general population (173). Three- to five-year post-transplant survivors reported more frequent affective, neurocognitive, and physical appearance issues. Headaches and depression were also more common when compared with patients earlier in their transplant course (173). These symptoms had a greater influence on women resulting in a lower percentage gain in quality of life than in men (174). Similar findings have been described (175) in a group of 10-year survivors and are likely due to the chronic use of immunosuppressive medications, transplant comorbidities, and the development of BOS in long-term survivors.

V. Which Patients Should and Which Should Not Be Considered for Surgery?

It is evident that several surgical approaches are available for the patient with COPD. Increasing data are allowing health care providers to decide which approach is optimal for an individual patient. We will initially discuss the three main surgical options (bullectomy, LVRS, and lung transplantation) individually and attempt to summarize the current state of the art for the surgical approach to a patient with COPD.

A. Bullectomy

Most investigators have attempted to identify optimal surgical candidates using pulmonary function tests and radiographic studies to identify compressed normal lung that is most likely to respond to bullectomy (176). These are summarized in Table 1.

Clinical Features

In general, ideal candidates experience persistent exercise limitation despite optimal medical therapy including pulmonary rehabilitation. Some series have suggested worse surgical result in older patients. Laros et al. (61) noted a mean age of 56 years in those patients who died of respiratory insufficiency after bullectomy compared with those who exhibited favorable long-term responses (mean age < 50 years). Similar results were published by Fitzgerald and colleagues (60). Some have suggested higher morbidity and worse long-term results in the presence of superimposed chronic bronchitis (60,61,65). As such, although imperfect, a history of chronic sputum production and recurrent respiratory infections may provide a suggestion of more

Table 1 Potential Indications and Contraindications for Classical Bullectomy

Parameter	Indications	Contraindications
Clinical	Young age ($<$ 50 years)	Age $>$ 50 years
	Rapid progressive dyspnea despite maximal medical therapy	Comorbid illness
	Ex–smoker	Cardiac disease
		Pulmonary hypertension
		$>$ 10% weight loss
		Frequent respiratory infections—chronic bronchitis
		Ongoing tobacco use
Physiological	Normal or slightly $\downarrow$ FVC	
	$FEV_1 > 40\%$ predicted	$FEV_1 < 35\%$ predicted
	Little bronchoreversibility	
	"High" trapped lung volume	"Low" trapped gas volume
	Normal or near normal DL_{CO}	Decreased DL_{CO}
	Normal PaO_2 and $PaCO_2$	
Imaging	CXR—bulla more than one-third hemithorax	CXR—vanishing lung syndrome poorly defined bullae
	CT—large and localized bulla with vascular crowding and normal, compressed pulmonary parenchyma around bulla	CT—multiple ill-defined bullae in underlying lung
	Angiography—vascular crowding with preserved distal vascular branching	Angiography—vague bullae; disrupted vasculature elsewhere
	Isotope scan—well-localized matching defect with normal uptake and washout for underlying lung	Isotope scan—absence of target zones, poor washout in remaining lung

Abbreviations: CT, computed tomography; CXR, chest roentgenogram; FEV_1, forced expiratory volume in one second; FVC, forced vital capacity ratio.
Source: Adapted from Ref. 177.

predominant airway disease (1). Similarly, most authors have reported poorest long-term outcome in those individuals with greater degrees of emphysema in the remaining lung.

Physiological Status

In general, patients with a "restrictive" picture by spirometry with simultaneous elevation of FRC and TLC (178) tend to experience more favorable results, while those with severe obstruction, particularly when associated with smaller bullae, have been suggested to experience poorer long-term results (178). For example, Nakahara and colleagues noted the best improvement in patients with an $FEV_1 > 40\%$ predicted (179). Significant bronchoreversibility has been proposed as an additional, relative contraindication (Table 1) (4,176,178). Elevation of the trapped gas volume has been seen in patient groups demonstrating better responses to classic bullectomy (60,178). The DL_{CO} has been suggested as a marker of greater underlying emphysema with two investigative groups suggesting a better response in those patients with higher DL_{CO} and lack of exertional desaturation (59,179). Absolute thresholds are not available, however.

Imaging

Multiple authors have reported inferior results in patients with bullae occupying more than one-third of the hemithorax, particularly for the long-term maintenance of functional improvement (60–62,180). In the past 15 years, computed tomography (CT) has become the imaging study of choice in the assessment of bullous structure and size. CT allows an assessment of the volume of air in bullae, the presence of compressed lung, and an examination of the structure of the remaining lung tissue (62,178,181,182). Some groups have advocated the use of radionuclide scans to assess the relative function of bullous and nonbullous areas, which may be particularly useful in identifying lung zones which appear normal or minimally involved on CT or chest radiograph (183).

B. Lung Volume Reduction Without Giant Bullae

Clinical Features

The clinical evaluation should be used to identify patients with predominantly emphysema (176). The presence of frequent respiratory infections and chronic, copious sputum production may be useful in identifying patients with primarily airway disease (184). In addition, clinical assessment should attempt to identify patient features predicting a higher mortality or likelihood of poor functional result (Table 2). For example, coronary artery disease is frequently seen in this patient population (185), although it should not be considered an absolute contraindication to surgery. Successful combined LVRS and cardiac surgery has been well documented (186,187). Similarly, pulmonary hypertension has been described as a relative contraindication for LVRS (188), although prohibitive pulmonary hypertension is infrequent in this patient population (189–192). The effect of milder pulmonary vascular abnormality has not been prospectively studied (17), although several groups have reported either no consistent change or an improvement in pulmonary artery pressure early after bilateral LVRS (99,100,193,194). Others have reported improved right ventricular function early after LVRS (98,101,195). Importantly, some have reported worsening resting pulmonary hypertension after LVRS (102).

Less favorable outcomes have been reported in the presence of α_1-antitrypsin deficiency (41,196,197). Cassina and colleagues noted similar short-term clinical and physiological responses in 12 patients with α_1-antitrypsin deficiency compared with 18 patients with α_1-antitrypsin replete individuals (116); long-term response (12–24 months) was clearly poorer in those with α_1-antitrypsin deficiency (116). Similarly, Gelb et al. described only modest spirometric improvement after lower lobe LVRS via VATS in six α_1-antitrypsin deficiency patients (198). Interestingly, one group has recently reported good long-term results in a group of emphysema patients with α_1-antitrypsin deficiency who were followed up to five years after thoracoscopic LVRS (199). NETT investigators reported inferior clinical outcomes in a small number of α_1-antitrypsin deficient individuals undergoing bilateral LVRS (197).

An impaired nutritional status as measured by a lower body mass index (BMI) or by decreased percentage of ideal body weight or fat-free mass index has been associated with increased perioperative complications (200,201). Importantly, clinical severity of disease has not proven a consistent contraindication (107,114,202,203).

Table 2 Potential Indications and Contraindications for LVRS

Parameter	Indications	Contraindications
Clinical	Age <75 years	Age >75–80 years
	Clinical picture consistent with emphysema	Comorbid illness that increases surgical mortality
	Dyspnea despite maximal medical treatment pulmonary rehabilitation	Clinically significant coronary artery disease
	Ex-smoker (>6 months)	Pulmonary hypertension (PA systolic > 45, PA mean >35 mmHg)
	Requiring <20 mg prednisone/day	Surgical constraints: Previous thoracic procedure Pleuradesis Chest wall deformity
Physiologic	FEV_1 after bronchodilator <45% predicted	$FEV_1 \leq 20\%$ predicted and $DL_{CO} \leq 20\%$ predicted
	Hyperinflation TLC >100% predicted RV >150% $PaO_2 > 45$ mmHg $PaCO_2 < 60$ mmHg	↑Inspiratory resistance
	Postrehabilitation six-minute walk distance >140 m	
	Low postrehabilitation maximal achieved cycle ergometry watts	
Imaging	CXR—Hyperinflation	Homogeneous emphysema and $FEV_1 \leq 20\%$ predicted
	CT—high resolution CT confirming severe emphysema, ideally with upper lobe predominance	Non-upper lobe predominant emphysema and high post-rehabilitation cycle ergometry maximal achieved wattage

Abbreviations: CT, computed tomography; CXR, chest roentgenogram; FEV_1, forced expiratory volume in one second; LVRS, lung volume reduction surgery; RV, residual volume; TLC, total lung capacity.
Source: Adapted from Ref. 177.

Physiological Features

Pulmonary function testing has proven instrumental in identifying optimal candidates for surgery (Table 2) (176). A lower limit of FEV_1 that identifies individuals at prohibitive risk has not been agreed upon, although the NETT investigators noted that a lower FEV_1 was independently predictive of greater postoperative pulmonary morbidity (204). Some have reported acceptable outcomes in patients with very severely decreased FEV_1 (<500 mL) (76,114,202,205). As the mechanism of improvement in spirometry relates to improvement in elastic recoil (206), patients with airflow obstruction from structural emphysema appear to be the ones who benefit most from LVRS. Ingenito and colleagues reported a relationship between low inspiratory resistance (reflecting less predominant airway disease) and short-term improvements in FEV_1 (207). These same investigators have confirmed that measurement of inspiratory resistance provides additional information to emphysema distribution as defined by perfusion scintigraphy (207). In fact, one group has recently confirmed that greater histopathological abnormalities of the smaller airways are associated with poorer short-term response to LVRS (208).

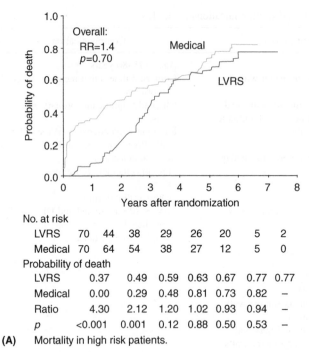

No. at risk

LVRS	70	44	38	29	26	20	5	2
Medical	70	64	54	38	27	12	5	0

Probability of death

LVRS	0.37		0.49	0.59	0.63	0.67	0.77	0.77
Medical	0.00		0.29	0.48	0.81	0.73	0.82	–
Ratio	4.30		2.12	1.20	1.02	0.93	0.94	–
p	<0.001		0.001	0.12	0.88	0.50	0.53	–

(A)   Mortality in high risk patients.

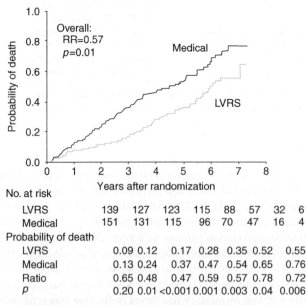

No. at risk

LVRS	139	127	123	115	88	57	32	6
Medical	151	131	115	96	70	47	16	4

Probability of death

LVRS	0.09	0.12	0.17	0.28	0.35	0.52	0.55
Medical	0.13	0.24	0.37	0.47	0.54	0.65	0.76
Ratio	0.65	0.48	0.47	0.59	0.57	0.78	0.72
p	0.20	0.01	<0.001	0.001	0.003	0.04	0.006

(B)   Mortality in patients with upper lobe predominant emphysema
and low, post-rehabilitation exercise capacity.

Figure 9   *(Caption on facing page)*

Although some have advocated LVRS only in those patients with a significant elevation of TLC (188), the RV, and RV/TLC ratio may be better predictors of response (209). Preliminary data have suggested that an elevated RV/TLC ratio may be the best physiological parameter to identify patients demonstrating improved quality of life, pulmonary function, and exercise capacity after bilateral LVRS (210). Importantly, the NETT did not identify lung volume as a predictor of mortality or functional improvement after bilateral LVRS (20).

Several groups have suggested that a very low DL_{CO} increases risk (81,106,211), while others have not confirmed these findings (205). Importantly, the NETT identified two subgroups of patients at particularly high risk of surgical mortality after bilateral LVRS (Fig. 9A) (20,75); patients with a post-bronchodilator $FEV_1 \le 20\%$ predicted and a $DL_{CO} \le 20\%$ predicted exhibited a much higher mortality with LVRS than with medical management (OR 2.98, 95% CI 1.3–7.7). This same group has confirmed that a lower DL_{CO} was independently associated with postoperative pulmonary morbidity (204).

Arterial blood gas abnormalities have been suggested as predictive of a bad outcome. Several investigators have suggested impaired outcome and higher mortality in patients with hypercapnia (95,106,43,212), while others have not confirmed this finding (114,213–216). The most definitive data come from the NETT where baseline $PaCO_2$ was not associated with impaired outcome despite over 30% of randomized patients exhibiting baseline hypercapnia (20).

Preoperative exercise capacity has been documented to be a predictor of outcome by numerous investigators (106,202,212). The most compelling data come from the NETT, where one of the primary endpoints was maximal achieved workload on a cycle ergometer while breathing 30% supplemental oxygen (20). A threshold of 40% of the baseline workload demonstrated a clear breakpoint in mortality for the overall study group; this corresponded to a workload of 25 W for females and 40 W for male patients (20). These thresholds, in conjunction with CT data, allowed a clear separation of non-high risk patients into four distinct categories (Fig. 10 and Table 3).

Imaging

Thoracic imaging is crucially important the evaluation of patients for LVRS (218), with most authorities considering topographic heterogeneity an important predictor of an optimal response from LVRS (17,18). CT has proven particularly useful (219–221). Several groups have suggested that the severity of emphysema on CT is associated with outcome of LVRS (222–224). The importance of emphysema heterogeneity has

---

Figure 9 (A,B) Kaplan–Meier estimates of the probability of death as a function of the number of months after randomization in the NETT. *p* Values were derived by Fisher's exact test for the comparison between groups over a median follow-up period of 4.3 years. High-risk patients were defined as those with an FEV_1 that was 20% or less of the predicted value and either homogeneous emphysema or a carbon monoxide diffusing capacity that was 20% or less of the predicted value. A low baseline exercise capacity was defined as a maximal workload at or below the sex-specific 40th percentile (25 W for women and 40 W for men); a high exercise capacity was defined as a workload above this threshold. This was an intention-to-treat analysis. *Abbreviations*: FEV_1, forced expiratory volume in one second; LVRS, lung volume reduction surgery; NETT, National Emphysema Treatment Trial. *Source*: From Ref. 75.

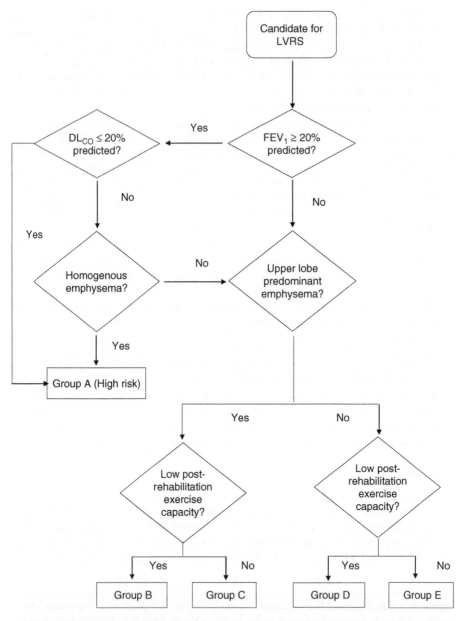

Figure 10 Diagnostic algorithm for patients being considered for LVRS based on data from the NETT. *Abbreviations*: FEV$_1$, forced expiratory volume in one second; LVRS, lung volume reduction surgery; NETT, National Emphysema Treatment Trial. *Source*: From Refs. 20, 217.

been suggested by many investigators (205,211,224–230). The most compelling data supporting the value of visual grading of emphysema distribution have been provided by NETT investigators (20). Radiologists at 17 participating clinical centers classified high resolution CT (HRCT) scans as predominantly exhibiting upper lobe or non-upper

Table 3 Results of Bilateral LVRS Compared to Medical Therapy in Patients with Severe Emphysema

| Patients | 90-Day mortality | | | Total mortality | | | |
	LVRS	Medical therapy	p Value	LVRS	Medical therapy	Risk ratio[a]	p value
Group A	20/70 (28.6)	0/70 (0)	<0.001	42/70	30/70	1.82	0.06
Group B	4/139 (2.9)	5/151 (3.3)	1.00	26/139	51/151	0.47	0.005
Group C	6/206 (2.9)	2/213 (0.9)	0.17	34/206	39/213	0.98	0.70
Group D	7/84 (8.3)	0/65 (0)	0.02	28/84	26/65	0.81	0.49
Group E	11/109 (10.1)	1/111 (0.9)	0.003	27/109	14/111	2.06	0.02

| Patients | Improvement in exercise capacity[b] | | | | Improvement in health-related quality of life[c] | | | |
	LVRS	Medical therapy	Odds ratio	p Value	LVRS	Medical therapy	Odds ratio	p value
Group A	4/58 (7)	1/48 (2)	3.48	0.37	6/58 (10)	0/48 (0)	—	0.03
Group B	25/84 (30)	0/92 (0)	—	<0.001	40/84 (48)	9/92 (10)	8.38	<0.001
Group C	17/115 (15)	4/138 (3)	5.81	0.001	47/115 (41)	15/138 (11)	5.67	<0.001
Group D	6/49 (12)	3/41 (7)	1.77	0.50	18/49 (37)	3/41 (7)	7.35	0.001
Group E	2/65 (3)	2/59 (3)	0.90	1.00	10/65 (15)	7/59 (12)	1.35	0.61

Values in parentheses indicate percentages. Groups A–E refer to the patients as defined in Figure 10.
[a] Risk ratio for total mortality in surgically versus medically treated patients during a mean follow-up of 29.2 months.
[b] Increase in the maximal workload of more than 10 W from the patient's postrehabilitation baseline value (24 months after randomization).
[c] Improvement in the health-related quality of life was defined as a decrease in the score on the St. George's Respiratory Questionnaire of more than 8 points (on a 100-point scale) from the patient's postrehabilitation baseline score (24 months after randomization).
Abbreviation: LVRS, lung volume reduction surgery.
Source: From Refs. 20, 217.

lobe emphysema based on visual scoring of disproportionate disease between non-anatomic thirds divided equally from the apex to the base (231). Using this method, in conjunction with the maximal achieved workload during oxygen supplemented maximal cycle ergometry, NETT investigators published several sentinel studies that clarified the role of CT imaging in the evaluation of patients for LVRS. An early manuscript identified an increased risk of surgical mortality in patients with severe obstruction ($FEV_1 \leq 20\%$ predicted) and either diffuse emphysema on HRCT or a $DL_{CO} \leq 20\%$ predicted (RR 3.9, 95% CI 1.9–9.0) (20). Patients with upper lobe predominant emphysema and a low post-rehabilitation exercise tolerance exhibited a decreased risk of mortality during long-term follow-up (RR 0.57, $p=0.01$) after LVRS (Fig. 9B) (75). Patients with non-upper lobe predominant emphysema and a high post-rehabilitation exercise capacity exhibited an increased risk of death during follow-up after LVRS which was not statistically significant (RR 1.10, $p=0.79$). Patients with upper lobe predominant emphysema and a high post-rehabilitation exercise capacity or patients with non-upper lobe predominant emphysema and a low post-rehabilitation exercise capacity did not have a survival advantage or disadvantage (20,75).

However, regarding this latter group of patients, homogeneous emphysema alone was found to confer increased odds of 90-day mortality, regardless of post-rehabilitation exercise capacity (OR 2.99, $p=0.009$) (204). Finally, patients with upper lobe predominant emphysema treated surgically were more likely to improve their exercise capacity compared to medically treated patients (Table 3). Figure 10 and Table 3 illustrate an approach to the evaluation of patients based on NETT data.

Unfortunately, the definition of emphysema heterogeneity has varied widely in the published literature (231). As such, many investigators have utilized quantitative CT methodology to define disease heterogeneity. Several groups have confirmed moderately strong correlations between several quantitative CT values and outcome measures (91,232). Nakano et al. reported a positive correlation between the amount of severe emphysema in the peripheral 50% of the lung and improvement in maximal achieved watts during cycle ergometry after LVRS (233). This same group examined the relationship between the number and size of emphysematous lesions and short-term response to LVRS (234). The power law exponent (D) represents the slope of the relationship between the log of the cumulative number of emphysematous lesions and the log of the emphysema lesion size. As such, a steep slope and thus large D represents lungs with predominantly small lesions while a shallow slope and small D suggests lungs with larger emphysematous lesions. A positive correlation was noted between the change in D and the change in maximal wattage achieved during cycle ergometry. The authors suggested that patients with larger, upper lobe lesions respond better to surgery than patients with small, uniformly distributed lesions (234).

Several groups have suggested that identifying heterogeneous perfusion during ventilation/perfusion scanning may predict outcome after LVRS (235–238). Thurnheer et al. compared semiquantitative perfusion scans and CT images, noting that functional improvement was better correlated with physiological hyperinflation and emphysema heterogeneity as assessed by CT compared to perfusion scintigraphy (118). Hunsaker et al. correlated LVRS outcomes with indexes of CT and ventilation/perfusion (V/Q) imaging (223). Patients with more heterogeneous emphysema, as determined by CT or V/Q, tended to show a greater magnitude and likelihood for improved FEV_1. Cederlund et al. noted little difference in emphysema heterogeneity classification based on CT or scintigraphy alone (239). The combination of the two was superior when contrasted with quantitative methodology as the "gold standard." It is likely that CT and scintigraphy demonstrate similar predictive ability in suggesting outcome after LVRS.

C. Lung Transplantation

Given the significant morbidity and mortality associated with lung transplantation careful patient selection is crucial to optimize outcome (240). In addition, controversy exists regarding whether a survival benefit is noted after lung transplantation for COPD (56,129,241–245). A summary of potential selection criteria is presented in Table 4.

Clinical Features

Candidates for lung transplantation should have end-stage pulmonary disease that is nonresponsive to maximal medical management, no other serious major organ system dysfunction or active systemic disease, no active extrapulmonary infection, have the ability to ambulate and participate in pulmonary rehabilitation, have strong social

Table 4 General and Disease-Specific Selection Guidelines for Candidate Selection for Lung Transplantation in COPD Patients

General selection guidelines	COPD disease-specific criteria
Relative contraindications	*Referral*
Age older than 65 years	BODE >5
Critical or unstable clinical condition	*Listing*
Severely limited functional status	BODE $>7–10$ or at least one of the following:
Colonization with highly resistant or highly virulent bacteria, fungi, or mycobacteria	History of hospitalizations for exacerbations associated with acute hypercapnia
Severe obesity (BMI >31 kg/m^2)	Pulmonary hypertension despite oxygen therapy
Severe or symptomatic osteoporosis	$FEV_1 < 20\%$ predicted and either $DL_{CO} < 20\%$
Mechanical ventilation	predicted or homogenous distribution of
Other medical conditions that have not resulted in end-stage organ damage should be optimally treated	emphysema
Absolute contraindications	
Malignancy in the last two years, with the exception of cutaneous (basal and squamous cell) tumors	
Untreatable advanced dysfunction of another organ system	
Non-curable chronic extrapulmonary infection including chronic active hepatitis B, hepatitis C, and HIV	
Significant chest wall/spinal deformity	
Documented nonadherence or inability to follow through with medical therapy or office follow-up	
Untreatable psychiatric or psychological condition	
Absence of consistent or reliable social support system	
Substance addiction that is either active or within the previous six months	

Abbreviations: BMI, body mass index; COPD, chronic obstructive pulmonary disease; FEV_1, forced expiratory volume in one second.
Source: Adapted from Ref. 240.

support systems, no evidence of malignancy for at least two to five years, no substance addiction (including tobacco use) for at least six months, and no untreatable psychiatric condition that would compromise compliance or the ability to "cope" with high stress situations (240). These criteria are usually designated as "absolute" contraindications, whereas several "relative" contraindications are transplant center dependent (Table 4).

    Older recipients have a significantly worse survival (37). The most recent update of the Pulmonary Scientific Council of the International Society for Heart and Lung Transplant suggests a potential upper limit for recipient age of greater than 65 years (240). A BMI of <17 kg/m^2 or >30 kg/m^2 has been associated with greater 90-day

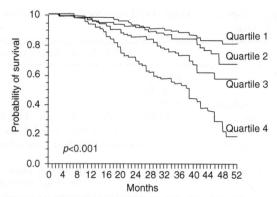

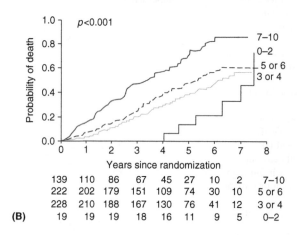

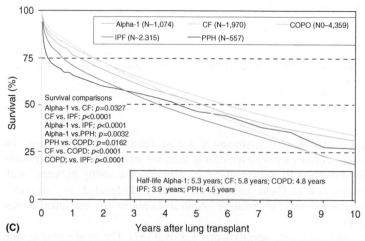

Figure 11 (*Caption on facing page*)

mortality (246,247). Kanasky et al. described a mortality rate three times higher in lung recipients with a BMI > 30 kg/m^2 (248). Therefore, these criteria may be considered contraindications for transplantation. Severe osteoporosis should also be considered prior to transplant listing as it is common in patients with end-stage lung disease (249). Accelerated bone loss as well as atraumatic fractures are associated with lung transplantation (250–252) which may lead to long-term complications. Mechanical ventilation, colonization with antibiotic resistant bacteria, fungi, or atypical mycobacteria; other medical conditions, including previous coronary artery bypass grafting, severe gastroesophageal reflux disease, or diabetes mellitus, are additional relative contraindications for lung transplant listing (240).

Physiologic

Physiological testing has been the most frequently used modality to assess prognosis in patients with COPD (253). As such, numerous investigators have documented that the FEV_1 after bronchodilator administration is an important predictor of mortality in COPD (254–258). Other predictors of mortality include weight loss (259,260), dyspnea (261), and exercise capacity (262). An acute exacerbation of COPD requiring hospitalization can be predictive for a poor outcome. One year mortality rates of 35% to 50% have been reported (263,264). Multivariate analysis of factors predicting death of patients on the United Network for Organ Sharing lung transplant waiting list confirmed these findings (265).

The field of prognostication in COPD has been advanced by recent data confirming that multidimensional approaches to stratifying disease severity is likely a better approach (266). The BODE score, which incorporates BMI, degree of airflow obstruction (FEV_1), and measurement of dyspnea and exercise capacity, predicts survival in COPD better than spirometry alone (267). Figure 11A illustrates how an increasing quartile of BODE score is associated with a worse prognosis in a large cohort of COPD patients. Similarly, in the NETT medically treated cohort, a group that in many ways resembles COPD patients eligible for transplantation, increasing BODE score is associated with impaired prognosis (Fig. 11B). Although comparisons must be made with great caution, one can contrast these estimates of survival with the most recent data presented from the International Society of Heart and Lung Transplant (ISHLT) registry (Fig. 1). It is evident that one can suggest that only COPD patients with greater BODE scores are likely to experience any survival

---

Figure 11 (A) Kaplan–Meier survival curves for four quartiles of the body mass index, degree of airflow obstruction, dyspnea, and exercise capacity index (BODE) for a cohort of 625 chronic obstructive pulmonary disease (COPD) patients. Quartile 1 is a score of 0–2, quartile 2 is a score of 3–4, quartile 3 is a score of 5–6, while quartile 4 is a score of 7–10. (B) Kaplan–Meier estimates of the probability of death as a function of the number of years after randomized patients for medically treated patients in the National Emphysema Treatment Trial (NETT) segregated by modified BODE index. The *p* value was derived from the log rank test for the comparison between subgroups over a median follow-up period of 3.9 years. The curve labels reflect the ranges of BODE scores. (C) Kaplan–Meier survival by diagnosis for adult lung transplantations performed between January 1994 and June 2004. *Source*: From Refs. 37, 267, 268.

benefit from transplantation (Table 4). Additional, data are required to better refine these concepts.

Imaging

Imaging techniques have a less defined role in the preoperative evaluation for lung transplantation. It seems intuitive that the presence of emphysema would be associated with a worse prognosis than chronic airflow obstruction primarily related to an airway process. The early work of the University of Arizona College of Medicine supports this hypothesis. These investigators examined the survival rate and rate of decline in FEV_1 during 10 years of follow-up in white, non-Mexican Americans with chronic airflow obstruction (269). Patients with clinical features most consistent with chronic asthmatic bronchitis (a primarily airway process) were contrasted with patients believed to have nonatopic, smoking-related obstructive disease (more consistent with emphysema). The authors found the rate of decline in FEV_1 to be greater, and survival to be decreased in patients with nonasthmatic airflow obstruction. The recent report of the NETT Research Group confirms that increasing emphysema volume and distribution independently impact long-term survival in a large cohort of medically treated patients with emphysema (268).

CT appears to alter the surgical approach to lung transplantation in selected patients. Kazerooni and colleagues retrospectively examined the results of preoperative chest radiography and CT in 190 transplant candidates (270). CT prompted a change in the determination of which lung was more severely diseased for 27 of 169 patients. Of the 45 patients who subsequently underwent transplantation CT prompted a change in the determination of which side to perform SLT in four. This same group has identified pulmonary nodules, suspicious for malignancy, in 8 of 190 patients evaluated for lung transplantation (271). As an active malignancy precludes transplantation, such a finding would clearly alter the candidacy of a patient for lung transplantation. Finally, the presence of unsuspected bronchiectasis could alter the decision to perform DLT in contrast to SLT.

D. Lung Transplantation vs. LVRS

Given the overlap of selection criteria for lung transplantation and LVRS, it is evident that careful consideration for the optimal surgical procedure needs to take place for individual COPD patients. The data from the NETT are particularly valuable in allowing the proposal of a detailed algorithm for decision making (Fig. 12). Recommendation for LVRS in patients with non-upper lobe predominant emphysema and low post-rehabilitation exercise capacity (Group D, Table 3) is tempered by the finding of increased risk for 90-day mortality in this subgroup (204), and consideration of LVRS for this subset of patients should be made carefully. Additional data are required to confirm the validity of this approach and to refine recommendations.

VI. Conclusions

The extensive literature has been published regarding surgical therapies for advanced COPD, with the most widely accepted directed at surgical relief of hyperinflation. Bullectomy and LVRS are established surgical techniques for a very limited number of

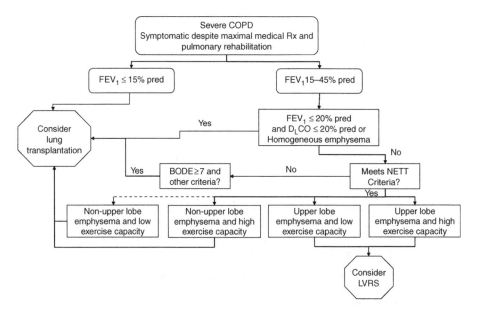

Figure 12 Potential algorithm for the consideration of lung volume reduction surgery (LVRS) and lung transplantation in patients with advanced COPD. NETT criterial include a clinical and radiological scenario consistent with bilateral emphysema, body mass index (BMI)$\leq$31.1 for men and 32.3 for women, prednisone dose $\leq$20 mg daily, $FEV_1 \leq$45% predicted, total lung capacity (TLC)$\geq$100% predicted, residual volume (RV)$\geq$150% predicted, $PaCO_2 \leq$60 mmHg ($\leq$55 mg at altitude), $PaO_2 \geq$45 mmHg ($\geq$30 mg at altitude), stable cardiac status, post-pulmonary rehabilitation six-minute walk distance $\geq$140 m and able to complete three minutes of unloaded pedaling in maximal, oxygen supplemented exercise test. The hashed line reflects uncertainty in long-term value of LVRS in this subgroup. *Abbreviations*: COPD, chronic obstructive pulmonary disease; FEV_1, forced expiratory volume in one second; NETT, National Emphysema Treatment Trial. *Source*: Modified from Refs. 71, 272.

patients. The patients with the poorest long-term outcomes appear to be those with the most abnormal respiratory function or greater extent of emphysema on imaging studies. Lung transplantation may serve as a viable therapeutic option for some of these COPD patients.

References

1. Martinez FJ. Diagnosing chronic obstructive pulmonary disease. The importance of differentiating asthma, emphysema and chronic bronchitis. Postgrad Med 1998; 103:112–25.
2. Pauwels RA, Buist AS, Calverley PMA, Jenkins CR, Hurd SS, GOLD Scientific Committee. Global strategy for the diagnosis, management, and prevention of chronic obstructive pulmonary disease. NHLBI/WHO Global Initiative for Chronic Obstructive Lung Disease (GOLD) Workshop Summary. Am J Respir Crit Care 2001; 163:1256–76.
3. Celli BR, MacNee W, and committee members. ATS/ERS Task Force. Standards for the diagnosis and treatment of patients with COPD: a summary of the ATS/ERS position paper. Eur Respir J 2004; 23:932–46.

4. Gaensler EA, Cugell DW, Knudson RJ, FitzGerald MX. Surgical management of emphysema. Clin Chest Med 1983; 4:443–63.
5. Deslauriers J. Surgical management of chronic obstructive pulmonary disease. Ann Thorac Surg 1995; 60:873–4.
6. Deslauriers J. History of surgery for emphysema. Semin Thorac Cardiovasc Surg 1996; 8:43–51.
7. Meyers BF, Patterson GA. Chronic obstructive pulmonary disease. 10: bullectomy, lung volume reduction surgery, and transplantation for patients with chronic obstructive pulmonary disease. Thorax 2003; 58:634–8.
8. Brantigan O, Kress M, Mueller E. A surgical approach to pulmonary emphysema. Am Rev Respir Dis 1959; 39:194–202.
9. Brantigan O, Mueller E. Surgical treatment of pulmonary emphysema. Am Surg 1957; 23:789–804.
10. Delarue NC, Woolf CR, Sanders DE, et al. Surgical treatment for pulmonary emphysema. Can J Surg 1977; 20:222–31.
11. Even P, Sors H, Safran D, Reynaud P, Venet A, Debesse B. Hemodynamique des bulles d'emphyseme un nouveau syndrome: la tamponade cardiaque emphysemateuse. Rev Fr Mal Respir 1980; 8:117–20.
12. Dahan M, Salerin F, Berjaud J, Renella Coll J, Gaillard J. Interet de l'exploration hemodynamique dans les indications chirurgicales des emphysemes. Ann Chir 1989; 43:669–72.
13. Crosa-Dorado VL, Pomi J, Perez-Penco EJ, Carriquiry G. Treatment of dyspnea in emphysema: pulmonary remodeling; hemo- and pneumostatic suturing of the emphysematous lung. Res Surg 1992; 4:152–5.
14. Wakabayashi A. Thoracoscopic laser pneumoplasty in the treatment of diffuse bullous emphysema. Ann Thorac Surg 1995; 60:936–42.
15. Wakabayashi A, Brenner M, Kayaleh RA, et al. Thoracoscopic carbon dioxide laser teratment of bullous emphysema. Lancet 1991; 337:881–3.
16. Cooper JD, Trulock EP, Triantafillou AN, et al. Bilateral pneumectomy (volume reduction) for chronic obstructive pulmonary disease. J Thorac Cardiovasc Surg 1995; 109:106–16.
17. Utz JP, Hubmayr RD, Deschamps C. Lung volume reduction surgery for emphysema: out on a limb without a NETT. Mayo Clin Proc 1998; 73:552–6.
18. Flaherty KR, Martinez FJ. Lung volume reduction surgery for emphysema. Clin Chest Med 2000; 21:819–48.
19. Benditt JO. Surgical therapies for chronic obstructive pulmonary disease. Respir Care 2004; 49:53–61.
20. National Emphysema Treatment Trial Research Group. A randomized trial comparing lung-volume-reduction surgery with medical therapy for severe emphysema. N Engl J Med 2003; 348:2059–73.
21. National Emphysema Treatment Trial Research Group. Safety and efficacy of median sternotomy versus video-assisted thoracic surgery for lung volume reduction surgery. J Thorac Cardiovasc Surg 2004; 127:1350–60.
22. Pompeo E, Marino M, Nofroni I, Matteucci G, Mineo TC. Reduction pneumoplasty versus respiratory rehabilitation in severe emphysema: a randomized study. Pulmonary Emphysema Research Group. Ann Thorac Surg 2000; 70:948–53 (discussion 954).
23. Goldstein RS, Todd TRJ, Guyatt GH, et al. Influence of lung volume reduction surgery (LVRS) on health related quality of life in patients with chronic obstructive pulmonary disease. Thorax 2003; 58:405–10.
24. Geddes D, Davies M, Koyama H, et al. Effect of lung-volume-reduction surgery in patients with severe emphysema. N Engl J Med 2000; 343:239–45.
25. Dunitz JM, Hertz MI. Surgical therapy for COPD: lung transplantation. Semin Respir Crit Care Med 1999; 20:365–73.
26. Veith FJ, Koerner SK. Problems in the management of lung transplant recipients. J Vasc Surg 1974; 8:273–82.
27. Veith FJ, Koerner SK, Siegelman SS, et al. Single lung transplantation in experimental and human emphysema. Ann Surg 1973; 178:463–76.
28. Wildevuur CRH, Benfield JR. A review of 23 human lung transplantation by 20 surgeons. Ann Thorac Surg 1970; 9:489–515.
29. Reitz BA, Wallwork JL, Hunt SA, et al. Heart–lung transplantation: successful therapy for patients with pulmonary vascular disease. N Engl J Med 1982; 306:557–64.
30. Toronto Lung Transplant Group. Unilateral lung transplantation for pulmonary fibrosis. N Engl J Med 1986; 314:1140–5.
31. Bates DV. The other lung. N Engl J Med 1970; 282:277–9.

32. Stevens PM, Johnson PC, Bell RL, Beall AC, Jenkins DE. Regional ventilation and perfusion after lung transplantation in patients with emphysema. N Engl J Med 1970; 282:245–9.

33. Cooper JD, Patterson GA, Grossman R, et al. Double-lung transplant for advanced chronic obstructive lung disease. Am Rev Respir Dis 1989; 139:303–7.

34. Patterson GA, Cooper JD, Dark JH, Jones MT. Experimental and clinical double lung transplantation. J Thorac Cardiovasc Surg 1988; 95:70–4.

35. Patterson GA, Cooper JD, Goldman B, et al. Technique of successful clinical double lung transplantation. Ann Thorac Surg 1988; 45:626–33.

36. Mal H, Andreassian B, Pamela F, et al. Unilateral lung transplantation in end-stage pulmonary emphysema. Am Rev Respir Dis 1989; 140:787–802.

37. Trulock EP, Edwards LB, Taylor DO, Boucek MM, Keck BM, Hertz MI. Registry of the International Society for Heart and Lung Transplantation: twenty-third official adult lung and Heart–lung transplantation report—2006. J Heart Lung Transplant 2006; 25:880–92.

38. Iwa T, Watanabe Y, Fukatani G. Simultaneous bilateral operations for bullous emphysema by median sternotomy. J Thorac Cardiovasc Surg 1981; 81:732–7.

39. Dartevelle P, Macchiarini P, Chapelier A. Operative technique of bullectomy. Chest Surg Clin N Am 1995; 5:735–49.

40. Liu HP, Chang CH, Lin PJ, Chu JJ, Hsieh MJ. An alternative technique in the management of bullous emphysema. Thoracoscopic endoloop ligation of bullae. Chest 1997; 111:489–93.

41. Cooper JD, Patterson GA, Sundaresan RS, et al. Results of 150 consecutive bilateral lung volume reduction procedures in patients with severe emphysema. J Thorac Cardiovasc Surg 1996; 112:1319–29 (discussion 1329–30).

42. Brenner M, Yusen R, McKenna R, Jr., et al. Lung volume reduction surgery for emphysema. Chest 1996; 110:205–18.

43. McKenna RJ, Jr., Brenner M, Gelb AF, et al. A randomized, prospective trial of stapled lung reduction versus laser bullectomy for diffuse emphysema. J Thorac Cardiovasc Surg 1996; 111:317–22.

44. McKenna RJ, Jr., Brenner M, Fischel RJ, Gelb AF. Should lung volume reduction for emphysema be unilateral or bilateral. J Thorac Cardiovasc Surg 1996; 112:1331–8.

45. Argenziano M, Thorashow B, Jellen PA, et al. Functional comparison of unilateral versus bilateral lung volume reduction surgery. Ann Thorac Surg 1997; 64:321–7.

46. Oey IF, Waller DA, Bal S, Singh SJ, Spyt TJ, Morgan MDL. Lung volume reduction surgery—a comparison of the long term outcome of unilateral vs bilateral approaches. Eur J Cardiothorac Surg 2002; 22:610–4.

47. Weill D, Keshavjee S. Lung transplantation for emphysema: two lungs or one. J Heart Lung Transplant 2001; 20:739–42.

48. Arcasoy SM, Kotloff RM. Lung transplantation. N Engl J Med 1999; 340:1081–91.

49. Force SD, Choong C, Meyers BF. Lung transplantation for emphysema. Chest Surg Clin N Am 2003; 13:651–67.

50. Trulock EP. Lung transplantation. Am J Respir Crit Care Med 1997; 152:947–52.

51. King MB, Savik K, Park SJ, et al. Similar outcomes after bilateral single lung transplantation for chronic obstructive pulmonary disease. J Heart Lung Transplant 1998; 17:59.

52. Sundaresan RS, Shiraishi Y, Trulock EP, et al. Single or bilateral lung transplantation for emphysema? J Thoracic Cardiovasc Surg 1996; 112:1485–95.

53. Meyer DM, Bennett LE, Novick RJ, Hosenpud JD. Single vs bilateral, sequential lung transplantation for end-stage emphysema: influence of recipient age on survival and secondary end-points. J Heart Lung Transplant 2001; 20:935–41.

54. Angles R, Tenorio L, Roman A, Soler J, Rochera M, de Latorre FJ. Lung transplantation for emphysema. Lung hyperinflation: incidence and outcome. Transpl Int 2005; 17:810–4.

55. de Perrot M, Chaparro C, McRae K, et al. Twenty-year experience of lung transplantation at a single center: influence of recipient diagnosis on long-term survival. J Thorac Cardiovasc Surg 2004; 127:1493–501.

56. Gunes A, Aboyoun CL, Morton JM, Plit M, Malouf MA, Glanville AR. Lung transplantation for chronic obstructive pulmonary disease at St Vincent's Hospital. Intern Med J 2006; 36:5–11.

57. Pochettino A, Kotloff RM, Rosengard BR, et al. Bilateral versus single lung transplantation for chronic obstructive pulmonary disease: intermediate-term results. Ann Thorac Surg 2000; 70:1813–9.

58. Orens JB, Shearon TH, Freudenburger RS, Conte JV, Bhorade SM, Ardehali A. Thoracic Organ Transplantation in the United States, 1995–2004. Am J Transplant 2006; 6:1188–97.

59. Hugh-Jones P, Whimster W. The etiology and management of disabling emphysema. Am Rev Respir Dis 1978; 117:343–78.
60. Fitzgerald M, Keelan P, Angell D. Long-term results of surgery for bullous emphysema. Surgery 1974; 68:566–82.
61. Laros CD, Gelissen HJ, Bergstein PG, et al. Bullectomy for giant bullae in emphysema. J Thorac Cardiovasc Surg 1986; 91:63–70.
62. Nickoladze GD. Functional results of surgery for bullous emphysema. Chest 1992; 101:119–22.
63. Potgieter PD, Benatar SR, Hewitson RP, Ferguson AD. Surgical treatment of bullous lung disease. Thorax 1981; 36:885–90.
64. Sung D, Payne W, Black L. Surgical management of giant bullae associated with obstructive airway disease. Surg Clin North Am 1973; 53:913–20.
65. Petro W, Hubner Ch, Greschuchna D, MaaBen W, Konietzko N. Bullectomy. Thorac Cardiovasc Surg 1983; 31:342–5.
66. Snider GL. Reduction pneumoplasty for giant bullous emphysema. Implications for surgical treatment of nonbullous emphysema. Chest 1996; 109:540–8.
67. Schipper PH, Meyers BF, Battafarano RJ, Guthrie TJ, Patterson GA, Cooper JD. Outcomes after resection of giant emphysematous bullae. Ann Thorac Surg 2004; 78:976–82.
68. Pearson MG, Ogilvie C. Surgical treatment of emphysematous bullae: late outcome. Thorax 1983; 38:134–7.
69. Palla A, Desideri M, Rossi G, et al. Elective surgery for giant bullous emphysema. A 5-year clinical and functional follow-up. Chest 2005; 128:2043–50.
70. Neviere R, Catto M, Bautin N, et al. Longitudinal changes in hyperinflation parameters and exercise capacity after giant bullous emphysema surery. J Thorac Cardiovasc Surg 2006; 132:1203–7.
71. National Emphysema Treatment Trial Research Group. Rationale and design of the National Emphysema Treatment Trial: a prospective randomized trial of lung volume reduction surgery. Chest 1999; 116:1750–61.
72. Lilm E, Ali A, Cartwright N, et al. Effect and duration of lung volume reduction surgery: mid-term results of the Brompton Trial. Thorac Cardiovasc Surg 2006; 54:188–92.
73. Miller JD, Malthaner RA, Goldsmith CH, et al. A randomized clinical trial of lung volume reduction surgery versus best medical care for patients with advanced emphysema: a two-year study from Canada. Ann Thorac Surg 2006; 81:314–21.
74. Hillerdal G, Lofdahl CG, Strom K, et al. Comparison of lung volume reduction surgery and physical training on health status and physiologic outcomes. A randomized controlled clinical trial. Chest 2005; 128:3489–99.
75. Naunheim KS, Wood DE, Mohsenifar Z, et al. Long-term follow-up of patients receiving lung-volume reduction surgery versus medical therapy for severe emphysema by the National Emphysema Treatment Trial Research Group. Ann Thorac Surg 2006; 82:431–43.
76. Eugene J, Dajee A, Kayaleh R, Gogia HS, Dos Santos C, Gazzaniga AB. Reduction pneumoplasty for patients with a forced expired volume in 1 second of 500 milliliters or less. Ann Thorac Surg 1997; 63:186–92.
77. Kotloff RM, Tino G, Bavaria JE, et al. Bilateral lung volume reduction surgery for advanced emphysema. A comparison of median sternotomy and thoracoscopic approaches. Chest 1996; 110:1399–406.
78. Yoshinaga Y, Iwasaki A, Kawahara K, Shirakusa T. Lung volume reduction surgery results in pulmonary emphysema. Changes in pulmonary function. Jpn J Thorac Cardiovasc Surg 1999; 47:445–51.
79. Nezu K, Kushibe K, Sawabata N, et al. Thoracoscopic lung volume reduction surgery for emphysema. Evaluation using ventilation–perfusion scintigraphy. Jpn J Thorac Cardiovasc Surg 1999; 47:267–72.
80. Lowdermilk GA, Keenan RJ, Landreneau RJ, et al. Comparison of clinical results for unilateral and bilateral thoracoscopic lung volume reduction. Ann Thorac Surg 2000; 69:1670–4.
81. Keenan RJ, Landrenau RJ, Sciurba FC, et al. Unilateral thoracoscopic surgical approach for diffuse emphysema. J Thorac Cardiovasc Surg 1996; 111:308–16.
82. Wisser W, Tschernko E, Senbaklavaci O, et al. Functional improvement after volume reduction: sternotomy versus videoendoscopic approach. Ann Thorac Surg 1997; 63:822–8.
83. Hazelrigg SR, Boley TM, Magee MJ, Lawyer CH, Henkle JQ. Comparison of staged thoracoscopy and median sternotomy for lung volume reduction surgery. Ann Thorac Surg 1998; 66:1134–9.
84. Ko CY, Waters PF. Lung volume reduction surgery: a cost and outcomes comparison of sternotomy versus thoracoscopy. Am Surg 1998; 64:1009–13.

85. Keller CA, Ruppel G, Hibbett A, Osterloh J, Naunheim KS. Thoracoscopic lung volume reduction surgery reduces dyspnea and improves exercise capacity in patients with emphysema. Am J Respir Crit Care Med 1997; 156:60–7.

86. Yusen RD, Trulock EP, Pohl MS, Biggar DG, The Washington University Emphysema Surgery Group. Results of lung volume reduction surgery in patients with emphysema. Semin Thorac Cardiovasc Surg 1996; 8:99–109.

87. Martinez FJ, Montes de Oca M, Whyte RI, Stetz J, Gay SE, Celli BR. Lung volume reduction improves dyspnea, dynamic hyperinflation and respiratory muscle function. Am J Respir Crit Care Med 1997; 155:1984–90.

88. Albert RK, Benditt JO, Hildebrandt J, Wood DE, Hlastala MP. Lung volume reduction surgery has variable effects on blood gases in patients with emphysema. Am J Respir Crit Care Med 1998; 158:71–6.

89. Roue C, Mal H, Sleiman C, et al. Lung volume reduction in patients with severe diffuse emphysema. A retrospective study. Chest 1996; 110:28–34.

90. Brenner M, McKenna RJ, Jr., Gelb AF, Fischel RJ, Wilson AF. Rate of FEV_1 change following lung volume reduction surgery. Chest 1998; 113:652–9.

91. Flaherty KR, Kazerooni EA, Curtis JL, et al. Short-term and long-term outcomes after bilateral lung volume reduction surgery: prediction by quantitative CT. Chest 2001; 119:1337–46.

92. Yusen RD, Lefrak SS, Gierada DS, et al. A prospective evaluation of lung volume reduction surgery in 200 consecutive patients. Chest 2003; 123:1026–37.

93. Benditt JO, Lewis S, Wood DE, Klima L, Albert RK. Lung volume reduction surgery improves maximal O_2 consumption, maximal minute ventilation, O_2 pulse, and dead space-to-tidal volume ratio during leg cycle ergometry. Am J Respir Crit Care Med 1997; 156:561–6.

94. Tschernko EM, Gruber EM, Jaksch P, et al. Ventilatory mechanics and gas exchange during exercise before and after lung volume reduction surgery. Am J Respir Crit Care Med 1998; 158:1424–31.

95. Ferguson GT, Fernandez E, Zamora MR, Pomerantz M, Buchholz J, Make BJ. Improved exercise performance following lung volume reduction surgery for emphysema. Am J Respir Crit Care Med 1998; 157:1195–203.

96. Criner GJ, Cordova FC, Furukawa S, et al. Prospective randomized trial comparing bilateral lung volume reduction surgery to pulmonary rehabilitation in severe chronic obstructive pulmonary disease. Am J Respir Crit Care Med 1999; 160:2018–27.

97. Dolmage TE, Waddell TK, Maltais F, et al. The influence of lung volume reduction surgery on exercise in patients with COPD. Eur Respir J 2004; 23:269–74.

98. Kubo K, Koizumi T, Fujimoto K, et al. Effects of lung volume reduction surgery on exercise pulmonary hemodynamics in severe emphysema. Chest 1998; 114:1575–82.

99. Oswald-Mammosser M, Kessler R, Massard G, Wihlm JM, Weitzenblum E, Lonsdorfer J. Effect of lung volume reduction surgery on gas exchange and pulmonary hemodynamics at rest and during exercise. Am J Respir Crit Care Med 1999; 158:1020–5.

100. Haniuda M, Kubo K, Fujimoto K, Aoki T, Yamanda T, Amano J. Different effects of lung volume reduction surgery and lobectomy on pulmonary circulation. Ann Surg 2000; 231:119–25.

101. Mineo TC, Pompeo E, Rogliani P, et al. Effect of lung volume reduction surgery for severe emphysema on right ventricular function. Am J Respir Crit Care 2002; 165:480–94.

102. Weg IL, Rossoff L, McKeon K, Graver LM, Scharf SM. Development of pulmonary hypertension after lung volume reduction surgery. Am J Respir Crit Care Med 1999; 159:552–6.

103. Cordova F, O'Brien G, Furukawa S, Kuzma AM, Travaline J, Criner GJ. Stability of improvement in exercise performance and quality of life following bilateral lung volume reduction surgery in severe COPD. Chest 1997; 112:907–15.

104. Naunheim KS, Keller CA, Krucylak PE, Singh A, Ruppel G, Osterloh JF. Unilateral video-assisted thoracic surgical lung reduction. Ann Thorac Surg 1996; 61:1092–8.

105. Eugene J, Ott RA, Gogia HS, Dos Santos C, Zeit R, Kayaleh RA. Video-thoracic surgery for treatment of end-stage bullous emphysema and chronic obstructive pulmonary disease. Am Surg 1995; 61:934–6.

106. Hazelrigg S, Boley T, Henkle J, et al. Thoracoscopic laser bullectomy: a prospective study with three-month results. J Thorac Cardiovasc Surg 1996; 112:319–27.

107. Bagley PH, Davis SM, O'Shea M, Coleman AM. Lung volume reduction surgery at a community hospital. Program development and outcomes. Chest 1997; 111:1552–9.

108. Cooper JD, Patterson GA. Lung volume reduction surgery for severe emphysema. Semin Thorac Cardiovasc Surg 1996; 8:52–60.

109. Daniel TM, Chan BBK, Bhaskar V, et al. Lung volume reduction surgery. Case selection, operative technique, and clinical results. Ann Surg 1996; 223:526–33.

110. Gaissert HA, Trulock EP, Cooper JD, Sundaresan RS, Patterson GA. Comparison of early functional results after volume reduction or lung transplantation for chronic obstructive pulmonary disease. J Thorac Cardiovasc Surg 1996; 111:296–307.

111. Bousamra M, II, Haasler GB, Lipchik RJ, et al. Functional and oximetric assessment of patients after lung reduction surgery. J Thorac Cardiovasc Surg 1997; 113:675–82.

112. McKenna RJ, Fischel RJ, Brenner M, Gelb AF. Combined operations for lung volume reduction surgery and lung cancer. Chest 1996; 110:885–8.

113. Miller DL, Dowling RD, Slater AD, McConnell JW. Combined lung volume reduction surgery and coronary artery bypass surgery. Chest 1996; 110(Suppl.):50S.

114. Argenziano M, Moazami N, Thomashow B, et al. Extended indications for lung volume reduction surgery in advanced emphysema. Ann Thorac Surg 1996; 62:1588–97.

115. Bingisser R, Zollinger A, Hauser M, Bloch KE, Russi EW, Weder W. Bilateral volume reduction surgery for diffuse pulmonary emphysema by video-assisted thoracoscopy. J Thorac Cardiovasc Surg 1996; 112:875–82.

116. Cassina PC, Teschler H, Konietzko N, Theegarten D, Stamatis G. Two-year results after lung volume reduction surgery in a-1-antitrypsin deficiency versus smoker's emphysema. Eur Respir J 1998; 12:1028–32.

117. Stammberger U, Bloch KE, Thurnheer R, Bingisser R, Weder W, Russi EW. Exercise performance and gas exchange after bilateral video-assisted thoracoscopic lung volume reduction for severe emphysema. Eur Respir J 1998; 12:785–92.

118. Thurnheer R, Engel H, Weder W, et al. Role of lung perfusion scintigraphy in relation to chest computed tomography and pulmonary function in the evaluation of candidates for lung volume reduction surgery. Am J Respir Crit Care Med 1999; 159:301–10.

119. Brenner M, McKenna RJ, Gelb AF, et al. Dyspnea response following bilateral thoracoscopic staple lung volume reduction surgery. Chest 1997; 112:916–23.

120. Sciurba FC, Rogers RM, Keenan RJ, et al. Improvement in pulmonary function and elastic recoil after lung-reduction surgery for diffuse emphysema. N Engl J Med 1996; 334:1095–9.

121. Scharf SM, Rossoff L, McKeon K, Graver LM, Graham C, Steinberg HN. Changes in pulmonary mechanics after lung volume reduction surgery. Lung 1998; 176:191–204.

122. Yusen RD, Morrow LE, Brown KL. Health-related quality of life after lung volume reduction surgery. Semin Thorac Cardiovasc Surg 2002; 14:403–12.

123. Mahler DA, Mackowiak JI. Evaluation of the short-form 36-item questionnaire to measure health-related quality of life in patients with COPD. Chest 1995; 6:1585–9.

124. Nishimura K, Tsukino M, Hajiro T. Health-related quality of life in patients with chronic obstructive pulmonary disease. Curr Opin Pulm Med 1998; 4:107–15.

125. Prieto L, Alonso J, Ferrer M, Anto JM, Group Quality of Life in COPD Study. Are results of the SF-36 Health Survey and the Nottingham Health Profile similar? A comparison in COPD patients. J Clin Epidemiol 1997; 50:463–73.

126. Anderson KL. Change in quality of life after lung volume reduction surgery. Am J Crit Care 1999; 8:389–96.

127. Moy ML, Ingenito EP, Mentzer SJ, Evans RB, Reilly JJ, Jr. Health-related quality of life improves following pulmonary rehabilitation and lung volume reduction surgery. Chest 1999; 115:383–9.

128. Norman M, Hillerdal G, Orre L, et al. Improved lung function and quality of life following increased elastic recoil after lung volume reduction surgery in emphysema. Respir Med 1998; 92:653–8.

129. Studer SM, Levy RD, McNeil K, Orens JB. Lung transplant outcomes; a review of survival, graft function, physiology, health-related quality of life and cost-effectiveness. Eur Respir J 2004; 24:674–85.

130. Levine SM, Anzueto A, Peters JI, et al. Medium term functional results of single-lung transplantation for endstage obstructive lung disease. Am J Respir Crit Care Med 1994; 150:398–402.

131. Kaiser LR, Cooper JD, Trulock EP, et al. The evolution of single lung transplantation for emphysema. J Thorac Cardiovasc Surg 1991; 102:333–41.

132. Patterson GA, Maurer JR, Williams TJ, Cardoso PG, Scavuzzo M, Todd TR. Comparison of outcomes of double and single lung transplantation for obstructive lung disease. J Thorac Cardiovasc Surg 1991; 101:623–32.

133. Low DE, Trulock EP, Kaiser LR, et al. Morbidity, mortality, and early results of single versus bilateral lung transplantation for emphysema. J Thorac Cardiovasc Surg 1992; 103:1119–26.

134. Cooper JD, Patterson GA, Trulock EP, Washington University Lung Transplant Group. Results of single and bilateral lung transplantaton in 131 consecutive recipients. J Thorac Cardiovasc Surg 1994; 107:460–71.

135. Mal H, Sleiman C, Jebrak G, et al. Functional results of single-lung transplantation for chronic obstructive lung disease. Am J Respir Crit Care Med 1994; 149:1476–81.

136. Briffa NP, Dennis C, Higenbottam T, et al. Single lung transplantation for end stage emphysema. Thorax 1995; 50:562–4.

137. Bjortuft O, Geiran OR, Fjeld J, Skovlund E, Johansen B, Boe J. Single lung transplantation for chronic obstructive pulmonary disease: pulmonary function and impact of bronchiolitis syndrome. Respir Med 1996; 90:553–9.

138. Bavaria JE, Kotloff R, Palevsky H, et al. Bilateral versus single lung transplantation for chronic obstructive pulmonary disease. J Thorac Cardiovasc Surg 1997; 113:520–8.

139. Brunsting LA, Lupinetti FM, Cascade PN, et al. Pulmonary function in single lung transplantation for chronic obstructive pulmonary disease. J Thorac Cardiovasc Surg 1994; 107:1337–45.

140. Cheriyan AF, Garrity ER, Pifarre R, Fahey PJ, Walsh JM. Reduced transplant lung volumes after single lung transplantation for chronic obstructive pulmonary disease. Am J Respir Crit Care Med 1995; 151:851–3.

141. Estenne M, Cassart M, Poncelet P, Gevenois PA. Volume of graft and native lung after single-lung transplantation for emphysema. Am J Respir Crit Care Med 1999; 159:641–5.

142. Boehler A, Estenne M. Post-transplant bronchiolitis obliterans. Eur Respir J 2003; 22:1007–18.

143. Chan A, Allen R. Bronchiolitis obliterans: an update. Curr Opin Pulm Med 2004; 10:133–41.

144. Estenne M, Maurer JR, Boehler A, et al. Bronchiolitis obliterans syndrome 2001: an update of the diagnostic criteria. J Heart Lung Transplant 2002; 21:297–310.

145. Al-Kattan K, Tadjkarimi S, Cox A, Banner N, Khagani A, Yacoub M. Evaluation of the long-term results of single versus Heart–lung transplantation for emphysema. J Heart Lung Transplant 1995; 14:824–31.

146. Snyder Laurie D, Palmer Scott M. Quality, quantity, or both? Life after lung transplantation Chest 2005; 128:1086–7.

147. Gerbase MW, Spiliopoulos A, Rochat T, Archinard M, Nicod LP. Health-related quality of life following single or bilateral lung transplantation: a 7-year comparison to functional outcome. Chest 2005; 128:1371–8.

148. Miyoshi S, Trulock EP, Schaefers HJ, Hsieh CM, Patterson GA, Cooper JD. Cardiopulmonary exercise testing after single and double lung transplantation. Chest 1990; 97:1130–6.

149. Gibbons WJ, Levine SM, Bryan CL, et al. Cardiopulmonary exercise responses after single lung transplantation for severe obstructive lung disease. Chest 1991; 100:106–11.

150. Williams TJ, Patterson GA, McClean PA, Zamel N, Maurer JR. Maximal exercise testing in single and double lung transplant recipients. Am Rev Respir Dis 1992; 145:101–5.

151. Levy RD, Ernst P, Levine SM, et al. Exercise performance after lung transplantation. J Heart Lung Transplant 1993; 12:27–33.

152. Orens JB, Becker FS, Lynch JP, III, Christensen PJ, Deeb GM, Martinez FJ. Cardiopulmonary exercise testing following allogeneic lung transplantation for different underlying disease states. Chest 1995; 107:144–9.

153. Schwaiblmair M, Reichenspurner H, Muller C, et al. Cardiopulmonary exercise testing before and after lung and Heart–lung transplantation. Am J Respir Crit Care Med 1999; 159:1277–83.

154. Kerber AC, Szidon P, Kesten S. Skeletal muscle dysfunction in lung transplantation. J Heart Lung Transplant 2000; 19:392–400.

155. Reinsma GD, ten Hacken NHT, Grevink RG, van der Bij W, Koeter GH, van Weert E. Limiting factors of exercise performance 1 year after lung transplantation. J Heart Lung Transplant 2006; 25:1310–6.

156. Williams TJ, Slater WR. Role of cardiopulmonary exercise testing in lung and Heart–lung transplantation. In: Weisman I, Zeballos R, eds. Clinical Exercise Testing. Basel: Karger, 2002:254–63 (Prog Respir Res).

157. Lands LC, Smountas AA, mesiano G, et al. Maximal exercise capacity and peripheral skeletal muscle function following lung transplantation. J Heart Lung Transplant 1999; 18:113–20.

158. Pantoja JG, Andrade FH, Stoki DS, Frost AE, Eschenbacher WL, Reid MB. Respiratory and limb muscle function in lung allograft recipients. Am J Respir Crit Care Med 1999; 160:1205–11.

159. Evans AB, Al-Himyary AJ, Hrovat MI, et al. Abnormal skeletal muscle oxidative capacity after lung transplantation by ^{31}P-MRS. Am J Respir Crit Care Med 1997; 155:615–21.

160. Tirdel GB, Girgis R, Fishman RS, Theodore J. Metabolic myopathy as a cause of the exercise limitation in lung transplant recipients. J Heart Lung Transplant 1998; 17:1231–7.
161. Wang XN, Williams TJ, McKenna MJ, et al. Skeletal muscle oxidative capacity, fiber type, and metabolites after lung transplantation. Am J Respir Crit Care Med 1999; 160:57–63.
162. McKenna MJ, Fraser SF, Li JL, et al. Impaired muscle Ca^{2+} and K^+ regulation contribute to poor exercise performance post-lung transplantation. J Appl Physiol 2003; 95:1606–16.
163. Hall MJ, Snell GI, Side EA, Esmore DS, Walters EH, Williams TJ. Exercise, potassium, and muscle deconditioning post-thoracic organ transplantation. J Appl Physiol 1994; 77:2784–90.
164. Hokanson JF, Mercier JG, Brooks GA. Cyclosporine A decreases rat skeletal muscle mitochondiral respiration in vitro. Am J Respir Crit Care Med 1995; 151:1848–51.
165. Mercier JG, Hokanson JF, Brooks GA. Effects of Cyclosporine A on skeletal muscle mitochondrial respiraton and endurance time in rats. Am J Respir Crit Care Med 1995; 151:1532–6.
166. Biring MS, Fournier M, Ross DJ, Lewis MI. Cellular adaptations of skeletal muscles to cyclosporin. J Appl Physiol 1998; 84:1967–75.
167. Cassivi SD, Meyers BF, Battafarano RJ, et al. Thirteen-year experience in lung transplantation for emphysema. Ann Thorac Surg 2002; 74:1663–9.
168. Gross CR, Savik K, Bolman RM, III, Hertz MI. Long-term health status and quality of life outcomes of lung transplant recipients. Chest 1995; 108:1587–93.
169. TenVergert EM, Essink-Bot ML, Geertsma A, van Enckevort PJ, de Boer WJ, van der Bij W. The effect of lung transplantation on health-related quality of life. A longitudinal study. Chest 1998; 113:358–64.
170. Cohen L, Littlefield C, Kelly P, Maurer J, Abbey S. Predictors of quality of life and adjustment after lung transplantation. Chest 1998; 113:633–44.
171. van Den Berg JW, Geertsma A, van der Bij W, et al. Bronchiolitis obliterans syndrome after lung transplantation and health-related quality of life. Am J Respir Crit Care Med 2000; 161:1937–41.
172. Anyanwu AC, McGuire A, Rogers CA, Murday AJ. Assessment of quality of life in lung transplantaion using a simple generic tool. Thorax 2001; 56:218–22.
173. Rodrigue JR, Baz MA, Kanasky WF, Jr., MacNaughton KL. Does lung transplantation improve health-related quality of life? The university of Florida experience J Heart Lung Transplant 2005; 24:755–63.
174. Rodrigue JR, Baz MA. Are there sex differences in health-related quality of life after lung transplantation for chronic obstructive pulmonary disease? J Heart Lung Transplant 2006; 25:120–5.
175. Rutherford RM, Fisher AJ, Hilton C, et al. Functional status and quality of life in patients surviving 10 years after lung transplantation. Am J Transplant 2005; 5:1099–104.
176. Martinez FJ, Chang A. Surgical therapy for chronic obstructive pulmonary disease. Semin Respir Crit Care Med 2005; 26:167–91.
177. www.thoracic.org/copd (last accessed February 17, 2007).
178. Gaensler EA, Jederlinic PJ, FitzGerald MX. Patient work-up for bullectomy. J Thorac Imaging 1986; 1:75–93.
179. Nakahara K, Nakaoka K, Ohno K, et al. Functional indications for bullectomy of giant bulla. Ann Thorac Surg 1983; 35:480–7.
180. Kinnear WJM, Tatterfield AE. Emphysematous bullae: surgery is best for large bullae and moderately impaired lung function. Br Med J 1990; 300:208–9.
181. Morgan MDL, Denison DM, Strickland B. Value of computed tomography for selecting patients with bullous lung disease for surgery. Thorax 1986; 41:855–62.
182. Carr DH, Pride NB. Computed tomography in pre-operative assessment of bullous emphysema. Clin Radiol 1984; 35:43–5.
183. Mehran RJ, Deslauriers J. Indications for surgery and patient work-up for bullectomy. Chest Surg Clin N Am 1995; 5:717–34.
184. Flaherty KR, Kazerooni EA, Martinez FJ. Differential diagnosis of chronic airflow obstruction. J Asthma 2000; 37:201–23.
185. Thurnheer R, Muntwyler J, Stammberger U, et al. Coronary artery disease in patients undergoing lung volume reduction surgery for emphysema. Chest 1997; 112:122–8.
186. Whyte RI, Bria W, Martinez FJ, Lewis P, Bolling SF. Combined lung volume reduction surgery and mitral valve reconstruction. Ann Thorac Surg 1998; 66:1414–6.
187. Schmid RA, Stammberger U, Hillinger S, et al. Lung volume reduction surgery combined with cardiac interventions. Eur J Cardiothorac Surg 1999; 15:585–91.
188. Lefrak SS, Yusen RD, Trulock EP, Pohl MS, Patterson A, Cooper JD. Recent advances in surgery for emphysema. Ann Rev Med 1997; 48:387–98.

189. Bach DS, Curtis JL, Christensen PJ, et al. Preoperative echocardiographic evaluation of patients referred for lung volume reduction surgery. Chest 1998; 114:972–80.
190. Bossone E, Martinez FJ, Whyte RI, Iannettoni MD, Armstrong WF, Bach DS. Dobutamine stress echocardiography for the preoperative evaluation of patients undergoing lung volume reduction surgery. J Thorac Cardiovasc Surg 1999; 118:542–6.
191. Scharf SM, Iqbal M, Keller C, et al. Hemodynamic characterization of patients with severe emphysema. Am J Respir Crit Care 2002; 166:314–22.
192. Thabut G, Dauriat G, Stern JB, et al. Pulmonary hemodynamics in advanced COPD candidates for lung volume reduction surgery or lung transplantation. Chest 2005; 127:1531–6.
193. Thurnheer R, Bingisser R, Stammberger U, et al. Effect of lung volume reduction surgery on pulmonary hemodynamics in severe pulmonary emphysema. Eur J Cardiothorac Surg 1998; 13:253–8.
194. Haniuda M, Kubo K, Fujimoto K, et al. Effects of pulmonary artery remodeling on pulmonary circulation after lung volume reduction surgery. Thorac Cardiovasc Surg 2003; 51:154–8.
195. Sciurba FC. Early and long-term functional outcomes following lung volume reduction surgery. Clin Chest Med 1997; 18:259–76.
196. Teschler H, Thompson AB, Stamatis G. Short- and long-term functional results after lung volume reduction surgery for severe emphysema. Eur Respir J 1999; 13:919–25.
197. Stoller JK, Gildea TR, Ries AL, Meli YM, Karafa MT, National Emphysema Treatment Trial Research Group. Lung volume reduction surgery in patients with emphysema and a-1 antitrypsin deficiency. Ann Thorac Surg 2007; 83:241–51.
198. Gelb AF, McKenna RJ, Brenner M, Fischel R, Zamel N. Lung function after bilateral lower lobe lung volume reduction surgery for a1-antitrypsin emphysema. Eur Respir J 1999; 14:928–33.
199. Tutic M, Bloch KE, Lardinois D, Brack T, Russi EW, Weder W. Long-term results after lung volume reduction surgery in patients with alpha-1 antitrypsin deficiency. J Thorac Cardiovasc Surg 2004; 128:408–13.
200. Mazolewski P, Turner JF, Baker M, Kurtz T, Little AG. The impact of nutritional status on the outcome of lung volume reduction surgery. A prospective study. Chest 1999; 116:693–6.
201. Nezu K, Yoshikawa M, Yoneda T, et al. The effect of nutritional status on morbidity in COPD patients undergoing bilateral lung reduction surgery. Thorac Cardiovasc Surg 2001; 49:216–20.
202. Naunheim KS, Hazelrigg SR, Kaiser LR, et al. Risk analysis for thoracoscopic lung volume reduction: a multi-institutional experience. Eur J Cardiothorac Surg 2000; 17:673–9.
203. Criner GJ, O'Brien G, Furukawa S, et al. Lung volume reduction surgery in ventilated-dependent COPD patients. Chest 1996; 110:877–84.
204. Naunheim KS, Wood DE, Krasna MJ, et al. Predictors of operative mortality and cardiopulmonary morbidity in the National Emphysema Treatment Trial. J Thorac Cardiovasc Surg 2006; 131:43–53.
205. McKenna RJ, Jr., Brenner M, Fischel RJ, et al. Patient selection criteria for lung volume reduction surgery. J Thorac Cardiovasc Surg 1997; 114:957–64 (discussion 964–7).
206. Gelb AF, Zamel N, McKenna RJ, Jr., Brenner M. Mechanism of short-term improvement in lung function after emphysema resection. Am J Respir Crit Care Med 1996; 154:945–51.
207. Ingenito EP, Loring SH, Moy ML, Mentzer SJ, Swanson SJ, Reilly JJ. Interpreting improvement in expiratory flows after lung volume reduction surgery in terms of flow limitation theory. Am J Respir Crit Care Med 2001; 163:1074–80.
208. Kim V, Criner GJ, Abdallah HY, Gaughan JP, Furukawa S, Solomides CC. Small airway morphometry and improvement in pulmonary function after lung volume reduction surgery. Am J Respir Crit Care Med 2005; 171:40–7.
209. Fessler HE, Permutt S. Lung volume reduction surgery and airflow limitation. Am J Respir Crit Care Med 1998; 157:715–22.
210. Leyenson V, Furukawa S, Kuzma AM, Cordova F, Travaline J, Criner GJ. Correlation of changes in quality of life after lung volume reduction surgery with changes in lung function, exercise, and gas exchange. Chest 2000; 118:728–35.
211. Brenner M, Kayaleh RA, Milne EN, et al. Thoracoscopic laser ablation of pulmonary bullae: radiographic selection and treatment response. J Thorac Cardiovasc Surg 1994; 107:883–90.
212. Szekely LA, Oelberg DA, Wright C, et al. Preoperative predictors of operative morbidity and mortality in COPD patients undergoing bilateral lung volume reduction surgery. Chest 1997; 111:550–8.
213. O'Brien GM, Furukawa S, Kuzma AM, Cordova F, Criner GJ. Improvements in lung function, exercise, and quality of life in hypercapnic COPD patients after lung volume reduction surgery. Chest 1999; 115:75–84.

214. Shade D, Jr., Cordova F, Lando Y, et al. Relationship between resting hypercapnia and physiologic parameters before and after lung volume reduction surgery in severe chronic obstructive pulmonary disease. Am J Respir Crit Care Med 1999; 159:1405–11.

215. Wisser W, Klepetko W, Senbaklavaci O, et al. Chronic hypercapnia should not exclude patients from lung volume reduction surgery. Eur J Cardiothorac Surg 1998; 14:107–12.

216. Mitsui K, Kurokawa Y, Kaiwa Y, et al. Thoracoscopic lung volume reduction surgery for pulmonary emphysema patients with severe hypercapnia. Jpn J Thorac Cardiovasc Surg 2001; 49:481–8.

217. Martinez FJ, Flaherty KR, Iannettoni M. Lung volume reduction surgery for emphysema. Chest Surg Clin N Am 2003; 13:669–85.

218. Gierada DS. Radiologic assessment of emphysema for lung volume reduction surgery. Semin Thorac Cardiovasc Surg 2002; 14:381–90.

219. Kazerooni EA. Radiologic evaluation of emphysema for lung volume reduction surgery. Clin Chest Med 1999; 20:845–61.

220. Goldin JG. Quantitative CT of the lung. Radiol Clin North Am 2002; 40:45–58.

221. Madani A, Keyzer C, Gevenois PA. Quantitative computed tomography assessment of lung structure and function in pulmonary emphysema. Eur Respir J 2001; 18:720–30.

222. Rogers RM, Coxson HO, Sciurba FC, Keenan RJ, Whittall KP, Hogg JC. Preoperative severity of emphysema predictive of improvement after lung volume reduction surgery: use of CT morphometry. Chest 2000; 118:1240–7.

223. Hunsaker AR, Ingenito EP, Reilly JJ, Costello P. Lung volume reduction surgery for emphysema: correlation of CT and V/Q imaging with physiologic mechanisms of improvement in lung function. Radiology 2002; 222:491–8.

224. Slone RM, Pilgram TK, Gierada DS, et al. Lung volume reduction surgery: comparison of preoperative radiologic features and clinical outcome. Radiology 1997; 204:685–93 (see comments).

225. Weder W, Thurnheer R, Stammberger U, Burge M, Russi EW, Bloch KE. Radiologic emphysema morphology is associated with outcome after surgical lung volume reduction. Ann Thorac Surg 1997; 64:313–20.

226. Wisser W, Klepetko W, Kontrus M, et al. Morphologic grading of the emphysematous lung and its relation to improvement after lung volume reduction surgery. Ann Thorac Surg 1998; 65:793–9.

227. Hamacher J, Bloch KE, Stammberger U, et al. Two years' outcome of lung volume reduction surgery in different morphologic emphysema types. Ann Thorac Surg 1999; 68:1792–8.

228. Wisser W, Senbaklavaci O, Ozpeker C, et al. Is long-term functional outcome after lung volume reduction surgery predictable? Eur J Cardiothorac Surg 2000; 17:666–72.

229. Pompeo E, Sergiacomi G, Nofroni I, Roscetti W, Simonetti G, Mineo TC. Morphologic grading of emphysema is useful in the selection of candidates for unilateral or bilateral reduction pneumoplasty. Eur J Cardiothorac Surg 2000; 17:680–6.

230. Bloch KE, Georgescu CL, Russi EW, Weder W. Gain and subsequent loss of lung function after lung volume reduction surgery in cases of severe emphysema with different morphologic patterns. J Thorc Cardiovasc Surg 2002; 123:845–54.

231. Sciurba FC. Preoperative predictors of outcome following lung volume reduction surgery. Thorax 2002; 57(Suppl. II):ii47–52.

232. Gierada DS, Slone RM, Bae KT, Yusen RD, Lefrak SS, Cooper JD. Pulmonary emphysema: comparison of preoperative quantitative CT and physiologic index values with clinical outcome after lung-volume reduction surgery. Radiology 1997; 205:235–42.

233. Nakano Y, Coxson HO, Bosan S, et al. Core to rind distribution of severe emphysema predicts outcome of lung volume reduction surgery. Am J Respir Crit Care Med 2001; 164:2195–9.

234. Coxson HO, Whittall KP, Nakano Y, et al. Selection of patients for lung volume reduction surgery using a power law analysis of the computed tomographic scan. Thorax 2003; 58:510–4.

235. Jamadar DA, Kazerooni EA, Martinez FJ, Whyte RI, Wahl RL. Semi-quantitative ventilation/perfusion scintigraphy and single photon emission computed tomography for evaluation of lung volume reduction surgery candidates: description and prediction of clinical outcome. Eur J Nuc Med 1999; 26:734–42.

236. Kotloff RM, Hansen-Flaschen J, Lipson DA, et al. Apical perfusion fraction as a predictor of short-term functional outcomes following bilateral lung volume reduction surgery. Chest 2001; 120:1609–15.

237. Wang SC, Fischer KC, Slone RM, et al. Perfusion scintigraphy in the evaluation for lung volume reduction surgery: correlation with clinical outcome. Radiology 1997; 205:243–8.

238. Hardoff R, Shitrit D, Tamir A, Steinmetz AP, Krausz Y, Kramer MR. Short- and long-term outcome of lung volume reduction surgery. The predictive value of the preoperative clinical status and lung scintigraphy. Respir Med 2006; 100:1041–9.
239. Cederlund K, Hogberg S, Jorfeldt L, et al. Lung perfusion scintigraphy prior to lung volume reduction surgery. Acta Radiol 2003; 44:246–51.
240. Orens JB, Estenne M, Arcasoy S, Conte JV, Corris P, Egan JJ, Egan T, Keshavjee S, Knoop C, Kotloff R, et al. International guidelines for the selection of lung transplant candidates: 2006 update—a consensus report from the pulmonary scientific council of the International Society for Heart and Lung Transplantation. J Heart Lung Transplant 2006; 25:745–55.
241. DeMeester J, Smits JMA, Persijn GG, Haverich A. Lung transplant waiting list: differential outcome of type of end-stage lung disease, one year after registration. J Heart Lung Transplant 1999; 18:563–71.
242. Demeester JD, Smits JMA, Persijn GG, Haverich A. Listing for lung transplantation: life expectancy and transplant effect, stratified by type of end-stage lung disease, the eurotransplant experience. J Heart Lung Transplant 2001; 20:518–24.
243. Hosenpud JD, Bennett LE, Keck BM, Edwards EB, Novick RJ. Effect of diagnosis on survival benefit of lung transplantation for end-stage lung disease. Lancet 1998; 351:24–7.
244. Charman SC, Sharples LD, McNeil KD, Wallwork J. Assessment of survival benefit after lung transplantation by patient diagnosis. J Heart Lung Transplant 2002; 21:226–32.
245. Stavem K, Bjortuft O, Borgan O, Geiran O, Boe J. Lung transplantation in patients with chronic obstructive pulmonary disease in a national cohort is without obvious survival benefit. J Heart Lung Transplant 2006; 25:75–84.
246. Madill J, Gutierrez C, Grossman J, et al. Nutritional assessment of the lung transplant patient: body mass index as a predictor of 90-day mortality following transplantation. J Heart Lung Transplant 2001; 20:288–96.
247. Culver DA, Mazzone PJ, Khandwala F, Blazey HC, DeCamp MM, Chapman JT. Discordant utility of ideal body weight and body mass index as predictors of mortality in lung transplant recipients. J Heart Lung Transplant 2005; 24:137–44.
248. Kanasky WF, Anton SD, Rodrigue JR, Perri MG, Szwed T, Baz MA. Impact of body weight on long-term survival after lung transplantation. Chest 2002; 121:401–6.
249. Tschopp O, Boehler A, Speich R, et al. Osteoporosis before lung transplantation: association with low body mass index, but not with underlying disease. Am J Transplant 2002; 2:167–72.
250. Shane E, Papadopoulos A, Staron RB, et al. Bone loss and fracture after lung transplantation. Transplantation 1999; 68:220–7.
251. Spira A, Gutierrez C, Chaparro C, Hutcheon MA, Chan CKN. Osteoporosis and lung transplantation: a prospective study. Chest 2000; 117:476–81.
252. Aris RM, Neuringer IP, Weiner MA, Egan TM, Ontjes D. Severe osteoporosis before and after lung transplantation. Chest 1996; 109:1176–83.
253. Martinez FJ, Kotloff R. Prognostication in chronic obstructive pulmonary disease: implications for lung transplantation. Semin Respir Crit Care Med 2001; 22:489–98.
254. Traver GA, Cline MG, Burrows B. Predictors of mortality in chronic obstructive pulmonary disease. A 15-year follow-up study. Am Rev Respir Dis 1979; 119:895–902.
255. Anthonisen NR, Wright EC, Hodgkin JE, IPPB Trial Group. Prognosis in chronic obstructive pulmonary disease. Am Rev Respir Dis 1986; 133:14–20.
256. Seersholm N, Dirksen A, Kok-Jensen A. Airway obstruction and two year survival in patients with severe alpha-1 antitrypsin deficiency. Eur Respir J 1994; 7:1985–7.
257. Seersholm N, Kok-Jensen A. Survival in relation to lung function and smoking cessation in patients with severe hereditary alpha1-antitrypsin deficiency. Am J Respir Crit Care Med 1995; 151:369–73.
258. The Alpha-1-Antitrypsin Deficiency Registry Study Group. Survival and FEV_1 decline in individuals with severe deficiency of a-1 antitrypsin. Am J Respir Crit Care Med 1998; 158:49–59.
259. Landbo C, Prescott E, Lange P, Vestbo J, Almdal TP. Prognostic value of nutritional status in chronic obstructive pulmonary disease. Am J Respir Crit Care Med 1999; 160:1856–61.
260. Gray-Donald K, Gibbons L, Shapiro SH, MacKlem PT, Martin JG. Nutritional status and mortality in chronic obstructive pulmonary disease. Am J Respir Crit Care Med 1996; 153:961–6.
261. Nishimura K, Izumi T, Tsukino M, Oga T, on Behalf of the Kansai COPD Registry and Research Group in Japan. Dyspnea is a better predictor of 5-year survival than airway obstruction in patients with COPD. Chest 2002; 121:1434–40.

262. Oga T, Nishimura K, Tsukino M, Sato S, Hajiro T. Analysis of the factors related to mortality in chronic obstructive pulmonary disease. Role of exercise capacity and health status. Am J Resp Crit Care Med 2002; 167:544–9.
263. Groenewegen KH, Schols AMWJ, Wouters E. Mortality and mortality-related factors after hospitalization for acute exacerbation of COPD. Chest 2003; 124:459–67.
264. Connors AF, Jr., Dawson NV, Thomas C, et al. Outcomes following acute exacerbation of severe chronic obstructive lung disease. Am J Respir Crit Care Med 1996; 154:959–67.
265. Egan TM, Murray S, Bustami RT, et al. Development of the new lung allocation system in the United States. Am J Transplant 2006; 6:1212–27.
266. Celli BR, Calverley PM, Rennard SI, et al. Proposal for a multidimensional staging system for chronic obstructive pulmonary disease. Respir Med 2005; 99:1546–54.
267. Celli BR, Cote CG, Marin JM, et al. The body-mass index, airflow obstruction, dyspnea, and exercise capacity index in chronic obstructive pulmonary disease. N Engl J Med 2004; 350:1005–12.
268. Martinez FJ, Foster G, Curtis JL, et al. Predictors of mortality in patients with emphysema and severe airflow obstruction. Am J Respir Crit Care Med 2006; 173:1324–36.
269. Burrows B, Bloom JW, Traver GA, Cline MG. The course and prognosis of different forms of chronic airways obstruction in a sample from the general population. N Engl J Med 1987; 317:1309–14.
270. Kazerooni EA, Chow LC, Whyte RI, Martinez FJ, Lynch JP. Preoperative examination of lung transplant candidates: value of chest CT compared with chest radiography. AJR Am J Roentgenol 1995; 165:1343–8.
271. Kazerooni EA, Hartker FW, Whyte RI, Martinez FJ, Lynch JP. Transthoracic needle aspiration in patients with severe emphysema. A study of lung transplant candidates. Chest 1996; 109:616–9.
272. Nathan SD. Lung transplantation. Disease-specific considerations for referral. Chest 2005; 127:1006–16.

23

Perioperative Medical Management for Patients with COPD: The Anesthesiologist's View

MARC LICKER and FRANÇOIS CLERGUE
Service d'Anesthésiologie, Hôpitaux Universitaires de Genève, Genève, Suisse

I. Introduction

A. COPD and Cardiovascular Disease in Surgical Patients

Nowadays, anesthesiologists are coping with larger numbers of high-risk respiratory patients as a consequence of prolonged life expectancy, increasing prevalence of chronic obstructive pulmonary disease (COPD) and greater needs for invasive diagnostic procedures and surgical interventions (1). The prevalence of COPD is even higher among some surgical candidates compared with age-matched population groups (e.g., 10–12% in cardiac surgery and 40% in thoracic surgery vs. 5–10% in the general population) (1–3). Since common risk factors (i.e., smoking, advanced age and sedentarity) are shared by both respiratory and cardiovascular diseases, a large proportion of COPD patients present with hypertension (34%), occlusive or aneurysmal arterial disease (12%), cardiac insufficiency (5%), arrhythmiac (4%), conduction blockade (10%), and/or ischemic heart disease (11%) (4,5).

Although mortality directly attributable to anesthesia is very low, probably around 1 in 250,000, the operative mortality risk averages 0.5% to 1%, paying a large tribute to myocardial infarction and heart failure, the leading causes of death in community-based populations (6–8). Not surprisingly, patients over the age of 40 are more likely to develop an acute coronary syndrome, heart failure, bronchopneumonia, or respiratory failure following major interventions, as a result of preexisting organ dysfunctions like ischemic heart disease, COPD, and renal insufficiency (9).

In the past, the clinical and prognostic relevance of postoperative pulmonary complications (PPCs) has been largely underestimated. Recent prospective cohort studies have highlighted that the incidence of respiratory failure (1–3%) and bronchopneumonia (1–5%) after noncardiac surgery was similar to the incidence of major cardiovascular complications (cardiac failure, 1–2%; myocardial infarction, 0–6%) (10–13). Both cardiac and pulmonary complications may concur in the same surgical patients (14). For instance, severe intraoperative bleeding directly increases the risk of myocardial ischemia/infarction, ventilator-induced pneumonia, sepsis and transfusion-related acute lung injury (ALI).

In addition to the short- and long-term death toll, both cardiac and pulmonary complications contribute significantly to hospital resource use, as a result of patient admission in intensive care units (ICUs), prolonged length of stay, application of "high-tech" monitoring tools, and use of expansive therapeutic treatment (15–17).

475

B. How to Define PPCs?

A prerequisite for assessing perioperative risk factors is a common agreement among clinicians on the most relevant criteria to describe specific disease conditions and outcome endpoints.

In the medical literature, the wide range in the incidence of PPCs (from 3% to 80%) reflects heterogenous population groups, inconsistencies in diagnostic or outcome endpoint definitions and incomplete data derived from retrospective studies (18,19). Although the development of respiratory dysfunction may lead to significant PPCs, it may also reflect the "natural" postoperative recovery processes. Transient and self-limiting reduction in spirometric values, impairment in respiratory muscle strength and mild alterations in gas exchange should be considered as part of the physiological responses to surgery. For instance, most patients undergoing cardiothoracic or abdominal operations present some degree of hypoxemia and diffuse microatelectasis that will barely impact on the postoperative clinical course. In contrast, pleural effusions, sustained bronchospasm or fever, lobar atelectasis, or hypoxemia, nonresponsive to supplemental oxygen may precede more serious adverse events like bronchopleural fistula, bronchopneumonia, ALI or respiratory failure requiring urgent medical interventions.

In an effort to standardize the reporting of adverse perioperative events, a group from the University Hospital of Zurich (Switzerland) has validated a five-grade scoring system based on the therapeutic consequences and residual disabilities related to surgical operations (20). Life-threatening complications requiring intermediate or intensive care facilities are distinguished from disorders treated on the ward. The duration of hospital stay is no longer used as a criterion for scaling morbidity but the need for pharmacological treatment or for any supportive/corrective interventions (physiotherapy, endoscopy, drainage, and re-interventions) and documentation of long-term disabilities are the cornerstones for objective ranking of postoperative complications (Table 1). Grade 1 complications include any deviation from the normal postoperative course with no need for medical interventions (except antiemetics, antipyretics, analgesics, electrolytes, and diuretics). Grades 2 and 3 involve complications requiring pharmacological treatment, blood transfusions or endoscopic, surgical or radiological interventions. Grade 4 includes life-threatening complications as well as single- or multiple organ failure requiring ICU admission; ultimately, Grade 5 relates to perioperative death. These objective and reliable outcome data are helpful to assess and improve quality of care and its cost efficiency (21).

Understanding the physiological response to surgical insults, identifying risk factors for mortality/morbidity and gaining control over health care processes are the preliminary steps before testing and implementing medical interventions aimed at improving postoperative outcome in COPD patients (22). Therefore, the first two parts of this review will be dedicated to the risk factors of postoperative cardiopulmonary complications and the respiratory consequences of surgery and anesthesia, irrespective of the presence or absence of COPD; then, we will propose guidelines for optimizing perioperative medical care in COPD patients. This chapter will mainly focus on the aspects of perioperative care, which specifically concern the anesthesiologist. The issue of operability in COPD subjects with lung cancer (or other potential indications of lung resection, e.g., aspergilloma) will not be specifically addressed; it requires an individual

Table 1 Grading of Postoperative Cardiopulmonary Complications

	Diagnostic criteria	Grade I	Grade II	Grade III	Grade IV
Cardiac Arrythmia	EKG, treatment with electrolytes, drugs an/or electrical shock	SVE, benign VE, sinus tachycardia, AF + electrolytes adjustment	+ Pharmacological treatment (anti-arrhythmic)	Tachyarrhythmia + electrical shock	Cardiac arrest + defibrillation and/or resuscitative maneuvers
Conduction blockade	EKG, treatment with pacemaker	AV 1st–2nd degree block	AV 2nd degree block (Wenckeback)	AV 3rd degree block + pacemaker	
Cardiac insufficiency	Chest X rays, drugs, echocardiography, ICU/HDU transfer, assist device	Asymptomatic	+ Diuretics, vasodilators	+ Transfer in HDU or ICU, inotropes	Low cardiac output syndrome, aortic balloon counterpulsation
Tampomade	Echocardiography, drainage			Pericardial drainage	Low cardiac output and drainage
Myocardial ischemia/infarct	EKG, troponin	Transient EKG changes: ST-segment, T wave	Troponin 0.1–1.5 ng/mL	Troponin > 1.5 ng	Troponin > 1.5 ng, unstable angina, arrhythmias, low cardiac output
Pulmonary Atelectasis	Chest X rays, CT-scan, treatment	+ Chest physiotherapy	+ CPAP	+ Bronchial fibroscopy	+ Respiratory failure
Bronchopneumonia	Temperature, WBC count, bacteriology, treatment		+ Antibiotics, on the ward	+ Antibiotics and supportive respiratory treatment	

(Continued)

Table 1 Grading of Postoperative Cardiopulmonary Complications (*Continued*)

	Diagnostic criteria	Grade I	Grade II	Grade III	Grade IV
Hypoxemia	SpO_2, PaO_2, $A\text{-}aDO_2$, PaO_2/FIO_2, chest X rays treatment	+Oxygen therapy	+Oxygen therapy	$PaO_2/FIO_2 < 220$+NIV ALI/ARDS	$PaO_2/FIO_2 < 220$+ intubation, mechanical ventilation, ALI/ARDS
Respiratory failure	Need for ventilatory support			+NIV	Intubation, mechanical ventilation
Bronchopleural fistula	Bronchoscopy, treatment		+Endoscopic treatment	+Surgical closure, empyema	
Pleural effusion	chest X rays, drainage	Mild	+Thoracic drainage		

Abbreviations: AF, atrial fibrillation; ALI, acute lung injury; ARDS, adult respiratory distress syndrome; AV, atrioventricular; CPAP, continuous positive airway pressure; CT, computed tomography; EKG, electrocardiogram; HDU, high dependency unit; ICU, intensive care unit; NIV, non-invasive ventilatory techniques; SVE, supra-ventricular extrasystole; VE, ventricular extrasystole.

Source: Adapted from Ref. 20.

multidisciplinary risk–benefit assessment involving the anesthesiologist as well as surgeons, respiratory physicians and oncologists.

II. Risk Factors for Postoperative Mortality and Cardiopulmonary Morbidity

A. Risk Stratification

Following major advances in surgical and anesthetic management, the operative mortality and morbidity rates have been considerably lowered over the past 20 years. For instance, after aortic abdominal reconstruction, operative mortality has dropped from 10% in the eighties to less than 3% in most reference hospital centers (23,24). In that context, the influence of patient- and procedure-related risk factors (e.g., age, sex, body mass index, smoking habit, pulmonary status, type and duration of anesthesia, surgical site) needs to be thoroughly re-evaluated with regard to their impact on postoperative cardiac and pulmonary outcomes.

Cardiac Risk Stratification

In 1999, Lee et al. (25). analyzed a large surgical database and identified five independent risk factors for major postoperative cardiac complications: (*i*) evidence for coronary artery disease, (*ii*) history of cerebrovascular disease (stroke, ischemic attack), (*iii*) moderate-to-severe renal insufficiency (serum creatinine greater than 180 μmol/L), (*iv*) diabetes mellitus, and (*v*) high-risk surgery (chest, abdominal, pelvic vascular). After further validation in other prospective studies (26–28), these five items have been incorporated in a Revised Cardiac Risk Index (RCRI) that has been adopted by the American College of Cardiology and American Heart Association (9,29).

Combined with the assessment of exercise tolerance [using metabolic equivalent (MET) scoring; 1 MET = basal metabolic rate], the RCRI is most useful to identify patients who should undergo further cardiac testing [i.e., stress echocardiography or electrocardiogram (EKG), myocardial scintigraphy, coronary angiography] and those who might benefit from preoperative revascularization and perioperative cardiac protective techniques (i.e., β-blockers, anti-agregants, statines) (30–32).

Importantly, recent data indicate that the risk-adjusted mortality following noncardiac surgery is much higher in patients with aortic stenosis (10–28%) or heart failure (11.7%) than in those with coronary artery disease (6.6%) (28,33–35). Degeneration and calcification of aortic cusps increases with age (the impairment occurring faster in patients with a bicuspid aortic valve), whereas heart failure is mainly the end stage of hypertensive, coronary, and valvular diseases. Because of the increase in life expectancy with modern therapies, the burden of these cardiovascular diseases is growing in COPD patients. Among adults older than 65 years, 2% to 9% suffer from aortic valve stenosis and the prevalence of congestive heart failure is 8% to 12% (36,37).

Hence, echocardiographic examination is mandatory in patients with poor exercise tolerance (<4 MET) and/or a history of acute pulmonary edema or abnormal clinical signs (heart murmur, fine crackles in basal lung areas, distended neck veins, peripheral edema). In addition, given the risk of sudden death and acute heart failure, postponing of elective surgery is obviously advisable in patients with recent cardiac symptoms (syncope, *angina pectoris*) and even in asymptomatic patients with high-grade aortic stenosis (mean transvalvular gradient >50 mmHg or valvular area <0.5 cm^2/m^2) (38). For those with heart failure [New York Heart Association (NYHA) class 3 and 4], lesser invasive and traumatic procedures should be preferentially selected and medical treatment should be carefully optimized by combining the administration of several drugs such as angiotensin converting enzyme inhibitors, angiotensin II receptor antagonists, β-blockers and/or diuretics (37). In selected cases of heart failure (e.g., bundle branch conduction blockade), ventricular re-synchronization with multi-lead electrical stimulation might improve short-term perioperative outcome as it has been shown to enhance cardiac performances while improving functional status (39).

Pulmonary Risk Factors

In two prospective studies, a Canadian group questioned the utility of preoperative respiratory-specific clinical assessment and lung function testing to predict the occurrence of PPCs (pneumonia, atelectasis requiring fibroscopy, mechanical ventilation, pneumothorax or pleural effusion requiring drainage) (2,40). Only 8% of surgical candidates were referred by the anesthesiologists to the internist's consultation and the occurrence of PPCs was related to five independent variables: age >65 years [Odds Ratio (OR) 5.9], a positive cough test (OR 3.8), smoking >40 pack-years (OR 1.9), the presence of a nasogastric tube (OR 7.7) and prolonged duration of anesthesia >2.5 hours (OR 3.3). The major limitations of these prospective investigations were related to the relatively small size of the population sample ($N = 1055$ and 272 patients), the low incidence of PPCs (2.8% and 8%) and the exclusion of patients with a high respiratory risk (e.g., sleep apnea syndrome, neuromuscular disease and severe COPD requiring a planned admission in ICU).

The first pulmonary risk indices predicting the occurrence of pneumonia and respiratory failure have been validated by analyzing two cohorts including more than 160,000 veterans undergoing noncardiac surgery (41,42). A pulmonary risk score was built by assigning points to several predictors of pneumonia (14 variables) and respiratory failure (12 variables; Table 2). The major contributors to PPCs were an advanced age (>70 years), the type of surgery (vascular, thoracic), the presence of COPD, renal failure or poor nutritional status as well as significant intraoperative blood loss (>4 units packed blood cells).

To date, the most useful information for preoperative pulmonary risk stratification has been gathered in a recent systematic review including 145 studies (cohort and case-control studies, case-series and randomized controlled trials) of whom 27 reported multivariate analysis. The overall incidence of PPC was 6.8% (ranging from 2% to 19%) (43). Not surprisingly, these clinical studies were heterogenous regarding the sample size (median: 148 patients per group), the study objectives, the definitions of PPC and the inclusion criteria. In contrast with cardiac risk stratification where the extent of coronary artery disease largely determines postoperative cardiac outcome, procedure-related risk factors largely dominate patient's related comorbidities to predict PPCs. Peripheral and orthopedic procedures are considered low-risk procedures whereas surgical interventions involving the thorax, the upper abdomen as well as the head and neck regions are more likely to interfere with respiratory function, particularly in the context of stress-induced immunodepression, large fluid administration, multiple transfusion and inadequate pain control. Among

Table 2 General Health Status Assessment

Variables	Class I	Class II	Class III	Class IV	Class V
ASA	Normal healthy, without organic, physiologic, or psychiatric disorders	Controlled medical condition without systemic effects (smoking without COPD, anemia, >70 yrs)	Medical condition with systemic effects and/or functional compromise (stable angina or heart failure, moderate BPCO)	Poorly controlled-medical condition potentially life-threatening (e.g., unstable angina, severe COPD)	Moribund, expected to survive less than 24 hrs postoperatively
Duke Activity Status Index	>8 MET run, swim, play tennis	5–7 MET yardwork, climb 4 flight of stairs	2–4 MET light housework, <3 flights of stairs	<2 MET walking 1–2 blocks, climb 1–2 flights of stairs, bedbound	

Abbreviations: ASA, American Society of Anesthesiologist; BPCO, chronic airflow obstruction; COPD, chronic obstructive pulmonary disease; MET, metabolic equivalent (1 ME = basal oxygen consumption).

patient-related predictors, the following items were found to be independently associated with PPCs: (*i*) advanced age (>70 years), (*ii*) the American Society of Anesthesiologist (ASA) physical status classification (ASA class ≥ 2), (*iii*) a history of congestive heart failure, (*iv*) the presence of COPD, (*v*) a poor functional status, and (*vi*) a low blood albumin level (<35 g/L) (Table 3).

B. Specific Risk Factors for Pulmonary Complications

COPD

Exacerbation of bronchial inflammation, stress-induced depression of the immune system and the increased muscular work of breathing during the postoperative period are thought to precipitate the onset of respiratory dysfunction leading to PPCs. Although cohort studies have demonstrated acceptable operative risk in COPD patients (44), the risk of PPCs (except atelectasis) parallels the severity of respiratory impairment [moderate, if forced expiratory volume in one second (FEV_1) 50–80%; severe, if FEV_1 <50%], particularly in patients with abnormal clinical findings (decreased breath sounds, wheezes, ronchi, prolonged expiration) and/or severe impairment of gas exchange (hypercarbia, hypoxemia requiring supplemental oxygen) (45–51). The worst prognosis is expected in cases of cor pulmonale and/or chronically fatigued respiratory muscles, leading to right heart failure and difficulties to wean from the ventilator (35,52).

In patients undergoing lung resection, a FEV_1 below 60% has been shown to carry a two to threefold increased risk for operative mortality and PPCs; besides the severity of COPD, the extent of lung resection, the presence of bronchial colonization and male sex are predictors of postoperative pneumonia (3,53). Besides, COPD patients have a two-to-three fold increased risk to develop noncardiogenic edema or post-pneumonectomy lung edema, a particular form of ALI (54). Major lung resection, a depressed antioxidant status (due to chemotherapy or chronic alcohol consumption), impaired lymphatic drainage and surgery-induced upregulation of inflammatory processes all render COPD patients more vulnerable to shear stress-related injuries at the alveolar-capillary membrane, as a result of mechanical positive pressure ventilation and/or excessive intravascular fluid loading.

Asthma

Recent asthma symptoms, current use of anti-asthma drugs and history of tracheal intubation for asthma have all been associated with the development of PPCs. In contrast, those patients with well-controlled asthma have a similar risk of PPCs than patients without asthma, regardless of the type of anesthesia (55). In Warner's study of over 1500 asthmatic patients, the rate of PPCs was similar for general and regional anesthesia, refuting the belief that regional anesthetic techniques were safer (56). Although infrequently associated with major PPCs, sustained or unrecognized bronchospasm induced by airway instrumentation can lead to life-threatening hypoxemia and its overzealous treatment with β-adrenergic agonists can cause fatal ventricular arrhythmias. In the closed claim study of the ASAs, severe bronchospasm resulted in death or irreversible brain damage in 90% of cases charged because of intraoperative respiratory problems (57).

Table 3 Multivariate Risk Indices for Postoperative Pneumonia, Respiratory Failure, and Cardiac Complications

Variables	Odds ratio (95% Cl) for PPC	Points for pneumonia	Points for respiratory failure	Odds ratio (95% Cl) for cardiac complications
Surgery type/site				
AAA repair	6.9 (2.7–17.4)	15	27	2.8 (1.6–4.9)
Thoracic	4.2 (2.9–6.2)	14	21	2.8 (1.6–4.9)
Neurosurgery	2.5 (1.8–3.5)	8	14	
Upper abdominal	2.9 (2.3–3.6)	10	14	2.8 (1.6–4.9)
Vascular	2.2 (1.8–2.7)	3	14	2.8 (1.6–4.9)
Head and neck	1.5 (1.3–1.7)	8	11	
Emergency surgery	2.2 (1.6–3.1)	3	11	
Prolonged surgery	2.3 (1.4–3.5)			
General anesthesia	1.8 (1.4–2.5)	4		
Transfusion > 4 units		4		
Age 60–69	2.1 (1.6–2.6)			
Age 70–79	3.0 (2.1–4.4)	13	6	
Age > 80		17	NA	
COPD	1.8 (1.4–2.2)	5	6	
Coronary artery disease		NA	NA	2.4 (1.3–4.2)
History of cardiac failure	2.9 (1.0–8.0)	NA	NA	1.9 (1.1–3.5)
History of stroke/TIA		4		3.2 (1.3–6.0)
Renal insufficiency[a]		3	8	3.0 (1.4–6.8)
ASA ≥ 3	2.6 (1.7–3.8)			
Functional dependency		10	7	
Weight loss 10%		7	NA	
Altered sensorium		4		
Smoking (< 1 yr)	1.3 (1.0–1.6)	3		
Steroid treatment		3		
Alcohol (≥ 2 drinks)		2		
Albumin < 3 g/dL	2.5	NA	9	

(Continued)

Table 3 Multivariate Risk Indices for Postoperative Pneumonia, Respiratory Failure, and Cardiac Complications (*Continued*)

Risk class (total)	Risk for pneumonia (%)	Risk for respiratory failure (%)
Class 1		
10–15 for pneumonia	0.24	
≤10 for resp. failure		0.50
Class 2		
16–25 for pneumonia	1.19	
11–19 for resp. failure		2.10
Class 3		
26–40 for pneumonia	4.0	
20–27 for resp. failure		5.3
Class 4		
41–55 for pneumonia	9.4	
28–40 for resp. failure		11.9
Class 5		
≥55 for pneumonia	15.8	
≥40 for resp. failure		30.9

[a] BUN >30 mg/dL (respiratory failure or pneumonia), creatinine >2 mg/dL (cardiac complications).
Abbreviations: AAA, aortic abdominal aneurysm; ASA, American Society of Anesthesiologist; CI, confidence interval; COPD, chronic obstructive pulmonary disease; PPC, postoperative pulmonary complication; TIA, transient ischemic attack.
Source: Adapted from Refs. 27–29, 41–43.

General Anesthesia

General anesthetic (GA) agents are known to interfere with respiratory muscle activity, central ventilatory drive as well as cellular components within the airways and alveolar compartments. The combined effects of supine position, GA and thoracic/abdominal incision are responsible for significant reduction in the functional residual capacity (FRC) and occurrence of atelectasis in the most dependent parts of the lung (58). Moreover, residual neuromuscular blockade persisting after anesthesia has been incriminated in deficient coughing and "silent" gastric content inhalation (59).

General anesthesia exceeding four hours has been identified as a strong predictor of PPCs (41,42,60). Indeed, prolonged exposure to GA agents may alter the immune status and gas exchange capacity by several mechanisms: decrease in the number and activity of alveolar macrophages, inhibition of the release of surfactant, increased permeability of the alveolar-capillary membrane, activation of the alveolar nitric-oxide synthase and cytokine inflammatory response, slowing of the muco-ciliary clearance and enhanced sensitivity of the pulmonary vasculature to neurohumoral mediators.

Upper airway instrumentation due to tracheal intubation and inhaled irritants (i.e., desflurane, disinfectants) may trigger vagally mediated reflex bronchoconstriction promoting expiratory collapse of the peripheral airways and incomplete lung alveolar emptying (61,62). Besides impaired gas exchange, lung hyperinflation with intrinsic positive end-expiratory pressure (PEEP) decreases systemic venous return, restricts cardiac filling and compromises cardiac performances according to the Franck–Starling relationship (63).

Obstructive Sleep Apnea Syndrome

A preoperative history of snoring or apnea during sleep and abnormalities in the oropharynx (large tonsils, retrognathia, maxillary hypoplasia) are strongly evocative of obstructive sleep apnea syndrome (OSAS), particularly in obese subjects. These individuals may also present difficulties with upper airway instrumentation (64).

Cardiovascular diseases such as hypertension, arrhythmias, congestive heart failure, coronary heart disease and stroke are often associated with OSAS. The occurrence of hypoxic episodes has been correlated with a greater propensity for ischemic myocardial and cerebral events. Very low concentrations of anesthetics [0.1 minimal alveolar concentration, (MAC)], sedatives and opiates may worsen obstructive sleep apnea (OSA) by decreasing pharyngeal muscle tone and attenuating the ventilatory and arousal responses to hypercarbia and upper airway obstruction (65,66). Accordingly, within the first days after surgery, patients with OAS are at greater risk for cardiac and cerebral ischemic damages secondary to repeated and prolonged hypoxemic events.

Age

After adjustment for concomitant illnesses, advanced age (>70 years) remains an independent predictor of operative mortality, PPCs and cardiac morbidity (67). The loss of physiological reserve and "silent" organ dysfunction make the elderly prone to develop cardiopulmonary complications when facing surgical or traumatic insults. For instance, the airway closing volume increases with age, as does the perfusion in lung units with low ventilation/perfusion ratios (V_A/Q), resulting in an increased venous admixture with, in turn, deterioration in blood oxygenation (58). Surprisingly, formation of atelectasis is independent of age, with children and teenagers showing as much atelectasis as elderly patients (68).

Obesity

Premature collapse of peripheral airways is most likely to occur in obese patients because of the restrictive ventilatory pattern and the elevated closing airway volume (69,70). Although the reduction in FRC facilitates the formation of atelectasis and aggravates postoperative hypoxemia, clinical investigations have consistently failed to document any association between mild-to-moderate obesity and severe PPCs, except in the subset of patients with OSA. In morbidly obese patients undergoing abdominal surgery (body mass index > 35 kg/m^2), the rate of atelectasis and pneumonia taken together is 29.3%, with an adjusted odds ratio of 2.8 [95% confidence interval (CI) 1.7–4.8] compared with non-obese patients (71). In addition to lung function impairment, the postoperative period is more frequently complicated with wound infection, venous thrombosis and pulmonary embolism in overweight patients.

General Status and Physical Fitness

The 5-grade ASA classification is applied worldwide by all anesthesiologists. This physical status scoring system was originally designed to estimate the risk of operative mortality. Subsequently, a number of studies have extended its use to predict postoperative outcome: patients belonging to ASA classes 3 and 4 being at higher risk for cardiopulmonary complications than ASA 1 and 2 patients (Table 2) (72).

Similarly, simple information from the patient's history and clinical examination such as altered senses, inability to climb at least two flights of stairs, and functional dependency (i.e., need for assistance in daily living) has been shown to be predictive of major postoperative cardiopulmonary complications. More sophisticated physiological assessment such as the determination of the anerobic threshold during exercise (maximal oxygen consumption, VO_2 max) and the six-minutes walking test also provides valuable prognostic information in borderline patients (73). Before lung resection, a VO_2 max less than 15 mL/kg per min, a walking distance less than 300 m or the inability to climb four flights of stairs are more effective than spirometric variables to predict cardiopulmonary complications. Besides compromised cardiac and pulmonary physiological reserves, severe reduction in exercise capacity may also reflect muscular deconditioning associated with chronic debilitating illnesses.

Smoking

Cigarette smoke contains more than 1000 components with wide-ranging effects on pulmonary, cardiovascular and immune functions, wound healing, hemostasis, drug metabolism and patient mental status, all of which influence the postoperative outcome (74–77). Smoking status is a consistent univariate risk factor for cardiac adverse events and a variety of pulmonary adverse events such as bronchospasm, laryngospasm, cough, and hypoxemia requiring ICU admission. In observational studies using multivariate analysis, current smoking (≥ 20 units pack year) has been identified as a modest risk factor for serious PPCs (OR 1.26 with 95% CI, 1.01–1.56) and tissue-healing problems but not for cardiac complications, although smoking behavior obviously influences the progression of vascular atheromatosis and long-term survival (43). Not only active smoking but also passive exposure to tobacco smoke in children and adults has been found to increase the risk of intra- and postoperative respiratory problems and even to prolong the effects of neuromuscular blocking agents (78,79).

Several mechanisms make smokers more susceptible to develop PPCs: excessive production of mucus, increased sensitivity of upper airways reflexes to chemical or anesthetic irritants (e.g., desflurane), slowed bronchial mucus clearance, alteration in surfactant synthesis, increase in pulmonary epithelial permeability as well as impaired macrophage, and natural killer cytotoxic activity. The number of pack years and the timing of smoking cessation may influence both the sensitivity and reactivity of the tracheobronchial tree, mucociliary transport, and the risk of PPCs (49,80). The impaired healing and increased dehiscence of anastomosis may result from the limited availability of oxygen within the healing tissues and the antiproliferative effects of nicotine on red blood cells, fibroblasts, and macrophages.

Interestingly, the dose requirements for anesthetic induction and postoperative opiate analgesia are slightly higher in smokers compared with non-smokers, whereas the incidence of nausea and vomiting is lower (Lysakowsky C. et al. Anaesthesia 2006 in press) (81,82). Although increased baseline stress is often reported among smokers, changes in perceived stress over the perioperative period and acute withdrawal symptoms are unrelated to the current smoking status (77,83).

Alcohol

A twofold increased risk of ALI has been observed among heavy alcohol consumers (more than 60 g of ethanol per day) admitted to medical ICU and those undergoing lung resection, compared with alcohol-free patients (54). Experimental data indicate that ethanol causes depletion of the pulmonary antioxidant glutathione, which in turn leads to decreased surfactant production, impaired alveolar liquid clearance, and alterations in epithelial cell permeability (84–86). Moreover, chronic alcoholics have a greater vulnerability to postoperative bleeding and infectious complications, as a consequence of (*i*) an impaired immune status (as exhibited by, e.g., a decrease in interleukin-6 to interleukin-10 ratio), (*ii*) nutritional deficits, and (*iii*) possible microaspiration in the context of autonomic neural dysfunction and alcohol withdrawal syndrome (87,88).

III. Respiratory Consequences of Anesthesia and Surgery

A. Anesthetic Techniques and Respiratory Function

Respiratory Mechanics and GA

In awake supine subjects, the contraction of the inspiratory muscles causes lung expansion and a downward shift of the diaphragm whereas during passive expiration, the diaphragm moves cranially as a result of lung elastic recoil, relaxation of the inspiratory muscles, and the hydrostatic pressure gradient generated by the abdominal content. Following induction of anesthesia,with or without muscular paralysis, all respiratory muscles being relaxed, there is a fall in FRC with a consistent cephalic shift of the dependent part of the diaphragm while the nondependent part slightly moves downwards or remains at the same position (Fig. 1) (89). With mechanical ventilation, the positive transpulmonary pressure causes the greatest displacement of the nondependent part, although with large tidal volume, all parts of the diaphragm move equally ("piston-like" motion). These anesthesia-induced diaphragmatic changes have been observed in healthy subjects as well as in COPD patients (90).

Using computed tomography (CT) and radiological chest imaging, atelectasis has been shown to develop in almost 90% of anesthetized patients, involving as much as 5% to 20% of the total lung area, predominantly in its dependent parts (58). By changing the position from upright to supine in healthy adults, the FRC is reduced by 0.8 to 1.0 L and there is a further decrease by 0.4 to 0.5 L after the induction of anesthesia. The reduction in FRC (from 3.5 to 2 L, near the residual volume) corresponds to the formation of atelectasis and areas of low ventilation–perfusion ratio (Fig. 1) that in turn reduce the compliance of the respiratory system (from a mean of 95 to 60 mL/cm H_2O) (58). Not surprisingly, the size of the atelectatic area has been shown to correlate with the decrease in FRC and with the arterial oxygen desaturation (91).

Some of the collapsed areas persist in the postoperative period and are compounded by limited respiratory motion due to insufficient pain control, injuries of respiratory muscles and/or neurally mediated diaphragmatic dysfunction after manipulation of abdominal viscera or intrathoracic interventions. Furthermore, increased "stiffness" of the thoracic/abdominal compartments and increased airway resistance due to lower lung volumes after major surgical procedures contribute to increase the work of breathing (58).

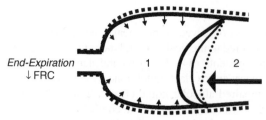

End-Expiration
↓FRC

1. Elastic lung recoil (passive; *small arrows*)
2. Abdominal forces (viscera, muscle contraction; *large arrow*)

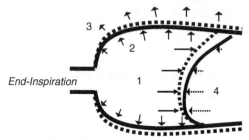

End-Inspiration

1. Contraction of inspiratory muscles
2. Mechanical ventilation (*small arrows*)
3. Elastic wall recoil (passive)
4. Abdominal forces (viscera, muscle contraction/tone)

Figure 1 Thoracic wall and diaphragmatic motion during breathing in awake (dotted line) and anesthetized (continuous line) subjects. *Abbreviation*: FRC, functional residual capacity.

GA Agents

GA agents modulate the respiratory function at three key levels: (*i*) the central medullar command and the neural reflex ventilatory pathways, (*ii*) the airways smooth muscle tone and mucociliary clearance, and (*iii*) the hypoxic pulmonary vasoconstriction (HPV) which controls the distribution of blood flow.

Hypnotic drugs, local anesthetics, and opiates attenuate both the central and peripheral chemosensitive reflexes, which induces a dose-dependent depression of the hypoxic and hypercapnic ventilatory responses (92–94). Given the preexistent impairment in carbon dioxide sensing mechanisms and surgical-induced alterations in sleeping patterns, patients with COPD, OAS, or genetic predisposition to a blunted carbon dioxide response are prone to develop episodes of apnea immediately after anesthesia and within the first days following major surgery (95). Thus, these higher-risk patients should be closely monitored (e.g., with pulse oximetry, respiratory frequency, and blood gas analysis) in step-down units where the effects of centrally acting sedative and analgesic drugs will be titrated to optimize patient's comfort while detecting sustained hypoxemia and the occurrence of apnea.

Inhalational anesthetic agents (halothane, isoflurane, desflurane, and sevoflurane) have been shown to induce direct relaxation of bronchial and vascular smooth muscle (96). In patients with bronchospastic disease, the beneficial effect of anesthesia-induced bronchodilatation resulting in reduced airway resistance and improved ventilation/ perfusion (V/Q) ratio outweighs the mild increase in intrapulmonary shunting due to partial inhibition of the HPV response. In isolated lung preparations with lobar atelectasis or hypoxic ventilation, volatile anesthetics given at twice the minimum alveolar concentration (2 MAC) have been shown to decrease the HPV response by 50% if the pulmonary flow was maintained constant; in these experimental conditions, redistribution of pulmonary blood flow towards poorly oxygenated regions contributes to widen the alveolar-arterial oxygen gradient (PA-aO$_2$) and to lower the arterial oxygen content (97). In clinical practice, only mild impairment in blood gas exchange are observed under inhalational anesthesia (with 1–1.5 MAC), because the direct anesthesia-induced inhibition of the HPV response is partially opposed by the reduced mixed venous oxygen pressure resulting from the negative inotropic effects of anesthesia (98). Of note, neither the bronchial smooth muscle activity nor the HPV response is influenced by hypnotics and local anesthetics.

Myorelaxants

As already mentioned, residual neuromuscular blockade is an independent predictor of PPCs and has been incriminated in alveolar hypoventilation and silent gastric regurgitation with microaspiration. Indeed, mild blockade of the muscarinic receptors with myorelaxants has been shown to attenuate the ventilatory response to hypoxia and to impair the contraction capacity of the pharyngo-laryngeal muscles, thereby interfering with the control of upper airways (99). In addition, volatile anesthetic agents and several pharmacological agents (e.g., magnesium and aminoglycosides) are known to enhance the effects of myorelaxants at the neuromuscular endplate by lowering the neural release of acetylcholine, inducing conformational change within the cholinergic receptor and/or altering intramuscular signaling (92,93,100–102). Prolonged neuromuscular blockade is also anticipated when long acting myorelaxants have been repeatedly administered, in patients with defective clearance pathways (hepatic or renal insufficiency) or neuromuscular disorders (i.e., myasthenia or, more often, deconditioning).

Regional Anesthesia

Spinal and epidural anesthesia at the lumbar level have no significant effects on respiratory function, except in morbidly obese patients where the neuraxial blockade has been shown to produce a 20% to 25% fall in forced expiratory volumes [FEV$_1$, forced vital capacity (FVC)] that may be associated with inefficient cough and inability to clear bronchial secretions (103–105).

With thoracic epidural analgesia (TEA) using high concentrations of local anesthetics (lidocaine 2%, bupivacaine 0.5%), paralysis of the intercostal and abdominal wall muscles are responsible for mild decreases in inspiratory and expiratory capacity (−16% to −20%) without affecting the HPV and the ventilatory response to hypoxia and hypercarbia (106,107). As far as the neuraxial blockade remains below the cervical level, the diaphragmatic function is unimpeded because the phrenic nerves originate at the cervical level (C3–C5). Interestingly, TEA conducted with lower concentrations of local anesthetics (lidocaine 0.5%, bupivacaine 0.1%) has been shown to decrease the airway resistance while minimizing the work of breathing and sparing the abdominal expiratory muscles in severe COPD patients (108). In addition to improvements in respiratory mechanics and optimization of pain control, TEA directly suppresses the sympathetic neural output, reduces by 20% the hypnotic requirements and has cardiac protective effects by improving coronary blood flow, lowering myocardial oxygen consumption, attenuating the platelet hyperaggregability, and raising the arrhythmic threshold (109–112).

Given the differential sensitivity of spinal and radicular nerves to anesthetic blockade, low concentrations of local anesthetics are preferentially combined with low doses of opiates in order to block afferent nociceptive inputs and efferent sympathetic output while preserving respiratory muscular activity, bronchial tone and HPV responses (107,113). In thoracic and upper abdominal surgery, continuous adminis-tration of a local anesthetics/opiate mixture via the thoracic epidural routes is currently the best strategy for dynamic pain control and modulation of the catabolic phase allowing early ambulation, oral feeding, and functional recovery (114–117).

Regarding peripheral nerve blockade, the supraclavicular techniques (i.e., intercalene) are contraindicated in patients with severe pulmonary disease since paralysis of the ipsilateral hemidiaphragm occurs in 100% of cases with consequent limitations of lung volumes (mean: -32% FEV_1, -30% FVC) (118). Preliminary studies have reported that the infraclavicular techniques,except the modified Raj approach, also produce mild-to-moderate impairment in respiratory function (119,120).

Interestingly, following systemic reabsorption, local anesthetics have been shown to exert mild stimulating ventilatory effects while reducing perception of nociceptive inputs (121).

B. Blood Gas Exchange

Despite the administration of 30% to 40% oxygen in the inspired gas, the $PA\text{-}aO_2$ gradient increases during GA, regardless of the type of anesthetic agent and the mode of ventilation (spontaneous or mechanically controlled). Breathing of pure oxygen may even further increase $PA\text{-}aO_2$ by promoting alveolar collapse as oxygen is transferred from poorly ventilated alveoli to the capillary blood (122).

The increase in $PA\text{-}aO_2$ has been mainly attributed to increased venous admixture ("shunting" effect) as a result of atelectasis, greater V_A/Q mismatch, and attenuation of the HPV response (123). Using a three-compartment lung model, "shrinkage" of the end-expiratory lung volume (FRC) following anesthesia is the main culprit for impaired blood gas exchange: the lung compartment with normal V_A/Q ratio becomes smaller whereas the compartments with airway closure (low V_A/Q units, "shunt-like") and parenchymal collapse (atelectasis, "true shunt") are getting larger (58).

On the second and third postoperative day, abnormal breathing patterns associated with sleep disturbances have been incriminated to produce recurrent nocturnal hypoxemic episodes which could be aggravated by analgesic and sedative drugs (124). Circulatory failure, sepsis, and hypermetabolic conditions represent non-respiratory causes of postoperative hypoxemia (11,54,125). For instance, elevated capillary hydrostatic pressure following ischemic heart failure and inflammatory damage of the alveolar-capillary barrier all produce interstitial lung edema and alveolar flooding resulting in poor diffusing capacity. Further impairment in lung O_2 transfer could be attributed to diaphragmatic contractile failure and low levels of mixed venous O_2 saturation concomitant with fever, shivering, or pain.

C. Anesthetic/Analgesic Techniques and COPD

Compared with healthy subjects, COPD patients exhibit a weaker HPV response and a dose-related depression of the ventilatory response to CO_2 and hypoxia in the presence of sedatives and opiates (126). Hence, postoperative cardiorespiratory arrest is feared in these patients with impaired respiratory chemosensitive reflexes, even with usual doses of opiates or benzodiazepines. More frequently, respiratory failure is related to ALI (sepsis, postpneumonectomy resection), heart failure, fluid overload, or diaphragmatic pump failure (deconditioned or chronically fatigued respiratory muscles) (52,54,127). Particularly, flattening and shortening of the diaphragm represent mechanical disadvantages compared with the dome-shaped diaphragm in healthy subjects.

Dynamic hyperinflation (wasted ventilation), premature closure of small airways, and alveolar collapse (shunt-like effects) can be aggravated by positive pressure ventilation, leading to further deterioration of the ventilation/perfusion mismatch and increased PA-aO_2 gradient (128–130). However, the extent of alveolar collapse and impairment in gas exchange during and following surgery are unrelated to the severity of preexistent lung disease (131,132). For instance, blood oxygenation is better maintained within the first 10 minutes of one-lung ventilation during thoracic surgery in patients with end-staged COPD compared with healthy control subjects (133). The lack of atelectasis formation and preservation of gas exchange in COPD patients under mechanical ventilation can be explained by several complementary mechanisms: (*i*) chronic airflow obstruction causing intrinsic positive end-expiratory pressure (PEEPi) and increased residual volume which may serve as a reservoir for oxygen, (*ii*) prevention of lung collapse by the loss of lung elastic recoil coupled to an increased stiffness of the chest wall, (*iii*) relaxation of the abdominal muscular tone with analgesia that promotes diaphragmatic caudal displacement and restores/maintains FRC, and (*iv*) length adaptation processes within the crural and costal parts of the diaphragmatic muscle, which partly maintains its contractile efficiency (90,134–136). In fact, chronically shortened diaphragms lose excess sarcomeres and with time, the remaining sarcomeres are restored to the proper optimal operating length, thereby generating virtual normal contraction at shortened length.

D. Influence of Major Surgery on Respiratory Function

The most important alterations in respiratory function are observed following upper abdominal and thoracic surgery whereas minor/short-lasting respiratory impairment occurs after lower abdominal and peripheral surgical procedures (38,137,138). In addition to standard pulmonary function tests (spirometry and plethysmography), imaging techniques (ultrasound, radiology and CT-scanning) and various physiological measurements [electromyography, esophageal, and gastric pressures (Pes, Pgas), thoracic and abdominal circumferences] have been applied in clinical and experimental studies to document postoperative respiratory dysfunction and to elucidate its underlying mechanisms (139).

The characteristic restrictive syndrome following thoracic and abdominal surgery/trauma consists in a marked reduction in lung volumes (-30% for FRC, -40% to -60% for FEV_1), with maximal changes during the first 24 hours and a progressive return towards preoperative levels within 8 to 10 days after surgery (38). Due to the fall in FRC and the increased stiffness of the respiratory system, the metabolic cost of breathing is largely increased. When the depressive central effects of

anesthetic agents have disappeared, the enhanced activity of respiratory control centers
is reflected by an elevated airway occlusion pressure. In addition to pain and anesthesia-
induced depression of respiratory centers, electrolytes imbalance (hypokalemia,
hypophosphatemia, and hypocalcemia), general debilitation and acute episodes of
circulatory failure or sepsis all compromise the contracting capacity of the respiratory
muscles. Infrequently, acute respiratory distress may result from intraoperative phrenic
nerve injuries due to compression, surgical dissection, tumor invasion or, ice cold-
fluids (140,141).

Although surgical patients maintain adequate minute ventilation, tidal volume is
smaller, the respiratory rate increases and there is a temporary shift from an abdominal
motion to a predominantly thoracic expansion (Fig. 2). Several studies involving patients
undergoing thoracic and abdominal surgery have repeatedly demonstrated a shallow
"thoracic" breathing pattern concomitant with a reduction in muscular diaphragmatic
activity which would presumably contribute to PPCs (142–144). Along the increasing
central drive to breath, the increased intercostal muscle activity outweighs the
diaphragmatic activity, resulting in a decreased Pga/Pes ratio and a reduced
diaphragmatic motion. Sustained tonic activity of the abdominal wall muscles during
the early phase of inspiration may prevent further caudal displacement of the diaphragm.
In some patients, sudden relaxation of the abdominal muscles at the onset of inspiration
has been shown to generate a paradoxical abdominal breathing cycle (145).

Numerous studies have addressed the issue of postoperative diaphragmatic
dysfunction, resulting either from the inhibition of phrenic nerve discharges by local
neural reflexes, anesthetic agents, and inflammatory mediators or from direct
impairment of the contractile capacity of the diaphragmatic myofibrilles.

Animal experiments have shown that abdominal/thoracic manipulations activate
afferent medullar pathways leading to a reflex inhibition of the phrenic nerve output and

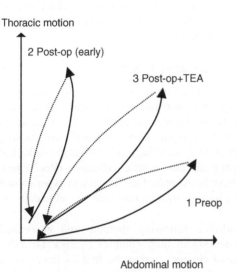

Figure 2 Time course of thoraco-abdominal breathing patterns following thoracic or
abdominal surgery and influence of TEA. *Abbreviation*: TEA, thoracic epidural blockade.

depression of the diaphragmatic muscular activity (146,147). Pain appears as an unlikely cause of this inhibition because provision of adequate analgesia with opiates only moderately improves the abnormal breathing pattern (148,149). Likewise, the central respiratory effects of anesthetic agents are short-lasting and the breathing pattern completely normalizes two to six hours after emergence from anesthesia in volunteers and patients undergoing peripheral or lower abdominal interventions.

Blocking both nociceptive and visceral neural afferences has been shown to reverse the abnormal breathing pattern. Indeed, provision of TEA (bupivacaine 0.5%) in patients recovering from abdominal surgery is accompanied by a decreased respiratory rate, increased tidal volume, and restored indices of diaphragmatic function (EMG diaphragmatic activity and transdiaphragmatic pressure) (150,151). In addition to interrupting the afferent inputs originating from the thorax and abdomen, TEA with high concentrations of local anesthetics also blocks the efferent output reaching the abdominal expiratory muscles and intercostals muscles (152). Hence, it has been speculated that the abdominal motor blockade would facilitate the downward diaphragmatic displacement by suppressing the interference of sustained tonic abdominal muscular activity with the indices of diaphragmatic activity rather than by changing the diaphragmatic activity by itself.

Clinical studies comparing the respiratory effects of laparoscopic and traditional "open" surgical approach support the hypothesis that alterations of indices of diaphragmatic function parallel the severity of surgical trauma. Not surprisingly, diaphragmatic function is less impaired and respiratory volumes are better preserved after a minimally invasive surgical approach with less inflammatory and neurohumoral responses (153–157).

In uncomplicated surgical cases, direct negative inotropic effects on the diaphragm have been ruled out on the basis of restored transdiaphragmatic pressure swings (Pgas/Pdi) during electrical stimulation of the phrenic nerves or when patients are simply asked to "take a deep breath" (158,159). However, following prolonged surgical stress or septic events, activation of the hypothalamic–pituitary–adrenal axis induces a catabolic process with respiratory muscle damage via the production of glucocorticoids and the release of cytokines, nitric oxide, and oxygen-derived free radicals (160,161). In such complicated cases, the fall in maximal diaphragmatic force parallels the reduction in muscular mass as a result of oxidative myofibrillar damage, increased protease activity and downregulation of insulin-like growth factor-I. In an attempt to limit this ongoing wasting process within the inspiratory muscles, the release of β-endorphin decreases the activation of respiratory muscles, by changing the pattern of breathing which becomes more rapid and shallow (162).

IV. Principles of Perioperative Anesthetic Care in COPD Patients

After major surgery, PPCs and cardiac complications are equally prevalent and clinically important regarding mortality/morbidity rates and hospital resource consumption. Care bundles, packages of the best evidence-based practices, are being introduced into several areas of medicine to speed up the recovery process and alleviate the costs of health care interventions. Fast-track anesthesia is advocated in all COPD patients to avoid the deleterious effects of prolonged mechanical ventilation and postoperative respiratory impairment can initially be treated by non-invasive ventilatory techniques (NIV) (163–165). As supported by the current medical knowledge, Table 4 summarizes several strategies aimed at reducing the risk of perioperative infections as well as cardiac and pulmonary complications in all surgery patients including those with COPD (165–167).

A. Preoperative Consultation

The preoperative anesthesiologist consultation addresses the following key questions: "Is this patient fit for surgery? Is it possible to improve the patient's condition? Are there alternate therapeutic modalities?" High-risk respiratory and cardiac patients can usually be identified on the basis of age, comorbidities, presenting disease, and proposed surgery. Selected additional investigations can be of help (168,169).

For cardiac risk stratification, the clinical preoperative workup should be targeted towards seven independent predictors of cardiac complications:

- the presence of severe aortic stenosis,
- heart failure (NYHA classes 3 and 4),
- and the five items of the RCRI (major surgery, coronary artery disease, renal insufficiency, history of stroke, and diabetes mellitus) (170).

In patients with an abnormal heart murmur, a limited exercise capacity or a history of heart failure, transthoracic echocardiography is a valuable, simple, and rapid

Table 4 Effects of Anesthesia on Respiratory Function

Lung volume
  Atelectasis in dependent lung areas
    ↙ FRC
    ↗ Closing volume
    ↙ Lung compliance
  In COPD patients: ↗ FRC and ↗ dead space (air trapping) due to incomplete expiratory emptying of the most diseased lung regions
Airways
  Bronchodilatation (volatile anesthetic agents)
    ↙ Tonic activity of the muscle controlling the upper airways
    ↙ Bronchial mucociliary clearance
    ↗ Airway resistance
Ventilatory control
    ↙ Ventilatory response to hypercarbia
    ↙ Ventilatory response to hypoxia
    ↙ Ventilatory response to acidosis
Pulmonary circulation
    ↙ Hypoxic vasoconstrictor response (volatile anesthetic agents)
Blood gas exchange
    ↗ $PA_{-a}O_2$ gradient due to mismatch in regional V_A/Q ratios
Immune function
    ↙ Bactericidal activity of alveolar and bronchial macrophages
    ↗ Release of pro-inflammatory cytokines

Abbreviations: COPD, chronic obstructive pulmonary disease; FRC, functional respiratory capacity; $PA_{-a}O_2$ gradient, alveolar-arterial oxygen gradient; V_A/Q ratios, ventilation–perfusion ratios.

diagnostic tool to rule out valvular abnormalities or pulmonary hypertension and to assess ventricular function (10,26,171–173).

For respiratory risk stratification, patients should be specifically asked about the intensity and frequency of dyspnea and cough attacks, the intensity of medical treatment, smoking habits, previous hospital admission, and recent infection (43). Procedure-related factors such as the site of incision, the duration of intervention, and transfusion needs should be discussed with the surgeon while taking into account the presenting pathology as well as the skills, expertise, and experience of the operating team. In addition to the patient history and clinical examination, routine chest X rays and functional laboratory testing are not helpful to further refine pulmonary risk assessment, except (*i*) when the diagnosis of lung disease is unclear, (*ii*) in case of clinical deterioration (i.e., poorly controlled asthma), and (*iii*) in patients scheduled to undergo lung resection. Hence, preoperative lung function testing should be prescribed only when the results add new information regarding the disease status and may influence the choice of anesthesia, monitoring, or surgical approach. A survey conducted by the ASAs has revealed that anesthesiologists ordered preoperative lung function tests in approximately 60% of surgical candidates presenting with restrictive of obstructive lung diseases: 68% of patients with asthma, 80% of patients with COPD, and 53% of patients with severe scoliosis (168).

B. Patient's Preparation

Rehabilitation

Muscular endurance training and re-nutrition enhance respiratory muscle strength and may facilitate weaning from the ventilator after major or prolonged operations. Multidisciplinary rehabilitation programs have been shown to be cost-effective treatments in severe COPD patients, compared with lung volume reduction surgery (174,175). The preoperative setting provides a "teaching window" for effective encouragement of exercise training, smoking and alcohol cessation, and instructions regarding chest physiotherapy. For instance, preoperative education on lung expansion maneuvers reduces pulmonary complications to a greater degree than when educative information is provided after surgery (176).

Medications

Preoperative inhaled β_2-adrenergic agonists (e.g., salbutamol) and anticholinergic agents (i.e., ipratropium) are continued up to the day of surgery in all symptomatic asthmatic and patients COPD with bronchial hyperresponsiveness. Combined short-term treatment with systemic or inhaled corticosteroids has been shown to "tune up" lung function and to decrease the incidence of wheezing following endotracheal intubation (177). Concerns regarding impaired wound healing and immunosuppression have been ruled out in a study conducted in asthmatic patients receiving prophylactic doses of corticosteroids (178). Antibiotics should only be prescribed when the aspect of sputum suggests an infection and, whenever possible, the surgical procedure should be postponed for at least 10 days. Although theophylline is effective to attenuate bronchospasm and to increase diaphragmatic contractility, it is no longer a first-line drug in the management of acute asthma and respiratory failure; moreover, it has the potential to produce fatal arrhythmias and convulsive episodes.

All COPD patients with coronary artery disease or cardiac risk factors should be considered to receive a pharmacological cardioprotective regimen involving antiadrenergic agents, platelet antiaggregants and/or statins (10,179,180). These medications should be continued or started preoperatively. Although β-blockers are contraindicated in case of moderate-to-severe bronchospastic disorders, a meta-analysis supports the safety of selective $β_1$-blockers in the majority of COPD patients since the FEV_1 remains stable and inhaled $β_2$ adrenergic agonists are still effective to alleviate exacerbations (181,182). Likewise, $α_2$ adrenergic agonists (i.e., clonidine, dexmedetomidine) are devoid of any bronchospastic effect and have been shown to prevent myocardial ischemia, to reduce anesthetic/analgesic requirements and to attenuate thermoregulatory shivering during the perioperative period (183–186). Accordingly, these agents might be beneficial in patients with combined bronchospastic and coronary artery diseases to decrease airway reactivity and to modulate the cardiac sympathetic tone (Table 5).

Smoking Cessation

Cessation of smoking shortly before cardiothoracic surgery (less than two months) has not been associated with a significant reduction in PPCs (80,187). A "hang-over" effect comparable to delirium and increased sputum production may actually increase the risk of PPCs, particularly of atelectasis and silent microaspiration. Attempts towards smoking cessation are successful in less than 30% of cases and the normalization of tissue-healing processes and reduction in PPCs require at least eight weeks of smoking cessation (74,188,189). Other overwhelming health benefits of quitting smoking are always worth mentioning to motivate patients, and accumulate with the increasing duration of abstinence: first, carboxyhemoglobin levels decrease and the excitatory effects of nicotine are abolished within 48 hours, respiratory symptoms improve after four to six weeks, FEV_1 increases within the first year whereas the risks for ischemic myocardial and cerebrovascular events are reduced after two to five years, and lower risk for cancer are observed after five to nine years (77).

C. Hospital Structures and Health Care Processes

Volume of Procedures and Structural Aspects

Besides specialized surgical/medical training, professional expertise and technical skills, the operative outcome is also largely influenced by the number of major procedures performed at a single institution: this emphasizes the critical importance of the organizational processes including a multidisciplinary coordinated team approach (190). In large-volume hospitals, better results in terms of patient satisfaction, mortality/morbidity data and cost containment can be achieved by adopting stringent safety practices, implementing protective strategies, standardizing the processes of care and defining clinical pathways for homogeneous groups of patients. In several leading American hospitals, health care quality-improvement projects are focused on specific targets such as the perioperative use of β-blockers, computerization of the medical and nursing files as well as 24 hours availability of high-dependency units. Hence, health authorities and insurance companies recommend to refer higher-risk patients and complex operations in these high-volume hospitals where all necessary supporting

Table 5 Strategies to Reduce the Risk of Major Postoperative Complications

	Strength of evidence	Type of complications studied
Risk reduction strategy for postoperative cardiac *complications*		
Clinical risk stratification	B	MI, CHF, arrhythmia, operative mortality
Smoking cessation	I	Misch
Drugs		
β-adrenergic antagonists	A and B	Misch, MI, CHF, arrhythmia, short- and long-term mortality
α₂-adrenergic agonists	B	Misch, MI, short-term mortality
Calcium-channel blockers	C	MI, CHF, arrhythmia, short-term mortality
Statines	C	MI, short- and long-term mortality
Aspirine	C	MI, short- and long-term mortality
Regional analgesis		
Thoracic epidural analgesia (intra-postoperative)	B	MI (mortality)
Spinal/epidural analgesia	C	Mortality, deep venous thrombosis, PTE, (MI, stroke)
Rewarming, normothermia	B	Misch
Hematocrit > 28%	C	Misch, serious cardiac adverse events
Right heart catheterization	D	Mortality, arrhythmia, thromboembolism
Risk reduction strategy for postoperative pulmonary *complications*		
Clinical risk stratification	C	Atelectasis, BPN, respiratory failure
Smoking cessation preoperatively	I	Postoperative ventilator support
Monitoring of neuromuscular blockade and/or short-acting myorelaxants	B	Atelectasis, BPN
Intraoperative neuraxial blockade versus general anesthesia	C	Mortality, BPN, respiratory failure
Patient-controlled versus on-demand analgesia	C	Pain score, overall complication, hospital length of stay
Neuraxial blockade post(intra-) operative	C	Miscellaneous PPCs
Laparoscopic versus open procedures	C	Spirometry, atelectasis, BPN, overall PPC
Selective nasogastric drainage	B	Atelectasis, BPN, bronchoaspiration
Postoperative lung expansion modalities	B	Atelectasis, BPN, bronchitis, severe hypoxemia

(Continued)

Table 5 Strategies to Reduce the Risk of Major Postoperative Complications (*Continued*)

	Strength of evidence	Type of complications studied
Risk reduction strategy for postoperative pulmonary complications		
Nutrition		
Routine parenteral or enteral nutrition	D	
Immunonutrition	I	
Right heart catheterization	D	Pneumonia
Risk reduction strategy for postoperative nonpulmonary infections		
Hand washing (medical and nursing team)	A	Wound infection
Antibiotic prophylaxis	A	Wound infection
Blood glucose control	B	Wound infection
Supplemental oxygen (intra-postop)	B	Wound infection
Rewarming, normothermia	C	Wound infection
Avoidance of indwelling catheters (central venous line, bladder)	C	Bacteriemia, catheter-related sepsis, urinary infection
Smoking cessation preoperative	C	Wound infection

Abbreviations: A, good evidence that the strategy reduces complications and that benefits outweighs harms; B, at least fair evidence that the strategy reduces complications; BPN, bronchopneumonia; C, at least fair evidence of positive impact although the harm and benefit balance is too close to justify a general recommendation; CHF, congestive heart failure; D, at least fair evidence that the strategy does not reduce complications or harm outweigh benefits; I, insufficient data to support any recommendation; MI, myocardial infarct; Misch, myocardial ischemia; PTE, pulmonary thromboembolism; PPC, postoperative pulmonary complication.

facilities are available and where evidence-based and cost-efficient medical interventions and nursing care are applied (191,192).

Minimally Invasive Procedures

Compared with the standard "open" operations, minimally invasive procedures such as endovascular aortic prothesis and laparoscopy produce lesser tissue damage with an attenuated neurohumoral and inflammatory response and in turn, reduced respiratory impaiment (156–159). Consequently, the minimally invasive approach confers major advantages including shorter hospital stay, earlier ambulation and feeding, lesser need for analgesic medications, and better preservation of lung functional volume (193–195). For patients undergoing "open" aortic abdominal reconstruction, the retro-peritoneal approach should be preferred in COPD patients since it produces less impairment in respiratory function and fewer PPCs (196).

Nasogastric Drainage

Routine nasogastric drainage fails to speed bowel recovery and may even increase the risk of silent aspiration and PPCs. Randomized controlled trials have shown that selective nasogastric drainage resulted in earlier bowel function and fewer PPCs compared with routine gastric drainage (197). Hence, the indications for nasogastric decompression should be limited to specific situations (i.e., acute abdomen, head trauma, and drug overdose) and in cases of postoperative nausea or vomiting, inability to tolerate oral fluid, or symptomatic abdominal distension.

D. Anesthetic Agents and Techniques

General Anesthesia

Whenever possible, central neuraxial, peripheral nerve blockade, or GA without tracheal intubation should be preferred in COPD patients. The new laryngeal masks offer the advantage of lesser upper airways irritation compared with endotracheal tubes, and various modes of spontaneous, pressure support, or volume-controlled ventilation can be adapted depending on the patient's respiratory status and intervention (62,198).

Following endotracheal intubation, wheezing is more likely to occur when barbiturates are used as anesthetic induction agents as compared with propofol, ketamine or volatile anesthetics (61,199–201). To attenuate the bronchoconstrictive reflex due to endotracheal intubation or suctioning, prophylactic treatment with lidocaine (intravenous or inhaled) and/or a β_2-adrenergic agonist is recommended in asthmatic and COPD patients (202–204). Intravenous lidocaine doses of 1 to 2 mg/kg of body weight have been shown to attenuate histamine-induced bronchoconstriction in asthmatic volunteers. Given by inhalation, lidocaine produces a mild direct airway irritation followed by attenuation of bronchial reactivity that occurs at lower plasma concentrations than following systemic administration.

As already pointed out, volatile anesthetics are effective bronchodilating agents with potential adverse effects regarding intrapulmonary shunting (96,205). For many years, they have been the preferred agents for anesthesia maintenance in COPD patients with few differences between the different agents (isoflurane, desflurane, and sevoflurane) with respect to their efficacy in treating intraoperative bronchospasm, except for desflurane which may induce coughing, bronchospasm, laryngospasm, and bronchial hypersecretion (201,206). In rare cases where hypoxemia is attributed to the inhibition of HPV response, the administration of volatile anesthetic should be interrupted and replaced by a continuous infusion of intravenous propofol or ketamine.

When muscle relaxants are needed, short-acting agents are titrated to maintain an adequate depth of muscular blockade as assessed by neuromuscular testing. Residual neuromuscular blockade should be reversed before tracheal extubation with the administration of cholinesterase inhibitors (prostigmine).

Controlled Mechanical Ventilation and Inspiratory Oxygen Fraction

Pressure support ventilation has become popular even outside the ICUs. Although it has the potential disadvantage of providing inadequate tidal volume in the case of sudden increases in airway resistance or decreased respiratory compliance, inspiratory air flow is distributed more homogeneously and at a lower mean distending pulmonary pressure. Yu et al. demonstrated that bi-level positive airway pressure (Bi-PAP) ventilation was beneficial in decreasing ventilation–perfusion mismatch and improving oxygenation when compared with conventional intermittent positive pressure ventilation (with or without PEEP) (207). In COPD patients with decreased elastic lung recoil and increased airway resistance, the ventilation settings should be precisely adjusted to maximize alveolar gas emptying and to avoid dynamic hyperinflation (low respiratory rate, inspiratory/expiratory ratio, and PEEPi; Fig. 3) (208).

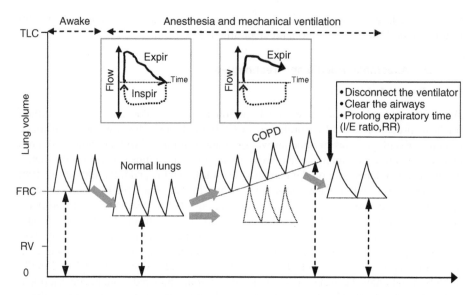

Figure 3 Progressive dynamic hyperinflation in COPD patients during mechanical ventilation and its treatment by opening the airway and adjusting the ventilatory settings. *Abbreviations*: COPD, chronic obstructive pulmonary disease; TLC, total lung capacity; FRC, functional residual capacity; RR, relative risk; RV, residual volume.

In patients with an ALI syndrome, limiting the tidal ventilatory volume (5–7 mL/kg) and optimizing PEEP levels have been shown to improve outcome and to attenuate the mechanical and biological stress acting at the alveolar-capillary level (209). These results support the view that a high plateau pressure may be a risk factor for ventilator-induced lung injury. Although no beneficial effects on the systemic and pulmonary inflammatory responses have been demonstrated in healthy lungs, similar protective ventilation settings including a pressure support mode and lung recruitment maneuvers are currently advocated in patients with respiratory diseases undergoing prolonged and major operations, particularly lung resection (54,210,211).

Besides i.v. antibiotic prophylaxis and maintenance of normothermia and normoglycemia, the delivery of high-percentage inhaled oxygen (80% intraoperatively and supplemental oxygen up to two hours after surgery) has been shown to lower the risk of wound infections by enhancing the bactericidal activity of inflammatory cells (212,213). Although formation of resorption atelectasis occurs in all patients breathing pure O_2 within seven minutes after anesthesia induction, atelectasis are much less frequent in the FIO_2 80% ventilated group and almost absent in those ventilated with 60% FIO_2 (214). Thus, prevention of complete alveolar gas resorption together with preservation of the bactericidal activity of inflammatory cells can be achieved by setting the inspiratory O_2 fraction between 50% and 80% and by performing periodic "vital capacity maneuvers" (215). These new proposals contrast with the current usual practice of setting the inspiratory O_2 fraction around 30% and applying a 5 cm H_2O PEEP.

Compared with PEEP, lung recruitment maneuvers are more effective to prevent or reverse intraoperative atelectasis. Re-opening 50% to 100% of atelectatic areas requires that a plateau airway pressure of 30 to 40 cm H_2O should be maintained for seven seconds in patients with healthy lungs (216). Such a large inflation corresponds to a maximum spontaneous inspiration (vital capacity) and may transiently compromise hemodynamics by influencing preload, afterload, and contractility of the ventricules. In morbidly obese patients, Wahlen et al. demonstrated the efficacy of alveolar recruitment to improve oxygenation, but these positive effects were short lived and associated with more frequent administration of vasopressors (217).

Regional Anesthesia and Analgesia

Provision of effective pain relief is a prerequisite for an accelerated postoperative recovery. Patient-controlled rather than "on demand" administration of i.v. opioids and central neuraxial or peripheral nerve blockade using local anesthetics (with or without opioids) are the cornerstone of modern analgesic strategies (116,218). By combining different analgesic agents (opioids, paracetamol, and non-steroidal anti-inflammatory drugs), the effectiveness of pain control may be further increased while drug-related side effects are minimized (219–221).

Despite criticisms on study protocols, heterogenous population samples, and statistical methods, several meta-analysis have supported the concept that regional anesthetic techniques improve surgical outcome not only through better pain control but also through attenuation of the neuroendocrine response to surgery, maintenance of the immune function, and improvement of tissue oxygenation (222–226). The use of intraoperative central neuraxial techniques (spinal/epidural) has been associated with reduced operative mortality rates and fewer episodes of deep vein thrombosis, pulmonary embolism and stroke as well as a lower need for blood transfusion. Likewise, maintenance of TEA for several days after major abdominal or thoracic surgery has been shown to reduce mortality as well as the incidence of myocardial infarcts, arrhythmia, atelectasis, bronchopneumonia, and respiratory failure. By blocking the afferent nociceptive stimuli and inhibiting the efferent sympathetic outflow, TEA affords cardiac and pulmonary protection as demonstrated by improvement in myocardial oxygen balance, inhibition of platelet hyperaggregability, limitation of myocardial infarct size, and preservation of diaphragmatic function. In patients with end-stage COPD, Gruber et al. demonstrated that TEA resulted in better ventilatory mechanics (work of breathing, inspiratory capacity, and forced expiratory volume) and maintenance of adequate gas exchange (227). Moreover, the time to extubation is shortened in patients with TEA as lower doses of depressant respiratory drugs are administered, more rapid recovery of bowel motility allows early resumption of oral intake and blunting of protein catabolism facilitates rapid mobilization, avoiding the consequences of bed confinement such as muscle wasting, fatigue, and venous thrombosis (115,228).

Compared with epidural analgesic techniques, a single shot of intrathecal morphine (0.2–1 mg) at the lumbar site is simpler, faster, and more reliable to produce adequate pain relief at the first attempt in non-experienced hands. However, a meta-analysis including 668 cardiac surgical patients did not demonstrate any benefit in terms of mortality and major cardiopulmonary complications (115). Due to the presence of opioid receptors in the substantia gelatinosa of the spinal cord, intrathecal morphine is 100 times more potent than systemic injection and has been shown to modulate the perioperative stress response, alleviate pain for the first 24 hours after surgery, and fasten extubation. The dose-related respiratory depressive effect of intrathecal morphine mandates a close monitoring within the first 24 hours after the injection of doses exceeding 0.5 mg (229–232).

Despite undisputable advantages, catastrophic complications have been attributed to central neuraxial techniques: cardiac arrests related to anesthetic overdose or concurrent sedation (2.5–6.4 per 10,000 spinal anesthesia; 0–2.5 per 10,000 epidural anesthesia) and spinal hematoma with paraplegic syndrome (1/1,150,000 with epidural anesthesia and 1/220,000 with spinal anesthesia) (233). Thus, for understandable reasons, fear of spinal hematoma and nerve injuries will continue to discourage the use of regional anesthetic techniques in low-risk patients in whom various combinations of parenteral opiates, non-steroidal anti-inflammatory drugs, and paracetamol should be preferred. In contrast, for higher risk patients, the risk–benefit analysis favors central neuraxial blockade. These important issues should be discussed preoperatively with each patient. For instance, surgical candidates undergoing major aortic surgery have an average 3% to 5% risk of myocardial infarction and 5% to 10% risk of PPCs. Considering the fact that central neuraxial blockade confers a median 30% to 50% relative risk reduction for cardiac and pulmonary complications, then one myocardial infarction and one PPC would be avoided for every 30 to 60 treated patients. Furthermore, for each person suffering a spinal hematoma (1 in 150,000), it may be estimated that TEA may prevent at least 40 to 100 deaths in the high-risk group of COPD patients undergoing major surgery.

E. Monitoring

Although no single monitoring device has been shown to improve outcome in the operating room and ICU, the combination of EKG, pulse oxymetry, blood pressure monitoring, and capnography is well designed to identify the most critical cardiopulmonary events that will trigger corrective interventions. Given the added risk and lack of benefits related to right heart catheterization, there is a trend towards minor invasive and more advanced monitoring (172). It is now widely accepted that measurement of cardiac output no longer requires a Swan–Ganz catheter as it is reliably assessed by transesophageal Doppler ultrasounds, arterial pulse contour analysis or lithium dilution technique. Although the validity of functional cardiovascular monitoring including extravascular lung water, ventricular contractility indices, and volumetric variables for cardiovascular filling status has been proven, future clinical studies are warranted to demonstrate the outcome benefits of goal-oriented hemodynamic treatments (234–236).

As moderate levels of hypothermia (34–35°C) have been associated with higher incidences of myocardial ischemia and wound infection, body temperature should be measured and kept above 36°C by preventing heat losses and using various warming devices (blanket, fluid infusion, and mattress) (237).

Monitoring the neuromuscular function is mandatory to ascertain both the depth of muscular relaxation and the functional recovery before tracheal extubation. The ability to raise the head for five seconds, to open the eyes on demand or to take a deep inspiratory breath are unreliable signs of neuromuscular recovery and should be complemented by routine neuromuscular testing (238). Different modes of electrical stimulation of a peripheral nerve have been proposed, of which the train-of-four and double-burst methods are widely used (239). Squeletal muscles vary greatly in their sensitivity to muscle relaxants: the diaphragm being the most resistant whereas the peripheral small muscles of the hands and feet, the upper airway, and pharyngeal muscles are more sensitive (99).

Improved processing of electroencephalographic signals and evoked potentials may be helpful to target an adequate depth of anesthesia. Preliminary evidence indicates that the administration of GAs guided by the bispectral index of the electroencephalogram lowers the risk for intraoperative awareness and improves the overall postoperative outcome (240,241). Indeed, two prospective studies including more than 6000 patients demonstrated that deeper maintenance of anesthetic levels was associated with higher one-year postoperative death rates in patients aged 40 years or more undergoing major noncardiac surgery (242,243). Interestingly, the risk of death within one year after surgery was expected to increase by nearly 20% for every hour with a bispectral index score of less than 45 (indicating excessive deep hypnotic levels).

F. Lung Expansion Maneuvers

To complement the effects of intraoperative vital capacity maneuvers, various techniques of respiratory physiotherapy such as incentive spirometry, deep breathing exercises, diaphragmatic breathing, intermittent positive-pressure breathing, continuous positive airway pressure (CPAP), or non-invasive ventilation (NIV) are currently applied to prevent the postoperative fall in functional lung volume and/or to re-open atelectatic areas (244,245). Although several bias limit the interpretation of most clinical studies (inclusion of low-risk groups, poorly defined clinical endpoints, and non-standardized respiratory interventions), a meta-analysis of 14 randomized controlled trials suggests that incentive spirometry and deep breathing exercises each reduces by about 50% the risk of postoperative complications; combining these techniques fails to confer additional benefit (246).

Patient's empowerment can be reinforced by an informative preoperative consultation including practical demonstration of prophylactic respiratory maneuvers which are aimed to reverse the diaphragmatic dysfunction consequent to upper abdominal and thoracic surgery (247–249). The positive impact of optimal analgesia without undue sedation and early mobilization should also be emphasized.

Prophylactic application of CPAP or NIV is equally effective but less cost efficient, as it requires more sophisticated devices and the availability of trained hospital personnel. The use of CPAP should be restricted for patients unable to perform deep breathing exercises (or incentive spirometry). Besides prevention of postoperative atelectasis, NIV with Bi-PAP has also been recommended in COPD patients with hypercapnic acute respiratory failure and those with cardiogenic pulmonary edema with the aim to unload the inspiratory muscles and to improve cardiac performances (250,251).

V. Conclusions

In the near future, anesthesiologists and surgeons will be confronted with an increasing number of patients with COPD and cardiovascular diseases. Thorough preoperative assessment based on clinical history and targeted physiological testing is required to identify high-risk patients who are prone to develop PPCs and cardiac adverse events that will markedly impact on hospital resource consumption, survival expectancy, and quality of life.

Besides patient's comorbidities, procedure-related factors (thoracic and upper abdominal interventions, prolonged surgery) are the main risk factors of PPCs as a consequence of severe impairment of respiratory function and surgical stress-induced immunosuppression.

There is growing evidence suggesting that preoperative patient's selection, perioperative optimization and monitoring of organ function, control of neuroendocrine and inflammatory responses, as well as standardization of health care processes of care are the cornerstones for improving patient safety and surgical outcome.

The recent success of minimally invasive procedures is reflected by the decrease in postoperative cardiopulmonary complications and shorter hospital stay as a result of lesser tissue trauma.

Several advances in anesthesia care have been shown to be particularly beneficial for COPD patients:

1. avoiding/minimizing airway instrumentation by using regional anesthetic blockade or laryngeal masks,
2. new volatile anesthetic agents with bronchodilating properties (e.g., sevoflurane),
3. prevention or treatment of atelectasis by lung recruitment maneuvers,
4. reversal of residual neuromuscular blockade under close monitoring,
5. multimodal analgesic regimen for blocking nociceptive inputs,
6. implementation of cardioprotective strategies (e.g., β-blockers, α_2-agonists, statines, TEA),
7. maintenance of normothermia, tight control of blood glucose and provision of supplemental oxygen to reduce wound infection rate.

References

1. Halbert RJ, Natoli JL, Gano A, Badamgarav E, Buist AS, Mannino DM. Global burden of COPD: systematic review and meta-analysis. Eur Respir J 2006; 28:523–32.
2. McAlister FA, Khan NA, Straus SE, et al. Accuracy of the preoperative assessment in predicting pulmonary risk after nonthoracic surgery. Am J Respir Crit Care Med 2003; 167(5):741–4.
3. Licker MJ, Widikker I, Robert J, et al. Operative mortality and respiratory complications after lung resection for cancer: impact of chronic obstructive pulmonary disease and time trends. Ann Thorac Surg 2006; 81(5):1830–7.
4. Huiart L, Ernst P, Suissa S. Cardiovascular morbidity and mortality in COPD. Chest 2005; 128(4):2640–6.
5. Sin DD, Wu L, Man SF. The relationship between reduced lung function and cardiovascular mortality: a population-based study and a systematic review of the literature. Chest 2005; 127(6):1952–9.
6. Lagasse RS. Anesthesia safety: model or myth? A review of the published literature and analysis of current original data Anesthesiology 2002; 97(6):1609–17.
7. Ergin A, Muntner P, Sherwin R, He J. Secular trends in cardiovascular disease mortality, incidence, and case fatality rates in adults in the United States. Am J Med 2004; 117(4):219–27.
8. Gordon HS, Johnson ML, Wray NP, et al. Mortality after noncardiac surgery: prediction from administrative versus clinical data. Med Care 2005; 43(2):159–67.
9. Kaafarani HM, Itani KM, Thornby J, Berger DH. Thirty-day and one-year predictors of death in noncardiac major surgical procedures. Am J Surg 2004; 188(5):495–9.

10. Kertai MD, Klein J, Bax JJ, Poldermans D. Predicting perioperative cardiac risk. Prog Cardiovasc Dis 2005; 47(4):240–57.
11. Fleischmann KE, Goldman L, Young B, Lee TH. Association between cardiac and noncardiac complications in patients undergoing noncardiac surgery: outcomes and effects on length of stay. Am J Med 2003; 115(7):515–20.
12. Older P, Hall A. Clinical review: how to identify high-risk surgical patients. Crit Care 2004; 8(5):369–72.
13. Pedersen T. Complications and death following anaesthesia. A prospective study with special reference to the influence of patient-, anaesthesia-, and surgery-related risk factors. Dan Med Bull 1994; 41(3):319–31.
14. Williams-Russo P, Charlson ME, MacKenzie CR, Gold JP, Shires GT. Predicting postoperative pulmonary complications. Is it a real problem? Arch Intern Med 1992; 152(6):1209–13.
15. van de Pol MA, van Houdenhoven M, Hans EW, et al. Influence of cardiac risk factors and medication on length of hospitalization in patients undergoing major vascular surgery. Am J Cardiol 2006; 97(10):1423–6.
16. Schweizer A, Khatchatourian G, Hohn L, Spiliopoulos A, Romand J, Licker M. Opening of a new postanesthesia care unit: impact on critical care utilization and complications following major vascular and thoracic surgery. J Clin Anesth 2002; 14(7):486–93.
17. Manku K, Bacchetti P, Leung JM. Prognostic significance of postoperative in-hospital complications in elderly patients. I. Long-term survival. Anesth Analg 2003; 96(2):583–9 (table of contents).
18. Fisher BW, Majumdar SR, McAlister FA. Predicting pulmonary complications after nonthoracic surgery: a systematic review of blinded studies. Am J Med 2002; 112(3):219–25.
19. Smetana GW. Preoperative pulmonary evaluation. N Engl J Med 1999; 340(12):937–44.
20. Dindo D, Demartines N, Clavien PA. Classification of surgical complications: a new proposal with evaluation in a cohort of 6336 patients and results of a survey. Ann Surg 2004; 240(2):205–13.
21. Bruce J, Russell EM, Mollison J, Krukowski ZH. The measurement and monitoring of surgical adverse events. Health Technol Assess 2001; 5(22):1–194.
22. Veen EJ, Janssen-Heijnen ML, Leenen LP, Roukema JA. The registration of complications in surgery: a learning curve. World J Surg 2005; 29(3):402–9.
23. Licker M, Khatchatourian G, Schweizer A, Bednarkiewicz M, Tassaux D, Chevalley C. The impact of a cardioprotective protocol on the incidence of cardiac complications after aortic abdominal surgery. Anesth Analg 2002; 95(6):1525–33 (table of contents).
24. Bonnet F, Marret E. Influence of anaesthetic and analgesic techniques on outcome after surgery. Br J Anaesth 2005; 95(1):52–8.
25. Lee TH, Marcantonio ER, Mangione CM, et al. Derivation and prospective validation of a simple index for prediction of cardiac risk of major noncardiac surgery. Circulation 1999; 100(10):1043–9.
26. Boersma E, Poldermans D, Bax JJ, et al. Predictors of cardiac events after major vascular surgery: role of clinical characteristics, dobutamine echocardiography, and beta-blocker therapy. J Am Med Assoc 2001; 285(14):1865–73.
27. Almanaseer Y, Mukherjee D, Kline-Rogers EM, et al. Implementation of the ACC/AHA guidelines for preoperative cardiac risk assessment in a general medicine preoperative clinic: improving efficiency and preserving outcomes. Cardiology 2005; 103(1):24–9.
28. Boersma E, Kertai MD, Schouten O, et al. Perioperative cardiovascular mortality in noncardiac surgery: validation of the Lee cardiac risk index. Am J Med 2005; 118(10):1134–41.
29. Eagle KA, Berger PB, Calkins H, et al. ACC/AHA guideline update for perioperative cardiovascular evaluation for noncardiac surgery—executive summary a report of the American College of Cardiology/American Heart Association Task Force on Practice Guidelines (Committee to Update the 1996 Guidelines on Perioperative Cardiovascular Evaluation for Noncardiac Surgery). Circulation 2002; 105(10):1257–67.
30. Fleisher LA, Beckman JA, Brown KA, et al. ACC/AHA 2006 guideline update on perioperative cardiovascular evaluation for noncardiac surgery: focused update on perioperative beta-blocker therapy: a report of the American College of Cardiology/American Heart Association Task Force on Practice Guidelines (Writing Committee to Update the 2002 Guidelines on Perioperative Cardiovascular Evaluation for Noncardiac Surgery): developed in collaboration with the American Society of Echocardiography, American Society of Nuclear Cardiology, Heart Rhythm Society, Society of Cardiovascular Anesthesiologists, Society for Cardiovascular Angiography and Interventions, and Society for Vascular Medicine and Biology. Circulation 2006; 113(22):2662–74.

31. Legner VJ, Doerner D, McCormick WC, Reilly DF. Clinician agreement with perioperative cardiovascular evaluation guidelines and clinical outcomes. Am J Cardiol 2006; 97(1):118–22.
32. Auerbach AD, Goldman L. beta-Blockers and reduction of cardiac events in noncardiac surgery: clinical applications. J Am Med Assoc 2002; 287(11):1445–7.
33. Kertai MD, Bountioukos M, Boersma E, et al. Aortic stenosis: an underestimated risk factor for perioperative complications in patients undergoing noncardiac surgery. Am J Med 2004; 116(1):8–13.
34. Hernandez AF, Whellan DJ, Stroud S, Sun JL, O'Connor CM, Jollis JG. Outcomes in heart failure patients after major noncardiac surgery. J Am Coll Cardiol 2004; 44(7):1446–53.
35. Ramakrishna G, Sprung J, Ravi BS, Chandrasekaran K, McGoon MD. Impact of pulmonary hypertension on the outcomes of noncardiac surgery: predictors of perioperative morbidity and mortality. J Am Coll Cardiol 2005; 45(10):1691–9.
36. Zahid M, Sonel AF, Saba S, Good CB. Perioperative risk of noncardiac surgery associated with aortic stenosis. Am J Cardiol 2005; 96(3):436–8.
37. Hernandez AF, Newby LK, O'Connor CM. Preoperative evaluation for major noncardiac surgery: focusing on heart failure. Arch Intern Med 2004; 164(16):1729–36.
38. Christ M, Sharkova Y, Geldner G, Maisch B. Preoperative and perioperative care for patients with suspected or established aortic stenosis facing noncardiac surgery. Chest 2005; 128(4):2944–53.
39. Abraham WT. Cardiac resynchronization therapy. Prog Cardiovasc Dis 2006; 48(4):232–8.
40. McAlister FA, Bertsch K, Man J, Bradley J, Jacka M. Incidence of and risk factors for pulmonary complications after nonthoracic surgery. Am J Respir Crit Care Med 2005; 171(5):514–7.
41. Arozullah AM, Khuri SF, Henderson WG, Daley J. Development and validation of a multifactorial risk index for predicting postoperative pneumonia after major noncardiac surgery. Ann Intern Med 2001; 135(10):847–57.
42. Arozullah AM, Daley J, Henderson WG, Khuri SF. Multifactorial risk index for predicting postoperative respiratory failure in men after major noncardiac surgery. The National Veterans Administration Surgical Quality Improvement Program. Ann Surg 2000; 232(2):242–53.
43. Smetana GW, Lawrence VA, Cornell JE. Preoperative pulmonary risk stratification for noncardiothoracic surgery: systematic review for the American College of Physicians. Ann Intern Med 2006; 144(8):581–95.
44. Kroenke K, Lawrence VA, Theroux JF, Tuley MR. Operative risk in patients with severe obstructive pulmonary disease. Arch Intern Med 1992; 152(5):967–71.
45. Svensson LG, Hess KR, Coselli JS, Safi HJ, Crawford ES. A prospective study of respiratory failure after high-risk surgery on the thoracoabdominal aorta. J Vasc Surg 1991; 14(3):271–82.
46. Pedersen T, Viby-Mogensen J, Ringsted C. Anaesthetic practice and postoperative pulmonary complications. Acta Anaesthesiol Scand 1992; 36(8):812–8.
47. Wong DH, Weber EC, Schell MJ, Wong AB, Anderson CT, Barker SJ. Factors associated with postoperative pulmonary complications in patients with severe chronic obstructive pulmonary disease. Anesth Analg 1995; 80(2):276–84.
48. Barisione G, Rovida S, Gazzaniga GM, Fontana L. Upper abdominal surgery: does a lung function test exist to predict early severe postoperative respiratory complications? Eur Respir J 1997; 10(6):1301–8.
49. Bluman LG, Mosca L, Newman N, Simon DG. Preoperative smoking habits and postoperative pulmonary complications. Chest 1998; 113(4):883–9.
50. Canturk NZ, Canturk Z, Okay E, Yirmibesoglu O, Eraldemir B. Risk of nosocomial infections and effects of total cholesterol, HDL cholesterol in surgical patients. Clin Nutr 2002; 21(5):431–6.
51. Ferguson MK, Durkin AE. Preoperative prediction of the risk of pulmonary complications after esophagectomy for cancer. J Thorac Cardiovasc Surg 2002; 123(4):661–9.
52. Jaber S, Delay JM, Chanques G, et al. Outcomes of patients with acute respiratory failure after abdominal surgery treated with noninvasive positive pressure ventilation. Chest 2005; 128(4):2688–95.
53. Schussler O, Alifano M, Dermine H, et al. Postoperative pneumonia after major lung resection. Am J Respir Crit Care Med 2006; 173(10):1161–9.
54. Licker M, de Perrot M, Spiliopoulos A, et al. Risk factors for acute lung injury after thoracic surgery for lung cancer. Anesth Analg 2003; 97(6):1558–65.
55. Tirumalasetty J, Grammer LC. Asthma, surgery, and general anesthesia: a review. J Asthma 2006; 43(4):251–4.
56. Warner DO, Warner MA, Barnes RD, et al. Perioperative respiratory complications in patients with asthma. Anesthesiology 1996; 85(3):460–7.
57. Peterson GN, Domino KB, Caplan RA, et al. Management of the difficult airway: a closed claims analysis. Anesthesiology 2005; 103:33–9.

58. Hedenstierna G, Edmark L. The effects of anesthesia and muscle paralysis on the respiratory system. Intensive Care Med 2005; 31(10):1327–35.

59. Berg H, Roed J, Viby-Mogensen J, et al. Residual neuromuscular block is a risk factor for postoperative pulmonary complications. A prospective, randomised, and blinded study of postoperative pulmonary complications after atracurium, vecuronium and pancuronium. Acta Anaesthesiol Scand 1997; 41(9):1095–103.

60. Smetana GW. Preoperative pulmonary evaluation: identifying and reducing risks for pulmonary complications. Cleve Clin J Med 2006; 73(Suppl. 1):S36–41.

61. Goff MJ, Arain SR, Ficke DJ, Uhrich TD, Ebert TJ. Absence of bronchodilation during desflurane anesthesia: a comparison to sevoflurane and thiopental. Anesthesiology 2000; 93(2):404–8.

62. Berry A, Brimacombe J, Keller C, Verghese C. Pulmonary airway resistance with the endotracheal tube versus laryngeal mask airway in paralyzed anesthetized adult patients. Anesthesiology 1999; 90(2):395–7.

63. Georgopoulos D, Mitrouska I, Markopoulou K, Patakas D, Anthonisen NR. Effects of breathing patterns on mechanically ventilated patients with chronic obstructive pulmonary disease and dynamic hyperinflation. Intensive Care Med 1995; 21(11):880–6.

64. den Herder C, Schmeck J, Appelboom DJ, de Vries N. Risks of general anaesthesia in people with obstructive sleep apnoea. Br Med J 2004; 329(7472):955–9.

65. Beydon L, Hassapopoulos J, Quera MA, et al. Risk factors for oxygen desaturation during sleep, after abdominal surgery. Br J Anaesth 1992; 69(2):137–42.

66. Rosenberg J, Wildschiodtz G, Pedersen MH, von Jessen F, Kehlet H. Late postoperative nocturnal episodic hypoxaemia and associated sleep pattern. Br J Anaesth 1994; 72(2):145–50.

67. Polanczyk CA, Marcantonio E, Goldman L, et al. Impact of age on perioperative complications and length of stay in patients undergoing noncardiac surgery. Ann Intern Med 2001; 134(8):637–43.

68. Gunnarsson L, Tokics L, Gustavsson H, Hedenstierna G. Influence of age on atelectasis formation and gas exchange impairment during general anaesthesia. Br J Anaesth 1991; 66(4):423–32.

69. von Ungern-Sternberg BS, Regli A, Schneider MC, Kunz F, Reber A. Effect of obesity and site of surgery on perioperative lung volumes. Br J Anaesth 2004; 92(2):202–7.

70. Sprung J, Whalley DG, Falcone T, Warner DO, Hubmayr RD, Hammel J. The impact of morbid obesity, pneumoperitoneum, and posture on respiratory system mechanics and oxygenation during laparoscopy. Anesth Analg 2002; 94(5):1345–50.

71. Flier S, Knape JT. How to inform a morbidly obese patient on the specific risk to develop postoperative pulmonary complications using evidence-based methodology. Eur J Anaesthesiol 2006; 23(2):154–9.

72. Wolters U, Wolf T, Stutzer H, Schroder T. ASA classification and perioperative variables as predictors of postoperative outcome. Br J Anaesth 1996; 77(2):217–22.

73. Win T, Jackson A, Sharples L, et al. Cardiopulmonary exercise tests and lung cancer surgical outcome. Chest 2005; 127(4):1159–65.

74. Moller AM, Villebro N, Pedersen T, Tonnesen H. Effect of preoperative smoking intervention on postoperative complications: a randomised clinical trial. Lancet 2002; 359(9301):114–7.

75. Delgado-Rodriguez M, Medina-Cuadros M, Martinez-Gallego G, et al. A prospective study of tobacco smoking as a predictor of complications in general surgery. Infect Control Hosp Epidemiol 2003; 24(1):37–43.

76. Malone DL, Genuit T, Tracy JK, Gannon C, Napolitano LM. Surgical site infections: reanalysis of risk factors. J Surg Res 2002; 103(1):89–95.

77. Warner DO. Perioperative abstinence from cigarettes: physiologic and clinical consequences. Anesthesiology 2006; 104(2):356–67.

78. Reisli R, Apilliogullari S, Reisli I, Tuncer S, Erol A, Okesli S. The effect of environmental tobacco smoke on the dose requirements of rocuronium in children. Paediatr Anaesth 2004; 14(3):247–50.

79. Drongowski RA, Lee D, Reynolds PI, et al. Increased respiratory symptoms following surgery in children exposed to environmental tobacco smoke. Paediatr Anaesth 2003; 13(4):304–10.

80. Warner MA, Offord KP, Warner ME, Lennon RL, Conover MA, Jansson-Schumacher U. Role of preoperative cessation of smoking and other factors in postoperative pulmonary complications: a blinded prospective study of coronary artery bypass patients. Mayo Clin Proc 1989; 64(6):609–16.

81. Creekmore FM, Lugo RA, Weiland KJ. Postoperative opiate analgesia requirements of smokers and nonsmokers. Ann Pharmacother 2004; 38(6):949–53.

82. Whalen F, Sprung J, Burkle CM, Schroeder DR, Warner DO. Recent smoking behavior and postoperative nausea and vomiting. Anesth Analg 2006; 103(1):70–5 (table of contents).

83. Warner DO, Patten CA, Ames SC, Offord K, Schroeder D. Smoking behavior and perceived stress in cigarette smokers undergoing elective surgery. Anesthesiology 2004; 100(5):1125–37.

84. Burnham EL, Moss M, Harris F, Brown LA. Elevated plasma and lung endothelial selectin levels in patients with acute respiratory distress syndrome and a history of chronic alcohol abuse. Crit Care Med 2004; 32(3):675–9.

85. Moss M, Parsons PE, Steinberg KP, et al. Chronic alcohol abuse is associated with an increased incidence of acute respiratory distress syndrome and severity of multiple organ dysfunction in patients with septic shock. Crit Care Med 2003; 31(3):869–77.

86. Guidot DM, Roman J. Chronic ethanol ingestion increases susceptibility to acute lung injury: role of oxidative stress and tissue remodeling. Chest 2002; 122(6 Suppl.):309S–14.

87. Paull DE, Updyke GM, Davis CA, Adebonojo SA. Complications and long-term survival for alcoholic patients with resectable lung cancer. Am J Surg 2004; 188(5):553–9.

88. Tonnesen H. Alcohol abuse and postoperative morbidity. Dan Med Bull 2003; 50(2):139–60.

89. Warner DO. Diaphragm function during anesthesia: still crazy after all these years. Anesthesiology 2002; 97(2):295–7.

90. Gunnarsson L, Tokics L, Lundquist H, et al. Chronic obstructive pulmonary disease and anaesthesia: formation of atelectasis and gas exchange impairment. Eur Respir J 1991; 4(9):1106–16.

91. Lindberg P, Gunnarsson L, Tokics L, et al. Atelectasis and lung function in the postoperative period. Acta Anaesthesiol Scand 1992; 36(6):546–53.

92. van den Elsen M, Dahan A, DeGoede J, Berkenbosch A, van Kleef J. Influences of subanesthetic isoflurane on ventilatory control in humans. Anesthesiology 1995; 83(3):478–90.

93. Dahan A, van den Elsen MJ, Berkenbosch A, et al. Effects of subanesthetic halothane on the ventilatory responses to hypercapnia and acute hypoxia in healthy volunteers. Anesthesiology 1994; 80(4):727–38.

94. van den Elsen M, Sarton E, Teppema L, Berkenbosch A, Dahan A. Influence of 0.1 minimum alveolar concentration of sevoflurane, desflurane and isoflurane on dynamic ventilatory response to hypercapnia in humans. Br J Anaesth 1998; 80(2):174–82.

95. Groeben H, Meier S, Tankersley CG, Mitzner W, Brown RH. Influence of volatile anaesthetics on hypercapnoeic ventilatory responses in mice with blunted respiratory drive. Br J Anaesth 2004; 92(5):697–703.

96. Rooke GA, Choi JH, Bishop MJ. The effect of isoflurane, halothane, sevoflurane, and thiopental/nitrous oxide on respiratory system resistance after tracheal intubation. Anesthesiology 1997; 86(6):1294–9.

97. Moudgil R, Michelakis ED, Archer SL. Hypoxic pulmonary vasoconstriction. J Appl Physiol 2005; 98(1):390–403.

98. Schwarzkopf K, Schreiber T, Bauer R, et al. The effects of increasing concentrations of isoflurane and desflurane on pulmonary perfusion and systemic oxygenation during one-lung ventilation in pigs. Anesth Analg 2001; 93(6):1434–8 (table of contents).

99. Eikermann M, Blobner M, Groeben H, et al. Postoperative upper airway obstruction after recovery of the train of four ratio of the adductor pollicis muscle from neuromuscular blockade. Anesth Analg 2006; 102(3):937–42.

100. Eriksson LI. Ventilation and neuromuscular blocking drugs. Acta Anaesthesiol Scand Suppl 1994; 102:11–5.

101. Eriksson LI, Sato M, Severinghaus JW. Effect of a vecuronium-induced partial neuromuscular block on hypoxic ventilatory response. Anesthesiology 1993; 78(4):693–9.

102. Wulf H, Ledowski T, Linstedt U, Proppe D, Sitzlack D. Neuromuscular blocking effects of rocuronium during desflurane, isoflurane, and sevoflurane anaesthesia. Can J Anaesth 1998; 45(6):526–32.

103. Regli A, von Ungern-Sternberg BS, Reber A, Schneider MC. Impact of spinal anaesthesia on perioperative lung volumes in obese and morbidly obese female patients. Anaesthesia 2006; 61(3):215–21.

104. von Ungern-Sternberg BS, Regli A, Reber A, Schneider MC. Comparison of perioperative spirometric data following spinal or general anaesthesia in normal-weight and overweight gynaecological patients. Acta Anaesthesiol Scand 2005; 49(7):940–8.

105. Hedenstierna G, Lofstrom J. Effect of anaesthesia on respiratory function after major lower extremity surgery. A comparison between bupivacaine spinal analgesia with low-dose morphine and general anaesthesia. Acta Anaesthesiol Scand 1985; 29(1):55–60.

106. Sakura S, Saito Y, Kosaka Y. The effects of epidural anaesthesia on ventilatory response to hypercapnia and hypoxia in elderly patients. Anesth Analg 1996; 82(2):306–11.

107. Ishibe Y, Shiokawa Y, Umeda T, Uno H, Nakamura M, Izumi T. The effect of thoracic epidural anesthesia on hypoxic pulmonary vasoconstriction in dogs: an analysis of the pressure-flow curve. Anesth Analg 1996; 82(5):1049–55.

108. Groeben H, Schafer B, Pavlakovic G, Silvanus MT, Peters J. Lung function under high thoracic segmental epidural anesthesia with ropivacaine or bupivacaine in patients with severe obstructive pulmonary disease undergoing breast surgery. Anesthesiology 2002; 96(3):536–41.
109. Hodgson PS, Liu SS. Epidural lidocaine decreases sevoflurane requirement for adequate depth of anesthesia as measured by the Bispectral Index monitor. Anesthesiology 2001; 94:799–803.
110. Licker M, Spiliopoulos A, Tschopp JM. Influence of thoracic epidural analgesia on cardiovascular autonomic control after thoracic surgery. Br J Anaesth 2003; 91(4):525–31.
111. Groban L, Zvara DA, Deal DD, Vernon JC, Carpenter RL. Thoracic epidural anesthesia reduces infarct size in a canine model of myocardial ischemia and reperfusion injury. J Cardiothorac Vasc Anesth 1999; 13(5):579–85.
112. Blomberg S, Emanuelsson H, Kvist H, et al. Effects of thoracic epidural anesthesia on coronary arteries and arterioles in patients with coronary artery disease. Anesthesiology 1990; 73(5):840–7.
113. Groeben H. Effects of high thoracic epidural anesthesia and local anesthetics on bronchial hyperreactivity. J Clin Monit Comput 2000; 16(5–6):457–63.
114. Groeben H, Schwalen A, Irsfeld S, Tarnow J, Lipfert P, Hopf HB. High thoracic epidural anesthesia does not alter airway resistance and attenuates the response to an inhalational provocation test in patients with bronchial hyperreactivity. Anesthesiology 1994; 81(4):868–74.
115. Liu SS, Block BM, Wu CL. Effects of perioperative central neuraxial analgesia on outcome after coronary artery bypass surgery: a meta-analysis. Anesthesiology 2004; 101(1):153–61.
116. Block BM, Liu SS, Rowlingson AJ, Cowan AR, Cowan JA, Jr., Wu CL. Efficacy of postoperative epidural analgesia: a meta-analysis. J Am Med Assoc 2003; 290(18):2455–63.
117. Rubin GJ, Hotopf M. Systematic review and meta-analysis of interventions for postoperative fatigue. Br J Surg 2002; 89(8):971–84.
118. Urmey WF, Gloeggler PJ. Pulmonary function changes during interscalene brachial plexus block: effects of decreasing local anesthetic injection volume. Reg Anesth 1993; 18(4):244–9.
119. Rettig HC, Gielen MJ, Boersma E, Klein J, Groen GJ. Vertical infraclavicular block of the brachial plexus: effects on hemidiaphragmatic movement and ventilatory function. Reg Anesth Pain Med 2005; 30(6):529–35.
120. Dullenkopf A, Blumenthal S, Theodorou P, Roos J, Perschak H, Borgeat A. Diaphragmatic excursion and respiratory function after the modified Raj technique of the infraclavicular plexus block. Reg Anesth Pain Med 2004; 29(2):110–4.
121. Labaille T, Clergue F, Samii K, et al. Ventilatory response to CO_2 following intravenous and epidural lidocaine. Anesthesiology 1985; 63:179–83.
122. Rothen HU, Sporre B, Engberg G, Wegenius G, Hogman M, Hedenstierna G. Influence of gas composition on recurrence of atelectasis after a reexpansion maneuver during general anesthesia. Anesthesiology 1995; 82(4):832–42.
123. Rothen HU, Sporre B, Engberg G, Wegenius G, Hedenstierna G. Airway closure, atelectasis and gas exchange during general anaesthesia. Br J Anaesth 1998; 81(5):681–6.
124. Rosenberg J, Rasmussen GI, Wojdemann KR, Kirkeby LT, Jorgensen LN, Kehlet H. Ventilatory pattern and associated episodic hypoxaemia in the late postoperative period in the general surgical ward. Anaesthesia 1999; 54(4):323–8.
125. Yende S, Wunderink R. Causes of prolonged mechanical ventilation after coronary artery bypass surgery. Chest 2002; 122(1):245–52.
126. Montes de Oca M, Celli BR. Mouth occlusion pressure, CO_2 response and hypercapnia in severe chronic obstructive pulmonary disease. Eur Respir J 1998; 12(3):666–71.
127. Dulu A, Pastores SM, Park B, et al. Prevalence and mortality of acute lung injury and ARDS after lung resection. Chest 2006; 130:73–8.
128. Alvisi V, Romanello A, Badet M, et al. Time course of expiratory flow limitation in COPD patients during acute respiratory failure requiring mechanical ventilation. Chest 2003; 123:1625–32.
129. Myles PS, Evans AB, Madder H, et al. Dynamic hyperinflation: comparison of jet ventilation versus conventional ventilation in patients with severe end-stage obstructive lung disease. Anaesth Intensive Care 1997; 25:471–5.
130. Bardoczky GI, d'Hollander AA, Rocmans P, et al. Respiratory mechanics and gas exchange during one-lung ventilation for thoracic surgery: the effects of end-inspiratory pause in stable COPD patients. J Cardiothorac Vasc Anesth 1998; 12:137–41.
131. Bardoczky GI, Szegedi LL, d'Hollander AA, et al. Two-lung and one-lung ventilation in patients with chronic obstructive pulmonary disease: the effects of position and $F(IO)_2$. Anesth Analg 2000; 90:35–41.

132. Guenoun T, Journois D, Silleran-Chassany J, et al. Prediction of arterial oxygen tension during one-lung ventilation: analysis of preoperative and intraoperative variables. J Cardiothorac Vasc Anesth 2002; 16(2):199–203.

133. Aschkenasy SV, Hofer CK, Zalunardo MP, et al. Patterns of changes in arterial PO_2 during one-lung ventilation: a comparison between patients with severe pulmonary emphysema and patients with preserved lung function. J Cardiothorac Vasc Anesth 2005; 19:479–84.

134. Kleinman BS, Frey K, VanDrunen M, et al. Motion of the diaphragm in patients with chronic obstructive pulmonary disease while spontaneously breathing versus during positive pressure breathing after anesthesia and neuromuscular blockade. Anesthesiology 2002; 97:298–305.

135. Gorman RB, McKenzie DK, Pride NB, et al. Diaphragm length during tidal breathing in patients with chronic obstructive pulmonary disease. Am J Respir Crit Care Med 2002; 166:1461–9.

136. Hedenstierna G, Rothen HU. Atelectasis formation during anesthesia: causes and measures to prevent it. J Clin Monit Comput 2000; 16:329–35.

137. Dureuil B, Cantineau JP, Desmonts JM. Effects of upper or lower abdominal surgery on diaphragmatic function. Br J Anaesth 1987; 59:1230–5.

138. Maeda H, Nakahara K, Ohno K, et al. Diaphragm function after pulmonary resection. Relationship to postoperative respiratory failure. Am Rev Respir Dis 1988; 137:678–81.

139. Nimmo AF, Drummond GB. Respiratory mechanics after abdominal surgery measured with continuous analysis of pressure, flow and volume signals. Br J Anaesth 1996; 77(3):317–26.

140. Deng Y, Byth K, Paterson HS. Phrenic nerve injury associated with high free right internal mammary artery harvesting. Ann Thorac Surg 2003; 76:459–63.

141. Licker M, Schweizer A, Hohn L, et al. Unexpected postoperative respiratory failure due to diaphragmatic paralysis. Anesthesiology 1997; 87:1239.

142. Clergue F, Whitelaw WA, Charles JC, et al. Inferences about respiratory muscle use after cardiac surgery from compartmental volume and pressure measurements. Anesthesiology 1995; 82:1318–27.

143. Ford GT, Rosenal TW, Clergue F, et al. Respiratory physiology in upper abdominal surgery. Clin Chest Med 1993; 14:237–52.

144. Berdah SV, Picaud R, Jammes Y. Surface diaphragmatic electromyogram changes after laparotomy. Clin Physiol Funct Imaging 2002; 22:157–60.

145. Kelly S, Zin WA, Decramer M, et al. Salutary effect of fall in abdominal pressure during diaphragm paralysis. J Appl Physiol 1984; 56:1320–4.

146. Road JD, Burgess KR, Whitelaw WA, et al. Diaphragm function and respiratory response after upper abdominal surgery in dogs. J Appl Physiol 1984; 57:576–82.

147. Sprung J, Barnas GM, Cheng EY, et al. Changes in functional residual capacity and regional diaphragm lengths after upper abdominal surgery in anesthetized dogs. Anesth Analg 1992; 75:977–82.

148. Simonneau G, Vivien A, Sartene R, et al. Diaphragm dysfunction induced by upper abdominal surgery. Role of postoperative pain. Am Rev Respir Dis 1983; 128:899–903.

149. Vassilakopoulos T, Mastora Z, Katsaounou P, et al. Contribution of pain to inspiratory muscle dysfunction after upper abdominal surgery: a randomized controlled trial. Am J Respir Crit Care Med 2000; 161:1372–5.

150. Pansard JL, Mankikian B, Bertrand M, et al. Effects of thoracic extradural block on diaphragmatic electrical activity and contractility after upper abdominal surgery. Anesthesiology 1993; 78:63–71.

151. Manikian B, Cantineau JP, Bertrand M, et al. Improvement of diaphragmatic function by a thoracic extradural block after upper abdominal surgery. Anesthesiology 1988; 68:379–86.

152. Polaner DM, Kimball WR, Fratacci MD, et al. Thoracic epidural anesthesia increases diaphragmatic shortening after thoracotomy in the awake lamb. Anesthesiology 1993; 79:808–16.

153. Ciofolo MJ, Clergue F, Seebacher J, et al. Ventilatory effects of laparoscopy under epidural anesthesia. Anesth Analg 1990; 70:357–61.

154. Sharma RR, Axelsson H, Oberg A, et al. Diaphragmatic activity after laparoscopic cholecystectomy. Anesthesiology 1999; 91:406–13.

155. Hasukic S, Mesic D, Dizdarevic E, et al. Pulmonary function after laparoscopic and open cholecystectomy. Surg Endosc 2002; 16:163–5.

156. Joris JL, Hinque VL, Laurent PE, et al. Pulmonary function and pain after gastroplasty performed via laparotomy or laparoscopy in morbidly obese patients. Br J Anaesth 1998; 80:283–8.

157. Putensen-Himmer G, Putensen C, Lammer H, et al. Comparison of postoperative respiratory function after laparoscopy or open laparotomy for cholecystectomy. Anesthesiology 1992; 77:675–80.

158. Dureuil B, Viires N, Cantineau JP, et al. Diaphragmatic contractility after upper abdominal surgery. J Appl Physiol 1986; 61:1775–80.

159. Chuter TA, Weissman C, Mathews DM, et al. Diaphragmatic breathing maneuvers and movement of the diaphragm after cholecystectomy. Chest 1990; 97:1110–4.
160. Vassilakopoulos T, Roussos C, Zakynthinos S. Is loaded breathing an inflammatory stimulus? Curr Opin Crit Care 2005; 11(1):1–9.
161. Vassilakopoulos T, Roussos C, Zakynthinos S. The immune response to resistive breathing. Eur Respir J 2004; 24:1033–43.
162. Barreiro E, de la Puente B, Minguella J, et al. Oxidative stress and respiratory muscle dysfunction in severe chronic obstructive pulmonary disease. Am J Respir Crit Care Med 2005; 171:1116–24.
163. Esteban A, Anzueto A, Frutos F, et al. Characteristics and outcomes in adult patients receiving mechanical ventilation: a 28-day international study. J Am Med Assoc 2002; 287(3):345–55.
164. Battisti A, Michotte JB, Tassaux D, van Gessel E, Jolliet P. Non-invasive ventilation in the recovery room for postoperative respiratory failure: a feasibility study. Swiss Med Wkly 2005; 135(23–24):339–43.
165. Lawrence VA, Cornell JE, Smetana GW. Strategies to reduce postoperative pulmonary complications after noncardiothoracic surgery: systematic review for the American College of Physicians. Ann Intern Med 2006; 144(8):596–608.
166. Buhre W, Rossaint R. Perioperative management and monitoring in anaesthesia. Lancet 2003; 362:1839–46.
167. Hedrick TL, Anastacio MM, Sawyer RG. Prevention of surgical site infections. Expert Rev Anti Infect Ther 2006; 4:223–33.
168. American Society of Anesthesiologists Task Force on Preanesthesia Evaluation. Practice advisory for preanesthesia evaluation: a report by the American Society of Anesthesiologists Task Force on Preanesthesia Evaluation. Anesthesiology 2002; 96:485–96.
169. Garcia-Miguel FJ, Serrano-Aguilar PG, Lopez-Bastida J. Preoperative assessment. Lancet 2003; 362(9397):1749–57.
170. Barak M, Ben-Abraham R, Katz Y. ACC/AHA guidelines for preoperative cardiovascular evaluation for noncardiac surgery: a critical point of view. Clin Cardiol 2006; 29(5):195–8.
171. Froehlich JB, Karavite D, Russman PL, et al. American College of Cardiology/American Heart Association preoperative assessment guidelines reduce resource utilization before aortic surgery. J Vasc Surg 2002; 36(4):758–63.
172. Polanczyk CA, Rohde LE, Goldman L, et al. Right heart catheterization and cardiac complications in patients undergoing noncardiac surgery: an observational study. J Am Med Assoc 2001; 286(3):309–14.
173. Rohde LE, Polanczyk CA, Goldman L, Cook EF, Lee RT, Lee TH. Usefulness of transthoracic echocardiography as a tool for risk stratification of patients undergoing major noncardiac surgery. Am J Cardiol 2001; 87(5):505–9.
174. Nici L, Donner C, Wouters E, et al. American Thoracic Society/European Respiratory Society statement on pulmonary rehabilitation. Am J Respir Crit Care Med 2006; 173(12):1390–413.
175. Salman GF, Mosier MC, Beasley BW, Calkins DR. Rehabilitation for patients with chronic obstructive pulmonary disease: meta-analysis of randomized controlled trials. J Gen Intern Med 2003; 18(3):213–21.
176. Castillo R, Haas A. Chest physical therapy: comparative efficacy of preoperative and postoperative in the elderly. Arch Phys Med Rehabil 1985; 66(6):376–9.
177. Silvanus MT, Groeben H, Peters J. Corticosteroids and inhaled salbutamol in patients with reversible airway obstruction markedly decrease the incidence of bronchospasm after tracheal intubation. Anesthesiology 2004; 100:1052–7.
178. Pien LC, Grammer LC, Patterson R. Minimal complications in a surgical population with severe asthma receiving prophylactic corticosteroids. J Allergy Clin Immunol 1988; 82:696–700.
179. Karthikeyan G, Bhargava B. Managing patients undergoing non-cardiac surgery: need to shift emphasis from risk stratification to risk modification. Heart 2006; 92(1):17–20.
180. McGory ML, Maggard MA, Ko CY. A meta-analysis of perioperative beta blockade: what is the actual risk reduction? Surgery 2005; 138(2):171–9.
181. Salpeter S, Ormiston T, Salpeter E. Cardioselective beta-blockers for chronic obstructive pulmonary disease. Cochrane Database Syst Rev 2005; (4):CD003566.
182. Salpeter SR, Ormiston TM, Salpeter EE. Cardiovascular effects of beta-agonists in patients with asthma and COPD: a meta-analysis. Chest 2004; 125:2309–21.
183. O'Connell F, Thomas VE, Fuller RW, et al. Effect of clonidine on induced cough and bronchoconstriction in guinea pigs and healthy humans. J Appl Physiol 1994; 76:1082–7.

184. Groeben H, Mitzner W, Brown RH. Effects of the alpha2-adrenoceptor agonist dexmedetomidine on bronchoconstriction in dogs. Anesthesiology 2004; 100(2):359–63.

185. Wallace AW, Galindez D, Salahieh A, et al. Effect of clonidine on cardiovascular morbidity and mortality after noncardiac surgery. Anesthesiology 2004; 101:284–93.

186. Wijeysundera DN, Naik JS, Beattie WS. Alpha-2 adrenergic agonists to prevent perioperative cardiovascular complications: a meta-analysis. Am J Med 2003; 114:742–52.

187. Barrera R, Shi W, Amar D, et al. Smoking and timing of cessation: impact on pulmonary complications after thoracotomy. Chest 2005; 127(6):1977–83.

188. Moller A, Tonnesen H. Risk reduction: perioperative smoking intervention. Best Pract Res Clin Anaesthesiol 2006; 20(2):237–48.

189. Moller A, Villebro N. Interventions for preoperative smoking cessation. Cochrane Database Syst Rev 2005; (3):CD002294.

190. Dimick JB, Birkmeyer JD, Upchurch GR, Jr. Measuring surgical quality: what's the role of provider volume? World J Surg 2005; 29:1217–21.

191. Birkmeyer NJ, Birkmeyer JD. Strategies for improving surgical quality—should payers reward excellence or effort? N Engl J Med 2006; 354:864–70.

192. Birkmeyer JD, Sun Y, Goldfaden A, Birkmeyer NJ, Stukel TA. Volume and process of care in high-risk cancer surgery. Cancer 2006; 106(11):2476–81.

193. Aziz O, Constantinides V, Tekkis PP, et al. Laparoscopic versus open surgery for rectal cancer: a meta-analysis. Ann Surg Oncol 2006; 13:413–24.

194. Rosman AS, Melis M, Fichera A. Metaanalysis of trials comparing laparoscopic and open surgery for Crohn's disease. Surg Endosc 2005; 19:1549–55.

195. Johnson N, Barlow D, Lethaby A, et al. Methods of hysterectomy: systematic review and meta-analysis of randomised controlled trials. Br Med J 2005; 330:1478.

196. Compton CN, Dillavou ED, Sheehan MK, et al. Is abdominal aortic aneurysm repair appropriate in oxygen-dependent chronic obstructive pulmonary disease patients? J Vasc Surg 2005; 42:650–3.

197. Nelson R, Tse B, Edwards S. Systematic review of prophylactic nasogastric decompression after abdominal operations. Br J Surg 2005; 92:673–80.

198. Kim ES, Bishop MJ. Endotracheal intubation, but not laryngeal mask airway insertion, produces reversible bronchoconstriction. Anesthesiology 1999; 90(2):391–4.

199. Brown RH, Wagner EM. Mechanisms of bronchoprotection by anesthetic induction agents: propofol versus ketamine. Anesthesiology 1999; 90(3):822–8.

200. Choi JH, Rooke GA, Wu SC, Bishop MJ. Reduction in post-intubation respiratory resistance by isoflurane and albuterol. Can J Anaesth 1997; 44(7):717–22.

201. Dikmen Y, Eminoglu E, Salihoglu Z, Demiroluk S. Pulmonary mechanics during isoflurane, sevoflurane and desflurane anaesthesia. Anaesthesia 2003; 58(8):745–8.

202. Scalfaro P, Sly PD, Sims C, Habre W. Salbutamol prevents the increase of respiratory resistance caused by tracheal intubation during sevoflurane anesthesia in asthmatic children. Anesth Analg 2001; 93(4):898–902.

203. Groeben H, Schlicht M, Stieglitz S, et al. Both local anesthetics and salbutamol pretreatment affect reflex bronchoconstriction in volunteers with asthma undergoing awake fiberoptic intubation. Anesthesiology 2002; 97:1445–50.

204. Groeben H, Grosswendt T, Silvanus M, et al. Lidocaine inhalation for local anaesthesia and attenuation of bronchial hyper-reactivity with least airway irritation. Effect of three different dose regimens. Eur J Anaesthesiol 2000; 17:672–9.

205. DeSouza G, deLisser EA, Turry P, Gold MI. Comparison of propofol with isoflurane for maintenance of anesthesia in patients with chronic obstructive pulmonary disease: use of pulmonary mechanics, peak flow rates, and blood gases. J Cardiothorac Vasc Anesth 1995; 9(1):24–8.

206. Volta CA, Alvisi V, Petrini S, et al. The effect of volatile anesthetics on respiratory system resistance in patients with chronic obstructive pulmonary disease. Anesth Analg 2005; 100:348–53.

207. Yu G, Yang K, Baker AB, Young I. The effect of bi-level positive airway pressure mechanical ventilation on gas exchange during general anaesthesia. Br J Anaesth 2006; 96(4):522–32.

208. Neumann P, Rothen HU, Berglund JE, Valtysson J, Magnusson A, Hedenstierna G. Positive end-expiratory pressure prevents atelectasis during general anaesthesia even in the presence of a high inspired oxygen concentration. Acta Anaesthesiol Scand 1999; 43(3):295–301.

209. Moran JL, Bersten AD, Solomon PJ. Meta-analysis of controlled trials of ventilator therapy in acute lung injury and acute respiratory distress syndrome: an alternative perspective. Intensive Care Med 2005; 31:227–35.

210. Ferrer M, Iglesia R, Roca J, et al. Pulmonary gas exchange response to weaning with pressure-support ventilation in exacerbated chronic obstructive pulmonary disease patients. Intensive Care Med 2002; 28:1595–9.

211. Fernandez-Perez ER, Keegan MT, Brown DR, et al. Intraoperative tidal volume as a risk factor for respiratory failure after pneumonectomy. Anesthesiology 2006; 105:14–8.

212. Belda FJ, Aguilera L, Garcia de la Asuncion J, et al. Supplemental perioperative oxygen and the risk of surgical wound infection: a randomized controlled trial. J Am Med Assoc 2005; 294:2035–42.

213. Pryor KO, Fahey TJ, III, Lien CA, et al. Surgical site infection and the routine use of perioperative hyperoxia in a general surgical population: a randomized controlled trial. J Am Med Assoc 2004; 291:79–87.

214. Edmark L, Kostova-Aherdan K, Enlund M, Hedenstierna G. Optimal oxygen concentration during induction of general anesthesia. Anesthesiology 2003; 98(1):28–33.

215. Oczenski W, Schwarz S, Fitzgerald RD. Vital capacity manoeuvre in general anaesthesia: useful or useless? Eur J Anaesthesiol 2004; 21(4):253–9.

216. Rothen HU, Neumann P, Berglund JE, et al. Dynamics of re-expansion of atelectasis during general anaesthesia. Br J Anaesth 1999; 82:551–6.

217. Whalen FX, Gajic O, Thompson GB, et al. The effects of the alveolar recruitment maneuver and positive end-expiratory pressure on arterial oxygenation during laparoscopic bariatric surgery. Anesth Analg 2006; 102(1):298–305.

218. Werawatganon T, Charuluxanun S. Patient controlled intravenous opioid analgesia versus continuous epidural analgesia for pain after intra-abdominal surgery. Cochrane Database Syst Rev 2005; (1):CD004088.

219. Remy C, Marret E, Bonnet F. Effects of acetaminophen on morphine side-effects and consumption after major surgery: meta-analysis of randomized controlled trials. Br J Anaesth 2005; 94:505–13.

220. Marret E, Kurdi O, Zufferey P, et al. Effects of nonsteroidal antiinflammatory drugs on patient-controlled analgesia morphine side effects: meta-analysis of randomized controlled trials. Anesthesiology 2005; 102:1249–60.

221. Elia N, Lysakowski C, Tramer MR. Does multimodal analgesia with acetaminophen, nonsteroidal antiinflammatory drugs, or selective cyclooxygenase-2 inhibitors and patient-controlled analgesia morphine offer advantages over morphine alone? Meta-analyses of randomized trials Anesthesiology 2005; 103:1296–304.

222. Beattie WS, Badner NH, Choi P. Epidural analgesia reduces postoperative myocardial infarction: a meta-analysis. Anesth Analg 2001; 93:853–8.

223. Brodner G, Mertes N, Van Aken H, et al. Epidural analgesia with local anesthetics after abdominal surgery: earlier motor recovery with 0.2% ropivacaine than 0.175% bupivacaine. Anesth Analg 1999; 88:128–33.

224. Rigg JR, Jamrozik K, Myles PS, et al. Epidural anaesthesia and analgesia and outcome of major surgery: a randomised trial. Lancet 2002; 359:1276–82.

225. Park WY, Thompson JS, Lee KK. Effect of epidural anesthesia and analgesia on perioperative outcome: a randomized, controlled Veterans Affairs cooperative study. Ann Surg 2001; 234:560–9 (discussion 569–71).

226. Buggy DJ, Doherty WL, Hart EM, et al. Postoperative wound oxygen tension with epidural or intravenous analgesia: a prospective, randomized, single-blind clinical trial. Anesthesiology 2002; 97:952–8.

227. Gruber EM, Tschernko EM, Kritzinger M, et al. The effects of thoracic epidural analgesia with bupivacaine 0.25% on ventilatory mechanics in patients with severe chronic obstructive pulmonary disease. Anesth Analg 2001; 92(4):1015–9.

228. Carli F, Mayo N, Klubien K, et al. Epidural analgesia enhances functional exercise capacity and health-related quality of life after colonic surgery: results of a randomized trial. Anesthesiology 2002; 97:540–9.

229. Clergue F, Montembault C, Despierres O, et al. Respiratory effects of intrathecal morphine after upper abdominal surgery. Anesthesiology 1984; 61:677–85.

230. Renaud B, Brichant JF, Clergue F, et al. Ventilatory effects of continuous epidural infusion of fentanyl. Anesth Analg 1988; 67:971–5.

231. Shapiro A, Zohar E, Zaslansky R, Hoppenstein D, Shabat S, Fredman B. The frequency and timing of respiratory depression in 1524 postoperative patients treated with systemic or neuraxial morphine. J Clin Anesth 2005; 17(7):537–42.

232. Bailey PL, Rhondeau S, Schafer PG, et al. Dose–response pharmacology of intrathecal morphine in human volunteers. Anesthesiology 1993; 79(1):49–59.
233. Horlocker TT, Wedel DJ, Benzon H, et al. Regional anesthesia in the anticoagulated patient: defining the risks (the second ASRA Consensus Conference on Neuraxial Anesthesia and Anticoagulation). Reg Anesth Pain Med 2003; 28(3):172–97.
234. Cholley BP, Payen D. Noninvasive techniques for measurements of cardiac output. Curr Opin Crit Care 2005; 11:424–9.
235. Bein B, Worthmann F, Tonner PH, et al. Comparison of esophageal Doppler, pulse contour analysis, and real-time pulmonary artery thermodilution for the continuous measurement of cardiac output. J Cardiothorac Vasc Anesth 2004; 18:185–9.
236. Rocco M, Spadetta G, Morelli A, et al. A comparative evaluation of thermodilution and partial CO_2 rebreathing techniques for cardiac output assessment in critically ill patients during assisted ventilation. Intensive Care Med 2004; 30:82–7.
237. Pestel GJ, Kurz A. Hypothermia—it's more than a toy. Curr Opin Anaesthesiol 2005; 18:151–6.
238. Pino RM. Residual neuromuscular blockade: a persistent clinical problem. Int Anesthesiol Clin 2006; 44:77–90.
239. Baillard C, Clec'h C, Catineau J, et al. Postoperative residual neuromuscular block: a survey of management. Br J Anaesth 2005; 95:622–6.
240. American Society of Anesthesiologists Task Force on Intraoperative Awareness. Practice advisory for intraoperative awareness and brain function monitoring: a report by the American Society of Anesthesiologists Task Force on Intraoperative Awareness. Anesthesiology 2006; 104:847–64.
241. Lennmarken C, Sandin R. Neuromonitoring for awareness during surgery. Lancet 2004; 363(9423):1747–8.
242. Monk TG, Saini V, Weldon BC, Sigl JC. Anesthetic management and one-year mortality after noncardiac surgery. Anesth Analg 2005; 100(1):4–10.
243. Ekman A, Lindholm ML, Lennmarken C, Sandin R. Reduction in the incidence of awareness using BIS monitoring. Acta Anaesthesiol Scand 2004; 48(1):20–6.
244. Cahalin LP, Braga M, Matsuo Y, et al. Efficacy of diaphragmatic breathing in persons with chronic obstructive pulmonary disease: a review of the literature. J Cardiopulm Rehabil 2002; 22:7–21.
245. Tobias JD. Noninvasive ventilation using bilevel positive airway pressure to treat impending respiratory failure in the postanesthesia care unit. J Clin Anesth 2000; 12(5):409–12.
246. Thomas JA, McIntosh JM. Are incentive spirometry, intermittent positive pressure breathing, and deep breathing exercises effective in the prevention of postoperative pulmonary complications after upper abdominal surgery? A systematic overview and meta-analysis Phys Ther 1994; 74:3–16.
247. Christensen EF, Schultz P, Jensen OV, et al. Postoperative pulmonary complications and lung function in high-risk patients: a comparison of three physiotherapy regimens after upper abdominal surgery in general anesthesia. Acta Anaesthesiol Scand 1991; 35:97–104.
248. Fagevik Olsen M, Hahn I, Nordgren S, et al. Randomized controlled trial of prophylactic chest physiotherapy in major abdominal surgery. Br J Surg 1997; 84:1535–8.
249. Mackay MR, Ellis E, Johnston C. Randomised clinical trial of physiotherapy after open abdominal surgery in high risk patients. Aust J Physiother 2005; 51:151–9.
250. Squadrone E, Frigerio P, Fogliati C, et al. Noninvasive vs invasive ventilation in COPD patients with severe acute respiratory failure deemed to require ventilatory assistance. Intensive Care Med 2004; 30(7):1303–10.
251. Valipour A, Cozzarini W, Burghuber OC. Non-invasive pressure support ventilation in patients with respiratory failure due to severe acute cardiogenic pulmonary edema. Respiration 2004; 71(2):144–51.

24

Providing Palliative and End-of-Life Care for Patients with COPD

DAVID H. AU
Health Services Research and Development, Veterans Administration Puget Sound
Health Care System, and Division of Pulmonary and Critical Care Medicine,
Department of Medicine, University of Washington, Seattle, Washington, U.S.A.

J. RANDALL CURTIS
Division of Pulmonary and Critical Care Medicine, Department of Medicine,
University of Washington, Seattle, Washington, U.S.A.

I. Introduction

Chronic obstructive pulmonary disease (COPD) is the fourth leading cause of death in the United States and the only major cause of death for which the age-adjusted mortality is increasing (1). This fact has lead some to estimate that COPD will become the third leading cause of death and fifth leading cause of disability worldwide by the year 2020 (2). COPD causes significant amount of burden to patients and their family caregivers as well as to the medical care system (3). There have been no new therapies for patients with COPD that have been proven to reduce mortality since the reports of a smoking cessation intervention (4) and the use of long-term oxygen therapy for severely hypoxemic patients (5). In this sense, all other modern therapies for the treatment of COPD could be considered palliative in that their benefits are derived largely from improvements in symptoms and functional status (6–8). However, the magnitude of the treatment effect, averaged across patients, usually approaches those considered to be the minimally clinically important different on symptoms and functional status and there are a significant number of individuals who remain significantly symptomatic despite maximal therapy (6–8).

The best way to improve palliative and end-of-life care among patients with COPD remains largely unexplored. There are a number of barriers that have contributed to this lack of attention which include uncertainty around trajectory toward death, lack of clinician efficacy regarding the delivery of end-of-life care, and misperceptions about patients' desires to discuss end-of-life care on the part of health care providers. Although there has been some recent attention directed to palliative and end-of-life care by professional societies (9), promotion of palliative and end-of-life care has been largely excluded from major guidelines regarding the management of COPD (10). The first step in delivering high-quality palliative and end-of-life care to patients with severe COPD is recognition that it is the responsibility of all clinicians and especially those with expertise in lung diseases to provide these services to individuals approaching death. It is also vitally important to acknowledge that end-of-life care is an integral and essential part of delivering high-quality health care, especially for patients with terminal or life-limiting illness such as severe COPD. The focus of this chapter is to provide a framework for clinicians that helps define high-quality end-of-life care, facilitates discussions and decision making about end-of-life care, and improves the care of patients with advanced COPD.

II. What Is Quality Palliative and End-of-Life Care?

The Institute of Medicine acknowledged that the concept of "good" and "bad" deaths cannot be singularly defined but that care that patients receive at the end of life should be influenced by individual experiences and beliefs, the available technology, and the individual's interactions with society and culture (11). Therefore, the Institute of Medicine defines an acceptable quality of experience at the end of life as "one that is free from avoidable distress and suffering for patients, families, and caregivers; in general accord with patients' and families' wishes; and reasonably consistent with clinical, cultural, and ethical standards" (11). Similarly, they define an unacceptable quality of dying and death as one that is "characterized by needless suffering, disregard for patient or family wishes or values, and a sense among participants or observers that norms of decency have been offended" (11). These definitions of a good and bad experience cannot be measured from a single individual's perspective, but rather incorporate the experience of the community of individuals who are involved with the patients' life. Unlike other commonly assessed measures of quality of care such as the proper prescribing and delivery of medications, assessing the quality of care at the end of life is multidimensional because it requires integration of the experiences of not only the patient but also individuals who are closely involved with them. Furthermore, in contrast to other measures of quality of care, there is a greater emphasis on ensuring concordance between the care that is desired and that which is delivered. This is especially true when balancing the tension that may exist between providing care directed at prolongation of life and palliating symptoms at the end of life.

The conceptual and pragmatic features of delivering a high quality of care at the end of life do not differ from the delivery of quality care in any other situation. The essential attributes include understanding the goals of care, communicating expectations about the results of therapy and prognoses, as well as understanding what therapies would be considered acceptable to those receiving the care. To be able to provide this care at the end of life, clinicians must have strong interpersonal skills that place value on patient autonomy while being able to provide care, integrate patient's value, and advise patients based on the best available evidence and their professional experience. Although these issues may seem readily apparent, medical education has not, until recently, provided emphasis on how to master these necessary skills. Without providing a structured educational approach to these issues, clinicians are left to develop these skills independently and this fact likely contributes to heterogeneity in the delivery of care at the end of life.

Curtis and colleagues developed a conceptual model that characterized domains of physicians' skills at providing high-quality end-of-life care based on a series of focus groups (12). Patients with severe COPD were included along with patients with advanced AIDS or metastatic cancer and their family members. Based on these focus groups, 12 domains of physician skills were identified and further grouped into five categories as shown in Figure 1 (12). Cognitive and affective skills were placed at the top of the model based on the importance placed on them by patients. Emotional support provided by physicians was consistently ranked the most important skill among all patients regardless of condition. Communication with patients (communication skills) was the second most highly desirable characteristic. Patient-centered values focused on physicians' attention to patient values, respect and humility, and supporting patient autonomy. Finally, patient-centered care systems focused on accessibility, continuity of care, and team communication and coordination. Each of the individual domains represents opportunities to evaluate and improve the quality of end-of-life care for not only those patients with COPD but also those with any chronic, life-limiting illness.

III. Do Patients with COPD Receive Less Palliative Care at the End of Life?

The Study to Understand Prognosis and Preferences for Outcomes and Treatments (SUPPORT), enrolled seriously ill, hospitalized patients with one of six life-limiting illnesses, including COPD (13). SUPPORT found that, compared to patients with lung cancer, patients with COPD were much more likely to die in the intensive care unit (ICU), on mechanical ventilation, and with dyspnea (14). These differences in care occurred despite the fact that most patients with COPD preferred treatment focused on comfort rather than on prolonging life. In fact, the SUPPORT investigators found that

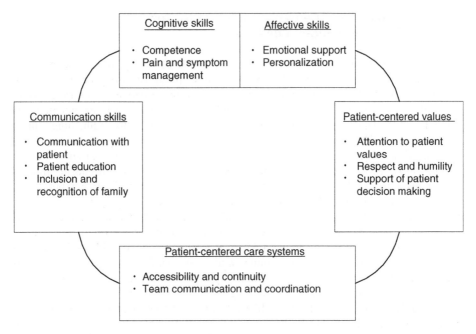

Figure 1 Conceptual model of the domains of physician skills at providing high-quality end-of-life care.

patients with lung cancer and patients with COPD were equally likely to prefer not to be intubated and not to receive cardiopulmonary resuscitation (CPR) (14). These differences in the delivery of palliative care for patients with COPD and lung cancer at the end of life have been replicated in a number of studies. A study in Britain found that patients with COPD were much less likely to die at home and much less likely to receive palliative care services than patients with lung cancer (15). In fact, comparison of symptoms for patients with advanced COPD or lung cancer suggests that they have similar physical and psychologic needs, yet patients with COPD are less likely to receive needed support (16). Additional studies from Britain documented the poor quality of palliative care and significant burden of symptoms among patients with COPD (17). Health care for these patients was often initiated in response to acute exacerbations rather than being initiated based on a previously developed plan for managing their disease (18). A recent study of patients with COPD or lung cancer in the U.S. Veterans Affairs health system confirmed that patients with COPD were much more likely to be admitted to an ICU and have greater lengths of stay in the ICU during their terminal hospitalization than patients with lung cancer (19). The investigators also found significant geographic variation in ICU utilization for patients with COPD that were not seen for patients with lung cancer (19). Although variation in care may be influenced by many factors including availability, access, and reimbursement issues, such geographic variation suggests a lack of consensus concerning the best approach to end-of-life care for patients with COPD. Taken together, these studies suggest that despite evidence that patients would like to receive similar care to patients with lung cancer, there were less palliative services provided to patients with COPD.

IV. Relationship Between the Trajectory Toward Death and End-of-Life Care

The differences in health care for patients with COPD compared to those with cancer may be due, in part, to the difficulty physicians have prognosticating for patients with COPD and especially in identifying with confidence those patients who are likely to die within six months. The prognostic models used in SUPPORT documented this difficulty (14). These models showed that, at five days prior to death, lung cancer patients were predicted to have less than 10% chance of surviving six months, while patients with COPD were predicted to have more than 50% chance of surviving six months (14). More recent efforts to identify disease-specific prognostic models for patents with COPD improve prognostic accuracy for groups of patients, but do not predict survival for individual patients with comparable accuracy as can be done for many patients with lung cancer (20). Recently, the BODE Index was developed and validated for patients with COPD (20). This index incorporates *B*ody mass index, severity of *O*bstruction, the modified Medical Research Council (MMRC) *D*yspnea scale, and *E*xercise by the six-minute walk test (Table 1). This measure had significantly better discrimination for mortality than forced expiratory volume in one second (FEV_1) alone; however, even among these patients, there was a limited ability to distinguish individuals who were likely to die in the subsequent six months. For example, among individuals with BODE scores of 7 to 10 that represented the 25% with the worse scores, 55% of patients were alive at three years. In the next highest stratum (scores of 5–6), approximately 75% were alive at three years. This suggests that, even

Table 1 BODE Index

Characteristic	Points on Score			
	0	1	2	3
FEV$_1$ (% predicted)	≥ 65	50–64	36–49	≤ 35
Distance walked (6 min, m)	≥ 350	250–349	150–249	≤ 149
MMRC dyspnea score	0–1	2	3	4
Body mass index	> 21	≤ 21		

Abbreviations: FEV$_1$, forced expiratory volume in one second; MMRC, modified Medical Research Council; BODE, body mass index, obstruction, dyspnea, exercise.

among very severe individuals, it is difficult to distinguish which patient is likely to meet standard criteria for hospice care in the United States (six-month survival or less). The uncertainty of prognosis must therefore play a much more prominent role in discussions of prognosis and end-of-life care for patients with COPD than for patients with lung cancer. It is consequently not surprising that physicians have a more difficult time knowing when to raise issues about end-of-life care for patients with COPD. Despite these difficulties in prognostication, the responsibility remains in the hands of physicians caring for patients with COPD to educate patients about their likely experiences and the types of care they may need toward the end of life. Having such discussions with patients is likely the best way to ensure that patients receive the best possible care that is in line with their informed preferences for care at the end of life.

V. Why Don't Physicians Discuss End-of-Life Care with Patients with Severe COPD?

In the outpatient setting, it is not surprising that physicians consistently note insufficient time during an appointment as a barrier to having discussion about end-of-life and advance care planning (21). Furthermore, in one study, two-thirds of physicians who reported infrequently discussing end-of-life care reported feeling inadequately prepared to have such discussions (17). Time issues coupled with insecurity about being able to perform these discussions are often sufficient to ensure physicians will avoid end-of-life discussions altogether. It is often necessary for patients to express a desire for these discussions and, as described below, this likely contributes to the relatively low reported prevalence of end-of-life care discussions between patients with severe COPD and their physicians. This would suggest that systems of care should be designed and implemented to trigger conversations about advanced care planning. These systems would need to provide the patient the opportunity to express their goals of care while providing this information succinctly to their surrogates and physicians. Another important system change is the need to improve how clinicians learn to perform high-quality end-of-life care planning with patients. Currently, most physicians learn in the model of apprenticeship, and there are few programs that exist within the medical training that allow for developing these skills in a systematic and effective way. These programs would likely work best if they allowed students to observe and then to confront uncomfortable situations in a controlled setting with close observation by individuals skilled with these discussions. In addition, the core elements should be based in part on areas that are in need of improvement. For example, we recently found that only a third of patients with oxygen-dependent COPD had discussed end-of-life care with their physicians and less than 25% of those physicians who did conduct such discussions had discussed some particularly important aspects of end-of-life care with their patients (22). These infrequently discussed aspects included talking about how long the patient might live, talking about what dying might be like, talking with family about what dying might be like, and asking patients about their spiritual or religious beliefs. We also examined those items that patients with COPD rated as being performed most poorly. These poorly performed items included talking about how long patients might have to live and asking about the patients' spiritual or religious beliefs. This study suggests that efforts targeted to improve the quality of communication about end-of-life care should include means to improve the quality of discussions about prognosis, dying, and spirituality.

Educational sessions also need to address common misperceptions of patient's lack of desire for discussions about end-of-life care. In a study examining provider and patient barriers to end-of-life communication, physicians commonly ascribed two barriers to patients which may not be true (21). These included that "discussing end-of-life care will take away their hope" and "the patient is not ready to talk about the care they want if they get sick." Previous results suggest that the majority of patients with COPD would like to have such discussions, but that these discussions do not occur regularly (23). These findings have been replicated in additional studies including a qualitative study of patients with severe COPD in Britain (17). This study showed that most patients wanted more information about their disease and prognosis and, despite general agreement by practitioners of the importance of these discussions, only 41% of these physicians reported "often" or "always" discussing prognosis with their patients with COPD. In our qualitative study comparing physician skills of patients with severe COPD, metastatic cancer, or advanced AIDS, patients with COPD were most likely to report wanting more information in the following five areas: diagnosis and disease process, treatment, prognosis, what dying might be like, and advance care planning (Table 2) (24). To highlight patients' overall need for additional knowledge of COPD, among 12 patient-rated physician skills at providing end-of-life care, patients rated providing education about COPD higher than skills such as clinician competence, attention to patient values, and personalization (12,24).

In clinical practice, an important minority of patients is uncomfortable with obtaining prognostic information and advanced care planning. In a survey of older patients with serious illnesses but limited life expectancy, over half (56%) of participants with COPD wanted to know their life expectancy and 44% did not (25). Results from SUPPORT suggest, however, that providers may be missing important

Table 2 Patient Reported Desirable Components to End-of-Life Communication

Their diagnoses and disease process
Role of treatment to improve symptoms, quality of life, and length of life
Prognosis for survival and quality of life
What dying might be like
Advance care planning for future medical care and exacerbations

Source: From Ref. 24.

information from those individuals who did not want to have discussions about end-of-life care. For example, SUPPORT investigators demonstrated that of the 58% of individuals who did not want to have discussion about CPR, 25% of them did not want to have CPR. Furthermore, of those individuals (88%) who did not want prolonged mechanical ventilation, 70% of them never had discussion about mechanical ventilation (26). These findings highlight important challenges for physicians. First, how does a physician distinguish patients who desire prognostic information from those who do not? Second, in the context of the findings from SUPPORT, how do physicians impart the need to communicate with patients if patients themselves are reticent to have such conversations? We suggest providing education and having conversations with all patients should be part of providing high-quality care and that being able to say that these types of conversations are a matter of "routine practice" diffuses some of the tension that may exist for both patients and providers. Physicians need to develop skills to gently address these issues with patients who are reticent to discuss them. Furthermore, it is our observation from interviews that we have performed that when physicians do a good job of discussing palliative care, patients perceive their physicians to be interested in them as an entire person, rather than just a person with a lung problem.

VI. Frequency and Timing of End-of-Life Discussions

Although the precise reasons explaining why patients with COPD receive less palliative care than those with lung cancer are not entirely clear, several studies have shown that only a minority of patients with moderate-to-severe COPD have discussed treatment preferences and end-of-life care issues with their physicians and yet most of these patients do want to discuss these issues (22,23,27). Further, the majority of these patients believe their physicians do not know their preferences for end-of-life care (23,27). A recent study found that when Canadian respirologists discussed mechanical ventilation for end-stage COPD, the discussions occurred late in the disease trajectory; they most commonly took place in the ICU, with only 23% occurring in the clinic or office (28). Eighty-four percent of physicians waited until dyspnea was severe and 75% of physicians waited until the FEV_1 was $< 30\%$ predicted. SUPPORT demonstrated that interventions designed to improve patient education and palliative care services performed at the time of admission to hospital did not improve quality of care and their findings suggest that seriously ill hospitalized patients are less likely to want to discuss end-of-life care than outpatients with severe COPD (13). These results suggest that discussions that occur in the hospital setting may come too late and that physicians should be raising these issues early and before patients are in the hospital.

When discussions occur in the setting of exacerbations or respiratory failure, they also limit the range of individuals who may actually benefit from these discussions. Among the most severely impaired individuals, respiratory failure is a common etiology for death, but for the majority of patients with COPD the cause of death is attributed to either cardiovascular disease or lung cancer (7,29). In these situations, COPD represents a coexisting condition that may modify outcome but may not be directly responsible for their deaths. Together, these studies suggest that physicians do not frequently discuss preferences for care at the end of life and when done, often limit discussion to individuals who are very severely impaired. This behavior limits discussions to the minority of individuals who have severe COPD and acute respiratory failure and neglects others who may also benefit from understanding how COPD may modify their treatment options. We believe that incorporating discussion into routine outpatient clinical care may improve patient's ability to adjust and anticipate future health status and health care needs.

VII. What Common Symptoms and Conditions Do Patients with COPD Experience at the End of Life?

In order for clinicians to effectively provide palliative and end-of-life care, they must be familiar with the symptoms that patients will commonly experience at the end of life. A recent systematic review determined the prevalence of 11 common symptoms in five advanced life-limiting conditions, including COPD (30). The results of the estimated prevalence among patients with COPD are shown in Table 3. Not surprisingly, the prevalence of breathlessness was the highest among patients with COPD with the prevalence estimated between 90% and 95%. Pain (prevalence 34–77%), fatigue (prevalence 68–80%), and insomnia (prevalence 55–65%) are under-appreciated and common symptoms and are only occasionally included in patient symptom scales for COPD (31). Anxiety and depression are especially prevalent among patients with COPD. These disorders are important to recognize because of their detrimental effects on health-related quality of life and because they are treatable. Anorexia that contributes to weight loss, an ominous predictor of survival, has a prevalence estimated between 35% and 67%, which is comparable to some estimates among patients dying with cancer, AIDS, and end-stage renal disease (30).

VIII. Palliative Treatments for Dyspnea and Other Symptoms

Treatment of most of the symptoms for patients with advanced COPD is similar to the treatment of these symptoms for other patients with advanced chronic illness and is beyond the scope of this chapter. Nonetheless, recognition and treatment of these symptoms is a key component of high-quality end-of-life care for patients with advanced COPD.

Table 3 Prevalence of Symptoms Among Patients with Chronic Obstructive Pulmonary Disease

Symptom	Number	Prevalence (%)
Breathlessness	372	90–95
Insomnia	150	55–65
Fatigue	285	68–80
Pain	372	34–74
Anxiety	1008	51–75
Confusion	309	18–33
Depression	150	37–71
Anorexia	150	35–67
Constipation	150	27–44

Dyspnea is a significant source of disability for persons with COPD and profoundly affects quality of life (32). Many of the treatments for dyspnea in severe COPD have been covered in other chapters in this volume, but it is important to address the treatment of dyspnea in settings where patients have received optimal bronchodilator, corticosteroid, and oxygen therapy and yet continue to suffer from chronic dyspnea. Patients who survive a hospitalization after an acute exacerbation of COPD often experience shortness of breath for the rest of their lives (33). In the last year of life, as many as 94% of patients with chronic lung disease experience dyspnea (16). SUPPORT investigators found that, compared to patients with lung cancer, patients with COPD were more likely to die with poor control of dyspnea (14). These studies not only demonstrate the prevalence of dyspnea, but also reaffirm the need to identify evidence-based treatments for this burdensome symptom for patients with severe COPD and ensure that patients receive these treatments. Bronchodilators, corticosteroids, and oxygen therapy are important components of therapy for dyspnea in COPD and have been covered elsewhere in this volume. We will address some additional therapies for refractory dyspnea in these patients.

A. Opiates

Opiates are an important part of the armamentarium for the treatment of dyspnea in the patient with severe COPD maximally treated with bronchodilators and other therapies; however, the benefit achieved with these agents is relatively modest. There have been a number of randomized trials and a recent meta-analysis which suggest that oral opiates can reduce the sensation of dyspnea (34). This meta-analysis also suggests that while oral and parental opiates can reduce the sensation of dyspnea, there are inadequate data to conclude that nebulized opiates are effective.

B. Other Pharmacological Agents for Dyspnea

A number of small studies have examined the role of other oral agents including benzodiazepines, phenothiazines, and busparone. These studies, recently analyzed in two reviews of treatment of dyspnea in severe COPD, were either negative or inconclusive, suggesting that these agents should not be routinely used for dyspnea in patients with COPD (35,36). Although antidepressants are not routinely used for the treatment of dyspnea among patients with COPD, it is important to note that treatment of depression can also reduce symptoms of dyspnea in patients with COPD and depression (37,38).

C. Nonpharmacological Treatments

There are a number of nonpharmacologic approaches that can have an important effect on dyspnea and other symptoms as well as quality of life. An example of such approaches includes pulmonary rehabilitation. Although different pulmonary rehabilitation programs include different components, randomized trials have clearly shown that pulmonary rehabilitation can improve dyspnea, exercise tolerance, and health-related quality of life (39–41). Important components of this nonpharmacologic therapy include teaching patients breathing techniques and other nonpharmacologic methods such as the use of fans and relaxation techniques which may help reduce sensations of anxiety and increase the perception of control when patients feel dyspneic.

D. Hospice

Another important treatment option for patients with severe COPD is referral to hospice. Hospice programs may be able to offer patients with COPD tremendous amount of psychologic, emotional, and spiritual support in their final months as well as intensive symptom assessment and management above what a hospital or office-based physician can offer. Hospice is under-utilized by patients with COPD (15). However, there are many patients with severe COPD for whom a physician may have reasonable confidence that the patient is likely to die within six months. If patients improve, they can be taken off the hospice benefit without penalty and still be eligible to return to hospice if they deteriorate again.

E. Coordinated Treatment Approach to Dyspnea

Most clinicians are familiar with the "Pain Ladder" promoted by the World Health Organization for a stepped treatment of pain. A recent review article proposed a "Dyspnea Ladder" into routine assessment of patients with progressing COPD (Fig. 2) (42). This approach may help clinicians assess the adequacy of dyspnea management and intensify treatment when the current treatment is not successful. Clinicians should balance benefits and side effects of any medication on an individual basis.

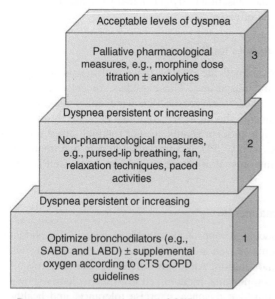

Dyspnea management in server COPD

Figure 2 The dyspnea ladder. *Abbreviations*: COPD, chronic obstructive pulmonary disease; CTS, Canadian Thoracic Society; LABD, long-acting bronchodilator; SABD, short-acting bronchodilator.

IX. Does Patient Health Status Influence the Desire for Life-Sustaining Treatment?

Previous studies suggest that, when confronted with making treatment recommendations for patients who are incapable of making their own decisions, physicians will often project their belief structure onto their patient's situation. Although this is certainly understandable and at times the only way to proceed, the concordance between physician and patient preferences are usually no better than chance alone (43). This concept is important because many patients with COPD have poor health status and physicians may incorrectly assume that poor health status may lead to a higher likelihood of refusing life-sustaining treatment (44–46). In contrast, in our study of patients with COPD who required long-term oxygen treatment, health status (as measured by the St. George's Respiratory Questionnaire) was not associated with end-of-life treatment preferences (45). These results are in agreement with two prior studies performed in elderly outpatients without severe comorbidity and among seriously ill, hospitalized patients with one of several chronic diseases (46,47). Since physicians underestimate patients' health-related quality of life compared with the patients' own assessments (47,48) and physicians' beliefs for patients' treatment preferences are influenced by the physicians' perception of the patients' quality of life (49), physicians should examine their own assumptions and elicit treatment preferences directly from patients. Furthermore, preferences for care will also likely be dependent on the burden of that care in relation to the expected outcome. For example, Fried and colleagues demonstrated that important differences in desiring life-sustaining therapy were based on patients' attitudes toward treatment burden, the potential outcomes of care, and the likelihood of those outcomes (50). Of particular importance to patients were both functional and cognitive states. In an important follow-up study, Fried demonstrated that these attitudes and preferences, which were based on treatment burden, outcomes of care including death, and the likelihood of outcomes, were stable over a two-year period (51). This suggests that when incorporating these three features, patient treatment preferences are likely stable over time and suggest that once performed, repeated assessment may need to occur infrequently for stable patients.

X. Decision Making in the Setting of Depression

As noted above, depression is a common coexisting condition among patients with COPD and may modify patients' treatment preferences. Depression has been associated with treatment preference in a number of studies. For example, in our study of 115 patients with oxygen-dependent COPD, we found that a higher burden of depressive symptoms was significantly associated with a preference against CPR (22). This association was similar to findings of two prior investigations, one from SUPPORT and one by Blank and colleagues, that assessed preferences for CPR, but not specifically for patients with COPD (13,52). It is important to remember that depression is a treatable disorder and observational studies suggest that patients with depression are likely to change their treatment preferences after depression resolves (53). In our study on the quality of communication for patients with oxygen-dependent COPD, depression was negatively associated with the quality of patient–physician communication about end-of-life care when compared with those without depression (45). It is not clear whether this finding reflects an effect of depression on patients' ratings of the quality of communication or whether the quality of patient–physician communication is negatively influenced by depression. There is little understanding of the ways in which depression and treatment preferences interact. Nonetheless, clinicians should consider a diagnosis of depression or anxiety disorder, develop a treatment plan for such psychiatric disorders, and consider the effect of these disorders on advance care planning as well as the importance of reassessing treatment preferences after treatment of depression or anxiety.

XI. The Role of Advance Directives

It is clear that in their current form, advance directives are largely ineffectual and may actually be a barrier to high-quality communication about end-of-life care because patients with an advance directive may mistakenly believe that they therefore do not need to have conversations with either surrogate decision makers or physicians (21). Advance directives have been shown not to modify the type or delivery of care (47,54,55) and do not affect decision making at the end of life (56–59). However, there is some evidence that advance directives can improve the family experience of end-of-life decision making (60). Despite the lack of effectiveness at changing the care patients receive, there are systems of care that are mandating that advance directives be completed and recorded in patients' medical record.

Because of the way that most standard advance care directives are worded, they lack the specificity required to be of clinical utility and most times lack the principal of expressing the patients' goals of care. Without understanding the patients' true goals of care, it is difficult to estimate whether any given therapy may be able to achieve those goals. As part of a conversation between patients, families, and physicians, advance directives may have an important role in end-of-life care. In particular, for patients who have experienced or witnessed mechanical ventilation in the past, physicians have the opportunity to use patients' prior experiences as a reference point for discussing potential future episodes of acute respiratory failure. Patients' prior experiences with mechanical ventilation or with relatives or friends who have required life support can be important facilitators to patient–physician communication about treatment preferences and end-of-life care. Prior authors have reported on the development of COPD-specific advance directives (61,62), although there have not been studies showing that these advance directives improve the quality of end-of-life care.

XII. Summary

Patients with COPD deserve high-quality palliative and end-of-life care. COPD is a common condition that causes significant morbidity and mortality in the United States and worldwide. The effects of COPD in terms of disability-adjusted life years in both industrialized and nonindustrialized countries are projected to increase. There is a growing body of literature to suggest that patients with COPD do not receive high-quality end-of-life care. Over the past several years, there has been significant progress made at understanding the barriers and facilitators to providing high-quality end-of-life care; however, there are many remaining unaddressed questions.

These include identifying effective strategies to improve medical education about how to deliver effective end-of-life care, to change both system and physician recognition about the importance of providing high-quality end-of-life care and how to modify physician behavior to incorporate end-of-life care planning into routine clinical practice.

Acknowledgments

Dr. Au is funded by the Department of Veterans Affairs Health Services Research and Development Advanced Research Career Development Award. Dr. Curtis is funded by a NIH K24 HL068593.

References

1. National Heart, Lung, Blood Institute. Morbidity and Mortality Chartbook on Cardiovascular, Lung and Blood Diseases. Bethesda, MD: U.S. Department of Health and Human Services/Public Health Service/National Institutes of Health, 2006.
2. Murray CJ, Lopez AD. Alternative projections of mortality and disability by cause 1990–2020: Global Burden of Disease Study. Lancet 1997; 349:1498–504.
3. Sullivan SD, Ramsey SD, Lee TA. The economic burden of COPD. Chest 2000; 117:5S–9.
4. Anthonisen NR, Skeans MA, Wise RA, Manfreda J, Kanner RE, Connett JE. The effects of a smoking cessation intervention on 14.5-year mortality: a randomized clinical trial. Ann Intern Med 2005; 142:233–9.
5. NOTT Study Group. Continuous or nocturnal oxygen therapy in hypoxemic chronic obstructive lung disease: a clinical trial. Nocturnal Oxygen Therapy Trial Group. Ann Intern Med 1980; 93:391–8.
6. Aaron SD, Vandemheen KL, Fergusson D, et al. Tiotropium in combination with placebo, salmeterol, or fluticasone–salmeterol for treatment of chronic obstructive pulmonary disease: a randomized trial. Ann Intern Med 2007; 146(8):545–55.
7. Calverley PM, Anderson JA, Celli B, et al. Salmeterol and fluticasone propionate and survival in chronic obstructive pulmonary disease. N Engl J Med 2007; 356:775–89.
8. Fishman A, Martinez F, Naunheim K, et al. A randomized trial comparing lung-volume-reduction surgery with medical therapy for severe emphysema. N Engl J Med 2003; 348:2059–73.
9. Standards for the Diagnosis and Management of Patients with COPD, 2007. (Accessed April 16, 2007 at http://www.thoracic.org/sections/copd/index.html)
10. Executive Summary: Global Strategy for the Diagnosis, Management, and Prevention of COPD, 2007. (Accessed April 16, 2007 at goldcopd.com)
11. Field MJ, Cassel CK. Approaching Death: Improving Care at the End of Life. Institue of Medicine Report. Washington, DC: National Academy Press, 1997.
12. Curtis JR, Wenrich MD, Carline JD, Shannon SE, Ambrozy DM, Ramsey PG. Understanding physicians' skills at providing end-of-life care perspectives of patients, families, and health care workers. J Gen Intern Med 2001; 16:41–9.
13. The SUPPORT Investigators. A controlled trial to improve care for seriously ill hospitalized patients. The study to understand prognoses and preferences for outcomes and risks of treatments (SUPPORT). The SUPPORT Principal Investigators. J Am Med Assoc 1995; 274:1591–8.
14. Claessens MT, Lynn J, Zhong Z, et al. Dying with lung cancer or chronic obstructive pulmonary disease: insights from SUPPORT. Study to understand prognoses and preferences for outcomes and risks of treatments. J Am Geriatr Soc 2000; 48:S146–53.
15. Gore JM, Brophy CJ, Greenstone MA. How well do we care for patients with end stage chronic obstructive pulmonary disease (COPD)? A comparison of palliative care and quality of life in COPD and lung cancer. Thorax 2000; 55:1000–6.
16. Edmonds P, Karlsen S, Khan S, Addington-Hall J. A comparison of the palliative care needs of patients dying from chronic respiratory diseases and lung cancer. Palliat Med 2001; 15:287–95.

17. Elkington H, White P, Higgs R, Pettinari CJ. GPs' views of discussions of prognosis in severe COPD. Fam Pract 2001; 18:440–4.
18. Skilbeck J, Mott L, Page H, Smith D, Hjelmeland-Ahmedzai S, Clark D. Palliative care in chronic obstructive airways disease: a needs assessment. Palliat Med 1998; 12:245–54.
19. Au DH, Udris EM, Fihn SD, McDonell MB, Curtis JR. Differences in health care utilization at the end of life among patients with chronic obstructive pulmonary disease and patients with lung cancer. Arch Intern Med 2006; 166:326–31.
20. Celli BR, Cote CG, Marin JM, et al. The body-mass index, airflow obstruction, dyspnea, and exercise capacity index in chronic obstructive pulmonary disease. N Engl J Med 2004; 350:1005–12.
21. Knauft E, Nielsen EL, Engelberg RA, Patrick DL, Curtis JR. Barriers and facilitators to end-of-life care communication for patients with COPD. Chest 2005; 127:2188–96.
22. Curtis JR, Engelberg RA, Nielsen EL, Au DH, Patrick DL. Patient–physician communication about end-of-life care for patients with severe COPD. Eur Respir J 2004; 24:200–5.
23. Heffner JE, Fahy B, Hilling L, Barbieri C. Attitudes regarding advance directives among patients in pulmonary rehabilitation. Am J Respir Crit Care Med 1996; 154:1735–40.
24. Curtis JR, Wenrich MD, Carline JD, Shannon SE, Ambrozy DM, Ramsey PG. Patients' perspectives on physician skill in end-of-life care: differences between patients with COPD, cancer, and AIDS. Chest 2002; 122:356–62.
25. Fried TR, Bradley EH, O'Leary J. Prognosis communication in serious illness: perceptions of older patients, caregivers, and clinicians. J Am Geriatr Soc 2003; 51:1398–403.
26. Hofmann JC, Wenger NS, Davis RB, et al. Patient preferences for communication with physicians about end-of-life decisions. SUPPORT Investigators. Study to understand prognoses and preference for outcomes and risks of treatment. Ann Intern Med 1997; 127:1–12.
27. Heffner JE, Fahy B, Hilling L, Barbieri C. Outcomes of advance directive education of pulmonary rehabilitation patients. Am J Respir Crit Care Med 1997; 155:1055–9.
28. McNeely PD, Hebert PC, Dales RE, et al. Deciding about mechanical ventilation in end-stage chronic obstructive pulmonary disease: how respirologists perceive their role. CMAJ 1997; 156:177–83.
29. Sin DD, Wu L, Anderson JA, et al. Inhaled corticosteroids and mortality in chronic obstructive pulmonary disease. Thorax 2005; 60:992–7.
30. Solano JP, Gomes B, Higginson IJ. A comparison of symptom prevalence in far advanced cancer, AIDS, heart disease, chronic obstructive pulmonary disease and renal disease. J Pain Symptom Manage 2006; 31:58–69.
31. Au DH, Blough DK, Kirchdoerfer L, Weiss KB, Udris EM, Sullivan SD. Development of a quantifiable symptom assessment tool for patients with chronic bronchitis: the chronic bronchitis symptoms assessment scale. COPD 2005; 2:209–16.
32. Curtis JR, Deyo RA, Hudson LD. Pulmonary rehabilitation in chronic respiratory insufficiency. 7. Health-related quality of life among patients with chronic obstructive pulmonary disease. Thorax 1994; 49:162–70.
33. Lynn J, Ely EW, Zhong Z, et al. Living and dying with chronic obstructive pulmonary disease. J Am Geriatr Soc 2000; 48:S91–100.
34. Jennings AL, Davies AN, Higgins JP, Gibbs JS, Broadley KE. A systematic review of the use of opioids in the management of dyspnoea. Thorax 2002; 57:939–44.
35. Manning HL. Dyspnea treatment. Respir Care 2000; 45:1342–50 (discussion 50–4).
36. Runo JR, Ely EW. Treating dyspnea in a patient with advanced chronic obstructive pulmonary disease. West J Med 2001; 175:197–201.
37. Borson S, Claypoole K, McDonald GJ. Depression and chronic obstructive pulmonary disease: treatment trials. Semin Clin Neuropsychiatry 1998; 3:115–30.
38. Borson S, McDonald GJ, Gayle T, Deffebach M, Lakshminarayan S, VanTuinen C. Improvement in mood, physical symptoms, and function with nortriptyline for depression in patients with chronic obstructive pulmonary disease. Psychosomatics 1992; 33:190–201.
39. Ries AL, Kaplan RM, Limberg TM, Prewitt LM. Effects of pulmonary rehabilitation on physiologic and psychosocial outcomes in patients with chronic obstructive pulmonary disease. Ann Intern Med 1995; 122:823–32.
40. Wijkstra PJ, Ten Vergert EM, van Altena R, et al. Long term benefits of rehabilitation at home on quality of life and exercise tolerance in patients with chronic obstructive pulmonary disease. Thorax 1995; 50:824–8.

41. Wijkstra PJ, Van Altena R, Kraan J, Otten V, Postma DS, Koeter GH. Quality of life in patients with chronic obstructive pulmonary disease improves after rehabilitation at home. Eur Respir J 1994; 7:269–73.
42. Rocker GM, Sinuff T, Horton R, Hernandez P. Advanced chronic obstructive pulmonary disease: innovative approaches to palliation. J Palliat Med 2007; 10:783–97.
43. Seckler AB, Meier DE, Mulvihill M, Paris BE. Substituted judgment: how accurate are proxy predictions? Ann Intern Med 1991; 115:92–8.
44. Levenson JW, McCarthy EP, Lynn J, Davis RB, Phillips RS. The last six months of life for patients with congestive heart failure. J Am Geriatr Soc 2000; 48:S101–9.
45. Stapleton RD, Nielsen EL, Engelberg RA, Patrick DL, Curtis JR. Association of depression and life-sustaining treatment preferences in patients with COPD. Chest 2005; 127:328–34.
46. Uhlmann RF, Pearlman RA. Perceived quality of life and preferences for life-sustaining treatment in older adults. Arch Intern Med 1991; 151:495–7.
47. Sprangers MA, Aaronson NK. The role of health care providers and significant others in evaluating the quality of life of patients with chronic disease: a review. J Clin Epidemiol 1992; 45:743–60.
48. Wilson KA, Dowling AJ, Abdolell M, Tannock IF. Perception of quality of life by patients, partners and treating physicians. Qual Life Res 2000; 9:1041–52.
49. Schneiderman LJ, Kaplan RM, Pearlman RA, Teetzel H. Do physicians' own preferences for life-sustaining treatment influence their perceptions of patients' preferences? J Clin Ethics 1993; 4:28–33.
50. Fried TR, Bradley EH, Towle VR, Allore H. Understanding the treatment preferences of seriously ill patients. N Engl J Med 2002; 346:1061–6.
51. Fried TR, Van Ness PH, Byers AL, Towle VR, O'Leary JR, Dubin JA. Changes in preferences for life-sustaining treatment among older persons with advanced illness. J Gen Intern Med 2007; 22:495–501.
52. Blank K, Robison J, Doherty E, Prigerson H, Duffy J, Schwartz HI. Life-sustaining treatment and assisted death choices in depressed older patients. J Am Geriatr Soc 2001; 49:153–61.
53. Rosenfeld KE, Wenger NS, Phillips RS, et al. Factors associated with change in resuscitation preference of seriously ill patients. The SUPPORT Investigators. Study to understand prognoses and preferences for outcomes and risks of treatments. Arch Intern Med 1996; 156:1558–64.
54. Danis M, Mutran E, Garrett JM, et al. A prospective study of the impact of patient preferences on life-sustaining treatment and hospital cost. Crit Care Med 1996; 24:1811–7.
55. Danis M, Southerland LI, Garrett JM, et al. A prospective study of advance directives for life-sustaining care. N Engl J Med 1991; 324:882–8.
56. Schneiderman LJ, Kronick R, Kaplan RM, Anderson JP, Langer RD. Effects of offering advance directives on medical treatments and costs. Ann Intern Med 1992; 117:599–606.
57. Teno J, Lynn J, Connors AF, Jr, et al. The illusion of end-of-life resource savings with advance directives. SUPPORT Investigators. Study to understand prognoses and preferences for outcomes and risks of treatment. J Am Geriatr Soc 1997; 45:513–8.
58. Teno J, Lynn J, Wenger N, et al. Advance directives for seriously ill hospitalized patients: effectiveness with the patient self-determination act and the SUPPORT intervention. SUPPORT Investigators. Study to understand prognoses and preferences for outcomes and risks of treatment. J Am Geriatr Soc 1997; 45:500–7.
59. Teno JM, Licks S, Lynn J, et al. Do advance directives provide instructions that direct care? SUPPORT Investigators. Study to understand prognoses and preferences for outcomes and risks of treatment. J Am Geriatr Soc 1997; 45:508–12.
60. Norris K, Merriman MP, Curtis JR, Asp C, Tuholske L, Byock IR. Next of kin perspectives of the experience of end-of-life care in a community setting. J Pain Symptom Manage (in press).
61. Dales RE, O'Connor A, Hebert P, Sullivan K, McKim D, Llewellyn-Thomas H. Intubation and mechanical ventilation for COPD: development of an instrument to elicit patient preferences. Chest 1999; 116:792–800.
62. Singer P. Advance directives in COPD. Monaldi Arch Chest Dis 1995; 50:62–3.

25

A Global Strategy for a Global Disease

CHRISTINE JENKINS
Woolcock Institute of Medical Research, University of Sydney, and Department of Thoracic Medicine, Concord Hospital, Sydney, Australia

I. Introduction

There is virtually no part of the world that is not affected by chronic obstructive pulmonary disease (COPD); therefore, efforts to address the serious impact of this disease have had a global dimension from very early on. Landmark reports on global health (1,2), highlighting the current burden of disease and predicting a dramatic rise in morbidity and mortality from COPD, have focused the minds of clinicians and public health physicians on the potential to turn these devastating statistics around. Epidemiologic data indicating the rise in the burden of COPD against a background of impressive falls in mortality and prevalence of other chronic diseases further emphasize the urgent need to implement strategies to curb the growth of COPD (3,4). The development of regional and global guidelines for COPD care has been one vital strategy in the promotion of lung health and the prevention and optimal management of COPD (5,6).

II. The First Global COPD Initiative and Guideline: GOLD

International clinical practice guidelines for the management of COPD date back approximately 20 years. They lagged behind the development of asthma guidelines, probably due to a widely prevalent nihilism about COPD that guidelines themselves have helped to change. The magnitude of the impact of COPD and its increasing prevalence were not appreciated and there was no confidence that this disease was both preventable and treatable. Clinical practice guidelines for COPD have mentioned this apparent neglect and have helped to change these views, and it is now recognized that good management of this disease is making a difference to its impact (7). Additionally, over the last 15 to 20 years, the principles underlying the optimal approach to guideline development have been refined and have significantly influenced the quality of the documents and recommendations produced (8–10). Guideline development has moved from a consensus approach, initially reflecting expert opinion, to a rigorous, standardized process involving evaluation and ranking of the evidence and the provision of information regarding the strength of the recommendation, feasibility, and, in some instances, the economic rationale (11). Based on the quality of the evidence, guideline users can now have some confidence regarding the strength of the recommendation, its relevance, and its likely cost implications for the local context (12,13).

The first global guidelines for COPD, and the only ones that continue to be so, were the product of the Global Initiative for Chronic Obstructive Lung Disease (GOLD) (5). GOLD began through the vision of a small group of concerned individuals who sought the support of the U.S. National Heart, Lung, and Blood Institute, and the involvement of the World Health Organization (WHO) to establish a representative group of COPD expert clinicians and researchers, to develop the first global COPD guideline. GOLD has grown significantly since then, and although the guideline is still a central plank in its activities, other activities such as the World COPD day and the engagement of the GOLD national leaders in promulgating and implementing the guidelines are crucial aspects of its ongoing work. GOLD works with healthcare professionals, public health officials, and nongovernment organizations around the world to raise awareness of COPD and to improve its prevention and treatment.

The GOLD guideline already has many of the desirable elements of a successful guideline (14,15). These include

- being user-friendly and concise (e.g., the GOLD pocket guide),
- using an explicit process for assessing the evidence,
- using an explicit process for recommendations,
- being relevant to patient care,
- being in several different and accessible formats (e.g., Web-based, executive summary, patient guide), and
- being adaptable to local conditions.

The GOLD Science Committee, which has the responsibility of reviewing published papers for consideration of inclusion in the GOLD guidelines, has established a rigorous process for assessing whether newly published papers provide evidence that should be included in the annually updated guideline and should change the GOLD recommendations. The new guideline copy is available on the GOLD Web site in its edited, marked-up version and a clean version for readers to quickly assess the new changes. This updating process has established a practical model for incorporating new information and has set a high standard for COPD guidelines.

However, guidelines alone will never meet all the needs of a strategic approach to addressing the local or global burden of COPD. Reducing disease burden, including mortality and morbidity, and enhancing awareness and preventative approaches to any major health threat require a coordinated, multifaceted approach to the implementation of guidelines over a sustained period of time (16,17). Systems change, removal of barriers to uptake, and sustained implementation strategies are essential to achieve optimal COPD outcomes influenced by best practice guidelines. Outside the immediate context of clinical care, engagement of public health administrators, policy makers, and funders is crucial to achieve widespread and consistent changes (18,19). Although without this engagement, dedicated, energetic, and effective local leaders can achieve change, such local efforts can sometimes be limited by their dependence on certain individuals who are the drivers of change, but who may not always be there. GOLD is a truly international venture and its reach has extended into many small, poor, and under-resourced countries with a high prevalence of COPD. Further, it has stimulated research and debate about COPD diagnosis, treatment, assessment of severity, and the targeting of public health initiatives to achieve maximum impact.

While global respiratory health may appear to be a grand vision, international initiatives such as GOLD and the burden of obstructive lung disease (BOLD), along with the work of international bodies such as the International Coalition for COPD (20), the WHO and the International Primary Care Airways Group (21), have all separately contributed to an increasingly international movement to address this disease. It is clear from studies conducted all over the world that many different factors contribute to the risk of developing COPD and that different solutions will be needed in different settings (22–25). While tobacco is the most readily identified and probably the most widely used cause of COPD, a range of other important factors can also be addressed to reduce the risk of developing COPD. These include industrial and motor vehicle emissions, biomass fuel burning, particularly in poorly ventilated houses, early life respiratory infection, and exposure to gases, dust, and fumes. Nevertheless, international efforts and global strategies can play an important role in setting standards and providing an impetus to local leaders and to initiate programs that are developed with local needs and resources in mind.

III. Subsequent Global Initiatives for COPD

Global initiatives to address COPD have increased since the very first GOLD workshop report in 2001. The Global Alliance Against Chronic Respiratory Disease (GARD) (26) is a voluntary alliance of internationally recognized organizations and agencies from developing and developed countries. It is an initiative of the WHO and aims to fight chronic respiratory disease (CRD), including COPD. The GARD Web site highlights the importance of CRD, indicating that 80 million people worldwide have moderate to severe COPD and that deaths from CRD will increase by an estimated 30% in the next 10 years if urgent action is not taken. It is these statistics which have captured people's attention and helped to develop the international coalitions that are currently growing in number and size. The objectives of GARD include (*i*) the standardization of data collection on CRD risk factors; (*ii*) encouragement of countries to implement health promotion and CRD prevention policies; and (*iii*) making recommendations of simple strategies for management of CRDs. GARD also promotes an integrated approach with other chronic diseases. GARD has established six working groups under the following topics:

1. burden, risk factors, and surveillance,
2. awareness and advocacy for action,
3. health promotion and prevention,
4. diagnosis of chronic respiratory disease and respiratory allergy,
5. control of CRD and allergy, and
6. pediatric asthma.

GARD will develop a standardized process for collecting data on CRD risk factors, disease burden, trends, quality, and affordability of care, as well as the economic burden imposed on families and countries alike. It acknowledges that addressing the global epidemic of CRD necessitates it becoming a public health priority in all countries. GARD will work to increase awareness and strengthen commitment for action across governments, the media, the general public, health-care professionals, and affected individuals. It will advise on the implementation of policies to reduce exposure to tobacco smoke, indoor and outdoor pollution, occupational hazards, and other risk factors and will recommend and promote simple, available, and affordable diagnostic tools for CRD. Finally, it will provide evidence-based training for health-care professionals on proper diagnosis of these conditions.

The International COPD Coalition (20) is another public advocacy coalition, focused primarily on people with COPD. The purpose and mission of the organization is to develop a network of COPD patient organizations worldwide, for health promotion among COPD patients, and COPD education through:

- planning, managing, and financing pilot projects to improve the health and access to care of COPD patients, with particular emphasis on developing countries and deprived;
- raising COPD awareness worldwide;
- providing support for preventive, diagnostic, and therapeutic measures for COPD as part of basic health care; and
- promoting better care for patients with COPD.

These purposes may be achieved in cooperation with recognized aid organizations, nongovernmental organizations, health authorities and ministries, health-care providers, and other interested international organizations.

IV. BOLD Project

The development of clinical practice guidelines has highlighted the urgent need for more research into COPD, particularly the need for more accurate epidemiologic data, in order to define the extent of the problem and to examine the circumstances that contribute to prevalence, severity, and outcomes in each region. The very first GOLD guidelines published as a workshop report in 2001 emphasized this. They made recommendations for future research and highlighted the need for "standardized methods for tracking trends in COPD prevalence, morbidity, and mortality over time so that countries can plan for future increases in the need for health-care services in view of predicted increases in COPD. This need is especially urgent in developing countries with limited health-care resources." In part, as a result of the momentum achieved at the time of the first GOLD workshop report, individuals with epidemiologic expertise recognized the urgency of this and initiated the BOLD (27) project, an undertaking that was ambitious in its scope, but which harnessed the energy and interest around the world among opinion leaders who recognized that basic epidemiologic data were needed before governments and clinicians could be persuaded that this disease could be neglected no longer. To prove this, figures were needed for broad population groups in order for advocacy to be successful and for the problem to be addressed in a systematic way through more effective prevention, diagnosis, management, and public health initiatives.

V. WHO Framework Convention on Tobacco Control

The WHO Web site (28) announces that "May 21st 2003 was a historic day for global public health. At the 56th World Health Assembly, WHO's 192 Member States unanimously adopted the world's first public health treaty, the WHO Framework Convention on Tobacco Control." Negotiated under the auspices of WHO, this new treaty is the first legal instrument designed to reduce tobacco-related deaths and disease around the world. Among its many measures, the treaty requires countries to (*i*) impose restrictions on tobacco advertizing, sponsorship, and promotion; (*ii*) establish new packaging and labeling of tobacco products; (*iii*) establish clean indoor air controls; and (*iv*) strengthen legislation to clamp down on tobacco smuggling.

The treaty obliges Party States to undertake a comprehensive ban on tobacco advertizing, promotion, and sponsorship, as far as their constitutions permit. It also encourages increasing tobacco taxes and requires cigarette manufacturers to increase the size of health warnings so that they take up at least 30% of the package cover. Parties whose constitution or constitutional principles do not allow them to undertake a comprehensive ban must apply a series of restrictions on all advertizing, promotion, and sponsorship. It came into force in February 2005 and has been signed by 168 countries. It is legally binding in 61 countries, representing 2.3 billion people.

VI. Translation into Practice

While the above developments are exciting in many respects, global guidelines pose particular problems in translation into relevant and user-friendly information for local implementation (29). It is widely accepted that optimal adoption of guidelines requires engagement of the health professionals "at the coal face"—those most likely to interpret and apply information (30). This principle of "bottom-up" engagement of health professionals in clinical practice guideline development cannot be feasibly employed when a global guideline is developed (31,32). By its very nature, a global guideline or even a regional guideline represents the interests and settings of a heterogeneous group of practitioners, patients, and caregivers. Global guideline development is essentially a "top-down" process, and widespread adoption of global guidelines is dependent on a robust process for dissemination and implementation, which involves progressive engagement of clinical leaders and respected peers to effectively translate the global guideline into the local context. Invariably, this means that global guidelines are first adopted at a national level and then modified locally to appropriately reflect the clinical practice environment, the resources available, and the varying nature of the disease as well as the availability of treatments (25). Subsequently, these guidelines can be reviewed and modified at a regional and local level to suit the practice environment and to meet local needs. At every level, it is essential that respected clinical leaders become advocates for the guideline and contributors to its translation into a relevant and authoritative document that has the respect of local clinicians and can feasibly be implemented (32,33).

For guidelines to be relevant and reflect the highest level of evidence, they must be regularly updated. This updating process is time consuming and resource hungry. It is able to be maintained only through the dedication of leaders in the field and the availability of resources to support their efforts. Inevitably, this effort represents an opportunity cost where these individuals could be working more effectively in a range of different activities to implement the guidelines. Currently, there is much redundancy in this effort and there is a persuasive argument that the duplication of effort is inefficient, distracts attention, reroutes resources, and delays the achievement of better outcomes for patients with COPD. One of the steps taken in Europe resulted in a generic methodology for guideline assessment, the Appraisal of Guidelines for ResEarch and Evaluation (AGREE) (10,34), and in the United States, the U.S. National Guideline Clearinghouse was established. In Australia and New Zealand, the national medical research bodies fund and promulgate guidelines for the development and implementation of clinical practice guidelines. These are all mechanisms for creating a standard for guidelines development that helps to promote best practice in guidelines formulation and implementation. While it is crucial that national research priorities and promotion of best clinical practice are underpinned by the appropriate development of evidence-based guidelines, the increasing proliferation of this guidelines may be somewhat less necessary now that the international access to the Internet and the ready availability of such resources to people around the world.

To address these issues, a multinational group of guideline experts has initiated the development of a non-profit organization promoting systematic guideline development and implementation and has created a searchable database, which now contains more than 2000 guideline resources. The purposes of this group, the Guidelines International Network (GIN) (35), are to promote the systematic development, dissemination, and implementation of clinical practice guidelines and to harmonize methodologies. Its membership is very broad and includes international partners representing government, public advocacy, professional colleges, health-care quality organizations, and major international coalitions including the AGREE collaboration and the WHO. The group has a website, which is a key tool supporting the network's activities and contains a searchable database for published and planned guidelines and related documents and tools. It contains evidence tables, search strategies, patient information, and advice for local adaptation of guidelines. Future plans include the development of methodologies for guideline adaptation and implementation.

By 2004, 52 organizations from 27 countries had joined the GIN, recognition that a "structured international partnership" is needed among leading guidelines groups to achieve the best possible outcome for guidelines development. The network continues to develop writing, implementation and evaluation tools and training, and a forum for resource and expertise sharing. With time, a unified process such as this should help to demonstrate that it is possible to develop international guidelines of the highest quality, from which local guidelines are distilled, modified, and implemented.

VII. Is One Global COPD Guideline Enough?

The leading COPD guidelines, GOLD (5), U.K.-National Institute for Clinical Excellence (12), and the American Thoracic Society-European Respiratory Society guidelines (36), represent the combined efforts of many dedicated individuals who are expert in particular areas of COPD pathophysiology, diagnosis, management, and patient education. But for a global disease like COPD, with a high and rising prevalence in virtually all parts of the world, a strong case can be made for the development of a global guideline, which is used as the source document from which local guidelines are developed and refined. There is no question that considerable efficiencies and synergies could be developed between the current leading guideline groups, in the creation of such a single international COPD guideline. It is to be hoped that the global vision for the recognition, prevention, and optimal management of COPD will help to facilitate a collaborative and cooperative program between these organizations. This would be in the interests of all those who wish to see the focus shift from the formulation of guidelines to their effective implementation: such a global guideline will help to avoid duplication of effort while freeing up scientists and practitioners to interpret the guideline in context and to put most of their energies into tailoring it to their local needs and resources. It is essential that this guideline is held in high regard and that it represents an up-to-date and relevant distillation of the highest level of knowledge and understanding of the disease.

Clearly, any global COPD guideline will require substantial adaptation to the widely varying local environments and settings for people around the world at risk of developing, or who already have, this disease. This task should appropriately fall to national and local bodies. The skills, tools, and expertise required for this translational task themselves need to be developed and promoted to enhance the efficiency of this process and avoid distortion of the guideline, which weakens its evidence base.

Some countries may need to expend minimal effort on guideline modification to suit their environments while others, due to limited resources or unique factors influencing the development or management of the disease, may need to undertake an extensive translation for relevance to their local setting.

VIII. Are There Deficiencies in Current International COPD Guidelines?

In the last decade, there has been a profusion of guidelines (37), many of which duplicate the central recommendations for the diagnosis and management of COPD. Although they appear in widely varying formats, not all are user-friendly and many contain dense information, which results in a document more akin to a textbook than a practical manual for critical care. Despite using a systematic approach to evaluating evidence, and incorporating these in many recommendations, in some guidelines, there remains no clear distinction between statements that are made on the basis of consensus and those that are supported by very strong evidence. Additionally, where evidence levels are provided, many guidelines still lack information regarding the strength of the recommendation. Guideline development is both an art and a science, not only necessitating rigorous attention to detail in interpreting evidence and making recommendations, but also requiring a sympathetic understanding of the difficulties in applying evidence in the everyday world of clinical practice.

Guidelines often lack explicit definitions and frequently treat the condition of interest as if it were not occurring in the context of complex co-morbid illness, crucial psychosocial issues, or interacting influences such as multiple drug therapies and compromised access to care (34,35). They are often based on randomized controlled trials from which patients with severe illness, co-morbidities, serious psychosocial issues, or advanced age are excluded. These trials also present their results as mean outcome data, making it difficult for clinicians and guideline developers to recognize the spectrum of patients who are included or the spectrum of outcomes achieved. For all these reasons, the recommendations contained in guidelines may require a platform or

Table 1 Comparison of the Presentation of Evidence in the Global Initiative for Chronic Obstructive Lung Disease (GOLD) and the American Thoracic Society (ATS)-European Respiratory Society (ERS) Guidelines for the Diagnosis and Treatment of Patients with Chronic Obstructive Pulmonary Disease

Criterion[a]	GOLD	ATS/ERS
Explicitly defining the question that the guideline or recommendation is addressing	This is partially done but not for all recommendations	For specific questions this is only partially done
Formulating eligibility criteria for evidence to be considered	Done	Not done
Conducting a systematic search for evidence	Done	Not done
Evaluating study quality, summarizing the studies (possibly through meta-analysis)	Not done (except for situations in which systematic reviews are cited). There is an overall lack of provision of effect estimates and estimates of uncertainty	Not done (except for situations in which systematic reviews are cited). There is an overall lack of provision of effect estimates and estimates of uncertainty
Evaluating the overall quality of evidence	Done	Not done (only for the section copied from GOLD)
Balancing the benefits and downsides of the alternative management strategies	Not done explicitly	Not done explicitly
Acknowledging values and preferences underlying the recommendations	Not done explicitly	Not done explicitly
Making a recommendation for action including a grading of that recommendation according to the balance of benefits and downsides, and the methodological quality of the evidence that leave no doubt as to the intention of the recommendation	Not done	Not done

[a] Based on Refs. 10,11,38,39

framework for interpretation to maximize their potential for effective implementation. Although this is a complex process, it can enable the translation of guideline documents into computer-based clinical decision-support systems. These can systematize guidelines, help to operationalize them, and integrate them into clinical pathways (Table 1) (40,41).

Table 2   The Appraisal of Guidelines for Research and Evaluation Tool for Appraising Clinical Practice Guidelines

Scope and purpose
  The overall objective(s) of the guideline is (are) specifically described
  The clinical question(s) covered by the guideline is (are) specifically described
  The patients to whom the guideline is meant to apply to are specifically described
  The recommendations are unambiguous
Stakeholder involvement
  The guideline development group includes individuals from all the relevant professional groups. The patients' views and preferences have been sought. The target users of the guideline are clearly defined. The guideline has been piloted among target users
Rigor of development
  Systematic methods were used to search for evidence. The criteria for selecting the evidence are clearly described. The methods used for formulating the recommendations are clearly described. The health benefits, side effects, and risks have been considered in formulating the recommendations. There is an explicit link between the recommendations and the supporting evidence. The guideline has been externally reviewed by experts prior to its publication. A procedure for updating the guideline is provided
Applicability
  The potential organizational barriers in applying the recommendations have been discussed. The potential cost implication of applying the recommendations has been considered. The guideline presents key review criteria for monitoring and/or audit purposes
Clarity and presentation
  The recommendations are unambiguous. The different options for management of the condition are clearly presented. Key recommendations are easily identifiable. The guideline is supported with tools for application. Quality Criterion
Editorial independence
  The guideline is editorially independent of the funding body. Conflicts of interest of guideline development members have been recorded

IX.   A Methodology for Appraising Clinical Practice Guidelines

A guideline should allow users to readily tick off a number of quality features against a standardized checklist. This is essential for users to have confidence that the adoption of a global or international guideline is appropriate as a benchmark and as a template for their own distillation of the recommendations into a local setting. It was with these concerns that the AGREE collaboration was formed. The AGREE tool (Table 2) (39) is a widely used, validated instrument for guideline appraisal. It addresses six domains that should be included in guideline development: scope and purpose, stakeholder involvement, rigor of development, clarity and presentation, applicability, and editorial independence.

X.   Should Guidelines Have a Standardized Format or Structure?

Currently, regional guidelines are highly varied in format. Several contain very detailed text with many references. Information is not necessary prioritized or readily accessible for clinical decisions. Algorithms may be complex even though they are intended to provide a clear clinical pathway. Some guidelines focus on clinical questions and, by doing so, often retain a high level of relevance, although complex issues may sometimes be oversimplified. There is a need for guidelines to reflect their cultural context in order to be readily accessible by health professionals in the local environment (42,43). The lack of availability of some medications, the high cost of others, differing levels of resources, and service delivery issues often necessitate the adaptation of regional or global guidelines to a local level.

Whether guidelines are global or local, there are principles regarding the presentation of information that any guideline needs to enshrine: guidelines should

- be simple and user-friendly,
- describe an explicit process for evaluating evidence,
- state the express process for determining the strength of evidence,
- state the strength of recommendation,
- make recommendations that are clear and concise,
- provide information that is accessible, and
- be adaptable to local conditions.

XI. What Are the Barriers to Effective Guideline Implementation?

It is well recognized that a gap exists between the information contained in clinical practice guidelines and the skills, knowledge, and expertise to implement them (42,43). Indeed, the evidence base for implementation is weaker than that for guidelines development. This is a paradox that needs to be addressed quite urgently. There are also international models of guideline translation to assist implementation, which have the potential to help bridge this gap between theory and practice most efficiently. To date, those responsible for implementing guidelines have used past experience and assumed knowledge to promulgate and implement change (35,43,44). Change management is a complex undertaking, which requires people with different skills to the clinicians who are usually participants in the guidelines development process. Most guideline implementation involves behavior change and not simply changes to infrastructure or the working environment, and these aspects of human activity create challenges that most clinicians are not skilled to manage. Guidelines implementation must therefore involve a wide range of professionals in the health-care environment in order to achieve better health outcomes (Table 3).

There is now a significant literature that highlights the strengths and weaknesses of particular approaches to developing and implementing guidelines (45). A global guideline needs to reflect this science, not only in regard to its content but also its

Table 3 Implementation: Setting Goals

What is the purpose of this activity?
What are the local needs?
Who is the target audience?
What are the barriers to success?
Are there incentives or disincentives?
How will this intervention be evaluated?
How will the results be disseminated?

Table 4 Planning an Implementation Activity

Identify desired goal
e.g., Prevention of development of COPD
Identify known risk factors
e.g., Smoking, occupational exposures, RTI, ETS
Identify targets
e.g., 10% reduction in teenage smoking
Identify strategies
e.g., Peer support education, point of sale fines
Measure outcome (indicator)
e.g., Uptake of smoking in teenagers

Abbreviations: COPD, chronic obstructive pulmonary disease; ETS, environmental tobacco smoke; RTI, respiratory tract infection.

format. In the case of clinical practice guidelines, the vehicle, whether it be an electronic resource or a hard-copy manual, is most likely to be read and applied when it is user-friendly and straightforward, fits with the resources and infrastructure available, and is supported and promoted by respected clinical leaders in the community.

Barriers to successful implementation of guidelines include complexity, cost, lack of expertise, and lack of practitioner confidence that the guideline is authoritative or that the recommendations will, if implemented, bring about the predicted outcome. Organizational barriers include ineffective strategies, lack of incentives, or active disincentives. Ultimately, to change practice, guidelines need to be accompanied by strategies to improve adherence to them—this is a very long-term goal (Table 4).

In a review of barriers to physician adherence to clinical practice guidelines (30), seven general categories of areas were identified. These include physician knowledge (lack of awareness or familiarity with the guideline), physician attitudes (lack of agreement, lack of self-efficacy, or outcome expectancy), and physician behavior (external barriers such as difficulty in reconciling patient preferences with guideline recommendations, contradictory guidelines, or environmental factors such as lack of time or resources, cost implications, and organizational constraints). It is crucial that these frequent barriers to the adoption of clinical practice guidelines are anticipated and, as much as possible, addressed in the process of implementing changes to clinical care.

Effective implementation should also employ proven techniques where there is evidence that interventions can change health practitioner behavior and patient outcomes (9,15,33,39,46). These include outreach visits, recalls and reminders, multifaceted interventions, audit and feedback, respected colleague support and endorsement, and interactive educational sessions. There are several strategies that have been shown to be helpful to change practice-and several that are generally not helpful. Effective implementation strategies are usually local (47). They can include any of the approaches listed below—there is evidence to support these approaches over passive dissemination and didactic teaching methods, which are usually relatively ineffective in changing behavior:

- engaging respected colleagues who are important local opinion leaders;
- enlisting support from allied health professionals;
- endorsement by professional colleges;

■ interactive educational activities;

■ "academic detailing"—personal visits to discuss the guideline/ change; and

■ locally adapted guidelines that acknowledge the existing infrastructure, are relevant to the local environment and respect the culture.

Participants in a consensus conference on guidelines for antithrombotic therapy participated in an online survey that was conducted to assess the feasibility, cost, and acceptability of a number of these interventions (39). These included computerized reminders, educational meetings, educational outreach visits, patient-mediated interventions, and audit and feedback. The results of this study indicated that the most feasible, acceptable, and least costly implementation strategies were the dissemination of educational material and educational meetings. There was high-quality evidence for a modest to moderate efficacious effect of computer reminders and patient-mediated interventions. Audit and feedback had only a modest effect on process of care and there were insufficient data for assessment of effect on patient outcomes. On the basis of this survey, the authors recommended that appreciable resources be devoted to compare computer reminders, dissemination of educational material, and patient-mediated interventions.

Collaboratives are another means by which implementation can occur (48). Collaboratives are proven change management approaches that have been used successfully in the United Kingdom, United States, and Scandinavian countries (49). The methodology is based on work initially conducted through the Institute for Healthcare Improvement in the United States (50). The aim of a collaborative is to identify, disseminate, and facilitate uptake of best practice across multiple sites over a relatively short time frame, generally 12 months. The collaborative methodology produces improvement by harnessing the collective wisdom of participants, an advisory panel of experts, and a literature review to develop strategies to aid implementation of evidence-based best practice. Skills workshops, progress reports, and hearing how colleagues have made changes and overcome problems can be motivating and provide practical ideas that can be implemented locally. Quality improvement cycles of "Plan, Do, Study, Act" are used by participants to test ideas and implement plans from the learning sessions in their local settings.

Plan-Do-Study-Act cycles for continuous quality improvement should involve the identification of targets that are agreed on by colleagues and collaborative participants. Targets should be linked to measurable outcomes, such as attendance at pulmonary rehabilitation, smoking cessation, self-management education, Emergency Department (ED) attendance, or admission rates. Targets could include, for example, >50% sustained smoking quit rates at 12 months, or prevention of readmissions by 10% reduction over six months, or performance of spirometry in all attending COPD patients.

XII. Evaluation of Implementation Strategies

As any implementation activity begins, targets for evaluation should be in place. These will vary depending on the setting. However, it is important to collect baseline data in the setting where the intervention is to be undertaken, ideally before the whole implementation process is underway, so that some useful "before and after" data are collected. The evaluation targets should be relatively simple, possibly using current sources of data collection—such as local or national databases if they exist—for hospital presentations and admissions, general practice (GP) consultations, and dispensing of medication.

Suggested outcome assessments include:

- hospital admission rates for COPD,
- readmission rates: within 14 or 28 days,
- out of hours GP or ED presentation rates for exacerbations of COPD,
- proportion of COPD patients referred for/given structured smoking cessation advice/nicotine replacement therapy/ongoing support,
- proportion of admitted or practice COPD patients who have ceased smoking in the last 12 months,
- proportion of COPD patients referred for/completing pulmonary rehabilitation, and
- proportion of practice/hospital COPD patients receiving skills and self-management education.

Targets can be set for each of these assessments—for instance, a 10% reduction in readmissions within 28 days over a year, or a 10% increase in the proportion of patients receiving skills and self-management education in a practice or hospital setting.

XIII. Advocacy

Clinical leaders and advocates should be mindful of the ways in which local and national health authorities can be informed of the scope of COPD as a health problem, the predictions about its increasing impact, the wide variety of causes, new treatments, and the potential to prevent the disease and change its natural history with effective tobacco and environmental control policies. Representatives of COPD lobby groups, patient care organizations, professional bodies of respiratory physicians, and allied health professionals need to be vigilant in relation to any opportunity to visit political leaders to raise awareness and influence the political process so that COPD is acknowledged as a major health issue which is to a very great extent preventable with appropriate public health messages and initiatives. The urgent need to recognize this and appropriately resource effective interventions at a national and local level should be highlighted at any opportunity. Governments and Health departments with strategic interests in managing an aging population and the complexities of chronic disease need to know that COPD is in many countries the only chronic illness that is increasing in mortality and morbidity. Strategies to address its high prevalence and burden can have significant cost and quality of life implications for the community.

XIV. Summary

COPD has been a seriously neglected disease for too long, and the major threat that it poses to world health is a result of decades of failure to recognize and address the many risk factors which contribute to its high prevalence and impact. The momentum that has gathered now is global, and both global and local strategies are likely to operate in parallel to turn the devastating statistics of this disease around. Integration of activities and a consistent, evidence-based approach to the development and implementation of best standards of care and prevention are likely to have the greatest benefit.

References

1. Murray CJL, Lopez AD. Evidence based health policy—lessons learned from the Global Burden of Disease Study. Science 1996; 274:740–3.
2. Lopez AD, Mathers CLD, Ezzotti M, Jamison DT, Murray CJL. Global and regional burden of disease and risk factors, 2001: systematic analysis of population health data. Lancet 2006; 367:1747–57.
3. Soriano JB, Maier WC, Egger P, et al. Recent trends in physician diagnosed COPD in women and men in the U.K. Thorax 2000; 55:789–94.
4. World Health Organisation. World Health Report. Geneva: WHO, 2000. (Accessed December 28, 2006 at www.who.int/whr/200/en/statistics.htm)
5. Pauwels RA, Buist AS, Calverley PMA, Jenkins CR, Hurd SS. Global strategy for the diagnosis, management and prevention of chronic obstructive pulmonary disease. Am J Respir Crit Care Med 2001; 163:1256–76.
6. Iqbal A, Schloss S, George D, Isonaka S. Worldwide guidelines for chronic obstructive pulmonary disease: a comparison of diagnosis and treatment recommendations. Respirology 2002; 7:233–9.
7. Celli B. Chronic obstructive pulmonary disease. From unjustified nihilism to evidence based optimism. Proc Am Thorac Soc 2006; 3:58–65.
8. Feder G. Guidelines for clinical guidelines. A simple pragmatic strategy for guideline development. Br Med J 1998; 317:427–8.
9. Hayes B, Haines A. Barriers and bridges to evidence based clinical practice. Br Med J 1998; 317:273–6.
10. Schunemann HJ, Jaeschke R, Cook DJ, et al. An official ATS statement: grading the quality of evidence and strengthen recommendations in ATS guidelines and recommendations. Am J Respir Crit Care Med 2006; 174:605–14.
11. Guyatt G, Baumann M, Pauker S, et al. Addressing resource allocation issues and recommendations from clinical practice guideline panels. Chest 2006; 129:182–7.
12. National Institute for Clinical Excellence (NICE). Chronic obstructive pulmonary disease: national clinical guideline for management of chronic obstructive pulmonary disease in adults in primary and secondary care. Thorax 2004; 59(Suppl. 1):1–196.
13. Halpin D. NICE guidance for COPD. Thorax 2004; 59:181–2.
14. Bero LA, Grilli RA, Grimshaw JM, et al. Closing the gap between research and practice: an overview of systematic reviews of interventions to promote the implementation of research findings. Br Med J 1998; 317:465–8.
15. Thompson R, Lavender M, Madhok R. How to ensure the guidelines are effective. Br Med J 1995; 311:237–42.
16. Riario-Sforza GC, Incorvara C, Pravettoni C, Dugmani N. Guidelines versus clinical practice in the treatment of COPD: a reappraisal. Eur Respir J 2006; 27:656.
17. Miravitlles M. Guidelines versus clinical practice in the treatment of chronic obstructive pulmonary disease. Eur Respir J 2002; 20:243–4.
18. Davis D, Taylor-Vassey A. Translating guidelines into practice: a systematic review of theoretic concepts, practical experience and research evidence in the adoption of clinical practice guidelines. Can Med Assoc J 1997; 157:408–16.
19. Partridge MR. Translating research into practice: how are guidelines implemented? Eur Respir J 2003; 21(Suppl. 39):23S–9.
20. International COPD coalition. (Accessed December 29, 2006 at http://www.internationalcopd.org/)
21. IPAG diagnosis and management handbook. Chronic airways diseases. A guide for primary care physicians. WONCA website http://www.globalfamilydoctor.com (last accessed August 29, 2007).
22. Haywood RS, Guyatt GH, Moore KA, et al. Canadian physicians attitudes about and preferences regarding clinical practice guidelines. Can Med Assoc J 1997; 156:1715–23.
23. Delva MD, Kirby JR, Knapper CK, Birthwhistle RV. Postal survey of approaches to learning among Ontario physicians: implications for continuing medical education. Br Med J 2002; 325:1–5.
24. Rutschmann OT, Janssens JP, Vermeulen B, Sarasin FP. Knowledge of guidelines for the management of COPD: a survey of primary care physicians. Respir Med 2004; 98:932–7.

25. Schachter KA, Cohen SJ. From research to practice: challenges to implementing national diabetes guidelines with five community health centers on the U.S.—Mexico border. Public Health Res Pract Policy 2005; 2:1–6.
26. The Global Alliance against Chronic Respiratory Diseases. (Accessed December 29, 2006 at http://www.who.int/respiratory/gard/en/)
27. The Burden of Obstructive Lung Disease. http://www.kpchr.org/boldcopd/apps/protocol.pdf (last accessed August 29, 2007).
28. WHO framework convention on tobacco control. (Accessed December 28, 2006 at http://www.who.int/features/2003/08/en/index.html)
29. Johnson GW. Clinicians attitudes to clinical practice guidelines. Med J Aust 2003; 178:354–5.
30. Cabana MD, Rand CS, Powe NR, et al. Why don't physicians follow clinical practice guidelines? J Am Med Assoc 1999; 282:1458–65.
31. Brindis RG, Sennett C. Physician adherence to clinical practice guidelines: does it really matter? Am Heart J 2003; 145:13–5.
32. Martens JD, Winkens AG, Van der Weijden T, et al. Does a joint development and dissemination of multidisciplinary guidelines improve prescribing behaviour: a pre-/post study with concurrent control group and a randomized trial. BMC Health Serv Res 2006; 6:145–52.
33. Eccles M, Grimshaw J, Walker A, Johnstone M, Pitts N. Changing the behaviour of health care professionals: the use of theory in promoting the uptake of research findings. J Clin Epidemiol 2005; 58:107–12.
34. Ollenschagler G, Marshall C, Qureshi S, et al. Improving the quality of healthcare: using international collaboration to inform guideline programs by founding the Guidelines International Network (GIN). Qual Saf Health Care 2004; 13:455–60.
35. Shiffman MRN, Michel G, Essaihi A, Thornquist E. Bridging the guideline implementation gap: a systematic, document centered approach to guideline implementation. J Am Med Inform Assoc 2004; 11:418–26.
36. ATS/ERS Taskforce. Standards for the diagnosis and treatment of patients with COPD: a summary of the ATS/ERS position paper. Eur Respir J 2004; 23:932–46.
37. Hibble A, Kanka D, Pencheon D, Pooles F. Guidelines in general practice: the new Tower of Babel? Br Med J 1998; 317:862–3.
38. Guyatt G, Drummond R. Users' Guides to the Medical Literature: A Manual for Evidence-Based Clinical Practice. Chicago, IL: AMA Press, 2002.
39. Schunemann HJ, Cook D, Grimshaw J, et al. Anti-thrombotic and thrombolytic therapy: from evidence to application. The seventh ACCP conference on antithrombotic and thrombolytic therapy. Chest 2004; 126:689S–96.
40. Classen DC. Clinical decision support systems to improve clinical practice and quality of care. J Am Med Assoc 1998; 280:1360–1.
41. Shea S, DuMouchel W, Bahamode L. A meta-analysis of 16 randomized controlled trials to evaluate computer-based clinical reminder systems for preventative care in the ambulatory setting. J Am Med Inform Assoc 1996; 3:399–409.
42. Phillips PA, Rubin GL, Morey PS. Evidence for evidence- based medicine at the coal face. Med J Aust 2000; 172:259–60.
43. Shiffman RN, Dixon J, Brandt C, et al. The guideline implementability appraisal (GLIA): development of an instrument to identify obstacles to guideline implementation. BMC Med Inform Decis Mak 2005; 5:23.
44. Roberts CM, Ryland I, Lowe D, et al. Audit of acute admissions of COPD: standards of care and management to the hospital setting. Eur Resp J 2001; 17:343–9.
45. Grimshaw JM, Thomas RP, McLennan G, et al. Effectiveness and efficiency of guideline dissemination and implementation strategies. Health Technol Assess 2004; 8(iii–iv):1–72.
46. Grol R. Successes and failures in the implementation of evidence based guidelines for clinical practice. Med Care 2001; 39:1154.
47. Barosi G. Strategies for dissemination and implementation of guidelines. Neurol Sci 2006; 27:S231–4.
48. Kilo CM. A framework for collaborative improvement: lessons learned from the Insititute for Healthcare Improvement's Breakthrough Series. Qual Manag Health Care 1998; 6:1–13.
49. Wagner EH, Glasgow RE, Davis C, et al. Quality improvement in chronic illness care: a collaborative approach. Jt Comm J Qual Improv 2001; 27:63–80.
50. Berwick DM. Eleven worthy aims for clinical leadership of health system reform. J Am Med Assoc 1994; 272(10):797–802.

26

Caring for the Patient with COPD: A Practical Summary of Guidelines for Clinicians

NICOLAS ROCHE and GÉRARD HUCHON
Pneumologie et Réanimation, Université Paris Descartes, Assistance Publique–Hôpitaux de Paris, Hôpital de l'Hôtel-Dieu, Paris, France

STEPHEN I. RENNARD
Department of Internal Medicine, University of Nebraska, Nebraska Medical Center, Omaha, Nebraska, U.S.A.

ROBERTO RODRÍGUEZ-ROISIN
Servei de Pneumologia, Hospital Clínic, Universitat de Barcelona, Barcelona, Spain

I. Introduction

The main aspects of chronic obstructive pulmonary disease (COPD) diagnosis, evaluation, and treatment are covered in detail in the preceding chapters. One difficult task for clinicians is to translate the corresponding scientific evidence into clinical practice; guidelines aim at helping them to do so, through a critical appraisal of available data by a multi-professional group of experts. The most recent and widely disseminated guidelines on COPD are the global initiative on obstructive lung diseases (GOLD) guidelines (1), which have been regularly updated following the initial report (2) and mention the level of scientific evidence supporting each recommendation. A few years before the last GOLD update, the American Thoracic Society and European Respiratory Society also issued international guidelines, which share most of their conclusions with the GOLD document (3). In many countries, adaptations of international guidelines have been developed, taking into account national specificity and constraints; the impact of these guidelines on quality of care and patients' outcomes has been seldom assessed, with variable but frequently disappointing results (4–20).

The purpose of the present chapter is neither to discuss methodological aspects of guidelines development and implementation (the reader will found relevant information on these aspects in the previous chapters), to review scientific evidence or challenge its interpretation by guidelines committees nor to compare the various available guidelines, but only to briefly summarize the main recommendations which can be found in the GOLD document (1). To help the reader, many tables and figures from this document have been reproduced. A few references have been added on topics which were not available when the guidelines were developed.

Based on a hypothetic clinical scenario, this chapter describes how guidelines may help answering practical questions that clinicians have to address when facing a patient with possible or certain COPD. These questions could also help respiratory physicians educating their general practitioners colleagues. They deal with:

- (early) diagnosis,
- initial assessment,
- pharmacological and non-pharmacological treatment,
- follow-up, and
- home, hospital assessment, and management of exacerbations.

It must be emphasized that, in the real life, a patient can enter the scenario at any stage, i.e., that the diagnosis may be suspected only when an exacerbation (which can be severe) occurs.

Situation 1. As a primary care physician, I know that the burden of COPD is a great cause of concern, and would like to help decrease it. I suppose that detecting COPD patients early is the first step.
Question 1.1: Is there really any advantage in early diagnosis of COPD?
COPD is a progressive disease that can decrease survival, induce a pronounced handicap, and generate important health care expenses. Early diagnosis can help:

- motivating the patient to quit smoking, thereby slowing disease progression,
- maintain or restore adequate physical exercise and nutritional intake before vicious cycles appear and amplify the handicap (Fig. 1).

Question 1.2: What should the target population be?
A diagnosis of COPD has to be considered in all individuals aged >40 years with any of the following indicators:

- exposure to tobacco smoke or domestic or occupational air pollution,
- chronic respiratory symptom(s): dyspnea, cough, sputum production.

In addition, the diagnosis also has to be considered in at risk patients with acute respiratory symptoms: COPD is (too) often detected when an acute respiratory episode occurs. In such cases, the clinician has to think about the possibility of COPD and go to "alternative situation 5" (see below).

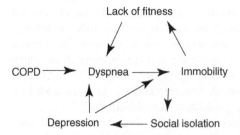

Figure 1 Vicious circles that have to be prevented and fought in chronic obstructive pulmonary disease patients. *Abbreviation*: COPD, chronic obstructive pulmonary disease.

Question 1.3: How should the diagnosis be confirmed or ruled out?

COPD is defined by airflow limitation.[a] Thus, the gold standard for the diagnosis and assessment is forced spirometry to measure pre- and post-bronchodilator forced expiratory volume in one second (FEV_1).

Situation 2. As a primary care or respiratory physician facing a patient in whom COPD was suspected and airflow obstruction has been confirmed by spirometry, I have to decide which other investigations are necessary.

Question 2.1: What are the goals of supplementary investigations once spirometry is performed?

Initial investigations aim at:

- confirming the diagnosis of COPD,
- characterizing the impact of COPD,
- determining disease's severity,
- assessing known or possible comorbid illnesses, and
- thereby forming the basis for treatment decisions and follow-up.

Question 2.2: In general, what are the other investigations to consider?

Investigations other than spirometry are not routinely recommended in all patients.

Therefore, the answer to this question depends on (*i*) the level of confidence about the diagnosis of COPD, (*ii*) the severity of airflow obstruction and symptoms, (*iii*) the presence or absence of suspected complications or comorbid illnesses, and (*iv*) the patient's medical history:

- if the clinical history is atypical, reversibility testing may help to distinguish COPD from asthma; high resolution computed tomography (CT)-scan may also help in the differential diagnosis;
- if airflow obstruction is severe ($FEV_1 < 50\%$), arterial blood gas measurement is recommended, as well as when acute or chronic respiratory failure of right heart failure are suspected clinically;
- if cardiac failure or lung cancer are suspected, chest X ray should be performed; and
- if the patient is of Caucasian descent and develops COPD at a young age (<45 years) or has a family history of the disease, screening for α_1 antitrypsin deficiency can be useful, at least to subsequently perform family screening and counseling.

Other investigations may be decided on an individual basis to assess comorbidities; they will be guided by risk factors and clinical presentation.

Question 2.3: How should disease severity be assessed?

The most widely used classification of severity relies on *post-bronchodilator* FEV_1 (Table 1). However, several other factors have an independent prognostic value, as shown in Table 2 (21–26). Therefore, composites indices have been developed, and are currently dominated by the BODE index, which is based on body mass index,

---

[a] Therefore, the previous Stage 0 (at risk subjects, with chronic bronchitis but without airflow obstruction) has been deleted from the most recent classification of chronic obstructive pulmonary disease.

Table 1 Classification of the Severity of Airflow Obstruction Based on Post-Bronchodilator Spirometric Values

	All: $FEV_1/FVC < 0.70$
Stage I: mild	$FEV_1 \geq 80\%$ predicted
Stage II: moderate	$50\% \leq FEV_1 < 80\%$ predicted
Stage III: severe	$30\% \leq FEV_1 < 50\%$ predicted
Stage IV: very severe	$FEV_1 < 30\%$ predicted or $FEV_1 < 50\%$ predicted plus chronic respiratory failure

Abbreviations: FEV_1, forced expiratory volume in one second; FVC, forced vital capacity.

FEV_1 (airflow obstruction), dyspnea Medical Research Council grade, and six-minute walking distance (Exercise; Table 3) (27). This index is better at predicting survival than FEV_1 alone. It may also be modified by some treatments, although evidence on this topic is still limited.

Whatsoever, individual assessment of disease severity has to be based on several components presented in Table 4, beginning with a thorough clinical assessment of symptoms (dyspnea, cough, and sputum production), activity limitations, quality of life, exacerbation frequency and severity, weight loss, psychiatric symptoms (depression and/or anxiety), known comorbidities.

Situation **3. Now that I know everything I need on my patient's condition, the next step is to decide which treatments might be useful.**
Question 3.1: What are the goals of treatment?

The goals of treatment are quite simple, as listed in Table 5. But reaching all of them is not that simple since only a few measures can definitely prevent disease progression (smoking cessation) and reduce mortality (smoking cessation, oxygen therapy in chronic respiratory failure, and lung volume reduction surgery in highly selected cases).

However, data from clinical trials should be a source of optimism, since the disease can no longer be considered as untreatable: nihilism is clearly not justified anymore.

Table 2 Non-Exhaustive List of Possible Prognostic Factors in Chronic Obstructive Pulmonary Disease

Persistence of smoking
Severity of dyspnea
Pulmonary hypertension and right heart failure
Arterial hypoxemia/hypercapnia
Weight loss
Muscle mass (21)
Exercise capacity/tolerance
Level of physical activity
Mucus hypersecretion (22)
Frequency of exacerbations
Health status impairment
Comorbidities including, e.g., anemia (23)
Cognitive function (24), depression
C-reactive protein serum level (25)

References have been added for factors not specifically mentioned in the global initiative on obstructive lung diseases document.

Table 3 Calculation of the BODE Index

Variable	0 point	1 point	2 points	3 points
FEV_1 (% predicted)	≥ 65	50–64	36–49	≤ 35
Six-minute walking distance (m)	≥ 350	250–349	150–249	≤ 149
MMRC dyspnea grade	0–1	2	3	4
Body-mass index	> 21	≤ 21		

Quartiles are:
1. score of 0 to 2 (4-year survival: about 85%).
2. score of 3 to 4 (4-year survival: about 70%).
3. score of 5 to 6 (4-year survival: about 60%).
4. score of 7 to 10 (4-year survival: about 20%).
Abbreviations: BODE index, *b*ody-mass index, severity of *o*bstruction *d*yspnea scale, and *e*xercise index; FEV_1, forced expiratory volume in one second; MMRC, modified Medical Research Council.
Source: From Ref. 27.

Question 3.2: What are the first interventions to consider?

Obviously, the first is reduction in avoidable risk factors, which can be separated into two categories: risk factors for long-term disease progression and risk factors for exacerbations.

The first step is to assess these factors, which are largely dominated by tobacco smoke. Exposure to occupational air pollution can also be involved. In some countries, domestic air pollution may play a role.

- Helping smokers to quit relies on counseling (the more intensive it is, the more successful it will be, but even brief counseling has positive results), nicotine replacement, bupropion, and now varenicline. The general strategy to help patients quitting smoking is shown in Table 6.
- When occupational or domestic exposures are detected in a patient with COPD, appropriate protection has to be implemented through masks or improvement in air quality. Education is of utmost importance to increase adherence to these measures and changes in professional situation or domestic environment may have to be envisaged.

Avoiding risk factors for exacerbations implicates:

- the use of vaccines, i.e., influenza vaccine for all COPD patients and pneumococcal vaccine for those aged > 65 years or < 65 years with an $FEV_1 < 40\%$ predicted; and

Table 4 Components of Severity Assessment in Patients with Chronic Obstructive Pulmonary Disease

Severity of symptoms
Severity of airflow limitation
Frequency and severity of exacerbations
Presence of one or more complications
Presence of respiratory failure
Presence of comorbid conditions
General health status
Number of medications needed to manage the disease

Table 5 Goals of Chronic Obstructive Pulmonary Disease Treatment

Relieve symptoms
Prevent disease progression
Improve exercise tolerance
Improve health status
Prevent and treat complications
Prevent and treat exacerbations
Reduce mortality

■ improving air quality and avoiding staying or exercising outdoors during pollution episodes.

Question 3.3: Which treatments should be prescribed?

The treatment of COPD includes pharmacological and non-pharmacological interventions. Treatment decisions should be based on the severity of the disease and symptoms (Fig. 2).

Question 3.4: Is it possible to firmly distinguish useful first and second-line pharmacological treatments from other agents?

With regard to pharmacological treatment, the following simple rules should be followed, based on data from clinical trials:

Firstly, the efficacy of some treatments has been convincingly demonstrated:

■ In patients with dyspnea, first line pharmacological agents are bronchodilators given on an as needed or regular basis, depending on the frequency of symptoms.

■ Short-acting inhaled β_2 agonists and anticholinergics can be used alone or in combination, their efficacy being individually assessed on symptoms (dyspnea), exercise tolerance, exacerbations, and health status. FEV_1 is not a reliable predictor of clinical efficacy. When one agent is insufficiently effective, it can be replaced by or associated with another agent. Combining bronchodilators may increase efficacy and decrease the risk of side-effects compared to increasing the dose of a single bronchodilator.

Table 6 General Strategy to Help Quitting Smoking

Ask	Systematically identify all tobacco users at every visit. Implement an office-wide system that ensures that, for *every* patient at *every* clinic visit, tobacco-use status is queried and documented
Advise	Strongly urge all tobacco users to quit. In a clear, strong, and personalized manner, urge every tobacco user to quit
Assess	Determine willingness to make a quit attempt. Ask every tobacco user if he or she is willing to make a quit attempt at this time (e.g., within the next 30 days)
Assist	Aid the patient in quitting. Help the patient with a quit plan; provide practical counseling; provide intra-treatment social support; help the patient obtain extra-treatment social support; recommend use of approved pharmacotherapy except in special circumstances; provide supplementary materials
Arrange	Schedule follow-up contact. Schedule follow-up contact, either in person or via telephone

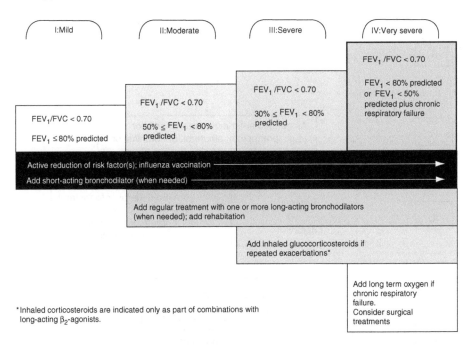

Figure 2 Severity-based long-term treatment of chronic obstructive pulmonary disease. *Abbreviations*: FEV₁, forced expiratory volume in one second; FVC, forced vital capacity.

- Long-acting β₂-agonists—(LABAs)- or anticholinergic (LAMA-) agents are more convenient for regular treatment.
- Oral xanthine derivatives are second line agents when inhaled bronchodilators are available, since their therapeutic ratio is small while they interact with several drugs and physiological variables.
- Inhaled corticosteroids should not be indicated unless given in combinations with LABAs in patients with FEV₁ <50% and repeated exacerbations. They have been shown to decrease exacerbation frequency and symptoms, and improve health status (ammendment after TOward a Revolution in COPD Health study).

Some authors have illustrated the main alternatives for bronchodilator treatments, as shown in Figure 3 (28).

Secondly, for other treatments the benefit/risk ratio is unfavorable or evidence is not sufficient:

- Long-term treatment with oral corticosteroids should be avoided since its efficacy has not been clearly demonstrated while major side-effects can be observed including impairment of muscle function.
- Similarly, anti-tussives and vasodilators may have deleterious effects (decreasing aurways protection by cough and impairing gas exchange, respectively).
- The efficacy of prophylactic use of antibiotics has not been demonstrated.

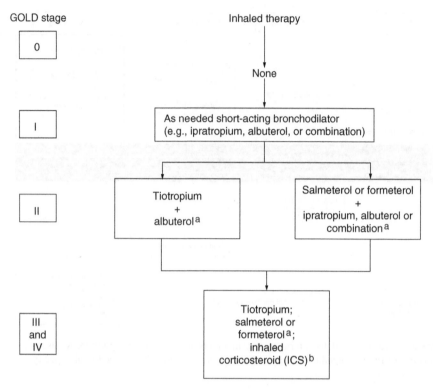

Figure 3 Algorithm for choosing pharmacological treatments in COPD. *Notes*: [a] A short-acting bronchodilator can be used for rescue medication. [b] ICSs are only in combination with LABAs in patients with FEV_1 <50% and repeated exacerbations. *Abbreviations*: COPD, chronic obstructive pulmonary disease; GOLD, global initiative for chronic obstructive lung disease; ICS, inhaled corticosteroid; LABA, long-acting β_2-agonist. *Source*: Modified from Ref. 28.

- Immunostimulators need to be further assessed.
- Mucoregulators could relieve symptoms in patients with viscous sputum, but evidence is limited.
- Leukotriene modifiers have also been insufficiently tested in COPD so that they are not recommended.

Question 3.5: Beyond smoking cessation, what non-pharmacological interventions could be useful?

Some non-pharmacological treatments are at least as important as pharmacological agents:

- Education is warranted in all patients to help smoking cessation and improve adherence to pharmacological and non-pharmacological treatment, knowledge and skills, ability to cope with illness, and health status while reducing use of health services.
- Rehabilitation provides many significant benefits listed in Table 7. It includes at least three components: exercise training, nutritional counseling,

Table 7 Benefits Provided by Pulmonary Rehabilitation, with Corresponding Levels of Evidence

Improves exercise capacity (Evidence A)
Reduces the perceived intensity of breathlessness (Evidence A)
Improves health-related quality of life (Evidence A)
Reduces the number of hospitalizations and days in the hospital (Evidence A)
Reduces anxiety and depression associated with chronic obstructive pulmonary disease (Evidence A)
Strength and endurance training of the upper limbs improves arm function (Evidence B)
Benefits extend well beyond the immediate period of training (Evidence B)
Improves survival (Evidence B)
Respiratory muscle training is beneficial, especially when combined with general exercise training (Evidence C)
Psychosocial intervention is helpful (Evidence C)

and education. Frequency of training is variable. Optimal length is at least 28 sessions of 10 to 45 minutes over at least six weeks.

■ When rehabilitation is not possible, patients should be advised to exercise on their own, at least 20 minutes daily.

Other non-pharmacological approaches may be of interest in selected subsets of patients only:

■ Oxygen therapy increases survival when PaO_2 is < 7.3 kPa (50 mmHg) or between 7.3 and 8.0 kPa (60 mmHg) with evidence of pulmonary hypertension or cor pulmonale, or polycythemia.
■ Benefits of long-term noninvasive pressure support ventilation remain to be firmly established, but this approach can be used in patients with pronounced daytime hypercapnia to decrease $PaCO_2$, improve dyspnea, and maybe decrease the risk of hospitalization.
■ Surgery is indicated only in highly selected subsets of patients:
  ■ Bullectomy in case of complicated large bullae (hemoptysis, infection, chest pain, compression of adjacent lung or mediastinal structures).
  ■ Lung volume reduction surgery in patients with severe COPD, marked hyperinflation, predominantly upper-lobe emphysema, and basal low exercise capacity. In such patients, advantages of lung volume reduction surgery have been found in terms of lung function, exercise capacity, quality of life, and even survival.
  ■ Lung transplantation in end-stage COPD.

***Situation* 4. Now that appropriate treatments are prescribed, follow-up needs to be planned.**

Question 4.1: What are the goals of follow-up?

As in all chronic diseases, the goals of follow-up are to assess:

■ exposure to risk factors,
■ disease progression,
■ development of complications,
■ exacerbations history,

- comorbidities,
- treatment changes, and
- knowledge and skills, ability to cope with the disease.

Thereby, follow-up will evaluate how the goals of treatment are met.

The first component of follow-up is obviously to discuss the above-mentioned items with the patient, as shown in Table 8.

Question 4.2: Which investigations should be repeated during follow-up and when?

Once-a-year spirometry will track the patient's decline in lung function. Spirometry is also needed if the patient's condition worsens significantly. In any case, it will lead to arterial blood gases measurement when FEV_1 falls below 50% predicted or when signs of respiratory failure or *cor pulmonale* are found.

Other investigations are decided on an individual basis:

- Chronic arterial hypoxemia can lead to polycythemia, but anemia can be also shown in 10% to 20% of the COPD series.
- Measuring carbon monoxide diffusion capacity and lung volumes can be useful in specific conditions, i.e., to assess more precisely the impact of the disease, when surgery is considered or when diagnostic uncertainties arise.

Table 8 Follow-up Clinical Evaluation of the Chronic Obstructive Pulmonary Disease Patient

Monitor exposure to risk factors
Has your exposure to risk factors changed since your last visit?
Since your last visit, have you quit smoking, or are you still smoking?
If you are still smoking, how many cigarettes/how much tobacco per day?
Would you like to quit smoking?
Has there been any change in your working environment?
Monitor disease progression and development of complications
How much can you do before you get short of breath? (Use an everyday example, such as walking up flights of stairs, up a hill, or on flat ground)
Has your breathlessness worsened, improved, or stayed the same since your last visit?
Have you had to reduce your activities because of your breathing or any other symptom?
Have any of your symptoms worsened since your last visit?
Have you experienced any new symptoms since your last visit?
Has your sleep been disrupted by breathlessness or other chest symptoms?
Since your last visit, have you missed any work/had to see a doctor because of your symptoms?
Monitor pharmacotherapy and other medical treatment
What medicines are you taking?
How often do you take each medicine?
How much do you take each time?
Have you missed or stopped taking any regular doses of your medicine for any reason?
Have you had trouble filling your prescriptions (e.g., for financial reasons, not on formulary)?
Please show me how you use your inhaler
Have you tried any other medicines or remedies?
Has your treatment been effective in controlling your symptoms?
Has your treatment caused you any problems?
Monitor exacerbation history
Since your last visit, have you had any episodes/times when your symptoms were a lot worse than usual?
If so, how long did the episode(s) last? What do you think caused the symptoms to get worse? What did you do to control the symptoms?

- Similarly, CT and ventilation–perfusion scanning are mainly useful when surgery is considered.
- Exercise testing is most often performed before, during and after pulmonary rehabilitation.
- Clinical follow-up will be used to detect signs of cor pulmonale (jugular vein enlargement, lower limb edema), then leading to investigations such as chest X ray, electrocardiography, or echocardiography.
- When dyspnea or hypercapnia is not fully explained by spirometric abnormalities, respiratory muscle function testing may be contributive.
- Similarly, when there is some discrepancy between the level of hypoxemia (or occurrence of right heart failure), and spirometry, sleep studies may be indicated.

Situation 5. Appropriate long-term treatment and follow-up have been arranged, but an acute exacerbation of symptoms occurs.

Alternative situation: the diagnosis of COPD is not known but the patient has risk factors (see Situation 1) and presents with an acute respiratory episode.

Question 5.1: What steps of management should be followed?

Exacerbations are not only a cause of morbidity, mortality, and health care expenses by themselves, but also impair quality of life and prognosis on the long term. Thus, their management should follow a rigorous standardized process:

- assessment of severity and other risk factors for poor outcome, guiding the decision regarding where the patient will be treated;
- treatment and assessment of treatment efficacy;
- discharge if the patient was hospitalized; and
- follow-up and, if required, revision of long-term treatment.

Question 5.2: In which case should the patient be referred to the hospital?

The criteria for home versus hospital care vary by health care setting. Nurse-administered "hospital-at-home" care associated with social support (if required) can be cost-effective in patients without acidotic respiratory failure. It can be arranged entirely in the community or following a visit to the emergency department with or without a short hospital stay.

Criteria to consider hospital referral are presented in Table 9.

Question 5.3: The patient can be managed at home. Which treatment should be prescribed?

The cornerstones of exacerbation treatment are (Fig. 4):

- short-acting inhaled bronchodilators (β_2 agonists or anticholinergics) administered with metered-dose inhaler with a spacer, hand held nebulizer or the patient's usual inhaler;
- antibiotics if sputum is purulent, and dyspnea and/or sputum volume are increased; and
- oral corticosteroids (30–40 mg/day, 7–10 days) if baseline FEV_1 is $<50\%$ predicted or if the patient's condition worsens despite initial treatment with bronchodilators and antibiotics.

Table 9 Criteria to Consider Hospital Referral for Chronic Obstructive Pulmonary Disease
Exacerbations

Marked increase in intensity of symptoms, such as sudden development of resting dyspnea
Severe underlying COPD
Onset of new physical signs (e.g., cyanosis, peripheral edema)
Failure of exacerbation to respond to initial medical management
Significant comorbidities
Frequent exacerbations
Newly occurring arrhythmias
Diagnostic uncertainty
Older age
Insufficient home support

Abbreviation: COPD, chronic obstructive pulmonary disease.

**Situation 6. The patient's condition worsens and dyspnea becomes severe. I now
work in the emergency department where he is referred.**
Question 6.1: Which investigations have to be performed?
    The purpose of investigations is to help assessing severity and looking for a cause
of the exacerbation:

■ Arterial blood gas measurement indicates respiratory failure when PaO_2 is <
   8.0 kPa (60 mmHg), and mechanical ventilation is required if respiratory
   acidosis is apparent, with pH < 7.36.

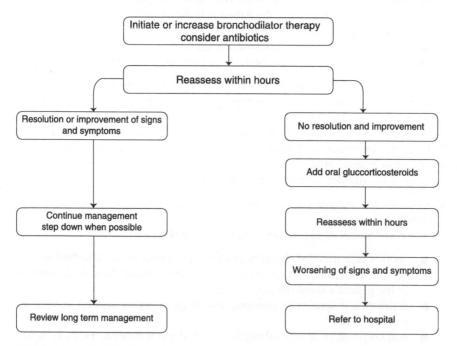

Figure 4 Home-based management of chronic obstructive pulmonary disease
exacerbations.

■ Chest X ray can help distinguishing an exacerbation from other diagnoses including pneumonia, pulmonary edema, pneumothorax, pleural effusion.

■ An electrocardiogram can show signs of right ventricular hypertrophy, arrhythmia or myocardial ischemia.

■ Routine blood tests are useful to assess red and white blood cell counts, electrolytes, glucose control, metabolic acid-base equilibrium.

■ More specific markers can be measured for differential and etiologic diagnosis: brain natriuretic peptide to identify congestive heart failure, procalcitonin to identify bacterial infection.

Other investigations will be discussed to rule out some differential diagnoses such as pulmonary embolism, based on clinical probability.

Question 6.2: When should intensive care unit (ICU) admission be considered?

Criteria for ICU admission are presented in Table 10. In some cases, depending on the patient's status, history, and local possibilities, ICU admission has to be considered earlier to ensure close monitoring or noninvasive ventilation (NIV).

Question 6.3: The exacerbation is severe but not life-threatening. How should it be managed?

Pharmacological therapy relies on the same agents as for home management, i.e., bronchodilators, antibiotic therapy if sputum is purulent.

Systemic corticosteroids (IV or oral) should be prescribed systematically.

Respiratory support (controlled oxygen therapy ± NIV) is the other cornerstone of hospital management (Table 11).

Question 6.4: If the patient's condition continues worsening, when should noninvasive or invasive ventilation be considered?

NIV provides success rates of 80% to 85%: it improves respiratory acidosis, decreases respiratory rate, and dyspnea, shortens hospital stay and reduces intubation rate and mortality. Selection criteria are shown in Table 12.

Failure of NIV is the main indication of invasive ventilation (Table 13).

Situation 7. The patient's condition finally improves.
Question 7.1: When can the patient be discharged?

Discharge criteria depend on the patient's condition, baseline status, rate of improvement. They are also influenced by home support and follow-up possibilities. General criteria are provided in Table 14.

Table 10 Criteria for Intensive Care Unit Admission of Patients with Chronic Obstructive Pulmonary Disease Exacerbations

Severe dyspnea that responds inadequately to initial emergency therapy
Changes in mental status (confusion, lethargy, coma)
Persistent or worsening hypoxemia ($PaO_2 < 5.3$ kPa, 40 mmHg), and/or severe/worsening hypercapnia ($PaCO_2 > 8.0$ kPa, 60 mmHg), and/or severe/worsening respiratory acidosis (pH < 7.25) despite supplemental oxygen and noninvasive ventilation
Need for invasive mechanical ventilation
Hemodynamic instability—need for vasopressors

Table 11 Treatment of Severe but not Life-Threatening Chronic Obstructive Pulmonary Disease Exacerbations in the Hospital

Assess severity of symptoms, blood gases, chest X ray
Administer controlled oxygen therapy and repeat arterial blood gas measurement after 30 to 60 minutes
Bronchodilators
Increase doses and/or frequency
Combine β_2-agonists and anticholinergics
Use spacers or air-driven nebulizers
Consider adding intravenous methylxanthines, if needed
Add oral or intravenous glucocorticosteroids
Consider antibiotics (oral or occasionally intravenous) when signs of bacterial infection
Consider noninvasive mechanical ventilation
At all times
Monitor fluid balance and nutrition
Consider subcutaneous heparin
Identify and treat associated conditions (e.g., heart failure, arrhythmias)
Closely monitor condition of the patient

Question 7.2: How should follow-up be arranged?

Exacerbation should be opportunities to intensify or revise long-term management, ensuring that all treatments directed at reducing exacerbation rate and severity are provided, as well as measures aiming at increasing the patient's autonomy for identification and early treatment of exacerbations.

All these measures should also be addressed before discharge. They include:

- Education, especially on:
    - how to recognize an exacerbation, assess its severity, and initiate its treatment,
    - smoking cessation if required,
    - knowledge of treatment regimen and importance of compliance, and
    - avoidable risk factors such as environmental, domestic or occupational air pollution

Table 12 Selection Criteria for Noninvasive Ventilation

Selection criteria
Moderate to severe dyspnea with use of accessory muscles and paradoxical abdominal motion
Moderate to severe acidosis (pH $\leq$ 7.35) and/or hypercapnia ($PaCO_2 > 6.0$ kPa, 45 mmHg) 386
Respiratory frequency > 25 breaths per minute
Exclusion criteria (any may be present)
Respiratory arrest
Cardiovascular instability (hypotension, arrhythmias, myocardial infarction)
Change in mental status; uncooperative patient
High aspiration risk
Viscous or copious secretions
Recent facial or gastroesophageal surgery
Craniofacial trauma
Fixed nasopharyngeal abnormalities
Burns
Extreme obesity

Table 13 Selection Criteria for Invasive Ventilation

Unable to tolerate NIV or NIV failure (or exclusion criteria, see Table 12)
Severe dyspnea with use of accessory muscles and paradoxical abdominal motion
Respiratory frequency >35 breaths per minute
Life-threatening hypoxemia
Severe acidosis (pH <7.25) and/or hypercapnia (PaCO$_2 > 8.0$ kPa, 60 mmHg)
Respiratory arrest
Somnolence, impaired mental status
Cardiovascular complications (hypotension, shock)
Other complications (metabolic abnormalities, sepsis, pneumonia, pulmonary embolism, barotrauma, and massive pleural effusion)

Abbreviation: NIV, noninvasive ventilation.

- Prescription of pharmacological agents (long-acting inhaled bronchodilators with inhaled corticosteroids if FEV$_1$ is $<50\%$ predicted):
  - inhaler technique,
  - vaccines,
  - rehabilitation,
  - social needs, and
  - need for long-term oxygen therapy or home nebulized treatments.

II. Conclusion

During the past 20 years or so, there has been a considerable increase in the scientific evidence available to guide the management of COPD. The mixture of rather heterogeneous entities became a single disease with better understood mechanisms and more and more effective treatments.

Thus, it is now possible to propose relatively simple rules of management that should decrease morbidity and perhaps mortality attributable to the disease.

Favoring the implementation or current guidelines is clearly a priority, as well as the fight against tobacco smoking. During the years to come, research will certainly provide clinicians with new therapeutic alternatives, which will be integrated in the regularly updated guidelines when a sufficient supporting level of evidence will be obtained.

Table 14 Discharge Criteria for Chronic Obstructive Pulmonary Disease Exacerbations

Inhaled β$_2$-agonist therapy is required no more frequently than every four hours
Patient, if previously ambulatory, is able to walk across room
Patient is able to eat and sleep without frequent awakening by dyspnea
Patient has been clinically stable for 12 to 24 hours
Arterial blood gases have been stable for 12 to 24 hours
Patient (or home caregiver) fully understands correct use of medications
Follow-up and home care arrangements have been completed (e.g., visiting nurse, oxygen delivery, meal provisions)
Patient, family, and physician are confident patient can manage successfully at home

References

1. Rabe KF, Hurd S, Anzueto A, et al. Global strategy for the diagnosis, management, and prevention of COPD-2006 Update. Am J Respir Crit Care Med 2007; May 16; [Epub ahead of print].
2. Pauwels RA, Buist AS, Calverley PM, Jenkins CR, Hurd SS. Global strategy for the diagnosis, management, and prevention of chronic obstructive pulmonary disease. NHLBI/WHO Global Initiative for Chronic Obstructive Lung Disease (GOLD) workshop summary. Am J Respir Crit Care Med 2001; 163:1256–76.
3. Celli BR, Macnee W. Standards for the diagnosis and treatment of patients with COPD: a summary of the ATS/ERS position paper. Eur Respir J 2004; 23:932–46.
4. Dheda K, Crawford A, Hagan G, Roberts CM. Implementation of British Thoracic Society guidelines for acute exacerbation of chronic obstructive pulmonary disease: impact on quality of life. Postgrad Med J 2004; 80:169–71.
5. Fritsch K, Jacot ML, Klarer A, et al. Adherence to the Swiss guidelines for management of COPD: experience of a Swiss teaching hospital. Swiss Med Wkly 2005; 135:116–21.
6. Harvey PA, Murphy MC, Dornom E, Berlowitz DJ, Lim WK, Jackson B. Implementing evidence-based guidelines: inpatient management of chronic obstructive pulmonary disease. Intern Med J 2005; 35:151–5.
7. Heffner JE, Ellis R. The guideline approach to chronic obstructive pulmonary disease: how effective? Respir Care 2003; 48:1257–66.
8. Iqbal A, Schloss S, George D, Isonaka S. Worldwide guidelines for chronic obstructive pulmonary disease: a comparison of diagnosis and treatment recommendations. Respirology 2002; 7:233–9.
9. Jindal SK, Gupta D, Aggarwal AN. Guidelines for management of chronic obstructive pulmonary disease (COPD) in India: a guide for physicians (2003). Indian J Chest Dis Allied Sci 2004; 46:137–53.
10. Kitamura S. COPD guideline of Japanese Respiratory Society. Nippon Rinsho 2003; 61:2077–81.
11. Laitinen LA, Koskela K. Chronic bronchitis and chronic obstructive pulmonary disease: finnish national guidelines for prevention and treatment 1998–2007. Respir Med 1999; 93:297–332.
12. O'Donnell DE, Aaron S, Bourbeau J, et al. Canadian Thoracic Society recommendations for management of chronic obstructive pulmonary disease—2003. Can Respir J 2003; 10(Suppl. A): 11A–65.
13. Price LC, Lowe D, Hosker H, Anstey K, Pearson M, Roberts CM. The U.K. National COPD Audit 2003: impact of hospital resources and organisation of care on patient outcome following admissions for acute COPD exacerbation. Thorax 2006; 61:837–42.
14. Roche N, Lepage T, Bourcereau J, Terrioux P. Guidelines versus clinical practice in the treatment of chronic obstructive pulmonary disease. Eur Respir J 2001; 18:903–8.
15. Russi EW, Leuenberger P, Brandli O, et al. Management of chronic obstructive pulmonary disease: the Swiss guidelines. Official Guidelines of the Swiss Respiratory Society. Swiss Med Wkly 2002; 132:67–78.
16. Tinelli C, Rezzani C, Biino G, et al. Evaluation of the efficacy of the Italian guidelines on COPD: a cluster randomized trial. Monaldi Arch Chest Dis 2003; 59:199–206.
17. Trakada G, Spiropoulos K. Chronic obstructive pulmonary disease management among primary healthcare physicians. Monaldi Arch Chest Dis 2000; 55:201–4.
18. Walters JA, Hansen E, Mudge P, Johns DP, Walters EH, Wood-Baker R. Barriers to the use of spirometry in general practice. Aust Fam Physician 2005; 34:201–3.
19. Ward MM, Yankey JW, Vaughn TE, et al. Provider adherence to COPD guidelines: relationship to organizational factors. J Eval Clin Pract 2005; 11:379–87.
20. Société de Pneumologie de Langue Française. Recommandations pour la prise en charge de la bronchopneumopathie chronique obstructive. Rev Mal Respir 2003; 20:294–329.
21. Marquis K, Debigare R, Lacasse Y, et al. Midthigh muscle cross-sectional area is a better predictor of mortality than body mass index in patients with chronic obstructive pulmonary disease. Am J Respir Crit Care Med 2002; 166:809–13.
22. Pistelli R, Lange P, Miller DL. Determinants of prognosis of COPD in the elderly: mucus hypersecretion, infections, cardiovascular comorbidity. Eur Respir J Suppl 2003; 40:10s–4.
23. Chambellan A, Chailleux E, Similowski T. Prognostic value of the hematocrit in patients with severe COPD receiving long-term oxygen therapy. Chest 2005; 128:1201–8.
24. Raffaele AI, Andrea C, Claudio P, et al. Drawing impairment predicts mortality in severe COPD. Chest 2006; 130:1687–94.

25. Dahl M, Vestbo J, Lange P, Bojesen SE, Tybjaerg-Hansen A, Nordestgaard BG. C-reactive protein as a predictor of prognosis in chronic obstructive pulmonary disease. Am J Respir Crit Care Med 2007; 175:250–5.
26. Garcia-Aymerich J, Lange P, Benet M, Schnohr P, Anto JM. Regular physical activity reduces hospital admission and mortality in chronic obstructive pulmonary disease: a population based cohort study. Thorax 2006; 61:772–8.
27. Celli BR, Cote CG, Marin JM, et al. The body-mass index, airflow obstruction, dyspnea, and exercise capacity index in chronic obstructive pulmonary disease. N Engl J Med 2004; 350:1005–12.
28. Tashkin DP, Cooper CB. The role of long-acting bronchodilators in the management of stable COPD. Chest 2004; 125:249–59.

Index

T - #0219 - 101024 - C0 - 234/156/33 [35] - CB - 9780849375873 - Gloss Lamination